PERSONS AT HIGH RISK OF CANCER
An Approach to
Cancer Etiology and Control

PERSONS AT HIGH RISK OF CANCER
An Approach to
Cancer Etiology and Control

PROCEEDINGS OF A CONFERENCE
Key Biscayne, Florida, December 10-12, 1974

SPONSORED BY
THE NATIONAL CANCER INSTITUTE*
AND THE AMERICAN CANCER SOCIETY

*Division of Cancer Control and Rehabilitation
and
Division of Cancer Cause and Prevention

ORGANIZING COMMITTEE

Joseph F. Fraumeni, Jr., Division of Cancer Cause and Prevention,
National Cancer Institute

Robert L. Woolridge, Division of Cancer Control and Rehabilitation,
National Cancer Institute

Stefano Vivona, American Cancer Society

PERSONS AT HIGH RISK OF CANCER
An Approach to
Cancer Etiology and Control

EDITED BY

JOSEPH F. FRAUMENI, JR.

NATIONAL CANCER INSTITUTE
BETHESDA, MARYLAND

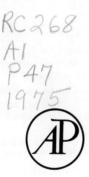

ACADEMIC PRESS, INC. NEW YORK SAN FRANCISCO LONDON 1975
A Subsidiary of Harcourt Brace Jovanovich, Publishers

ACADEMIC PRESS, INC.
111 Fifth Avenue, New York, New York 10003

United Kingdom Edition published by
ACADEMIC PRESS, INC. (LONDON) LTD.
24/28 Oval Road, London NW1

Library of Congress Cataloging in Publication Data
Main entry under title:

Persons at high risk of cancer.

1. Cancer—Prevention—Congresses.   2.   Carcino-
genesis—Congresses.   3.   Epidemiology—Congresses.
I.   Fraumeni, Joseph F.   II.   United States.   National
Cancer Institute.   Division of Cancer Control and Reha-
bilitation.   III.   United States.   National Cancer
Institute.   Division of Cancer Cause and Prevention.
IV.   American Cancer Society.
RC268.P47   616.9'94'071   75-34186
ISBN 0—12—265950—3

CONTENTS

LIST OF PARTICIPANTS

*David E. Anderson, Ph. D.
Department of Biology
University of Texas System Cancer Center
M.D. Anderson Hospital and Tumor Institute
Houston, Texas

J. Bradley Arthaud, M.D.
Department of Epidemiology
University of Texas System Cancer Center
M.D. Anderson Hospital and Tumor Institute
Houston, Texas

Anita K. Bahn, M.D., Sc. D.
Department of Community Medicine
University of Pennsylvania School of Medicine
Philadelphia, Pennsylvania

*John W. Berg, M.D.
Iowa Cancer Epidemiology Research Center
University of Iowa
Iowa City, Iowa

William A. Blattner, M.D.
Epidemiology Branch
National Cancer Institute
Bethesda, Maryland

William J. Blot, Ph. D.
Epidemiology Branch
National Cancer Institute
Bethesda, Maryland

*Lester Breslow, M.D.
The Center for Health Sciences
University of California School of Public Health
Los Angeles, California

*Glyn G. Caldwell, M.D.
Cancer and Birth Defects Division
Bureau of Epidemiology
Center for Disease Control
Atlanta, Georgia

Seymour S. Cohen, Ph. D.
Department of Microbiology
University of Colorado
Denver, Colorado

*Philip Cole, M.D.
Department of Epidemiology
Harvard School of Public Health
Boston, Massachusetts

Genrose D. Copley, M.D.
Division of Cancer Research Resources and Centers
National Cancer Institute
Bethesda, Maryland

John L. Cutler, M.D.
Division of Cancer Control and Rehabilitation
National Cancer Institute
Bethesda, Maryland

*Sidney J. Cutler, D. Sc.
Biometry Branch
National Cancer Institute
Bethesda, Maryland

*J. N. P. Davies, M.D.
Department of Pathology
Albany Medical College
Albany, New York

Robert Depue, Ph. D.
Division of Cancer Cause and Prevention
National Cancer Institute
Bethesda, Maryland

Diane J. Fink, M.D.
Division of Cancer Control and Rehabilitation
National Cancer Institute
Bethesda, Maryland

W. Gary Flamm, Ph. D.
Division of Cancer Cause and Prevention
National Cancer Institute
Bethesda, Maryland

ix

*Joseph F. Fraumeni, Jr., M.D.
Epidemiology Branch
National Cancer Institute
Bethesda, Maryland

John R. Goldsmith, M.D.
Field Studies and Statistics
National Cancer Institute
Bethesda, Maryland

Peter Greenwald, M.D.
Bureau of Cancer Control
New York State Department of Health
Albany, New York

Vincent F. Guinee, M.D.
Department of Epidemiology
University of Texas System Cancer Center
M.D. Anderson Hospital and Tumor Institute
Houston, Texas

*William M. Haenszel
Biometry Branch
National Cancer Institute
Bethesda, Maryland

*E. Cuyler Hammond, Sc. D.
American Cancer Society
New York, New York

G. Denman Hammond, M.D.
University of Southern California
School of Medicine
Los Angeles, California

Juliet Hananian, M.D.
Mailman Center for Child Development
University of Miami
Miami, Florida

*Clark W. Heath, Jr., M.D.
Cancer and Birth Defects Division
Bureau of Epidemiology
Center for Disease Control
Atlanta, Georgia

*Brian E. Henderson, M.D.
Department of Pathology
University of Southern California
School of Medicine
Los Angeles, California

*John Higginson, M.D.
International Agency for Research on
Cancer
Lyon, France

John P. Hills
Council on Environmental Quality
Washington, D. C.

Takeshi Hirayama, M.D.
Epidemiology Division
National Cancer Center Research Institute
Tokyo, Japan

Tomio Hirohata, M.D.
Epidemiology and Demography Unit
Cancer Center of Hawaii
University of Hawaii
Honolulu, Hawaii

Masaharu Hitosugi, M.D.
Epidemiology Branch
National Cancer Institute
Bethesda, Maryland

*Robert N. Hoover, M.D.
Epidemiology Branch
National Cancer Institute
Bethesda, Maryland

Lorne Houten, Ph. D.
Department of Biostatistics
Roswell Park Memorial Institute
Buffalo, New York

+George B. Hutchison, M.D.
Department of Epidemiology
Harvard School of Public Health
Boston, Massachusetts

*Seymour Jablon
Follow-Up Agency
National Academy of Sciences
Washington, D. C.

Andrew Z. Keller, D.M.D.
Epidemiologic Research
Veterans Administration Central Office
Washington, D. C.

*John H. Kersey, M.D.
Department of Laboratory Medicine and
Pathology
University of Minnesota
Minneapolis, Minnesota

Irving I. Kessler, M.D.
Department of Epidemiology
School of Hygiene and Public Health
Johns Hopkins University
Baltimore, Maryland

Ruth L. Kirschstein, M.D.
National Institute of General Medical Sciences
Bethesda, Maryland

*Alfred G. Knudson, Jr., M.D., Ph. D.
Graduate School of Biomedical Sciences
University of Texas Health Science Center
Houston, Texas

*Leopold G. Koss, M.D.
Department of Pathology
Albert Einstein College of Medicine
Montefiore Hospital and Medical Center
Bronx, New York

Herman F. Kraybill, Ph. D.
Division of Cancer Cause and Prevention
National Cancer Institute
Bethesda, Maryland

Donald V. Lassiter, Ph. D.
Occupational Safety and Health Administration
U. S. Department of Labor
Washington, D. C.

Richard Lemen
Division of Field Studies and Clinical
Investigations
National Institute for Occupational Safety
and Health
Cincinnati, Ohio

Frederick P. Li, M.D.
Epidemiology Branch
National Cancer Institute
(Boston Field Station)
Sidney Farber Cancer Center
Boston, Massachusetts

Martin Lipkin, M.D.
Memorial Sloan-Kettering Cancer Center
New York, New York

Henry T. Lynch, M.D.
Department of Preventive Medicine and Public
Health
Creighton University
Omaha, Nebraska

Thomas Mack, M.D.
Departments of Pathology, and Community
Medicine and Public Health
University of Southern California
School of Medicine
Los Angeles, California

*Brian MacMahon, M.D.
Department of Epidemiology
Harvard School of Public Health
Boston, Massachusetts

Winfred F. Malone, Ph. D.
Division of Cancer Control and Rehabilitation
National Cancer Institute
Bethesda, Maryland

*Thomas J. Mason, Ph. D.
Epidemiology Branch
National Cancer Institute
Bethesda, Maryland

James L. McQueen, Ph. D.
Division of Cancer Control and Rehabilitation
National Cancer Institute
Bethesda, Maryland

Anna T. Meadows, M.D.
Division of Oncology
Children's Hospital of Philadelphia
Philadelphia, Pennsylvania

*A. B. Miller, M.B.
Epidemiology Unit
National Cancer Institute of Canada
Toronto, Ontario, Canada

+Daniel G. Miller, M.D.
Preventive Medicine Institute
Strang Clinic
New York, New York

Elizabeth C. Miller, Ph. D.
McArdle Laboratory for Cancer Research
University of Wisconsin
Madison, Wisconsin

James A. Miller, Ph. D.
McArdle Laboratory for Cancer Research
University of Wisconsin
Madison, Wisconsin

*Robert W. Miller, M.D.
Epidemiology Branch
National Cancer Institute
Bethesda, Maryland

Alan S. Morrison, M.D.
Department of Epidemiology
Harvard School of Public Health
Boston, Massachusetts

*Calum S. Muir, M.B.
International Agency for Research on
Cancer
Lyon, France

*John J. Mulvihill, M.D.
Epidemiology Branch
National Cancer Institute
Bethesda, Maryland

Norton Nelson, Ph. D.
Institute of Environmental Medicine
New York University Medical Center
New York, New York

+Guy R. Newell, M.D.
Deputy Director
National Cancer Institute
Bethesda, Maryland

+Gregory T. O'Conor, M.D.
International Affairs
National Cancer Institute
Bethesda, Maryland

*James A. Peters, D.V.M.
Division of Cancer Cause and Prevention
National Cancer Institute
Bethesda, Maryland

Roland L. Phillips, M.D.
Department of Epidemiology
Loma Linda University
Loma Linda, California

*Malcolm C. Pike, Ph. D.
Departments of Community
Medicine and Pediatrics
University of Southern California
School of Medicine
Los Angeles, California

William A. Priester, D.V.M.
Epidemiology Branch
National Cancer Institute
Bethesda, Maryland

Alan S. Rabson, M.D.
Division of Cancer Biology and Diagnosis
National Cancer Institute
Bethesda, Maryland

+Rulon W. Rawson, M.D.
University of Texas System Cancer Center
M.D. Anderson Hospital and Tumor Institute
Houston, Texas

George P. Rosemond, M.D.
Department of Surgery
Temple University Health Sciences Center
Philadelphia, Pennsylvania
(President, American Cancer Society)

*Kenneth J. Rothman, Dr. P.H.
Department of Epidemiology
Harvard School of Public Health
Boston, Massachusetts

Umberto Saffiotti, M.D.
Carcinogenesis
National Cancer Institute
Bethesda, Maryland

*Marvin A. Schneiderman, Ph. D.
Field Studies and Statistics
National Cancer Institute
Bethesda, Maryland

*Bruce S. Schoenberg, M.D.
Departments of Neurology, and Medical
   Statistics and Epidemiology
Mayo Medical School
Rochester, Minnesota

*David Schottenfeld, M.D.
Memorial Hospital for Cancer and Allied
   Diseases
New York, New York

*Irving J. Selikoff, M.D.
Department of Community Medicine
Mount Sinai School of Medicine
New York, New York

Sam Shapiro
Health Services Research and Development
   Center
Johns Hopkins Medical Institutions
Baltimore, Maryland

*Michael B. Shimkin, M.D.
Department of Community Medicine
University of California, San Diego
La Jolla, California

+Philippe Shubik, D.M., D. Phil.
Eppley Institute for Research in Cancer
University of Nebraska
Omaha, Nebraska

*Beatrice D. Spector
Department of Laboratory Medicine and
   Pathology
University of Minnesota Medical School
Minneapolis, Minnesota

Bernard Talbot, M.D.
Viral Leukemia and Lymphoma Branch
National Cancer Institute
Bethesda, Maryland

*A. C. Templeton, M.D.
Department of Pathology
St. Vincent Hospital
Worcester, Massachusetts

Josef Vana, M.D.
Department of Epidemiology
Roswell Park Memorial Institute
Buffalo, New York

Nicholas J. Vianna, M.D.
Bureau of Cancer Control
New York State Department of Health
Albany, New York

Stefano Vivona, M.D.
American Cancer Society
New York, New York

*John Wakefield, Ph. D.
University Hospital of South Manchester
Christie Hospital
Manchester, England

Robert L. Woolridge, D. Sc.
Division of Cancer Control and Rehabilitation
National Cancer Institute
Bethesda, Maryland

*Ernst L. Wynder, M.D.
American Health Foundation
New York, New York

* Contributing author

+ Session chairman

PREFACE

There is increasing recognition that the identification of high-risk groups provides a key to the ultimate reduction of cancer incidence and mortality through opportunities for surveillance, early detection and treatment, etiologic research and preventive measures. This volume is based on a conference convened by the National Cancer Institute and the American Cancer Society and held in Key Biscayne, Florida, December 10-12, 1974. The purpose of the conference was to define the present state of knowledge of risk factors in cancer and to explore ways of applying this information for the protection and further identification of high-risk groups.

We have tried to present in 32 chapters a comprehensive view of cancer risk factors. Following the format of the conference, the book is divided into six parts. The first two parts represent a survey of antecedent host and environmental factors that are known or suspected to increase a person's risk of developing cancer. Consideration is given both to causal factors and to precancerous or precursor manifestations. The third part covers demographic features of cancer (e.g., age, sex, race, locale) that influence the distribution of risk factors, and facilitate their identification and modification by control programs. The utility of high-risk groups for surveillance and preventive measures is illustrated in the fourth part, while strategies to enlarge and sharpen our knowledge of risk factors are presented in the fifth. The final part consists of reports from two groups meeting during the conference to identify special opportunities for work in the areas of cancer etiology and control.

Contributions to the delineation of high-risk groups may come from the clinic, the laboratory, or field studies. To promote interchange at the conference, 90 participants were invited from various fields, including epidemiology, genetics, environmental and occupational health, chemical and viral carcinogenesis, immunology, and clinical oncology. The interaction among disciplines is reflected in many reports and discussion summaries concerned with cancer etiology. Although high-risk groups presently account for only a small portion of many cancers, they point the way to further research to elucidate risk factors of a fundamental nature that lie under the surface. Recent developments suggest that etiologic advances will depend heavily on laboratory studies to develop subclinical measures of risk and on increased collaboration between epidemiologists and experimentalists. Furthermore, the multifactorial nature of some high-risk groups will require sophisticated methods to identify interactions between environmental exposures or between environmental and host factors. At present, epidemiologic studies of high-risk groups are often high-risk ventures: slow, complicated, tedious, expensive. More rapid progress will require not only greater training and research support of epidemiologists, but special efforts to strengthen the resources and freshen the tactics of cancer epidemiology.

Throughout the book attention is given to the potential and the limitations of high-risk groups in intervention programs to reduce morbidity and mortality from cancer. Before a major impact can be made on clinical and public health practice, it is clear that advances will be needed in risk identification. More effective criteria of risk are also needed; whereas the commonly used "relative risk" (ratio of cancer rates with and without the antecedent risk factor) is the key measure in etiologically oriented studies, the infrequently used "absolute or attributable risk" (percentage of the total cancer rate attributed to a risk factor) is more relevant to the feasibility of control projects. However, the two approaches should be closely linked. In particular, as we learn more about cancer risk factors through etiologic research, it will be possible to expand control programs and direct them with precision to segments of the population that are most likely to benefit.

Joseph F. Fraumeni, Jr.

ACKNOWLEDGMENTS

This book is based on a conference supported by the National Cancer Institute (Division of Cancer Control and Rehabilitation, and Division of Cancer Cause and Prevention) and the American Cancer Society. Primary credit goes to the contributing authors for the high quality of their reports. I am indebted to Drs. Robert L. Woolridge and Stefano Vivona for help in planning the meeting, Drs. Marvin A. Schneiderman and Robert W. Miller for advice and guidance, and Donna Peterson for organizing the many details involved in producing the conference and book. The sessions were expertly moderated by the following chairmen: Drs. Rulon W. Rawson, James A. Peters, George B. Hutchison, Gregory T. O'Conor, Daniel G. Miller, Guy R. Newell, and Philippe Shubik. I am grateful to the rapporteurs who recorded and summarized the discussion following each presentation, to members of working groups that evaluated opportunities for cancer etiology and control, and to Gregory W. Lewis, Janis E. Baker, and the staff of JRB Associates, Inc., for administrative and logistic support. I also wish to express thanks and appreciation to Edwin A. Haugh, Patricia Bryant, Doris M. Chaney, and Constance P. Watson of JRB Associates, Inc., for editorial assistance and preparation of a subject index.

Joseph F. Fraumeni, Jr.

PERSONS AT HIGH RISK OF CANCER
An Approach to
Cancer Etiology and Control

HOST FACTORS

CONGENITAL AND GENETIC DISEASES

John J. Mulvihill, M.D.

Clinical Genetics Section
Epidemiology Branch, National Cancer Institute
Bethesda, Maryland

INTRODUCTION

Certain people are at high risk for cancer because of their genes. Since other reviews of genetic factors in human cancer are available [1-5], this chapter summarizes recent developments, with emphasis on the importance of genetics to clinical oncology and to the biology and prevention of cancer.

Genetic factors may be considered in three groups:

1) *Chromosomal,* with genetic imbalance because entire lengths of genetic material are absent or present in excess.

2) *Single-gene* locus, with disease arising from mutation either in one allele as in a dominant trait, or in paired alleles as in a recessive trait.

3) *Polygenic,* implying that many genes interact, perhaps with environmental factors, to cause disease, with no one factor or gene playing a major role. (This group is considered in Chapter 2 of this volume [6].)

CHROMOSOMAL DISORDERS IN CANCER

Asymmetrical mitosis could be chiefly considered for the origins of tumors. . . . My theory is able to explain above all the defective histologic form and the altered biochemical behavior of tumor cells. Are there any means of reaching a trustworthy decision as to the worthiness of the views presented here? The most obvious would be to devote renewed attention to the counting of chromosomes, if possible with better techniques [7].

The author thanks Ms. S. Trimble and Dr. J.F. Fraumeni, Jr., for library and bibliographic support; Miss W. Wade and Mrs. J. Pearson for editorial and secretarial work; and Dr. J. Whang-Peng for helpful criticism of an early draft. Literature review ended December 1974.

For 60 years Boveri's hypothesis that malignancy was caused by chromosomal imbalance has awaited proof through better techniques for studying chromosomes. A quantum advance came with Caspersson's technique of labeling chromosomes with fluorescent compounds [8]. Until then, the 46 human chromosomes were classified solely by overall size and shape, with little to distinguish one from the other in the same group. At least four standard techniques for staining permit identification of each chromosome, and even parts of chromosomes, by the pattern of differential staining called banding [9]. Karyotypes with banding led to new insights into clinical conditions which were known to be associated with chromosomal anomalies but were poorly understood because of the limitations of techniques. Also, minute but consistent errors, not previously demonstrable, were reported.

Numerous reviews of cancer cytogenetics are available [10-15], but all antedate wide use of banding techniques. The following account deals first with recent findings in the cytogenetics of certain neoplasms, especially leukemia, then summarizes their meaning to cancer etiology; and finally, highlights advances in the interrelationship of chromosomes, cancer, and congenital defects.

The Leukemias

Chronic Myelocytic Leukemia (CML)

Most patients with CML have a small marker chromosome in the leukemic cells. When first discovered [16], this marker was correctly considered a G group chromosome that had lost part of its long arms. Specifically, it was thought likely to be chromosome 21, the same one that was trisomic in individuals with Down's syndrome. New techniques showed that the Philadelphia chromosome (Ph[1]), as the marker in CML became known, was *not* the same one found in triplicate in Down's syndrome, but rather chromosome 22 [17]. Furthermore, often Ph[1] was not just a loss of the long arms of chromosome 22 but actually a translocation of this segment to the long arms of chromosome 9 [18, 19]. The possibility arises, to be resolved by further technical refinements, that minute parts of chromosome 9 or 22 are lost in translocation. In fact, if chromosomal loss is the basis of CML, then the deletion probably involves the long arms of chromosome 22, since translocation to 9 is not invariable; sometimes it is translocated to other chromosomes [20], sometimes just the long-arm deletion is seen [21].

Seventy to ninety percent of patients with CML have Ph[1] [22-24]; those without it have a different natural history and response to treatment, and perhaps etiology. Lately, a third group of about 30 CML patients have emerged [24, 25]. All are men who are older, survive longer, and have Ph[1]; in addition, the Y chromosome is lost from the leukemic cell line. Since the Y chromosome is frequently lost in older but apparently normal men, this subgroup of CML may also have a different etiology, perhaps involving premature aging of the bone marrow [25].

Ph[1] occasionally is seen in diseases other than CML: polycythemia vera, myeloid metaplasia, erythroleukemia, and acute myelocytic leukemia (AML) [11]. Some cases of AML may resemble the well-documented case of a 43-year-old man who, when seen for mild leukocytosis, had Ph[1] in 22 percent of marrow metaphases [26]. He was well for over 5 years, and then died of acute leukemia. Other apparently normal individuals with Ph[1], though incompletely reported, are a 29-year-old woman and her two young sons [27]. Although normal at last report, they may yet develop leukemia because the mother's father and his two sibs died of CML, and their father had an unknown type of leukemia.

Chronic Lymphatic Leukemia (CLL)

Another marker chromosome, the Christchurch chromosome, was found in two sibs with CLL as well as in normal relatives, segregating as a Mendelian dominant trait [28]. When 68 years old, a third sib developed lymphosarcoma and simultaneous CLL, and later two basal-cell carcinomas of the face; she died at age 74 of acute plasma-cell leukemia [29]. A familial Christchurch chromosome, a deletion of the short arms of chromosome 22, was found in two patients with acute leukemia, one of whom had Down's syndrome [30, 31]. Since the cell types were discordant and the three families were ascertained because of the malignancy, the etiologic relationship of the Christchurch chromosome and CLL remains unclear.

Acute Leukemia

Since CML carries a high risk for acute leukemia, it has been termed a "preleukemic condition" [32, 33]. As CML becomes acute, the karyotype changes. Typically, more chromosomes are acquired, especially in the C and G groups, and simultaneously, the histochemical reaction of leukemic marrow cells alters. Myeloblasts, which do not react with periodic acid-Schiff stain normally or in CML, begin to stain positively. About 30 to 50 percent of patients with AML have abnormal karyotypes, although old techniques did not reveal a consistent abnormality in any large number of cases [34-36]. Nonetheless, several patients had a very complex aneuploidy, consisting of loss of chromosomes from the C and G groups (including sex chromosomes) and additional chromosomes in groups D and E [37]. Again, banding techniques have made sense out of these bewildering anomalies. At least four reported patients have one specific karyotype [45,X,t(8q–,21q+) (q22;q22)] that can account for changes in all four groups (C, D, E, and G) [38,39]. Chromosome 8 may be a frequent breaking site in AML; an additional patient had translocation of the long arms of chromosome 8 to 17 instead of 21 [40]. Trisomy in the C group, to which chromosome 8 belongs, was also seen in surveys of acute leukemia and in CML patients entering blastic episodes. With banding techniques, trisomy 8 has been recognized in four patients with AML [41,42] and in four with sideroblastic anemia, a condition with known leukemic potential [42]. (One of the latter also had meningioma.)

Other Neoplasms

Cytogenetic abnormalities in other tumors are generally nonspecific [43]; recent studies associated meningioma with an absent number 22 and Burkitt lymphoma with an extra band on the long arms of chromosome 14 [44,45].

Etiologic Implications of Tumor Cytogenetics

Clinicians depend on chromosomal analysis to help in 1) diagnosis (e.g., differentiating CML from other myeloproliferative conditions or leukemoid reactions) and 2) prognosis (e.g., in response to therapy). Biomedical scientists, for their part, use cytogenetic findings to form and test hypotheses concerning carcinogenesis. These theories can be considered under five headings presented here in order of ascending controversy.

Clonal Origin of Cancer

The hypothesis is that clinical neoplasm, as a rule, derives from one cell that acquires malignant potential and proliferates to the time of clinical diagnosis [46, 47]. The specific association of Ph^1 with CML provides one of the strongest supports for the single-cell origin of human neoplasm, although much evidence exists beyond cytogenetics. Stepwise changes in the karyotype accompanies worsening of disease; that is, as serial samples of a patient's tumor are karyotyped during advancing disease, progression is seen from such simple chromosomal anomalies as Ph^1 to more complex ones. Each new karyotype appears to be derived from a prior simpler one.

This progression has been termed "stem-cell evolution" [48] and may be very important to therapy. Some clinical oncologists reason that *early* CML should be aggressively treated in an effort to eliminate Ph^1, a life-threatening task not yet accomplished, to my knowledge, and perhaps difficult to justify in a disease that may remain quiescent for years.

Parental Origin of Cancer

Banding techniques revealed previously unsuspected differences among karyotypes of normal individuals [49]. This polymorphic nature of normal chromosomes is not associated with any disease, and is so extensive that a person's karyotype may be as unique and private as his fingerprints. Slight differences between chromosome 22 of parents allow identification of the parental chromosome giving rise to Ph[1] in an offspring with CML. One case each of maternal and paternal origin of the marker has been demonstrated [50]. This approach is, in fact, a logical extension of the theory of clonal origin.

Etiology-Specific Karyotype

One fresh synthesis of cytogenetic data on human cancer is the hypothesis set forth independently by Mitelman et al. [51] and Rowley [52]: similar karyotypes, irrespective of the histologic type of tumor in which they occur, signify a similar etiologic agent. As a corollary, the theory resolves the problem of why human tumors of similar histology often have dissimilar karyotypes. It is well recognized that similar tumors may have diverse etiologies. The hypothesis states that the chromosomal diversity of histologically identical tumors merely reflects the diversity of etiologic agents.

Evidence for this theory is drawn from the association of Ph[1] with CML plus several other myeloproliferative disorders—these would be expected to have similar etiology. On the other hand, all conditions with Ph[1] would be expected to have a different etiology from Ph[1]-negative CML. Stronger evidence comes from experimental carcinogenesis with specific agents. Sarcomas induced in Chinese hamsters and rats by dissimilar agents [Rous sarcoma virus and 7,12-dimethylbenz[a]anthracene (DMBA)] are indistinguishable by histology but have very different karyotypes. However, *differing* tumor types in rats, such as leukemia and sarcoma, when induced by the *same* agent (DMBA again) have similar chromosomal changes [51].

These observations suggest that etiologic studies in man may need to group tumors by similarities of karyotype, not histology.

Genetics of Carcinogenesis

Since CML occurs when only one Ph[1] is present, it has been likened to a Mendelian dominant trait, although the marker is acquired and not heritable. The dominant expression of a single Ph[1] may also represent usually recessive genes whose action is unopposed because of the deletion. So argues Ohno [53, 54], addressing the question, "What advantage is aneuploidy to malignant cells?" Briefly, his reasoning begins with the demonstration that the deleted material (representing 0.5 percent of the total genetic material [55]) probably contains genes for functions other than leukogenesis, even perhaps genes for enzymes crucial for intermediary metabolism, such as 6-phosphogluconate dehydrogenase. Next, he shows that among the billion or so progenitor cells in the bone marrow, approximately one Ph[1] cell may arise daily, on the assumption that chromosome breaks are as frequent as point mutation. CML is not so common as that, but the deletion does allow an unopposed set of genes.

The exposed genes may be lethal and no neoplasm would ensue; or, the mutation may give the cell a selective advantage, perhaps by allowing continuous production of certain enzymes not usually made by a properly differentiating cell.

The selective advantage of Ph^1 in myeloid cells does not always produce fulminant disease, but the addition of a second Ph^1 or other chromosomal aberration does. Since the grotesque karyotypes of most advanced tumors are hyperploid (that is, with more chromosome material than normal), it could be that the advantageous recessive genes are duplicated, providing insurance against any subsequent "harmful" mutation such as back mutation. At the same time, unneeded chromosomes, like the Y or the second X chromosome, can be lost.

Anomalies of E group chromosomes have been especially common in leukemia and the solid tumors [56,57]. This observation is a possible example of Ohno's theory that malignant cells enjoy selective advantage by virtue of their special karyology. One of the E group chromosomes, number 17, contains the gene for the enzyme thymidine kinase, especially important in the metabolism of nucleic acid precursors and the base analogues used in chemotherapy. Possibly, mutations involving such an enzyme account for the nonrandom frequency of E group anomalies in human tumors.

Epiphenomena vs. Initial Event

These arguments constitute a plausible hypothesis that chromosomal aberrations contribute to tumor *progression.* The role of chromosomal change in the *initiation* of neoplasia is more contestable. On one hand, aberrant karyotypes of neoplasms may be epiphenomena, that is, features that are genuinely associated but nonetheless secondary. On the other hand, chromosomal errors can be considered as a primary etiologic event. The argument, far from settled, is summarized in Table 1 from multiple sources [12,15,58].

CANCER AND CONGENITAL DEFECTS

Strong support for a significant etiologic relationship between chromosomal defects and cancer comes from their common association with congenital defects [59-61].

Syndromes with Cancer of Possible Single-Gene Origin

Wilms' Tumor and Congenital Defects

Wilms' tumor, sometimes occurring alone as an autosomal dominant trait [62], is also associated with certain birth defects in four syndromes of unknown

TABLE 1
Relation of chromosome anomalies to carcinogenesis

As epiphenomena—secondary events	As etiologic event
Animal tumors, spontaneous or induced are usually diploid	Uniform karyotype for canine venereal tumor is universal
Anomalies are not seen in every human neoplasm	Ph[1] is noted in some preleukemic states
Anomalies are not consistent for even one cell type	Preneoplastic lesions (e.g., cervical dysplasia and intestinal polyps) are often diploid when benign and aneuploid when atypia predominates
Anomalies are not consistent even in one patient	
Ph[1] was not seen even one month before diagnosis of CML	Patients with chromosomal breaks, whether of genetic or environmental origin, have high risk for leukemia
Monozygotic twins discordant for CML are similarly discordant for Ph[1]	Several congenital syndromes with high risk for malignancy have aneuploidy

etiology [63,64]. All have urogenital malformations, but an additional feature in one is hemihypertrophy. Another syndrome has nonfamilial aniridia, perhaps with microcephaly, mental deficiency, and external ear defects. The third syndrome, reported in five patients, is Wilms' tumor, pseudohermaphroditism, and a nephron disorder [65]. The fourth is the visceral cytomegaly syndrome of Wiedemann and Beckwith, consisting of large tongue, omphalocele, and large viscera resulting from cells that are large in size and number [66]. This syndrome and hemihypertrophy alone have occurred in children with Wilms' tumor, primary hepatic cancer, and adrenocortical neoplasia.

In each syndrome, the coexistence of birth defects and neoplasia suggests a common etiologic mechanism perhaps in early gestation. The features of these syndromes may be scattered throughout a family, as in the report of hemihypertrophy in a mother whose three children had Wilms' tumor and a fourth had renal duplication [67].

In one patient with the Wilms' tumor-aniridia syndrome, computer technology combined with banding techniques revealed a minute deletion on the short arm of chromosome 8 representing no more than 15 percent of that chromosome [68]. If this observation is found in further cases, it will be the *second* time a chromosomal aberration has been found in a malformation syndrome that includes a neoplasm that can have autosomal dominant inheritance when it occurs alone.

Retinoblastoma and 13q- Syndrome

The *first* was retinoblastoma, which is a frequent feature of the 13q- syndrome of multiple malformations including mental and physical retardation, microcephaly, cardiac and eye defects, and various skeletal anomalies, especially hypoplastic thumbs [69]. In these patients, chromosome 13 may be in a ring or have various deletions of the long arms. Chromosomal banding patterns suggest that patients with the 13q- syndrome are divided into three groups [70]: those with high risk for retinoblastoma and only minor malformations have a deletion in q21; those with major malformations and less chance of retinoblastoma have a deletion of q34–q33 or q32–q31, depending on the pattern of malformations (Figure 1). The syndrome is rare, with about 50 reported cases, but may be an informative intersection of genetics, teratogenesis, and carcinogenesis.

The 13 q - syndromes

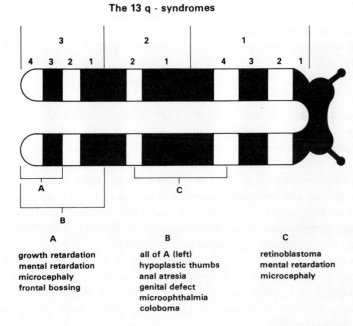

A	B	C
growth retardation	all of A (left)	retinoblastoma
mental retardation	hypoplastic thumbs	mental retardation
microcephaly	anal atresia	microcephaly
frontal bossing	genital defect	
	microophthalmia	
	coloboma	

FIGURE 1. In the 13q- syndrome, the pattern of birth defects and the frequency of retinoblastoma seem related to the site and extent of the chromosomal deletion (redrawn from [70, 71]).

There are two additional recent developments in retinoblastoma. The first is the double mutation explanation of etiology set forth by Knudson [72] and summarized in the next chapter [6]. This interpretation is clinically important in counseling patients and their parents. Unilateral sporadic retinoblastoma has low heritability, whereas bilateral retinoblastoma is much more often transmitted from parent to child [73]. A second finding is that survivors of bilateral retinoblastoma have an increased risk of second primary tumor, particularly osteosarcoma [74,75]. Some of these tumors arise in fields of therapeutic radiation; others arise in the leg, far from any radiation, and may manifest an inborn susceptibility to certain neoplasms. Indeed, there are pedigrees of retinoblastoma patients that include relatives with sarcoma but not retinoblastoma [76].

Cancer in Syndromes with Extra Chromosomes

Leukemia in Down's Syndrome

The rate of leukemia in patients with Down's syndrome is at least 11 times normal, but may be much higher [77]. The same cell types occur as in normal individuals of that age: in children, acute lymphoblastic leukemia is most common, whereas in newborn infants, myeloblastic leukemia predominates. In both age groups, chronic leukemia is rare [78].

The risk seems related to age, with fewer than 20 adults but about 200 children reported with Down's syndrome and leukemia. Another peculiarity is the great frequency of "pseudoleukemia" in newborn infants with Down's syndrome. The condition is morphologically indistinguishable from myelocytic leukemia, but is self-limited.

Perhaps because of small numbers, it is not known whether Down's syndrome predisposes to other malignancies, despite reports on patients with brain and testicular tumors and retinoblastoma [77].

Breast Cancer in Klinefelter's Syndrome

The risk of breast cancer in Klinefelter's syndrome approaches the risk in normal women, about 66 times the risk in normal men [79]. Conversely, Klinefelter's syndrome was found in 3.3 percent of men with breast cancer, compared to 0.2 percent in newborn infants [80]. Despite early suspicions, leukemia and lymphoma are probably not increased [81], but such autoimmune disease as systemic lupus erythematosus may be [82]. Perhaps the extra X chromosome of Klinefelter's syndrome leads to an excess of diseases usually predominant in females.

Cancer in Gonadal Dysgenesis

Gonadal Malignancy

Little can be added to Schellhas' review [83], which substantiates earlier conclusions by Teter [84]: the risk of gonadal malignancy in gonadal dysgenesis is about 25 percent. Of 72 cases tabulated from surgical series, 11 gonadoblastomas and 7 dysgerminomas were found. All had some cell lines with a Y chromosome. These observations, summarized in Figure 2, suggest that the Y chromosome predisposes the dysgenetic gonad to malignancy. For clinicians of patients with gonadal dysgenesis, the findings urge discovery of those patients with a Y chromosome cell line. For experimentalists, the challenge is to understand pathogenesis.

Y CHROMOSOME PREDISPOSES TO MALIGNANCY IN GONADAL DYSGENESIS

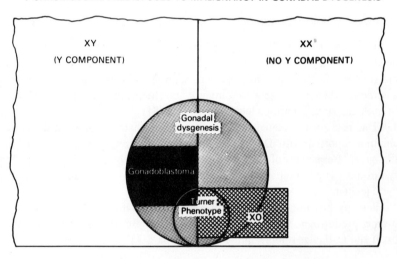

FIGURE 2.   The relation between sex chromosome constitution, gonadal dysgenesis, and gonadoblastoma. *Rectangle* represents the universe with regard to sex chromosome constitution: males with a Y chromosome, females without it. *Circles* straddling these groups contain individuals with ambiguous genitalia and gonadal dysgenesis, including the classic Turner phenotype. Those with 45,XO karyotype have, as a rule, little risk for gonadal malignancy. Rather the presence of a Y chromosome, even if confined just to a gonadal cell line, is associated with a high frequency of gonadoblastoma. (From [85], with publisher's permission.)

Nongonadal Tumors

The classic Turner's syndrome (primary amenorrhea, short stature, webbed neck, shield chest, cubitus valgus) includes benign tumors, such as multiple pigmented nevi, keloid formation, congenital hygroma colli, and, on occasion, hemangioma, phlebectasia, or telangiectasia causing intestinal hemorrhage [86]. A survey of cases in the literature and records at three medical centers documented a tendency toward unusual tumors of neural crest origins (ganglioneuroma, carcinoid tumor, schwannoma, and melanoma) in addition to various brain and pituitary tumors [87]; subsequent case reports support the suggestion (Table 2). Four patients with Turner's syndrome and uterine carcinoma were reported, all after prolonged estrogenic therapy [87,93]. Uterine cancer after estrogen use occurred in two other patients with X chromosomal anomalies, but neither had Turner's syndrome [93].

TABLE 2

Turner's syndrome with nongonadal neoplasms, 1970-1974[a]

Reference	Age (yrs)	Neoplasm	Karyotype
88	57	Nevoid basal-cell carcinoma syndrome	45,X
89	60	Meningioma	45,X/46,XX/47,XXX
90	47	"Cerebral tumor"	— —
91	16	Epithelioid sarcoma	45,X/46,XX
92	20	Acute lymphocytic leukemia	45,X
93	29	Adenosquamous carcinoma of uterus (20 years of estrogen therapy)	45,X

[a]To supplement Table 2 in [87].

Testicular Cancer in Cryptorchidism

The facts of this relationship are [94]: 1) Cryptorchid testes, found in about 2 percent of term male infants [95], have 33 times the normal risk of malignancy. 2) Risk increases with degree of maldescent, being four times greater with abdominal than inguinal testes. 3) In 20 to 25 percent of patients with unilateral cryptorchidism, the neoplastic testis is the properly descended one. 4) If orchiopexy is done before the age of six years, risk of malignancy may return to normal [96]; otherwise, it continues elevated after surgery.

The facts indicate that both general and local host factors predispose the undescended testes to malignancy. Testicular dysgenesis often occurs in the nonneoplastic tissue of cancerous testes [97]. Similarly, testicular biopsies taken at prepubertal orchiopexy show diminished or no spermatogonia [98]. All studies, however, fail to distinguish among various causes of cryptorchidism. Different risks of malignancy may accompany cryptorchidism in Noonan's syndrome compared to that associated with low gonadotropin levels.

Sacrococcygeal Teratomas and Pelvic Anomalies

In 19 boys with teratoma of the testis, the only birth defect found to excess was cryptorchidism in four of them, and perhaps inguinal hernia [99]. By contrast, major malformations of the lower spine were found in 10 of 91 patients with sacrococcygeal teratoma; furthermore, rare duplications of the lower intestinal and urogenital tracts occurred in 3 of 72 girls.

CANCER IN SINGLE-GENE DISORDERS

Unlike chromosomes, single genes must be looked at *indirectly,* by their consequences and analysis of pedigrees. This section considers first the human conditions caused by a single gene that are associated with a high risk for malignancy and with excessive chromosomal fragility. Next, a table of Mendelian conditions associated with neoplasia is presented, and examples are drawn from the table to illustrate the typical pattern in progress of understanding human disease.

Excess Chromosomal Breaks and High Risk of Cancer

At least five Mendelian conditions have chromosomal fragility: ataxia-telangiectasia, Fanconi's anemia, Bloom's syndrome, Kostmann's infantile genetic agranulocytosis, glutathione reductase deficiency [100].

Ataxia-telangiectasia

Despite popular notion, observations are inconclusive on chromosomal breaks in autosomal recessive ataxia-telangiectasia, whose clinical and neoplastic manifestations are discussed elsewhere [101-103]. Although breaks are seen in affected adults, they probably occur to excess only in children [104]. In 19 patients, in vitro clones of lymphocytes with translocations were documented and three had identical translocations between chromosomes 14 [104-107]. Serial analysis of one patient showed an increase of the translocation clone from 1 to 78 percent over 4 years until death from pulmonary insufficiency at age 23 [108]. The in vivo emergence of a lymphocytic line with selective advantage obviously suggests the clone could eventually become malignant. The risk of malignancy remains unknown when only one defective gene is present, as in heterozygotes.

Other Syndromes with Chromosomal Fragility

The spectrum of the autosomal recessive *Fanconi's anemia* has widened on three fronts: 1) In addition to myelomonocytic leukemia and squamous cell carcinoma [109,110], hepatic neoplasm is probably a feature of the syndrome. Of six such reported patients [111], all but one had treatment with androgenic steroids, which has also been incriminated in cases of hepatoma complicating idiopathic aplastic anemia [112]. 2) Heterozygotes may have an increased risk of malignancy [113]. Of 104 deaths in relatives of 8 unrelated patients with Fanconi's anemia, 24 malignant neoplasms were recorded on death certificates compared to 17.1 expected by proportional mortality. There were three leukemias and three lingual or tonsillar carcinomas, but no hepatomas. 3) Poon et al. [114] proposed a specific enzyme deficiency, namely, an exonuclease that removes DNA cross-links before normal repair of DNA. The discovery (in one patient) was based on observations that the chromosomal fragility in Fanconi's anemia arises from undue susceptibility to agents which specifically increase the amount of DNA cross-linking, like ultraviolet radiation and mitomycin C [115,116]. If Poon's finding is repeated, a second human disease with genetic malignancy will have a defect in DNA repair mechanisms, the first being xeroderma pigmentosum [117].

Among 50 patients with the autosomal recessive *Bloom's syndrome*, nine neoplasms have occurred in eight patients: four acute leukemias, two sigmoid carcinomas (one patient also had esophageal cancer at age 39), one squamous cell carcinoma of tongue, and one reticulum cell sarcoma [118]. In four parents (obligate heterozygotes for the gene) five neoplasms have occurred: two breast cancers, one myeloid metaplasia, one melanoma, and one double primary cancer (colon and stomach). The characteristic chromosomal aberration of Bloom's syndrome is the quadriradial configuration, although other breaks and rearrangements are seen.

In a tantalizing personal communication, H. D. Waller was said to know of 10 deaths from leukemia in 100 patients with *glutathione reductase deficiency* [100]. One case of acute monocytic leukemia is reported among seven patients with *Kostmann's infantile genetic agranulocytosis* who survived beyond 3 years of age [119].

Man's Genetic Repertory of Cancer

Syndromes of chromosomal fragility are but one type of disease of single-gene origin that predisposes to cancer. Fraumeni [3,120] termed such genetic diseases, "hereditary syndromes," and arbitrarily divided them into: 1) *hereditary neoplasms* in which the mutant gene is directly expressed as a tumor, and 2) *preneoplastic states* in which tumor arises from an precursor lesion. Four categories of preneoplastic states are dominantly inherited *hamarto-matous syndromes* and recessive *genodermatoses* and syndromes of *chromosomal fragility* and *immune deficiency*.

Fraumeni accepts for his classification only a score of well-proved genetic syndromes, but their number may be much larger. Known human mutations currently comprise 866 proved single-gene traits and 1,010 others with suggestive but inconclusive evidence of Mendelian behavior [121]. From these, I have extracted 161 conditions (9 percent) and added several others in which malignant or benign neoplasia or tumor was a sole feature, frequent concomitant or just a rare complication (Table 3).

The point of the table is its length. It is not complete; certain entries are contestable and others are missing, e.g., reference to all known familial aggregations of neoplasms of similar or diverse cell types. Generally arranged by major organ system, the table emphasizes that many Mendelian traits with tumors of a variety of cell types are known. A second point is that even the commonest types of cancer—colon, breast, skin—can be part of genetic syndromes. The clinician who diagnoses the *cancer* but not the *syndrome* of which it is a manifestation makes an incomplete diagnosis. This disservice to the patient may also extend to his relatives who may be denied the possible benefits of advice for cancer prevention and early detection. Although the conditions are rare, they deserve wider recognition by clinicians.

Recent advances in selected conditions from Table 3 illustrate four typical phases in the uneven pace of understanding genetic disease in man.

Phase 1: Clinical Delineation

As recounted earlier, Wilms' tumor is a feature of at least four syndromes distinguished by the different constellations of associated conditions. Such splitting recognizes the possible existence of as many etiologies as nosologic entities.

Similar heterogeneity exists among *thymoma* patients, who frequently have one or more additional diseases, such as myasthenia gravis, acquired pure red cell aplasia, and a host of other conditions felt to have an autoimmune or endocrinologic basis [143]. In one report, cancer, especially lymphoma, occurred in 21 percent of thymoma patients [144]. Although the high frequency was not confirmed by one study [145], another [146] showed excess malignancy in 1,243 patients with myasthenia gravis, except among those surviving three or more years after thymectomy. To date, there is no genetic basis for the emerging thymoma syndromes, despite reports of familial aggregation, especially of the associated autoimmune disorders.

TABLE 3

Neoplasia as single gene traits or as a feature or complication of other Mendelian disorders
(modified from [121] with additions)

Catalog No. or [reference]	Neoplasm or disorder	Inheritance	Associated neoplasms
A Phacomatoses			
16220	von Recklinghausen's neurofibromatosis	AD[a]	Fibrosarcoma, neuroma, schwannoma, meningioma, polyps, optic glioma, pheochromocytoma
19110	Tuberous sclerosis	AD[a]	Adenoma sebaceum, periungual fibroma, glial tumors, rhabdomyoma of heart, renal tumor, lung cysts
19330 23480	von Hippel-Lindau syndrome	AD[a] AR	Retinal angioma, cerebellar hemangioblastoma, other hemangiomas, pheochromocytoma, hyper-nephroma, cysts
18530	Sturge-Weber syndrome	AD	Angioma of numerous organs
B. Nervous System			
18020	Retinoblastoma, bilateral	AD[a]	Sarcoma
10100	Acoustic neuroma, bilateral	AD[a]	
25670 [122]	Neuroblastoma	AR AD	

Perhaps, meningioma, 15610-AD; glioma, 13780-AD; pseudoglioma, 26420-AR; pinealoma, 26220-AR; choroid plexus papilloma, 26050-AR; chordoma, 21540-AR; hypothalamic hamartoma, 21180-AR; congenital cerebral granulomas, 30630-XR.

C. Endocrine			
13110	Multiple endocrine adenomatosis I (Werner's syndrome)	AD[a]	Adenomas of islet cells, malignant schwannoma, parathyroid, pituitary and adrenal glands, nonappendiceal carcinoid

TABLE 3 (continued)

C. Endocrine (continued)

17140	Multiple endocrine adenomatosis II (Sipple's syndrome)	AD[a]	Medullary carcinoma of thyroid, parathyroid adenoma, pheochromocytoma
16230	Mucosal neuromas and endocrine adenomatosis	AD[a]	Pheochromocytoma, medullary carcinoma of the thyroid, neurofibroma, submucosal neuromas of tongue, lips, eyelids
16800	Paraganglioma (chemodectoma)	AD[a]	
17130	Pheochromocytoma	AD	
14500	Hyperparathyroidism	AD	Parathyroid adenoma, chief cell hyperplasia
10390	Dexamethasone-sensitive aldosteronism	AD	Multiple adrenocortical adenomas
13880	Thyroid goiter and dyshormonogenesis	AD	Benign goiter
27440-90		AR[a]	

Perhaps, intestinal carcinoid, 11490-AD; amenorrhea-galactorrhea syndrome with pituitary adenoma, 10460-AD; Bartter's syndrome, 24120-AR[a]

D. Mesoderm (soft tissue)

10940	Nevoid basal cell carcinoma syndrome	AD[a]	Basal cell carcinoma, medulloblastoma, jaw cysts, and ovarian fibroma and carcinoma
[123-125]	Multiple hamartoma syndrome (Cowden's disease)	AD[a]	Papillomatosis of lip and mouth, hypertrophic and cystic breast with early cancer, thyroid adenoma and carcinoma, bone and liver cysts, lipoma, polyps, meningioma
15110	LEOPARD syndrome	AD[a]	Multiple lentigines
13530	Gingival fibromatosis ± hypertrichosis or other anomalies	AD[a]	
13540		AD[a]	
13550		AD	

18

TABLE 3 (continued)

D. Mesoderm (soft tissue) (continued)

22860	Juvenile fibromatosis	AR	Multiple subcutaneous tumors
21660	Familial cutaneous collagenoma	AR	Multiple skin nodules
15080	Multiple leiomyomas	AD^a	Cutaneous, uterine, and/or esophageal leiomyomas
24610		AR	
15070		AD	
15190	Multiple lipomatosis, sometimes site specific, neck or conjunctiva	AD^a	Skin cancer
15170		AD	
15180			
25770	Goldenhar's syndrome	AR	Lipodermoid of conjunctiva, hemangioma
24810	Macrosomia adiposa congenita	AR	Obese soon after birth, eosinophilia, adrenocortical adenoma

E. Alimentary Tract

17510	Familial polyposis coli	AD^a	Intestinal polyps, carcinoma of colon
17530	Gardner's syndrome	AD^a	Intestinal polyps, osteomas, fibromas, sebaceous cysts, carcinoma of colon, ampulla of Vater, pancreas, thyroid and adrenal
17520	Peutz-Jeghers' syndrome	AD^a	Intestinal polyps, ovarian (granulosa cell) tumor
[126]	Colorectal carcinoma	AD^a	
16780	Hereditary pancreatitis	AD^a	Carcinoma of pancreas
14850	Tylosis with esophageal cancer	AD^a	Carcinoma of esophagus
24730	Hepatocellular carcinoma	AR	
11890	Familial, juvenile and neonatal cirrhosis	AD	Hepatocellular carcinoma
21560		AR^a	
23510		AR	
23520			

TABLE 3 (continued)

E. Alimentary Tract (continued)

14160	Hemochromatosis	AD^a	Hepatocellular carcinoma
23510		AR^a	
23520			

Perhaps, solitary discrete polyps [127]-AD; Turcot's syndrome, 27630-AR; polyposis-sarcoma [128]-AD; esophageal cancer [129]-AR; gastric cancer [130]-AR

F. Urogenital

23330	Gonadal dysgenesis, hermaphroditism, Reifenstein's	AR^a	Gonadoblastoma, dysgerminoma
23560	syndrome, testicular feminization	AR	
23340		XR^a	
31370		XR	
31230			
31210			
30610			
16700	Ovarian tumors	AD	
27780	Wilms' tumor	AR	
[62]		AD	
14340	Hydronephrosis, familial	AD	Congenital sarcoma of kidney

Perhaps, renal cell carcinoma, 14470-AD; ureteral cancer, 19160-AD; bladder cancer [131]-AD

G. Pulmonary

13500	Fibrocystic pulmonary dysplasia	AD^a	Bronchial adenocarcinoma
[132]	Aryl hydrocarbon hydroxylase inducibility	Codominant	Bronchogenic carcinoma

H. Vascular

13800	Multiple glomus tumors	AD^a	
18730	Hereditary hemorrhagic telangiectasia of Rendu-Osler-Weber	AD^a	Angioma

TABLE 3 (continued)

H. Vascular (continued)

15340	Lymphedema with distichia	AD[a]	Lymphangiosarcoma of edematous limb

Perhaps, Kaposi's sarcoma, 14800-AD; blue rubber-bleb nevus, 11220-AD[a]; and various other angiomatous conditions, 10590-AD,AR,XR, 14080, 14090, 15350, 18720, 24700, 27250, 30160

I. Skeletal

13370	Multiple exostosis	AD[a]	Osteosarcoma, chondrosarcoma
13360		AD	
12830			
11840	Cherubism	AD[a]	Fibrous dysplasia of jaws, giant-cell tumor
12390	Fibrous dysplasia	AD	Osteosarcoma, medullary fibrosarcoma
13560			
16730	Paget's disease of bone	AD	Osteosarcoma

Perhaps, osteosarcoma, 25950-AR, and chondrosarcoma, 21530-AR, isolated or complicating multiple enchondromatosis alone (Ollier's syndrome) or with hemangioma (Maffucci's syndrome), 16600-AD; Ewing's sarcoma [133]-AD

J. Skin and Appendages (also references [134–136])

21200	Breast cancer	AR	
[137]		AD	
15490	Mastocytosis	AD	
15560	Malignant melanoma	AD	
15570			
24940	Neurocutaneous melanosis	AR	Malignant melanoma of skin and meninges
16290	Nevi (pigmented and halo)	AD[a]	Malignant melanoma
23430		AR	
20310	Albinism	AR[a]	Skin cancer
20320			

TABLE 3 (continued)

J. Skin and Appendages (continued)

27870	Xeroderma pigmentosum, xerodermoid	AR[a]	Skin cancer
27880	pigmentosum (including DeSanctis-	AD	
19440	Cacchione syndrome)		
13170	Epidermolysis bullosa dystrophica	AD[a]	Skin cancer arising in scars
22660		AR[a]	
17590	Disseminated superficial actinic porokeratosis	AR[a]	Skin cancer
[138]	Multiple sebaceous gland tumors and visceral	AR	Diverse gastrointestinal and urogenital cancers
	carcinoma (Torre's syndrome)		
10190	Acrokeratosis verruciformis, van den Bosch's	AD[a]	Warty hyperkeratosis
31450	syndrome	XR[a]	
12420	Darier-White disease	AD[a]	Keratotic papules
18160	Scleroatrophy and keratosis of limbs	AD[a]	Skin and bowel cancer
12760	Pachyonychia congenita	AD[a]	Hyperkeratosis, cutaneous horns, leukoplakia
30560	Focal dermal hypoplasia (Goltz's syndrome)	XD[a]	Mucocutaneous papillomas
13270	Multiple trichoepithelioma	AD[a]	
31310	(Spiegler-Brooke's tumors)	XD	
13280	Self-healing squamous epithelioma	AD[a]	
18450	Steatocystoma multiplex ± pachyonychia congenita	AD[a]	
18460			

Perhaps, epidermodysplasia verruciformis with basal-cell carcinoma, 22640-AR; familial cutaneous papillomatosis, 16790-AD; pilomatrixoma, 13260-AD; multiple syringioma, 18660-AD; keloids alone, 14810-AD, or as part of syndrome with torticollis, cryptorchidism, and renal dysplasia, 31430-XR

K. Lymphatic and Hematopoietic

24640	Histiocytic reticulosis, generalized or neural only	AR[a]
26770	(Letterer-Siwe disease)	AR
24750		
24760		

TABLE 3 (continued)

K. Lymphatic and Hematopoietic (continued)

23590	Familial lipochrome histiocytosis	AR[a]	
20270	Kostmann's infantile genetic agranulocytosis	AR[a]	Acute monocytic leukemia (chromosomal breaks)
26330	Polycythemia vera	AR	Acute myelocytic leukemia (may have Philadelphia chromosome)
23190	Glutathione reductase deficiency	AR[a]	Leukemia (chromosomal breaks)

Perhaps, malignant reticuloendotheliosis, 31250-XR[a]; the four leukemias, 25470, 15140, [139,140]-AD,AR; Hodgkin's disease, 23600, [141]-AR,AD; mycosis fungoides, 25440-AR; multiple myeloma, 25450-AR

L. Immunodeficiency

30030	Bruton's agammaglobulinemia	XR[a]	Leukemia, lymphoreticular
30100	Wiskott-Aldrich syndrome	XR[a]	Lymphoreticular
20890	Ataxia-telangiectasia	AR[a]	Lymphoreticular, leukemia, carcinoma of stomach, brain tumors (chromosomal breaks)
21450	Chédiak-Higashi syndrome	AR[a]	Pseudolymphoma

M. Multiple System

21090	Bloom's syndrome	AR[a]	Leukemia, intestinal cancer (chromosomal breaks)
22790	Fanconi's anemia	AR[a]	Acute myelomonocytic leukemia, squamous cell carcinoma of mucocutaneous junctions, hepatic carcinoma or adenoma (chromosomal breaks)
30500	Dyskeratosis congenita (Zinsser-Cole-Engman syndrome)	XR[a]	Leukoplakia with squamous cell carcinoma
26840	Rothmund-Thomson syndrome	AR[a]	Squamous cell carcinoma
27770	Werner's syndrome	AR[a]	Sarcoma
16670	Osteopoikilosis	AD[a]	Nevi

23

TABLE 3 (continued)

N. Inborn Errors of Metabolism

30150	Angiokeratoma diffusa (Fabry's syndrome)	XR	
27670	Tyrosinemia, hypermethioninemia, galactosemia,	AR[a]	Postcirrhotic hepatoma
23890	Wilson's disease, glycogen storage disease, type IV	AR	
23040			
27790			
23250			
[142]	α_1-antitrypsin deficiency	Codominant	Hepatoma
30780	Vitamin D-resistant rickets	XR[a]	Parathyroid adenoma

[a]Mode of inheritance is judged to be proved. (AD = autosomal dominant, AR = autosomal recessive, XD = X-linked dominant, XR = X-linked recessive)

Phase 2: Recognition of Genetic Factors

Striking familial aggregations of cancer occur, especially as part of patterns of conditions in one individual or his extended family. Colorectal cancer, for example, has been documented in pedigrees of up to four generations as an autosomal dominant; however, *familial colorectal cancer* is often explained by the polyposis syndromes, such as multiple familial polyposis and Gardner's syndrome [126]. Colorectal cancer can also be associated with other tumors both as a double primary neoplasm in a single patient, and as one of several tumor types in a family, as in Lynch's familial adenocarcinoma syndrome (colon-endometrium) [147], Turcot's syndrome (colonic polyposis-brain tumor), and perhaps other patterns of colonic neoplasm with sarcomas or lymphomas [148]. Thus, as a *genetic* disease, colorectal cancer is seen, on occasion, as a single condition, but more often as part of a nonrandom association of benign or malignant diseases either in the patient or his family.

Familial breast cancer may obey the same rule. Certain pedigrees suggest a dominant trait with breast cancer alone or in association with mammary fibrocystic disease or with other types of neoplasms, like female genital cancer, sarcoma, and polyposis [137,149]. The last combination — breast cancer-polyposis — has emerged as a single-gene trait called Cowden's disease (after the first patient) or the multiple hamartoma syndrome, for it also consists of mucocutaneous warts, multiple lipomas, angiomas, and thyroid tumors [123-125].

Phase 3: Laboratory Studies

After clinical and genetic observations have defined a disease entity, the laboratory offers the chance for understanding its basic biology or pathogenesis. Genetic markers, like erythrocytic antigens or enzymes, may be studied in large case collections, as in reports associating blood group A with gastric cancer or HL-A2 with Hodgkin's disease [150]. In familial aggregations, markers might be tested in hopes of adding to human genetic linkage groups.

The hope of finding a correctable defect of a single enzyme that can be plausibly linked to carcinogenesis has not been realized. But deserved fanfare and anticipation surround developments in two conditions—one very rare, the other very common. Patients with the first, xeroderma pigmentosum, are extremely sun-sensitive and prone to fatal skin cancers. Their fibroblasts and epidermal cells poorly repair DNA damage after ultraviolet radiation, specifically in excising pyrimidine dimer [117].

The more common condition is lung cancer. Intermediate and high levels of inducibility of the enzyme aryl hydrocarbon hydroxylase were found in mitogen-stimulated lymphocytes of 96 percent of lung cancer patients compared with 56 percent of individuals with other types of cancer or none at all [132]. Since this enzyme forms carcinogenic epoxides from a variety of polycyclic hydrocarbons, like those found in tobacco smoke, individuals with high levels of inducibility of enzyme may be especially susceptible to inhaled precursors of carcinogenic compounds. One gene locus may control the level of inducibility in man as it does in mice [151]. Altogether the findings, if confirmed by another research group, may explain some of the heritability of human lung cancer [152].

Other inborn variations in metabolism, like glycogen-storage disease and hemochromatosis, may account for certain cases of familial hepatoma, especially following cirrhosis [153, 154]. Genetically determined deficiency of the enzyme α_1-antitrypsin recently joined the list. Familial aggregations of emphysema and adult cirrhosis or infantile hepatitis are associated with α_1-antitrypsin deficiency as a result of the Z allele, both in the homozygous and heterozygous states [155]. Liver cancer occurred in at least seven homozygous and four heterozygous individuals, accompanied not always with cirrhosis, but invariably with nonglycogen glycoprotein cytoplasmic globules that may be pathognomonic of the Z allele [142,156-158]. The same globules were found in livers from 10 percent of patients with hepatoma [155, 156]. Although α_1-antitrypsin could not be assayed in these retrospective series, the suggestion remains that a fair proportion of hepatomas occurs in persons with the Z allele whose frequency is as high as 2.4 percent in the population.

Phase 4: Reclassification, Lumping, and Splitting

The nosologic cycle continues as genetic and laboratory studies reveal new criteria permitting recognition of previously unsuspected heterogeneity or similarity.

For example, the same assay that identified the endonuclease defect in *xeroderma pigmentosum* also recognized new differences among clinically identical patients. In some patients, different enzymes may be defective; for co-cultivation of fibroblasts from certain pairs of patients *corrects* the in vitro molecular defect [117]. Similarly, subgroups within Fanconi's anemia may emerge based on the presence or absence of certain birth defects and perhaps the frequencies of chromosomal breakage and fibroblast transformation by simian virus 40 [159,160]. At the same time, similarities between Fanconi's anemia and dyskeratosis congenita suggest they may be combined as one nosologic entity [161].

Splitting and unraveling of syndromes, though necessary, may thwart identification of a common biologic thread. The recognition of a genuinely unifying concept is a rare event. One such synthesis, that has survived scrutiny and time, is Miller's enumeration of the genetic and acquired disorders of chromosomal fragility associated with leukemia [162].

A more recent synthesis deserving study is the concept of "neurocristopathy" [163]. Bolande coined the word to include diverse diseases involving tissue derived from the embryonic neural crest. This structure is identified only in early embryos, because it soon vanishes as cells migrate to form definitive pigmentary cells (skin and iris) and the autonomic nervous system as well as diverse cell types of the endocrine system, such as islet cells of the pancreas. Neoplasms of neural crest tissue include chemodectoma, pheochromocytoma, neuroblastoma, carcinoid, and medullary carcinoma of the thyroid. They may occur either singly or in various combinations, such as neurofibromatosis, the multiple endocrine adenomatoses, and the multiple mucosal neuroma syndrome.

Support for the concept comes, in part, from classical embryology and from similar ultrastructural and histochemical features of various adult tissues indicating the presence of small polypeptide hormones with a neurohumoral function [164]. Added support for the neural crest origin of neurofibromatosis may be the presence of high levels of nerve growth factor in patients with the condition [165]. The findings, obtained by tedious bioassay, could not be repeated by another group [166].

SUGGESTIONS FOR FURTHER WORK

The keystone to future work, I propose, is the further clinical, laboratory, and epidemiologic delineation of congenital, genetic, and familial syndromes that predispose to cancer. Such an effort to discover host factors requires collaboration among clinicians who have the patients, laboratory scientists with in vitro approaches, and epidemiologists with statistical and population resources. Selected medical genetics clinics may be suitable settings for such efforts. My personal opinions about future opportunities are:

1) Collaborative clinical studies: Further delineate congenital, genetic, and familial syndromes predisposing to cancer; identify preneoplastic lesions in such syndromes; relate genetic markers to malignancy; search for human mutagens.

2) Laboratory studies: Apply banding and computer technology in karyotyping selected tumors and patients; study molecular and cellular manifestations of human neoplastic syndromes, e.g., by hybridization of cells and nucleic acids; discover models of human neoplastic syndromes in inbred and domestic animals.

3) Epidemiologic studies: Study cancer experience of inbred groups; expand use of existing resources with record linkage if possible, e.g., registries of cancer, birth defects and twins; establish registries of rare events, e.g., rare cell types, adult cell types in children, long-term survivors, offspring

of cancer patients; determine frequency of cancer in heterozygotes of selected recessive traits.

4) Efforts for cancer control and prevention: Educate professionals and laymen in the known genetic basis of cancer and the need for attention to family medical history; extend cancer surveillance and screening to family, especially at diagnosis of syndrome predisposing to cancer, diagnosis of unusual array of tumors among relatives, or at birth of child to long-term survivor; evaluate methods of early diagnoses in high-risk patients; examine possible role of medical genetics clinics.

CONCLUSIONS

More cancers probably can be ascribed with certitude to genetic etiologies than to recognized environmental agents, although the causes of most human cancer are unknown. The Ph[1] chromosome in CML and the absent chromosome 22 in meningioma are consistent chromosomal markers of neoplasia. Whether they initiate malignancy or are just epiphenomena is unresolved; but, tumor progression seems favored by increasing chromosomal aberrations. Banding techniques and computer technology have disclosed specific chromosomal markers in AML, the Wilms' tumor-aniridia syndrome, and retinoblastoma in the 13q− syndrome. Clinicians depend on karyotypes in diagnosis and prognosis; researchers generate and test useful hypotheses concerning, e.g., the clonal origin of cancer, the possibility of etiology-specific karyotypes, and the necessary presence of the Y chromosome in the origins of gonadoblastoma.

Of the known single-gene traits in man, 161 (9 percent) have neoplastic or preneoplastic manifestations or complications. Five Mendelian diseases that have chromosomal fragility are of special interest because they represent gross defects of DNA associated with malignancy and produced by a pair of mutant genes. The malignancies associated with hereditary disease affect every organ system and are often histologically identical to the most frequent human cancers. More such conditions are likely to be discovered as collaborative efforts recognize clinical, genetic, and laboratory manifestations of heterogeneity in existing diseases. Such syndrome delineation is the foundation for future progress in the role of host factors in cancer.

REFERENCES

1. Symposium on fundamental cancer research, 1969. *Genetic Concepts and Neoplasia.* Williams & Wilkins, Baltimore, 1970.

2. Jackson, L.G. Genetics in neoplastic diseases. *In* Goodman, R.M., ed. *Genetic Disorders of Man,* Little, Brown, Boston, 1970, pp. 943-979.

3. Fraumeni, J.F., Jr. I-2. Genetic Factors. *In* Holland, J.F., and Frei, E. III, eds. *Cancer Medicine.* Lea & Febiger, Philadelphia, 1973, pp. 7-15.

4. Lawler, S.D. Cancer. *In* Sorsby, A., ed. *Clinical Genetics,* 2nd ed. Butterworth, London, 1973, pp. 568-589.

5. Lynch, H.T., and Kaplan, A.R. Cancer genetic problems: Host-environmental considerations. *Prog. Exp. Tumor Res.* *19:*333-352, 1974.

6. Anderson, D.E. Familial susceptibility. This volume, 1975.

7. Boveri, T. *Zur Frage der Entstehung maligner Tumoren.* Gustav Fischer, Jena, 1914.

8. Caspersson, T., Farber, S., Foley, G.E., et al. Chemical differentiation along metaphase chromosomes. *Exp. Cell Res.* *49:*219-222, 1968.

9. Yunis, J.J., ed. *Human Chromosome Methodology,* 2nd ed. Academic Press, New York, 1974.

10. Sandberg, A.A., and Hossfeld D.K. Chromosomal abnormalities in human neoplasia. *Annu. Rev. Med.* *21:*379-408, 1970.

11. Woodliff, H.J. *Leukaemia Cytogenetics.* Year Book Medical Publishers, Chicago, 1971.

12. Koller, P.C. The role of chromosomes in cancer biology. *Recent Results Cancer Res.* *38:*1-122, 1972.

13. Sandberg, A.A., and Hossfeld, D.K. II-4. Chromosomes in the pathogenesis of human cancer and leukemia. *In* Holland, J.F., and Frei, E. III, eds. *Cancer Medicine.* Lea & Febiger, Philadelphia, 1973, pp. 151-177.

14. Bishun, N.P., Raven, R.W., and Williams, D.C. Chromosomes and cancer, *J. Surg. Oncol.* *6:*163-181, 1974.

15. German, J., ed. *Chromosomes and Cancer.* John Wiley & Sons, New York, 1974.

16. Nowell, P.C., and Hungerford, D.A. A minute chromosome in human chronic granulocytic leukemia. *Science 132:*1497, 1960.

17. Caspersson, T., Gahrton, G., Lindsten, J., et al. Identification of the Philadelphia chromosome as a number 22 by quinacrine mustard fluorescence analysis. *Exp. Cell Res.* *63:*238-240, 1970.

18. Rowley, J.D. A new consistent chromosomal abnormality in chronic myelogenous leukaemia identified by quinacrine fluorescence and giemsa staining. *Nature (Lond.) 243:* 290-293, 1973.

19. Whang-Peng, J., Lee, E.C., and Knutsen, T.A. Genesis of the Ph[1] chromosome. *J. Natl. Cancer Inst. 52:*1035-1036, 1974.

20. Hayata, I., Kakati, S., and Sandberg, A.A. A new translocation related to the Philadelphia chromosome. *Lancet 2:*1385, 1973.

21. Mitelman, F. Heterogeneity of Ph[1] in chronic myeloid leukaemia. *Hereditas 76:* 315-316, 1974.

22. Whang-Peng, J., Canellos, G.P., Carbone, P.P., et al. Clinical implications of cytogenetic variants in chronic myelocytic leukemia. *Blood 32:*755-766, 1968.

23. Ezdinli, E.Z., Sokal, J.E., Crosswhite, L., et al. Philadelphia-chromosome-positive and -negative chronic myelocytic leukemia. *Ann. Intern. Med. 72:*175-182, 1970.

24. Shiffman, N.J., Stecker, E., Conen, P.E., et al. Males with chronic myeloid leukemia and the 45,XO,Ph[1] chromosome pattern. *Can. Med. Assoc. J. 110:*1151-1154, 1974.

25. Lawler, S.D., Lobb, D.S., and Wiltshaw, E. Philadelphia-chromosome positive bone-marrow cells showing loss of the Y in males with chronic myeloid leukaemia. *Br. J. Haematol. 27:*247-252, 1974.

26. Canellos, G.P., and Whang-Peng, J. Philadelphia-chromosome-positive preleukaemic state. *Lancet:2:*1227-1229, 1972.

27. Nusbacher, J., and Hirschhorn, K. Autosomal anomalies in man. *Adv. Teratol. 3:* 11-63, 1968.

28. Gunz, F.W., Fitzgerald, P.H., and Adams, A. An abnormal chromosome in chronic lymphocytic leukaemia. *Br. Med. J. 2:*1097-1099, 1962.

29. Fitzgerald, P.H., Rastrick, J.M., and Hamer, J.W. Acute plasma cell leukaemia following chronic lymphatic leukaemia: Transformation or two separate diseases? *Br. J. Haematol. 25;*171-177, 1973.

30. Goh, K. Smaller G(Gp–) and t(Gp–;Dp+) chromosomes: A familial study with one member having acute leukemia. *Am J. Dis. Child. 115:*732-738, 1968.

31. Juberg, R.C., and Jones, B. The Christchurch chromosome (Gp–): Mongolism, erythroleukemia and an inherited Gp– chromosome (Christchurch). *N. Engl. J. Med. 282:* 292-297, 1970.

32. Mastrangelo, R., Zuelzer, W.W., and Thompson, R.I. The significance of the Ph[1] chromosome in acute myeloblastic leukemia: Serial cytogenetic studies in a critical case. *Pediatrics 40:*834-841, 1967.

33. Pedersen, B. The blastic crisis of chronic myeloid leukemia: Acute transformation of a preleukaemic condition? *Br. J. Haematol. 25:*141-145, 1973.

34. Sandberg, A.A., Takagi, N., Sofuni, T., et al. Chromosomes and causation of human cancer and leukemia. V. Karyotypic aspects of acute leukemia. *Cancer 22:* 1268-1282, 1968.

35. Gunz, F.W., Bach, B.I., Crossen, P.E., et al. Relevance of the cytogenetic status in acute leukemia in adults. *J. Natl. Cancer Inst. 50:*55-61, 1973.

36. Trujillo, J.M., Cork, A., Hart, J.S., et al. Clinical implications of aneuploid cytogenetic profiles in adult acute leukemia. *Cancer 33:*824-834, 1974.

37. Hart, J.S., Trujillo, J.M., Freireich, E.J., et al. Cytogenetic studies and their clinical correlates in adults with acute leukemia. *Ann. Intern. Med. 75:*353-360, 1971.

38. Rowley, J.D. Identification of a translocation with quinacrine fluorescence in a patient with acute leukemia. *Ann. Genet. 16:*109-112, 1973.

39. Sakurai, M., Oshimura, M., Kakati, S., et al. 8-21 translocation and missing sex chromosomes in acute leukaemia. *Lancet 2:*227-228, 1974.

40. Rowley, J.D. Missing sex chromosomes and translocations in acute leukaemia. *Lancet 2:*835-836, 1974.

41. ——. Chromosomal patterns in myelocytic leukemia. *N. Engl. J. Med. 289:*220-221, 1973.

42. Jonasson, J., Gahrton, G., Lindsten, J., et al. Trisomy 8 in acute myeloblastic leukemia and sideroachrestic anemia. *Blood 43:*557-563, 1974.

43. Atkin, N.B. Chromosomes in human malignant tumors: A review and assessment. *In* German, J., ed. *Chromosomes and Cancer.* John Wiley & Sons, New York, 1974, pp. 375-422.

44. Mark, J. The human meningioma: A benign tumor with specific chromosome characteristics. *In* German, J., ed. *Chromosomes and Cancer.* John Wiley & Sons, New York, 1974, pp. 497-517.

45. Manolov, G., and Manolova, Y. Marker band in one chromosome 14 from Burkitt lymphomas. *Nature (Lond.) 237:*33-34, 1972.

46. Gartler, S.M. Utilization of mosaic systems in the study of the origin and progression of tumors. *In* German, J., ed. *Chromosomes and Cancer.* John Wiley & Sons, New York, 1974, pp. 313-334.

47. Fialkow, P.J. The origin and development of human tumors studied with cell markers. *N. Engl. J. Med. 291:*26-35, 1974.

48. Hauschka, T.S. The chromosomes in ontogeny and oncogeny. *Cancer Res. 21:* 957-974, 1961.

49. Van Dyke, D.L., Palmer, C.G., and Nance, W.E. Chromosome polymorphism and twin zygosity (Abstract). *Am. J. Hum. Genet. 26:*88A, 1974.

50. Gahrton, G., Lindsten, J., and Zech, L. Clonal origin of the Philadelphia chromosome from either the paternal or the maternal chromosome number 22. *Blood 43:*837-840, 1974.

51. Mitelman, F., Mark, J., Levan, G., et al. Tumor etiology and chromosome pattern. *Science 176:*1340-1341, 1972.

52. Rowley, J.D. Do human tumors show a chromosome pattern specific for each etiologic agent? *J. Natl. Cancer Inst. 52:*315-320, 1974.

53. Ohno, S. Genetic implication of karyological instability of malignant somatic cells. *Physiol. Rev. 51:*496-526, 1971.

54. ——. Aneuploidy as a possible means employed by malignant cells to express recessive phenotypes. *In* German, J., ed. *Chromosomes and Cancer,* John Wiley & Sons, New York, 1974, pp. 77-94.

55. Rudkin, G.T., Hungerford, D.A., and Nowell, P.C. DNA contents of chromosome Ph[1] and chromosome 21 in human chronic granulocytic leukemia. *Science 144:*1229-1232, 1964.

56. Spiers, A.S.D., and Baikie, A.G. A special role of the group 17, 18 chromosomes in reticuloendothelial neoplasia. *Br. J. Cancer 24:*77-91, 1970.

57. Minkler, J.L., Gofman, J.W., and Tandy, R.K. A specific common chromosomal pathway for the origin of human malignancy—II. *Br. J. Cancer 24:*726-740, 1970.

58. Sandberg, A.A. Chromosome changes in human malignant tumors: An evaluation. *Recent Results Cancer Res. 44:*75-85, 1974.

59. Miller, R.W. Relation between cancer and congenital defects in man. *N. Engl. J. Med. 275:* 87-93, 1966.

60. Warkany, J. *Congenital Malformations. Notes and Comments.* Year Book Medical Publishers, Chicago, 1971, pp. 1199-1220.

61. Bolande, R.P. Relationships between teratogenesis and oncogenesis. *In* Perrin, E.V.D., Finegold, M.J., and Brunson, J.G., eds. *Pathobiology.* Williams & Wilkins, Baltimore, 1973, pp. 114-134.

62. Knudson, A.G., Jr., and Strong, L.C. Mutation and cancer. A model for Wilms' tumor of the kidney. *J. Natl. Cancer Inst. 48:*313-324, 1972.

63. Miller, R.W., Fraumeni, J.F., Jr., and Manning, M.D. Association of Wilms' tumor with aniridia, hemihypertrophy and other congenital malformations. *N. Engl. J. Med. 270:* 922-927, 1964.

64. Pendergrass, T.W. Congenital anomalies in children with Wilms' tumor: A new survey. *Cancer.* In press, 1975.

65. Barakat, A.Y., Papadopoulou, Z.L., Chandra, R.S., et al. Pseudohermaphroditism, nephron disorder and Wilms' tumor: A unifying concept. *Pediatrics 54:*366-369, 1974.

66. Beckwith, J.B. Macroglossia, omphalocele, adrenal cytomegaly, gigantism, and hyperplastic visceromegaly. *Birth Defects 5:*188-196, 1969.

67. Meadows, A.T., Lichtenfeld, J.L., and Koop, C.E. Wilms's tumor in three children of a woman with congenital hemihypertrophy. *N. Engl. J. Med. 291:*23-25, 1974.

68. Ladda, R., Atkins, L., Littlefield, J., et al. Computer-assisted analysis of chromosomal abnormalities: Detection of a deletion in aniridia/Wilms' tumor syndrome. *Science 185:*784-787, 1974.

69. Grace, E., Drennan, J., Colver, D., et al. The 13q– deletion syndrome. *J. Med. Genet. 8:*351-357, 1971.

70. Niebuhr, E., and Ottosen, J. Ring chromosome D (13) associated with multiple congenital malformations. *Ann. Genet. 16:*157-166, 1973.

71. Orye, E., Delbeke, M.J., and Vandenabeele, B. Retinoblastoma and long arm deletion of chromosome 13. Attempts to define the deleted segment. *Clin. Genet. 5:*457-464, 1974.

72. Knudson, A.G., Jr. Mutation and cancer: Statistical study of retinoblastoma. *Proc. Natl. Acad. Sci. USA 68:*820-823, 1971.

73. Sorsby, A. Bilateral retinoblastoma: A dominantly inherited affection. *Br. Med. J.* *2:*580-583, 1972.

74. Jensen, R.D., and Miller, R.W. Retinoblastoma: Epidemiologic characteristics. *N. Engl. J. Med.* *285:*307-311, 1971.

75. Kitchin, F.D., and Ellsworth, R.M. Pleiotropic effects of the gene for retinoblastoma. *J. Med. Genet.* *11:*244-246, 1974.

76. Gordon, H. Family studies in retinoblastoma. *Birth Defects 10:*185-190, 1974.

77. Miller, R.W. Neoplasia and Down's syndrome. *Ann. N.Y. Acad. Sci. 171:*637-644, 1970.

78. Rosner, F., and Lee, S.L. Down's syndrome and acute leukemia: Myeloblastic or lymphoblastic? Report of forty-three cases and review of the literature. *Am. J. Med. 53:* 203-218, 1972.

79. Jackson, A.W., Muldal, S., Ockey, C.H., et al. Carcinoma of male breast in association with the Klinefelter syndrome. *Br. Med. J. 1:*223-225, 1965.

80. Harnden, D.G., Maclean, N., and Langlands, A.O. Carcinoma of the breast and Klinefelter's syndrome. *J. Med. Genet. 8:*460-461, 1971.

81. Sohn, K-Y., and Boggs, D.R. Klinefelter's syndrome, LSD usage and acute lymphoblastic leukemia. *Clin. Genet. 6:*20-22, 1974.

82. Tsung, S.H., and Heckman, M.G. Klinefelter syndrome, immunological disorders, and malignant neoplasm: Report of a case. *Arch. Pathol. 98:*351-354, 1974.

83. Schellhas, H.F. Malignant potential of the dysgenetic gonad. Part I & Part II. *Obstet. Gynecol. 44:*298-309, 455-462, 1974.

84. Teter, J. A new concept of classification of gonadal tumours arising from germ cells (gonocytoma) and their histogenesis. *Gynaecologia 150:*84-102, 1960.

85. Mulvihill, J.J., Wade, W.M., and Miller, R.W. Gonadoblastoma in dysgenetic gonads with a Y chromosome. *Lancet 1:*863, 1975.

86. Schultz, L.S., Assimacopoulos, C.A., and Lillehei, R.C. Turner's syndrome with associated gastrointestinal hemorrhage: A case report. *Surgery 68:*485-488, 1970.

87. Wertelecki, W., Fraumeni, J.F., Jr., and Mulvihill, J.J. Nongonadal neoplasia in Turner's syndrome. *Cancer 26:*485-488, 1970.

88. Andreev, V.C., and Zlatkov, N.B., Basal cell nevus syndrome and Turner's syndrome in a patient. *Int. J. Dermatol. 10:*13-16, 1971.

89. Ayraud, N., Duplay, J., Grellier, P., et al.: Karyotype 45,X/46,XX/47,XXX et tumeur du systeme nerveux. Deux observations. *Nouv. Presse Med. 1:*2902-2903, 1972.

90. Buchanan, G. Turner's and Noonan's syndromes. *Br. Med. J. 2:*225, 1974.

91. Males, J.L., and Lain, K.C. Epithelioid sarcoma in XO/XX Turner's syndrome. *Arch. Pathol. 94:*214-216, 1972.

92. Pawliger, D.F., Barrow, M., and Noyes, W.D. Acute leukaemia and Turner's syndrome. *Lancet 1:*1345, 1970.

93. Cutler, B.S., Forbes, A.P., Ingersoll, F.M., et al. Endometrial carcinoma after stilbestrol therapy in gonadal dysgenesis. *N. Engl. J. Med. 287:*628-631, 1972.

94. Charny, C.W., and Wolgin, W. *Cryptorchism.* Hoeber-Harper, New York, 1957, pp. 61-71.

95. Santesteban, A. Cryptorchidism in the newborn. *Pediatrics 51:*310-311, 1973.

96. Gehring, G.G., Rodriguez, F.R., and Woodhead, D.M. Malignant degeneration of cryptorchid testes following orchiopexy. *J. Urol. 112:*354-356, 1974.

97. Ashley, D.J.B., and Mostofi, F.K. The spermatogenic function of tumor-bearing testes. *J. Urol. 81:*773-779, 1959.

98. Dougall, A.J., Maclean, N., and Wilkinson, A.W. Histology of the maldescended testis at operation. *Lancet 1:*771-774, 1974.

99. Fraumeni, J.F., Jr., Li, F.P., and Dalager, N. Teratomas in children: Epidemiologic features. *J. Natl. Cancer Inst. 51:*1425-1430, 1973.

100. Schroeder, T.M., and Kurth, R. Spontaneous chromosomal breakage and high incidence of leukemia in inherited disease. *Blood 37:*96-112, 1971.

101. Sedgwick, R.P., and Boder, E. Ataxia-telangiectasia. *In* Vinken, P.J., and Bruyn, G.W., eds. *Handbook of Clinical Neurology, The Phakomatoses.* North-Holland Publishing, Amsterdam, 1972, pp. 267-339.

102. Kersey, J.H., Spector B.D., and Good, R.A. Primary immunodeficiency diseases and cancer: The immunodeficiency-cancer registry. *Int. J. Cancer 12:*333-347, 1973.

103. Kersey, J.H. Immune deficiency diseases. This volume, 1975.

104. Harnden, D.G. Ataxia telangiectasia syndrome: Cytogenetic and cancer aspects. *In* German, J., ed. *Chromosomes and Cancer.* John Wiley & Sons, New York, 1974, pp. 619-636.

105. Hecht, F., and McCaw, B.K. Chromosomally marked lymphocyte clones in ataxia-telangiectasia. *Lancet 1:*563-564, 1974.

106. Bochkov, N.P., Lopukhin, Y.M., Kuleshov, N.P., et al. Cytogenetic study of patients with ataxia-telangiectasia. *Humangenetik 24:*115-128, 1974.

107. Rary, J.M., Bender, M.A., and Kelly, T.E. Cytogenetic studies of ataxia-telangiectasia (Abstract). *Am J. Hum. Genet. 26:*70A, 1974.

108. Hecht, F., McCaw, B.K., and Koler, R.D. Ataxia-telangiectasia – Clonal growth of translocation lymphocytes. *N. Engl. J. Med. 289:*286-291, 1973.

109. Dosik, H., Hsu, L.Y., Todaro, G.J., et al. Leukemia in Fanconi's anemia: Cytogenetic and tumor virus susceptibility studies. *Blood 36:*341-352, 1970.

110. Swift, M., Zimmerman, D., and McDonough, E.R. Squamous cell carcinomas in Fanconi's anemia. *J.A.M.A. 216:*325-327, 1971.

111. Mulvihill, J.M., Ridolfi, R.L., Schultz, F.R., et al. Hepatic adenoma in Fanconi anemia treated with oxymetholone. *J. Pediatr.* In press, 1975.

112. Meadows, A.T., Naiman, J.L., and Valdes-Dapena, M. Hepatoma associated with androgen therapy for aplastic anemia. *J. Pediatr. 84:*109-110, 1974.

113. Swift, M. Fanconi's anaemia in the genetics of neoplasia. *Nature (Lond.) 230:* 370-373, 1971.

114. Poon, P.K., O'Brien, R.L., and Parker, J.W. Defective DNA repair in Fanconi's anaemia. *Nature (Lond.) 250:*223-225, 1974.

115. Sasaki, M.S., and Tonomura, A. A high susceptibility of Fanconi's anemia to chromosome breakage by DNA cross-linking agents. *Cancer Res. 33:*1829-1836, 1973.

116. Finkelberg, R., Thompson, M.W., and Siminovitch, L. Survival after treatment with EMS, gamma-rays, and mitomycin C of skin fibroblasts from patients with Fanconi's anemia (Abstract). *Am. J. Hum. Genet. 26:*30A, 1974.

117. Robbins, J.H., Kraemer, K.H., Lutzner, M.A., et al. Xeroderma pigmentosum. An inherited disease with sun sensitivity, multiple cutaneous neoplasms, and abnormal DNA repair. *Ann. Intern. Med. 80:*221-248, 1974.

118. German, J. Bloom's syndrome. II. The prototype of human genetic disorders predisposing to chromosome instability and cancer. *In* German, J., ed. *Chromosomes and Cancer.* John Wiley & Sons, New York, 1974, pp. 601-617.

119. Gilman, P.A., Jackson, D.P., and Guild, H.G. Congenital agranulocytosis: Prolonged survival and terminal acute leukemia. *Blood 36:*576-585, 1970.

120. Fraumeni, J.F., Jr. Genetic determinants of cancer. *In* Doll, R., and Vodopija, I., eds. *Host Environment Interactions in the Etiology of Cancer in Man.* I.A.R.C. Scientific Publications No. 7. I.A.R.C. Lyon, 1973, pp. 49-55.

121. McKusick, V.A. *Mendelian Inheritance in Man. Catalogs of Autosomal Dominant, Autosomal Recessive, and X-linked Phenotypes,* 3rd ed. The John Hopkins Press, Baltimore, 1971.

122. Knudson, A.G., Jr., and Strong, L.C. Mutation and cancer: Neuroblastoma and pheochromocytoma. *Am. J. Hum. Genet. 24:*514-532, 1972.

123. Lloyd, K.M., II, and Dennis, M. Cowden's disease. A possible new symptom complex with multiple system involvement. *Ann. Intern, Med. 58:*136-142, 1963.

124. Weary, P.E., Gorlin, R.J., Gentry, W.C., Jr., et al. Multiple hamartoma syndrome (Cowden's disease). *Arch. Dermatol. 106:*682-690, 1972.

125. Gentry, W.C., Jr., Eskritt, N.R., and Gorlin, R.J. Multiple hamartoma syndrome (Cowden's disease). *Arch. Dermatol. 109:*521-525, 1974.

126. Wennstrom, J., Pierce, E.R., and McKusick, V.A. Hereditary benign and malignant lesions of the large bowel. *Cancer 34:*850-857, 1974.

127. Woolf, C.M., Richards R.C., and Gardner, E.J. Occasional discrete polyps of the colon and rectum showing an inherited tendency in a kindred. *Cancer 8:*403-408, 1955.

128. Fraumeni, J.F., Jr., Vogel, C.L., and Easton, J.M. Sarcomas and multiple polyposis in a kindred. A genetic variety of hereditary polyposis? *Arch. Intern. Med. 121:*57-61, 1968.

129. Pour, P., and Ghadirian, P. Familial cancer of the esophagus in Iran. *Cancer 33:* 1649-1652, 1974.

130. Creagan, E.T., and Fraumeni, J.F., Jr. Familial gastric cancer and immunologic abnormalities. *Cancer 32:*1325-1331, 1973.

131. Fraumeni, J.F., Jr., and Thomas, L.B. Malignant bladder tumors in a man and his three sons. *J.A.M.A. 201:*507-509, 1967.

132. Kellermann, G., Shaw, C.R., and Luyten-Kellerman, M. Aryl hydrocarbon hydroxylase inducibility and bronchogenic carcinoma. *N. Engl. J. Med. 289:*934-937, 1973.

133. Hutter, R.V.P., Francis, K.C., and Foote, F.W., Jr. Ewing's sarcoma in siblings. Report of the second known occurrence. *Am. J. Surg. 107:*598-603, 1964.

134. Newbold, P.C.H. Pre-cancer and the skin. *Br. J. Dermatol. 86:*417-434, 1972.

135. Dunham, L.J. Cancer in man at site of prior benign lesion of skin or mucous membrane: A review. *Cancer Res. 32:*1359-1374, 1972.

136. Reed, W.B., Boder, E., and Gardner, M. Congenital and genetic skin disorders with tumor formation. *Birth Defects 10:*265-284, 1974.

137. Anderson, D.E. Genetic study of breast cancer: Identification of a high risk group. *Cancer 34:*1090-1097, 1974.

138. Jakobiec, F.A. Sebaceous adenoma of the eyelid and visceral malignancy. *Am. J. Ophthalmol. 78:*952-960, 1974.

139. Snyder, A.L., Li, F.P., Henderson, E.S., et al. Possible inherited leukaemogenic factors in familial acute myelogenous leukaemia. *Lancet 1:*586-589, 1970.

140. Lundmark, K.M., Thilén, A., and Vahlquist, B. Familial leukaemia – three cases of acute leukaemia in four siblings. *Acta Paediatr. Scand. (Suppl.) 172:*200-205, 1967.

141. Fraumeni, J.F., Jr. Family studies in Hodgkin's disease. *Cancer Res. 34:*1164-1165, 1974.

142. Eriksson, S., and Hägerstrand, I. Cirrhosis and malignant hepatoma in alpha$_1$-antitrypsin deficiency. *Acta Med. Scand. 195:*451-458, 1974.

143. Souadjian, J.V., Enriquez, P., Silverstein, M.N., et al. The spectrum of diseases associated with thymoma. Coincidence or syndrome? *Arch. Intern. Med. 134:*374-379, 1974.

144. Souadjian, J.V., Silverstein, M.N., and Titus, J.L. Thymoma and cancer. *Cancer 22:*1221-1225, 1968.

145. Vessey, M.P., and Doll, R. Thymectomy and cancer–A follow-up study. *Br. J. Cancer 26:*53-58, 1972.

146. Papatestas. A.E., Osserman, K.E., and Kark, A.E. The relationship between thymus and oncogenesis. A study of the incidence of non thymic malignancy in myasthenia gravis. *Br. J. Cancer 25:*635-645, 1971.

147. Lynch, H.T., Guirgis, H., Swartz, M., et al. Genetics and colon cancer. *Arch. Surg. 106:*669-675, 1973.

148. Miller, R.W. Deaths from childhood leukemia and solid tumors among twins and other sibs in the United States, 1960-67. *J. Natl. Cancer Inst. 46:*203-209, 1971.

149. Li, F.P., and Fraumeni, J.F., Jr. Soft-tissue sarcomas, breast cancer, and other neoplasms. A familial syndrome? *Ann. Intern. Med. 71:*747-752, 1969.

150. Bodmer, W.F. Genetic factors in Hodgkin's disease: Association with a disease-susceptibility locus (DSA) in the HL-A region. *Natl. Cancer Inst. Monogr. 36:*127-134, 1973.

151. Nebert, D.W., and Gielen, J.E: Genetic regulation of aryl hydrocarbon hydroxylase induction in the mouse, *Fed. Proc. 31:*1315-1325, 1972.

152. Tokuhata, G.K. Familial factors in human lung cancer and smoking. *Am. J. Public Health 54:*24-32, 1964.

153. Fraumeni, J.F., Jr., Miller, R.W., and Hill, J.A. Primary carcinoma of the liver in childhood: An epidemiologic study. *J. Natl. Cancer Inst. 40:*1087-1099, 1968.

154. Hines, C., Jr., Davis, W.D., Jr., and Ferrante, W.A. Hepatoma developing in hemochromatosis in spite of adequate treatment by multiple phlebotomies. *Am. J. Dig. Dis. 16:*349-355, 1971.

155. Brunt, P.W. Progress report. Antitrypsin and the liver. *Gut 15:*573-580, 1974.

156. Berg, N.O., and Eriksson, S. Liver disease in adults with alpha$_1$-antitrypsin deficiency. *N. Engl. J. Med. 287:*1264-1267, 1972.

157. Rawlings, W., Jr., Moss, J., Cooper, H.S., et al. Hepatocellular carcinoma and partial deficiency of alpha$_1$-antitrypsin (MZ). *Ann. Intern. Med. 81:*771-773, 1974.

158. Lieberman, J. Emphysema, cirrhosis, and hepatoma with alpha$_1$-antitrypsin deficiency. *Ann. Intern. Med. 81:*850-852, 1974.

159. Hirschman, R.J., Shulman, N.R., Abuelo, J.G., et al. Chromosomal aberrations in two cases of inherited aplastic anemia with unusual clinical features. *Ann. Intern. Med. 71:*107-117, 1969.

160. Abels, D., and Reed, W.B. Fanconi-like syndrome. Immunologic deficiency, pancytopenia, and cutaneous malignancies. *Arch. Dermatol. 107:*419-423, 1973.

161. Steier, W., Van Voolen, G.A., and Selmanowitz, V.J. Dyskeratosis congenita: Relationship to Fanconi's anemia. *Blood 39:*510-521, 1972.

162. Miller, R.W. Persons with exceptionally high risk of leukemia. *Cancer Res. 27:* 2420-2423, 1967.

163. Bolande, R.P. The neurocristopathies. A unifying concept of disease arising in neural crest maldevelopment. *Hum. Pathol. 5:*409-429, 1974.

164. Pearse, A.G.E., and Polak, J.M. Endocrine tumours of neural crest origin: Neurolophomas, apudomas and the apud concept. *Med. Biol. 52:*3-18, 1974.

165. Schenkein, I., Bueker, E.D., Helson, L., et al.: Increased nerve-growth-stimulating activity in disseminated neurofibromatosis. *N. Engl. J. Med. 290:*613-614, 1974.

166. Tischler, A.S. A study of serum nerve growth stimulating activity in patients with neurofibromatosis utilizing a modified bioassay technique. *Exp. Neurol. 44:*440-447, 1974.

DISCUSSION

Dr. Knudson pointed out that only in the 13q-deletion syndrome is there evidence that the chromosome defect clearly is a precursor of the tumor. Whether other neoplasms have distinct chromosomal defects remains to be answered. **Dr. R. W. Miller** questioned the leukemogenic potential of the Philadelphia chromosome (Ph^1) in chronic myelocytic leukemia. **Dr. Knudson** agreed this translocation might be leukemogenic. However, the mutation is found only in the leukemic clone of cells, rather than all body cells as in the 13q- syndrome. Thus, one cannot prove the defect is responsible for the leukemia. **Dr. Miller** wondered if the mere rearrangement of genetic material, as in translocation, might be carcinogenic, and **Dr. Knudson** agreed there might be such a positional effect.

Dr. Bahn, agreeing that genetic factors are important in childhood cancer, asked for a numerical estimate of the importance of heredity in adult cancers. **Dr. Mulvihill** indicated that the cancer burden in populations owing to single-gene disorders is small, but that the interaction of genetic with environmental factors is probably of great importance. It is worthwhile to recognize genetically susceptible individuals, so that special efforts may be made to control environmental factors with which they might come into contact.

Dr. Koss discussed a chromosome study of 100 adult patients having various cancers prior to treatment. No karyotypic abnormalities were found beyond what one would expect in the population at large; but with advances in cytogenetic techniques, a higher yield of chromosome defects might be found. He also questioned the nature of the statistical relationship between male breast cancer and Klinefelter's syndrome. Only a small percentage of male breast-cancer patients have the chromosomal disorder, whereas most patients with Klinefelter's syndrome do not develop the neoplasm. **Dr. Mulvihill** responded that the frequency of the XXY syndrome in newborns is 0.2 percent, whereas the frequency of Klinefelter's syndrome among male breast-cancer patients is 3.3 percent. **Dr. Mulvihill** also reviewed Ohno's hypothesis of the selective advantage conferred by certain karyotypes, namely, those genes favorable to cancer development or metastases are often duplicated, whereas the genes not needed for the neoplastic process are lost. In many patients with chronic myelocytic leukemia and Ph^1, the appearance of a blastic phase is associated with increasingly bizarre karyotypes.

Dr. Saffiotti, referring to Dr. Mulvihill's introductory statement that some people develop cancer because of their genes, stated that all people do so in the sense that the species susceptibility to develop tumors must be genetically determined. He asked whether individuals with known genetic conditions are more vulnerable to chemical and physical carcinogens. **Dr. Mulvihill** related two examples of this interaction. Children with the basal-cell nevus syndrome are prone to medulloblastomas. After radiotherapy, crops of basal-cell carcinoma have appeared in the field of radiation. Also, patients with lung cancer seem to have more active levels of aryl hydrocarbon hydroxylase, a genetically determined enzyme, which may speed the conversion of environmental agents to potent carcinogens.

Dr. Schneiderman commented on the possibility that a classification of cancer might be based on karyotype rather than site or tissue of origin. Citing the work of Dr. Janet Rowley, **Dr. Mulvihill** responded that a similar karyotype might indicate a similar etiology regardless of histology. However, **Dr. Higginson** referred to experimental work by Yoshida in which 40 liver tumors induced by the same carcinogen yielded 40 different karyotypes, emphasizing that a karyotypic abnormality must be present prior to tumor development to prove a causal relation.

Anna T. Meadows

2

FAMILIAL SUSCEPTIBILITY

David E. Anderson, Ph. D.

The University of Texas System Cancer Center
M. D. Anderson Hospital and Tumor Institute
Houston, Texas

The aggregation of cancer in families is a well-documented phenomenon, dating back to the 17th century [1]. More recent evidence [2], accumulated primarily during the first half of this century, indicates that a family history of a neoplasm can double a person's risk for developing that neoplasm. However, some question still centers on the etiological significance of familial aggregation, whether it represents inherited susceptibility or common exposure to known or unknown environmental carcinogenic influences. Although some familial occurrences could have an environmental basis, there is now abundant evidence of a genetic component in the origin of many site-specific neoplasms. The question is no longer whether cancer susceptibility in man can be inherited, but rather, how do susceptibility genes act and interact with environmental influences and how may gene carriers be identified?

RETROSPECTIVE STUDIES

Generally, one of three methods has been used in genetic investigations of human cancer—retrospective studies, comparison of monozygotic and dizygotic

Supported in part by grants CA05831 from the National Cancer Institute and GM-19513 C-1 from the National Institute of General Medical Sciences. The author is also indebted to Dr. Louise C. Strong for her many fruitful ideas and comments during the preparation of this manuscript.

twins, and pedigree studies. The retrospective approach compares the morbidity and/or mortality rates in first-degree relatives of cancer patients with the rates in control relatives [2-4]. This approach is prone to methodologic deficiencies [5], particularly in the comparability of the experimental and control groups. To circumvent this problem, some studies compared the morbidity and/or mortality rates in the experimental groups with expected rates derived from population statistics. But, regardless of the nature or source of the data, a significant twofold to fourfold excess of cancer of the stomach [3,6-8], breast [2,4,9], large intestine [8], uterus [10], and lung [11] was demonstrated in relatives of patients over control relatives or that experienced by the general population. Increased risks were also observed for childhood brain tumors and sarcomas [12]. No significant excesses have been reported for esophageal or cervical carcinoma [2,6], and the results for prostatic cancer and leukemia have been equivocal [2,12]. A recent study of leukemia in Japan [13] utilized the unique approach of comparing the degree of consanguinity among the parents of sibling patients and nonfamilial leukemia patients. In 20 families with familial leukemia, 20 percent of the parents were first cousins and 10 percent were first cousins once removed or second cousins. In 200 families with nonfamilial leukemia, only 4.5 percent of the parents were first cousins. Although the number of families in the experimental group was small, the results suggest that genetic factors have an important function in the etiology of leukemia occurring in siblings.

The increased risks observed for siblings or other relatives of patients with cancer of the stomach, breast, large intestine, uterus, and lung, and with childhood brain tumors and sarcomas were also attributed to a genetic influence. This influence was apparently specific in its effect, since it enhanced the susceptibility of relatives only to the type of cancer present in the patient and not to cancer in general [2]. The magnitude of the risks, being relatively small, was considered to reflect a polygenic mechanism, likely involving several genes interacting with environmental factors with a larger overall effect. Environmental factors were discounted as being responsible for the excesses by showing that the patients' spouses [6-9] or spouses and their matched controls [7] did not exhibit an excess of the neoplasm under investigation. Another means of dismissing the possibility of an environmental factor was by controlling that factor in comparisons of relatives and controls. Tokuhata and Lilienfeld [11], for example, in a study of lung cancer, dissociated smoking from the familial effect. In the absence of smoking, the relative lung cancer mortality rate among first-degree relatives of lung cancer patients was four times higher than that among control relatives; in the absence of the familial factor, the lung cancer mortality rate among smokers was five times higher than among nonsmokers. The combined effect of smoking and familial factors resulted in a fourteenfold excess in lung cancer mortality compared with control relatives who did not smoke. Air pollution was discounted as being responsible for the increased risks because the control group was matched to the experimental group by neighborhood, thus both should have had similar exposures.

These previous studies were based on cancers occurring at a given site (e.g., lung, breast), and an assumption common to all studies was that the cancer under investigation was a single, homogeneous disease entity. It is well known that cancers occurring at a given site are classifiable into various histologic types, and each of these different types may involve different etiological mechanisms [14]. Breast cancer has long been, and still is, considered by many to be a single disease; however, pathologic, clinical, epidemiologic, and genetic evidence points to an etiologically heterogeneous disease [15-21]. If the neoplasm in question were indeed heterogeneous as evidence now strongly suggests, and not homogeneous as previously assumed, then the effect of such an assumption would be to dilute the measure of the genetic effect and would thus lead to a relatively low-risk estimate, as observed in previous surveys.

That this may well have occurred in the past is demonstrated by more recent studies on breast cancer. Previous studies [22] have consistently indicated a twofold to threefold increased risk for the disease in first-degree relatives of patients. However, when the disease was assumed to be heterogeneous and the patients were classified into presumably more homogeneous groupings based on age at onset, multiplicity of disease, and type of family history, the risks for relatives of some groups of patients increased from the usual twofold to threefold level to higher levels, ranging from ninefold to forty-sevenfold [20, 21]. The high risks occurred in premenopausal relatives of patients with premenopausal and/or bilateral disease whose mothers were also affected, whereas risks that were lower, but still higher than those in controls, occurred in relatives of patients with postmenopausal and/or unilateral disease whose mothers were unaffected. It is likely that increases in risk would also be observed for groups of colonic cancer patients if they were classified according to age at onset, histologic type, and, importantly, the site at which colonic cancers developed (e.g., right side including the transverse colon versus the left side). Colonic adenocarcinoma in unselected patients develops most often in the rectosigmoid and cecal areas; but in patients with impressive familial aggregations of colonic adenocarcinoma occurring independently of polyposis, the neoplasms are distributed more randomly throughout the colon and slightly favor the right side and transverse colon [23]. Differences in risk might also be observed in gastric cancer if a distinction were made between the diffuse and intestinal forms of this neoplasm [24], and in Hodgkin's disease (HD) if consideration were given to the age at onset and histologic type of the neoplasm [25-27]. Leukemia might be similar in this regard since the risks are higher for chronic lymphocytic leukemia [28] than for leukemia in general [2] and are associated with an early average age at diagnosis [12,13].

COMPARISONS OF TWINS

Studies of monozygotic and dizygotic twins also suffer from the problem of heterogeneity, perhaps more so than retrospective studies, because early comparisons of twins were based on cancer in general, regardless of the site and type. One of the major difficulties in twin studies has been the inability to generate sufficient numbers of unselected twins with and without a given type of cancer where zygosity is certain. Another problem is that twins share common pre- and postnatal environmental influences. Although the method is highly promising for indicating the relative importance of genetic versus nongenetic factors, it has provided little new information compared with that provided by retrospective studies of relatives of patients. A general conclusion would be that the concordance rate of cancer occurrence in monozygotic twins is about double the rate in dizygotic twins for cancer of the stomach, breast, and intestine, and for leukemia [12,29-33]. That higher concordance rates might be observed if a classification were made for age at onset is strongly suggested by the findings of Miller [12] and MacMahon and Levy [34]. These reports indicated that the concordance rates (17 to 25 percent) among monozygotic twins for childhood acute leukemia far exceeded random expectation. The ages at diagnosis of concordant affected twins were also earlier than for childhood leukemia generally [33]. The Japanese consanguinity study [13] indicated a similar trend, since the ages at onset among familial leukemia patients were much earlier (median, 6 years) when their parents were first cousins than when the parents were more distantly related or were not related (median, 27 years).

PEDIGREE STUDIES

The evaluation of single families or pedigrees is perhaps the most satisfactory and meaningful approach for demonstrating a genetic basis for cancer susceptibility. The method bypasses the problem of heterogeneity and the need for controls, but it may be criticized on the grounds that the resulting data are biased. Families frequently come to the attention of the investigator because they contain an impressive array of familial cases, but they are genetically meaningful when they are not selected and aggregation is detected by continued study of the family. The pedigree approach also provides data amenable to tests of genetic hypotheses; i.e., autosomal or sex-linked; dominant, recessive, or more complex patterns of inheritance; and linkage relationships. In addition, this approach provides relatively homogeneous data of clinical and basic research interest that cannot be readily collected or answered from series of patients or twins whose disease may have heterogeneous etiologies.

A variety of neoplasms whose familial distribution patterns are consistent with Mendelian inheritance patterns have been identified by this approach.

Knudson, Strong, and Anderson [33] concluded that virtually all cancers in man occur in a heritable (autosomal dominant) form as well as in a non-heritable form. Mulvihill [35] summarized 161 genetic conditions that involved either a malignant or benign tumor as the sole feature, frequent feature, or a rare complication. These neoplasms demonstrating impressive familial aggregations of a specific neoplasm are characterized by early average ages at onset or diagnosis. These average ages may be several years or decades earlier than the average age at onset of that same neoplasm in the general population. For example, a dominantly inherited form of basal cell carcinoma, as illustrated by the nevoid basal cell carcinoma syndrome, has early onset averaging about 20 years of age (Figure 1). This is markedly earlier than the average age of 50 years usually observed for basal cell carcinoma. Medullary thyroid carcinoma is generally first detected around 45 to 50 years of age, whereas one heritable form, Sipple's syndrome, is first detected around 30 years of age [33,36]. A heritable form of colonic adenocarcinoma occurring independently of and not in association with any preexisting polypoid disease, namely hereditary adenocarcinomatosis, is first detected at about 40 years of age, again well below the detection age of colonic adenocarcinoma in general [36]. Similar differences apply to malignant melanoma and breast cancer, where the disease in familial patients is first detected between 35 and 40 years of age, much earlier than that in unselected patients [21,37]. A relationship between a familial basis and age at onset is also indicated by the Japanese consanguinity study [13], where the ages at onset were much earlier in familial leukemia patients whose parents were closely related than in patients with more distantly related or nonrelated parents.

These early occurrences, whatever the cancer, might be considered the consequence of early detection, since family members might tend to seek early medical attention for a specific neoplasm once it has occurred in a close relative. However, the first cases in a family have early ages at occurrence as do later cases, and both are earlier on the average than the age usually encountered. Furthermore, early detection should not be a factor in comparisons of various categories of familial patients [13,21]. An early age at onset among relatives thus appears to be a biologic characteristic of neoplasms involving a heritable component.

Another characteristic of familial-occurring tumors is their tendency to develop at multiple sites in the same organ or bilaterally in paired organs [33, 36]. As shown in Table 1, the frequencies of multiple primary tumors were clearly much higher in familial than in unselected patients. The frequencies were likely underestimated in some instances since multiplicity was measured by the occurrence of bilateral tumors or tumors at multiple sites. Little or no information was available on the occurrence of multiple tumor foci or multicentric tumors in a single organ. Since familial tumors have an early age at

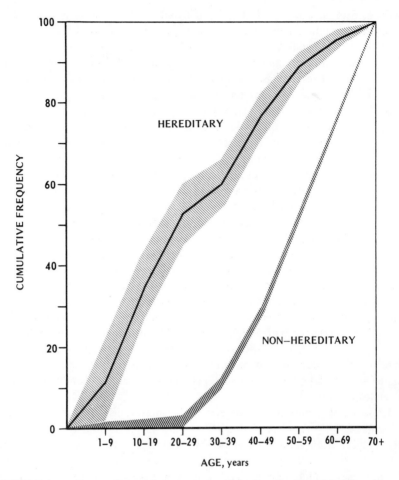

FIGURE 1.   Age at diagnosis in patients with the nevoid basal cell carcinoma
syndrome, a hereditary form of basal-cell carcinoma, compared
with patients having basal-cell carcinoma in general, which is for
the most part nonhereditary.

onset, the high frequency of multiple tumors might be attributed to a long period
of risk. But this apparently is not the case because the second or third primary
malignancy in a patient occurs earlier on the average than that same tumor type
in the general population. These characteristics of an early average age at onset
and a tendency for tumors to develop at multiple sites also have been observed
in inbred strains of mice with high degrees of genetic susceptibility to certain
tumors.

Another characteristic of familial neoplasms, primarily those in which the

TABLE 1

Percent frequency of multiple primary tumors in patients with familial
forms of neoplasms as compared with unselected patients

Type of cancer	Familial	Unselected	Reference
Adenocarcinomatosis	20	9	1
Breast cancer	15	3	19
Chemodectomas	34	5	59
Melanoma	14	2	37
Neuroblastoma	23	5	47
Nevoid basal cell cancer	98	4	63
Pheochromocytoma (simple)	40-44	12	47
Pheochromocytoma and medullary thyroid carcinoma	75-80	12	47
Retinoblastoma	27	0	45
Wilms' tumor	21	7	46

genetic effect on tumor development is strong, is their limited range of phenotypic expression [33,36]. Affected family members tend to develop the same
type of neoplasm in a single site or tissue system, as in hereditary forms of non-
chromaffin paraganglioma and malignant melanoma; or a single histologic type
may occur in various sites or organs, as in hereditary adenocarcinomatosis; or
different types may occur in an organ system, as in Sipple's syndrome or multiple
endocrine adenomatosis. In those cases where the genetic effect on tumor
development is indirect, i.e., the genetic effect is directed primarily to the
development of a disease state and tumors develop secondarily in a significant
fraction of patients [36], the resulting tumors are more varied in histologic
type. But the majority are still confined to a tissue system, such as the
reticuloendothelial system in the various inherited immunodeficiency diseases
[38] or inherited diseases characterized by chromosome instability [33,35,36].
However, one hereditary condition has been reported [39], and others may yet
be described, where diverse types of neoplasms develop in different organ
systems, such as the occurrence of breast cancer in association with leukemia,
sarcoma, brain tumor, and possibly other neoplasms. Even in this case, the
underlying metabolic, biochemical, or cellular defect may be relatively specific.
Studies are still required to determine the empiric risks of certain tumor constellations in relatives and thereby better define hereditary cancer syndromes
[35].

These characteristics of tumor specificity, early average age at onset, and
the tendency for tumors to develop at multiple sites thus serve to distinguish
between familial occurrences having genetic causation versus those arising from

environmental exposure [1,33,36]. These same characteristics may also apply to some tumors arising as a consequence of exposure to environmental carcinogens, such as mesothelioma among asbestos workers and leukemia as a consequence of radiation or benzene exposure, but such occurrences should be identifiable through the uniqueness of the tumor type and/or adequate medical and occupational histories. Highly variable ages at onset of diverse single-occurring tumor types among relatives, including distant relatives, would be suggestive of heterogeneous etiology; similarity among relatives in the time when a specific neoplasm develops, as observed for Hodgkin's disease [40], would be suggestive of common exposure to an environmental agent(s).

The numerous familial neoplasms that are considered to involve a heritable component point to a high degree of genetic heterogeneity for certain neoplasms. Adenocarcinoma of the colon, for example, may arise through a variety of different and presumably distinct hereditary mechanisms—polyposis coli, Gardner's syndrome, Peutz-Jegher's syndrome, discrete polyps, or other polypoid diseases [41], hereditary adenocarcinomatosis, hereditary gastrocolonic cancer, and hereditary colonic cancer [23]. Breast cancer may involve at least five hereditary types—an early site-specific type [21,42], a late site-specific type [43], an early type associated with leukemia, brain tumors, and sarcoma [39], a type associated with ovarian cancer [44], and perhaps one or more types with a more recessive or complex inheritance pattern [21]. Genetic heterogeneity also applies to ovarian adenocarcinomas and other ovarian neoplasms, pheochromocytoma, malignant melanoma, and several other types of neoplasms.

TWO-STEP MUTATION MODEL

Knudson [45] advanced a model to explain the occurrence of heritable and nonheritable tumors. His model proposed that all tumors derive from a single cell and are the consequence of two mutational events. The first event may be prezygotic or postzygotic, and the second is always postzygotic. When the first event is prezygotic and occurs in a germinal cell, it may thus be transmitted via the zygote and will occur in every cell of the recipient and be hereditary. The carrier of this mutant gene may then develop zero, one, two, or more tumors in accordance with a Poisson distribution. When the first mutation is postzygotic and occurs in a somatic cell, the mutant will be confined to a single cell and all subsequent daughter cells and will not be hereditary. Since one mutation has occurred in the heritable type and is present in all cells, only a single second event is necessary for tumor development. Consequently, the heritable type will be early and frequently multiple in occurrence. The nonheritable type, however, requires two infrequent mutational events in a single cell for tumor development and as such will be late and single in occurrence.

The model has been applied to retinoblastoma [45], Wilms' tumor [46], and neuroblastoma and pheochromocytoma [47], with excellent agreement between the observed and expected numbers of gene carriers with zero, one, two, or more tumors. The gene carriers were found to have an excess of multiple tumors and an early age at onset compared with patients with the nonheritable forms of the same tumors, as expected with the model. Furthermore, the fraction of surviving patients with a heritable form was constant over a given period, implying that a single event was occurring at a constant rate in a declining population of embryonal cells, in agreement with a single-hit hypothesis. The nonhereditary cases, however, showed a more curvilinear decline with time, implying a two-hit curve. The proposal was made that perhaps all bilateral or multiple cases of childhood cancers are the consequence of a germinal mutation.

This model may also have applicability to adult cancers [33]. They are similar to childhood cancers in that they occur in heritable and nonheritable forms. The heritable adult forms also have significantly earlier average ages at onset than the same neoplasm in the general population, and they exhibit a distinct tendency to develop at multiple sites, features which are expected with the two-step model. The model has not been applied to tumors involving an indirect genetic effect, i.e., where a neoplasm appears to develop secondarily in some fraction of individuals with an inherited disease. The immunodeficiency diseases, all of which are recessively inherited, would be examples of such conditions [38]. Consequently, whether the two-step or a more complex model has applicability to such tumors is still in need of investigation. The hypothesis of Burnet [48] regarding the interaction of DNA repair and the accumulation of mutations during informational transfer of DNA in xeroderma pigmentosum and progeria suggests a more complex model in such cases.

The model has been used to estimate the relative frequencies of some hereditary and nonhereditary neoplasms. Hereditary retinoblastoma was estimated to account for 40 percent of all cases of this tumor [45]. The hereditary fraction for Wilms' tumor was 38 percent [46], and for neuroblastoma, 22 percent [47]. The hypotheses involved in the model were also applied to estimate the fraction of hereditary cases of one adult cancer, i.e., breast cancer. The assumption was made that all bilateral cases of breast cancer were hereditary. If the bilaterality rate is generally 3 percent, and is 10 percent in familial cases, then 30 percent of all breast cancer cases should be of the hereditary type [33]. The fractions of hereditary cases among other adult cancers have not as yet been estimated. But some notion of magnitude of a minimal estimate can be determined from the percentage of patients with verified family histories of a given neoplasm among all patients with that neoplasm. These types of estimates indicate an extremely low fraction for esophageal cancer [23], 5 percent for malignant melanoma [37], and 15 to 20 percent for colonic cancer [23]. So in addition to their occurrence at virtually all major sites and their heterogeneity within sites, cancers involving a heritable component may individually and in the aggregate be more frequent than is generally suspected.

SUGGESTIONS FOR THE FUTURE

There are preciously few clues regarding the nature of the genetic effect that leads to the development of a neoplasm(s). Immune deficiency diseases, which are recessively inherited and predispose to reticuloendothelial malignancies, implicate the immune mechanism. In support of this hypothesis are the cases of immune dysfunction observed in families with chronic lymphocytic leukemia [49] and HD [50], a possible genetic defect of T-lymphocytes in a family with stomach cancer [51], and the possible association between HD and the "4c"-related set of HL-A antigens [27]. Kurita et al. [13] proposed that subsequent genetic studies of leukemia should concentrate on the immunogenetic aspects. The genetic effect on these malignancies seems to be related to the production of a defective or immature cell whose immune or surveillance function is impaired, and/or a cell with an enhanced likelihood of undergoing malignant transformation on subsequent exposure to some environmental stimulus. Bloom's syndrome and Fanconi's anemia, which are characterized by chromosome imbalance and instability and an increased frequency of leukemia, may be similar in this regard [52].

A somewhat related mechanism may apply to xeroderma pigmentosum, also recessively inherited, in which the cells of an affected individual are homozygous for a mutation leading to deficiency of an enzyme required during an early stage of DNA repair following damage by ultraviolet light [53]. Since the skin is primarily exposed to ultraviolet light, a variety of cutaneous neoplasms invariably develop in patients with this disorder. Burnet [48] recently proposed that DNA repair in xeroderma pigmentosum is only indirect evidence of the mechanism underlying the disease; the real mechanism is the incorporation of informational errors in physiologically completely repaired DNA. He hypothesized that cutaneous malignancies are ascribable to somatic mutations accumulating from the inheritance of error-prone key enzymes concerned with informational transfer of DNA.

With regard to familial neoplasms where the genetic effect on tumor development is seemingly more direct, i.e., the only phenotypic manifestation of susceptibility is the development of a tumor, little or no evidence is available concerning the mechanisms of gene action. One possibility, however, is the proposal of Lemon [54] regarding susceptibility to breast cancer. He postulated a genetic basis for impaired 17β-estradiol and estrone hydroxylation to estriol by 16α-hydroxylase, based on the variation in urinary excretion quotients of estriol/(estrone + 17β-estradiol) and the plasma clearance rates for estrone and estradiol among Caucasian women. At least three population clusters of excretion quotients and clearance rates were observed. These clusters were attributed to a genetic segregation of a mutant allele which reduced 16α-hydroxylase activity. Breast cancer patients aggregated into the two lowest estriol excretion groups and into the group with the lowest clearance rate and were thus assumed to be homozygous or heterozygous for the mutant 16α-hydroxylase allele. More recently, Lemon and Reilly [55] directly assayed the leukocyte estradiol hydroxylase activity (percent per 100μ g DNA). Three population clusters were again identified, and 18 of 31 breast cancer cases (58 percent) exhibited absent or low estradiol hydroxylating activity.

Another hydroxylase, aryl hydrocarbon hydroxylase (AHH), plays a primary role in modifying exogenous carcinogens into their proximate or active forms. The inducibility of this enzyme also exhibited three population clusters, a finding that was interpreted as indicating the segregation of a single autosomal locus [56]. Most patients with bronchogenic carcinoma (96 percent) showed intermediate or high AHH inducibility levels compared with 52 percent in the normal population, whereas only 4 percent of the patients showed low inducibility contrasted with 48 percent in the normal population [57]. Further studies are required to assess the interaction between the aryl hydrocarbon and 16α-hydroxylase systems, their genetic characteristics, and their involvement in the development of breast and lung cancer, or other cancers.

Studies of families with neoplasms involving a hereditary component would be particularly useful for experimental studies of carcinogenesis. The inherited molecular or biochemical mechanism should be relatively homogeneous and consistent in all patients with a given genetic entity and thus be more easily identifiable than the mechanism in a series of heterogeneous patients. Knowledge of such a mechanism would have obvious utility for subsequently identifying high-risk individuals in families. But in the absence of information on the underlying mechanism, high-risk individuals might still be identified through pedigree analysis, by noting which individuals are in direct line of descent of susceptibility genes or belong to sibships in which such genes are apparently segregating. High-risk individuals, particularly for leukemia, might be identified through in vitro transformation of fibroblasts by simian virus 40 (SV40) [58]. Genetic and chromosome markers could also be used for this purpose, provided there were a phenotypic and/or linkage relationship between a given genetic marker and a genetic condition or neoplasm. However, no useful phenotypic associations or linkage relationships have yet been identified. Neoplasms with a hereditary basis also have important practical relevance for early cancer detection in high-risk family members, whether by periodic screening examinations for breast, uterine, or gastrointestinal cancer [59], radioimmunoassay of calcitonin in medullary thyroid carcinoma [60], serum calcium and gastrin determinations in the multiple endocrine adenomatosis syndrome [61], or urinary catecholamines in neuroblastoma [62]. Periodic examinations of individuals at high risk for heritable tumors will more likely result in the detection of tumors at an earlier and more easily treatable stage than if detection were delayed until the development of signs and symptoms. Members of high-risk families should also be counseled concerning the possible genetic transmission of cancer susceptibility genes and the risks for subsequent tumor development.

SUMMARY

A genetic basis for many human cancers has been convincingly demonstrated by retrospective studies, comparisons of twins, and pedigree analyses. Retrospective and twin studies have been beset with methodological problems, including the important problem of etiological heterogeneity of cancers occurring at a specific site. Pedigree analysis is the most meaningful approach, since it permits testing of specific genetic hypotheses, provides material for basic and clinical studies, helps identify high-risk individuals, and avoids and helps clarify the problem of clinical and genetic heterogeneity among site-specific or histologically similar neoplasms. Genetic heterogeneity is common for specific histologic types of neoplasms, implying that a given neoplasm may arise through a variety of etiologic mechanisms.

Virtually all cancers developing in man have been identified as occurring in a heritable and nonheritable form. The tumors involving a heritable component occur at earlier ages and at multiple sites more frequently than do nonheritable cancers and are also more frequent than is generally suspected. The neoplasms studied to date with a dominant inheritance pattern agree with a two-step mutation model, but the mechanisms through which susceptibility genes act and interact with environmental factors in carcinogenesis are largely unknown.

REFERENCES

1. Lynch, H.T. Hereditary factors in carcinoma. *In Recent Results in Cancer Research*. Vol. 12. Springer-Verlag, New York, 1967, 186 pp.
2. Clemmesen, J. Statistical studies in the aetiology of malignant neoplasms. I. Review and results. *Acta Pathol. Microbiol. Scand. Supp. 174:*1–543, 1965.
3. Woolf, C.M. Investigations on genetic aspects of carcinoma of the stomach and breast. *Univ. Calif. Publ. Public Health 2:*265–350, 1955.
4. Anderson, V.E., Goodman, H.O., and Reed, S. *Variables Related to Human Breast Cancer*. Univ. Minnesota Press, Minneapolis, 1958, 172 pp.
5. Graham, S., and Lilienfeld, A.M. Genetic studies of gastric cancer in humans: An appraisal. *Cancer 11:*945–958, 1958.
6. Woolf, C.M. A further study on the familial aspects of carcinoma of the stomach. *Am. J. Hum. Genet. 8:*102–109, 1956.
7. Woolf, C.M. The incidence of cancer in the spouses of stomach cancer patients. *Cancer 14:*199–200, 1961.

8. Macklin, M.T. Inheritance of cancer of the stomach and large intestine in man. *J. Natl. Cancer Inst. 24:*551–571, 1960.

9. Macklin, M.T. Comparison of the number of breast cancer deaths observed in relatives of breast-cancer patients, and the number expected on the basis of mortality rates. *J. Natl. Cancer Inst. 22:*927–951, 1959.

10. Murphy, D.P. *Heredity in Uterine Cancer.* Harvard Univ. Press, Cambridge, Mass., 1952, 128 pp.

11. Tokuhata, G.K., and Lilienfeld, A.M. Familial aggregation of lung cancer in humans. *J. Natl. Cancer Inst. 30:*289–312, 1963.

12. Miller, R.W. Deaths from childhood leukemia and solid tumors among twins and other sibs in the United States, 1960-67. *J. Natl. Cancer Inst. 46:*203–209, 1971.

13. Kurita, S., Kamei Y., and Ota K. Genetic studies on familial leukemia. *Cancer 34:* 1098–1101, 1974.

14. Doll, R. Cancer in five continents. *Proc. R. Soc. Med. 65:*49–55, 1972.

15. Lilienfeld, A.M. The epidemiology of breast cancer. *Cancer Res. 23:*1503–1513, 1963.

16. de Waard, F., Baanders-van Halewijn, E.A., and Huizinga, J. The bimodal age distribution of patients with mammary carcinoma: Evidence for the existence of two types of human breast cancer. *Cancer 17:*141–151, 1964.

17. von Berndt, H., and Landmann, R. Zwei epidemiologische typen des mamma-karzinoms. *Arch. Geschwulstforsch. 33:*157–168, 1969.

18. Hems, G. Epidemiological characteristics of breast cancer in middle and late age. *Br. J. Cancer 24:*226–234, 1970.

19. Anderson, D.E. Genetic considerations in breast cancer. *In Breast Cancer: Early and Late.* Year Book Medical Publishers, Chicago, 1970, pp. 27–36.

20. Anderson, D.E. A genetic study of human breast cancer. *J. Natl. Cancer Inst. 48:* 1029–1034, 1972.

21. Anderson, D.E. Genetic study of breast cancer: Identification of a high risk group. *Cancer 34:*1090–1097, 1974.

22. Post, R.H. Breast cancer, lactation, and genetics. *Eugen. Q. 13:*1–29, 1966.

23. Anderson, D.E., and Strong, L.C. Genetics of gastrointestinal tumors. *In Proceedings of the 11th International Cancer Congress.* Excerpta Med. Int. Congr. Ser. In press, 1975.

24. Muñoz, N., Correa, P., Cuello, C., et al. Histologic types of gastric carcinoma in high- and low-risk areas. *Int. J. Cancer 3:*809–818, 1968.

25. Razis, D.V., Diamond, H.D., and Craver, L.F. Familial Hodgkin's disease: Its significance and implications. *Ann. Intern. Med. 51:*933–971, 1959.

26. Cole, P., MacMahon, B., and Aisenberg, A. Mortality from Hodgkin's disease in the United States: Evidence for the multiple-aetiology hypothesis. *Lancet 2:*1371–1375, 1968.

27. Bodmer, W.F. Genetic factors in Hodgkin's disease: Association with a disease-susceptibility locus (DSA) in the HL-A region. *Natl. Cancer Inst. Monogr. 37:*127–134, 1973.

28. Gunz, F.W., and Veale, A.M.O. Leukemia in close relatives—accident or predisposition? *J. Natl. Cancer Inst. 42:*517–524, 1969.

29. Macklin, M.T. An analysis of tumors in monozygous and dizygous twins: With a report of fifteen unpublished cases. *J. Hered. 31:*277–290, 1940.

30. Hauge, M., Harvald, B., Fischer, M., et al. The Danish twin register. *Acta Genet. Med. Gemellol. 17:*315–331, 1968.

31. Keith, L., and Brown, E. Epidemiologic study of leukemia in twins (1938-1969). *Acta Genet. Med. Gemellol. 20:*9–22, 1971.

32. Jarvik, L., and Falek, A. Comparative data on cancer in aging twins. *Cancer 15:* 1009-1018, 1962.

33. Knudson, A.G., Strong, L.C., and Anderson, D.E. Heredity and cancer in man. *Prog. Med. Genet. 9:*113–158, 1973.

34. MacMahon, B., and Levy, M. Prenatal origin of childhood leukemia: Evidence from twins. *N. Engl. J. Med. 270:*1082–1085, 1964.

35. Mulvihill, J.J. Congenital and genetic diseases. This volume, 1975.

36. Anderson, D.E. Genetic varieties of neoplasia. *In Genetic Concepts and Neoplasia.* Williams & Wilkins, Baltimore, 1970, pp. 85–104.

37. Anderson, D.E. Inheritance of a genetic type of melanoma in man. *In Pigmentation: Its Genesis and Biologic Control.* Appleton-Century-Crofts, Meredith Corp., New York, 1972, pp. 401–413.

38. Kersey, J.H., and Spector, B.D. Immune deficiency diseases. This volume, 1975.

39. Li, F.P., and Fraumeni, J.F., Jr. Soft-tissue sarcomas, breast cancer, and other neoplasms. A familial syndrome? *Ann. Intern. Med. 71:*747–752, 1969.

40. Vianna, N.G., Davies, J.N.P., Polan, A.K., et al. Familial Hodgkin's disease: An environmental and genetic disorder. *Lancet 2:*854–857, 1974.

41. McConnell, R.B. *The Genetics of Gastro-Intestinal Disorders,* Oxford Univ. Press, London, 1966, 282 pp.

42. Gardner, E.J., and Stephens, F.E. Breast cancer in one family group. *Am. J. Hum. Genet. 2:*30–40, 1950.

43. Woolf, C.M., and Gardner, E.J. The familial distribution of breast cancer in a Utah kindred. *Cancer 4:*515–520, 1951.

44. Lynch, H.T., and Krush, A.J. Carcinoma of the breast and ovary in three families. *Surg. Gynecol. Obst. 133:*644–648, 1971.

45. Knudson, A.G. Mutation and cancer: Statistical study of retinoblastoma. *Proc. Natl. Acad. Sci., USA 68:*820–823, 1971.

46. Knudson, A.G., and Strong, L.C. Mutation and cancer: A model for Wilms' tumor of the kidney. *J. Natl. Cancer Inst. 48:*313–324, 1972.

47. Knudson, A.G., and Strong, L.C. Mutation and cancer: Neuroblastoma and pheochromocytoma. *Am. J. Hum. Genet. 24:*514–532, 1972.

48. Burnet, F.M. Intrinsic mutagenesis, an interpretation of the pathogenesis of xeroderma pigmentosum. *Lancet 2:*495–498, 1974.

49. Fraumeni, J.F., Jr., Vogel, C.L., and De Vita, V.T. Familial chronic lymphocytic leukemia. *Ann. Intern. Med. 71:*279–284, 1969.

50. Creagan, E.T., and Fraumeni,J.F., Jr. Familial Hodgkin's disease. *Lancet 2:*547, 1972.

51. Creagan, E.T., and Fraumeni, J.F., Jr. Familial gastric cancer and immunologic abnormalities. *Cancer 32:*1325–1331, 1973.

52. German, J. Genes which increase chromosomal instability in somatic cells and predispose to cancer. *Prog. Med. Genet. 8:*61–101, 1972.

53. Cleaver, J.R. Defective repair replication of DNA in xeroderma pigmentosum. *Nature (Lond.) 218:*652–656, 1968.

54. Lemon, H.M. Genetic predisposition to carcinoma of the breast: Multiple human genotypes for estrogen 16 alpha hydroxylase activity in Caucasians. *J. Surg. Oncol. 4:*255–273, 1972.

55. Lemon, H.M., and Reilly, D. Genotypic variations in Caucasian leukocyte estradiol 16 hydroxylase activity: A measurable deterrent of breast cancer risk? *Nebr. State Med. J. 59:*151–155, 1974.

56. Kellermann, G., Luyten-Kellermann, M., and Shaw, C.R. Genetic variation of aryl hydrocarbon hydroxylase in human lymphocytes. *Am. J. Hum. Genet. 25:*327-331, 1973.
57. Kellermann, G., Shaw, C.R., and Luyten-Kellermann, M. Aryl hydrocarbon hydroxylase inducibility and bronchogenic carcinoma. *N. Engl. J. Med. 289:*934-937, 1973.
58. Miller, R.W., and Todaro, G.J. Viral transformation of cells from persons at high risk of cancer. *Lancet 1:*81-82, 1969.
59. Anderson, D.E. The role of genetics in human cancer. *Ca Cancer J. Clin. 24:*130-136, 1974.
60. Block, M.F., Jackson, C.E., and Tahjian, A.D., Jr. Medullary thyroid carcinoma detected by serum calcitonin assay. *Arch. Surg. 104:*579-586, 1972.
61. Snyder, N., Scurry, M., and Hughes, W. Hypergastrinemia in familial multiple endocrine adenomatosis. *Ann. Intern. Med. 80:*321-325, 1974.
62. Gerson, J., Chatten, J., and Eisman, S. Familial neuroblastoma—a follow up. *N. Engl. J. Med. 290:*1487, 1973.

DISCUSSION

Dr. E. C. Hammond referred to the mouse model in which milk-transmitted virus causes breast cancer in a genetically and hormonally susceptible host. He wondered if one could separate genetic effect from the horizontal transmission of a virus through milk in the etiology of human breast cancer. **Dr. Anderson** replied that despite the RNA/DNA homology studies of Spiegelman and others, and the detection of viruslike particles in human milk by Moore using electron microscopy, there are not convincing data that daughters of women with breast cancer are at increased risk because of a virus. A virus might be integrated into the DNA of either the mother or father and transmitted as any other genetic trait, but we have no way of distinguishing this possibility. **Dr. Knudson** commented that rather than considering the mutation hypothesis versus the viral hypothesis, it may be better to assume both are correct. In this manner, mutation may play a role in the integration or function of a tumor virus. In murine mammary tumors, host genes are an important factor in determining viral effects: if a human mammary tumor virus does exist, host genes may likewise be important in tumor production.

Dr. R. W. Miller stated that about 80 to 90 percent of cancers are reported to be caused by environmental factors and asked if genetic studies are out of the mainstream of cancer research. **Dr. Anderson** replied that small, in-depth family studies may be as revealing as large population studies. In large series of cancer patients diverse etiologies are involved, whereas in high-risk families a homogeneous genetic defect may be identified that has implications to the population at large. **Dr. Miller** requested amplification of this idea in relation to xeroderma pigmentosum. **Dr. Anderson** replied that DNA repair in xeroderma pigmentosum is not the only abnormality in these patients, since the accumulation of mutations during information transfer of defective DNA to RNA may be responsible for tumor development. The defective DNA repair mechanism may thus permit the incorporation of mutations in information transfer. The defect identified by studies on xeroderma may play a role in the origins of other neoplasms as well.

In regard to the relative significance of environmental versus hereditary determinants, **Dr. O'Conor** asked about the apparent excess of retinoblastoma (a heritable tumor) in underdeveloped countries. In reply, Dr. Miller commented on the substantial geographic variation in the frequency of many childhood tumors. In underdeveloped countries, however, some deep tumors are not as clinically evident as retinoblastoma, which may appear to have an increased relative frequency. Also, in Japan, there is a twelve-fold increase in the incidence of pinealoma compared with the rest of the world. However, if the rate remains high in Japanese who migrate to other countries, genetic susceptibility would be suggested. In comparison, both African and U.S. blacks have a low risk of Ewing's sarcoma compared with the white population. This deficiency may represent genetic resistance to a particular neoplasm.

Glyn G. Caldwell

3

IMMUNE DEFICIENCY DISEASES

John H. Kersey, M.D., and Beatrice D. Spector

Department of Laboratory Medicine and Pathology
University of Minnesota
Minneapolis, Minnesota

Much evidence has accumulated indicating an intimate relationship between immune deficiency and cancer. As reviewed recently [1], immunodeficiency produced in experimental animals frequently increases the risk of cancer. Similarly, humans with genetically induced or drug induced immunodeficiency often develop cancer more frequently and with a shorter latency period than age-matched control populations. The types of malignancies that develop in immunodeficient humans are somewhat unique [2-5] and are the primary subject of this review.

CANCER IN RENAL TRANSPLANT RECIPIENTS

Humans who receive renal transplants require long-term treatment with immunosuppressive drugs to prevent graft rejection. A significant proportion of patients develop cancer in the months and years following transplantation [2-4, 6,7]. The bulk of these malignancies are lymphoreticular with an especially high incidence of de novo brain tumors [4]. The risk of epithelial malignancies of the skin also is increased [6].

Supported in part by Public Health Service contracts NO1-CP-33357 and NO1-CP-43384 from the National Cancer Institute.

55

CANCER IN PERSONS WITH IMMUNODEFICIENCY SYNDROMES

Of special interest is the group of primary immunodeficiency disorders; most are genetically determined, either as X-linked or autosomal recessive traits. Data collected in the past few years suggest that these patients are at greatly increased risk of cancer [2, 5, 8]. To facilitate the collection and analysis of data related to malignancies that develop in these rare disorders, an Immunodeficiency-Cancer Registry was established in 1971. Data from almost 200 patients with immunodeficiency and malignancy have beeen analyzed [5].

The primary immunodeficiency disorders include those involving thymus-derived (T) lymphocytes and bone marrow-derived (B) lymphocytes [9]. Bruton's agammaglobulinemia, for example, appears to involve defects of B-lymphocytes exclusively. The disease, inherited in an X-linked manner, is limited to males. Affected males either have no B-lymphocytes or abnormal ones, and lack the immunoglobulins responsible for humoral defenses against encapsulated organisms. Thus, these boys are frequently infected with *Hemophilus, Pseudomonas,* and *Diplococcus pneumoniae.* The B-cell system is also involved in IgM deficiency, a disease associated with increased susceptibility to bacterial infection. Similarly, patients with IgA deficiency are prone to infections as well as autoimmune disorders.

Most of the primary immunodeficiency syndromes associated with increased cancer risk are combined immunodeficiency diseases; i.e., they involve components of both T- and B-cell systems [9]. Included are severe combined immune deficiency of infancy, a disorder that generally results in death from infection in early infancy. Immunologic abnormalities in the Wiskott-Aldrich syndrome, an X-linked disorder, are associated with eczema and platelet abnormalities. These boys often die from bleeding or infection when they are in their late teens. Ataxia-telangiectasia (A-T) combines defects in the lymphoid system, central nervous system, skin, and blood vessels. Overwhelming pulmonary infection or degenerative disease of the central nervous system [10] are the most frequent causes of death. Variable (late-onset) immunodeficiency is unpredictable in age of onset and expression and is often not seen until adult years.

As indicated in Figure 1, the age distribution of cancer in patients with these disorders largely reflects the age at onset of the primary immunodeficiency disorders. Thus, malignancies are seen mainly in children. Few individuals with most forms of primary immunodeficiency diseases survive to adulthood since they generally die very early of infections or malignancy. The predominance of adult cases in variable immunodeficiency reflects the fact that this disease generally develops in adults.

We attempted to determine the incidence of cancer in patients with primary immunodeficiency diseases through correspondence with physicians who care for these patients. Table 1 shows the overall lifetime risk of fatal malignancy is

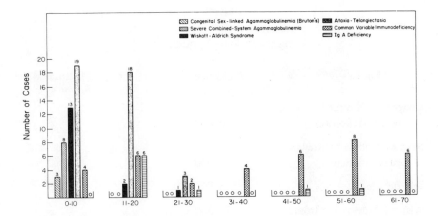

FIGURE 1.   Number of individuals with immunodeficiency syndromes known
to have developed cancer at various ages.

approximately 7 percent [5]. When the data are adjusted for years at risk, we
estimate that the risk is approximately 100 times that of the general population.
Up to August 1974, 196 persons with primary immune deficiencies are known
to have developed malignancy (Table 2).

PREDOMINANCE OF LYMPHORETICULAR NEOPLASMS

Malignancies arising in persons with immunodeficiency syndromes have
been reported to the Immunodeficiency-Cancer Registry in the following proportions by histologic type: epithelial 20 percent, lymphoreticular 55 percent,
leukemias 17 percent, mesenchymal tumors 3 percent, central nervous system
tumors 5 percent (Table 2). This distribution is significantly different than the
pattern of age-matched cases with malignancy in the general population. Solid
lymphoreticular malignancies (including reticulum cell sarcoma and lymphosarcoma) are relatively uncommon in children generally, but predominate in
children with primary immunodeficiency syndromes [11]. In a survey of
adults 20 years and older, those with primary immunodeficiencies had pro-
portionally more lymphoreticular and stomach tumors than the age-matched
population, but they did not seem at greater risk for other common tumors such
as lung, breast and colon [12]. However, these preliminary data are based on
small numbers and difficult to evaluate at this time.

IMMUNE DEFECTS IN INDIVIDUALS WITH CANCER

Abnormal humoral and cell-mediated immune function is frequently found
in cancer patients [1]. These immunologic abnormalities often are correlated

TABLE 1
Evidence of malignancy in primary
immunodeficiency syndromes [5]

Disease	Incidence	Estimated risk %
Congenital X-linked immunodeficiency	6/100	6
Severe combined system immunodeficiency	9/400	2
IgM deficiency	6/70	8
Wiskott-Aldrich syndrome	24/300	8
Ataxia-telangiectasia	52/500	10
Common variable immunodeficiency	41/500	8
Total	138/1870	7

with the extent of cancer and may be secondary to the malignant process. They also are associated with a variety of tumor types, including lymphomas, Hodgkin's disease, and solid tumors such as carcinomas of the breast and colon [1]. Of continuing interest is the question of the cancer patients' prior immunologic status, i.e., whether persons who develop these varying forms of cancer have subclinical and preexisting immunologic defects. Prospective studies of individuals suspected of being at increased risk should provide answers to this critical question.

POSSIBLE INCREASED CANCER RISK IN CARRIERS OF IMMUNODEFICIENCY GENES

The studies reported by the Immunodeficiency-Cancer Registry support the hypothesis that individuals who are homozygous for certain immunodeficiency genes develop cancer more frequently than age-matched controls. The risk of malignancy in persons who are heterozygous for immunodeficiency genes is a related question that should clarify both the role of genetic influences in oncogenesis and, more specifically, the association between immunodeficiency and cancer. While immunodeficiency genes in the homozygous form are quite rare, the gene frequency is high, perhaps as frequent as one per hundred for A-T [12].

TABLE 2

Summary of tumor histologies in reported cases of primary immunodeficiency diseases and cancer[a]

HISTOLOGIC TYPES

Immunodeficiency disease type	Epithelial	Lymphoreticular	Leukemia	Mesenchymal	Nervous System	Total
Bruton's agammaglobulinemia	0	6 (46)[b]	7 (54)	0	0	13
Severe combined system	0	7 (64)	4 (36)	0	0	11
Wiskott-Aldrich syndrome	0	23 (82)	3 (11)	1 (3.5)	1 (3.5)	28
Ataxia-telangiectasia	8 (12)	37 (57)	15 (23)	1 (2)	4 (6)	65
IgM deficiency	1 (15)	5 (70)	0	1 (15)	0	7
Variable immunodeficiency	21 (40)	26 (47)	4 (8)	1 (2)	1 (2)	53
IgA deficiency	10 (53)	4 (22)	0	2 (10)	3 (15)	19[c]
Total	40 (20)	108 (55)	33 (17)	6 (3)	9 (5)	196

[a]Through August 15, 1974.
[b]Numbers in parentheses indicate percent histologic type for each primary immunodeficiency disease.
[c]Occurring in 14 individuals.

TABLE 3

Mortality from cancer of various types
in children under 15 years of age [11]

Tumor type	Unselected children (%)[a]	With primary immunodeficiency diseases[b]	
		All areas (%)	U.S. only (%)
Leukemia (all types)	48	25 (16)	25 (10)
Central nervous system	16	4 (2)	3 (1)
Lymphoreticular (reticulum cell sarcoma, lympho-sarcoma, etc.)	8	67 (40)	69 (27)
Bone	4	2 (1)	0 (0)
Other	24	2 (1)	3 (1)
Totals		(60)	(39)

[a]Death certificates of 29,457 children in the United States for the period 1960-1966, Miller, R.W. *J. Pediatr.* 75:685–689, 1969.
[b]From Immunodeficiency-Cancer Registry; number of patients in parentheses.

In a review of 14 A-T families, Epstein et al. [14] found tumors in 21 family members. All of the tumors were in second-order relatives, but it was not possible to determine the number who were heterozygous for the A-T gene. However, five tumors were stomach carcinomas: a tumor known to be associated with A-T in the homozygous form. No immunologic data were available on the persons with cancer, although a number of first-order relatives were found to be immunodeficient.

Cancer history and quantitative immunoglobulin assays were performed in another A-T family by Haerer et al. [15]. Stomach cancer was reported in two A-T siblings and their mother. Before development of gastric adenocarcinoma the mother was reported to have normal immunoglobulins.

Another preliminary study [16] suggested that pancreatic carcinoma is 15 times more frequent in persons presumed to be heterozygous for A-T than in control relatives. Immunologic data were not available, and the association between immunodeficiency and cancer in family members is not conclusive.

Immunologic abnormalities have been observed in a few families with multiple malignancies. Fraumeni et al. [17] reported a family in which 3 of 13 siblings had chronic lymphatic leukemia (CLL). Abnormalities of cell-mediated and humoral immunity were observed in individuals with CLL and several "healthy" siblings. One of the latter, who had selective IgM deficiency, later developed carcinoma of the lung. In another family, four of nine siblings had malignant lymphoma, while a fifth sibling developed Waldenström's macroglobulinemia with lung adenocarcinoma. Other family members had Hodgkin's disease, lung adenocarcinoma, and acute lymphoblastic leukemia (ALL) [18]. Immunologic defects were found in both affected and healthy members of this family.

We recently observed [19] a family in which two siblings and a paternal aunt developed ALL. Studies of histocompatibility antigens revealed a paternally transmitted chromosome that was detected in the one child surviving with ALL and in two healthy siblings. All persons studied who carried this chromosome also had fewer T-lymphocytes by the rosette assay. This may be the first reported instance of a histocompatibility antigen-linked immune response gene defect. In the mouse, histocompatibility antigen-linked genes are clearly important in susceptibility or resistance to cancer, especially when virally induced [1]. Studies in additional families should help elucidate the significance of this defect in the control of human cancer.

EXPERIMENTAL MODELS LINKING IMMUNODEFICIENCY AND CANCER

Experiments relating immunodeficiency and DNA virus-induced tumors were first reported by Vandeputte et al. [20] who demonstrated that neonatally thymectomized rats inoculated with polyoma virus developed significantly more sarcomas, especially in kidney and bone, than did nonthymectomized controls. Using a hamster model, Defendi et al. [21] reported increased oncogenicity of polyoma virus in thymectomized animals. Allison and Taylor [22] found that neonatally thymectomized rats of two strains inoculated with another DNA virus (simian virus 40) developed more tumors after a shorter latent period than did nonthymectomized control rats. Later studies of experimental immuno-deficiency and DNA virus-induced tumors utilized antilymphocyte serum (ALS). Allison et al. [23] indicated that tumors could be readily induced by adeno-virus in susceptible CBA mice by use of either ALS or neonatal thymectomy. Allison and Law [24] reported additional experiments with C3H mice in which neonatal ALS treatment and polyoma virus inoculation caused a high fre-quency of parotid tumors. These and other studies showed that ALS treatment was often more effective than neonatal thymectomy in enhancing the develop-ment of polyoma-induced neoplasms.

Work with RNA viruses was initiated by McEndy, Boon, and Furth [25] who demonstrated that thymectomy in mice often inhibited leukemogenesis. They showed that thymectomy of young adults from the high leukemic AKR strain drastically reduced the incidence of lymphoid leukemia. The viral etiology of lymphoma in AKR mice was largely established by Gross[26] who demonstrated transmission by cell-free extracts. The thymic dependency of Gross passage A lymphoma has been a matter of great interest. Evidence provided by Kaplan et al. [27], Siegler and Rich [28], and Goodman and Block [29] established that, in at least certain strains of mice, the first histologic changes of lymphoma occur focally within the thymus.

Peterson et al. [30] and Dent et al. [31] demonstrated that Gross passage A virus is immunosuppressive. These data suggest a complex interrelationship between a virus, which is both immunosuppressive and oncogenic, and a target organ, the thymus, which is itself of major immunologic significance. Furthermore, Allison and Law [24] showed that ALS greatly increased the incidence of Moloney virus-induced leukemias and sarcomas, whereas thymectomy significantly reduced the incidence of these cancers.

Early studies in the chicken [32,33] indicated that thymectomy had no effect on the development of virally induced visceral lymphomatosis. Of special interest, however, was the prevention of virus-induced lymphomatosis when bursectomy was performed at 1 and 28 days of age. These and later studies [33,34] indicated that the lymphomas regularly originate in bursal follicles, and thus are of B-(bursal-dependent) cell origin. In contrast, thymectomy increased the incidence and decreased the latent period of soft-tissue sarcomas induced by the Carr-Zilber strain of Rous sarcoma virus (RSV) in the chicken [28].

Recent studies by McArthur et al. [35] revealed that bursectomy did not influence growth of sarcomas induced by Bryan-strain RSV. Bursectomy is known to markedly depress antibody formation, while cell-mediated immunity remains intact.

In the early 1950's, Malmgren et al. [36] demonstrated that chemical carcinogens also could be immunosuppressive. Prehn [37] further showed that 3-methylcholanthrene (MCA) interferes with an immune reaction in the doses commonly used. Stutman [38] found that strain I mice which are relatively resistant to tumor development after receiving a subcutaneous injection of MCA are also resistant to the immunosuppressive effects of the drug.

In an extensive review of the influence of neonatal thymectomy and ALS treatment on chemical carcinogenesis, Mäkelä [39] showed that immunosuppressive influences often increase the incidence and shorten incubation periods of chemically induced malignancies.

THE NUDE MOUSE AS AN EXPERIMENTAL MODEL OF
GENETICALLY DETERMINED IMMUNODEFICIENCY

Mice that are homozygous for the "nude" gene are markedly deficient in cell-mediated (T-cell) immunity, but do not have an increased incidence of spontaneous neoplasms [40]. Also, nude mice apparently are not prone to chemically induced neoplasms [41]. On the other hand, the risk of tumors following polyoma virus infection may be enhanced in these mice [42].

POSSIBLE MECHANISMS LINKING HUMAN IMMUNODEFICIENCY AND CANCER

Data from both experimental animals and humans indicate that immunodeficiency predisposes to cancer. The pathogenetic mechanisms responsible for this susceptibility are probably complex.

In humans, lymphoreticular neoplasms clearly predominate in both primary and drug-induced immunodeficiency. The possible causes for the lymphoid malignancies include the following:

1) Increased malignant transformation of lymphoid cells caused by: a) Intrinsic defects in lymphoid cells (e.g., chromosomal breaks), or b) Increased activity of endogenous and exogenous oncogenic viruses.

2) Decreased activity of the lymphoid system to recognize and destroy malignant lymphoid cells, caused by: a) Defective recognition, or b) Defective response following recognition.

Perhaps of major significance is the fact that the system which is defective (i.e., the lymphoid system) is the primary site for most malignancies. This may reflect intrinsic abnormalities, such as chromosomal breaks and rearrangements which are sometimes seen in immunodeficiency syndromes [43] and may predispose to malignant transformation. Likewise, chronic antigenic stimulation with resultant cellular proliferation, may enhance transformation. The role of exogenous or endogenous oncogenic viruses remains unclear. Immunodeficiency produced in experimental animals with neonatal thymectomy, ALS, or graft-versus-host reaction often activates endogenous oncogenic viruses and predisposes to infection with exogenous oncogenic viruses [1,44,45]. Of interest is the recent isolation of a DNA-containing papova virus from a lymphoid tumor that arose in a patient with the Wiskott-Aldrich syndrome [46]. Although we cannot now define the precise role of viruses and other factors in tumor formation, further experimental studies should lead to a better understanding of pathogenetic mechanisms.

There has been much interest lately in the hypothesis that a major function of the immune system is to provide "surveillance" against malignant cells that develop on perhaps a daily basis [47]. In its simplest form this hypothesis predicts that, in immunodeficiency diseases, the risk of malignancies will increase but the distribution by histologic type will remain unchanged. In other words, we would expect more of the same tumor types found in the general population in immunodeficient states. However, in patients with both primary and drug-induced immunodeficiency associated with renal transplantation, the distribution of malignancies is, as previously discussed, clearly different from the general population. Also, in most experimental systems, immunodeficiency results either in a predominance of lymphoid tumors [1] or, frequently, in no increase of malignancy [40,41].

PROSPECTS

More epidemiologic and experimental research is necessary to define the apparently complex relationship between the immune apparatus and malignant adaptation. Undoubtedly, many studies will center on the intimate relation between lymphoid malignancies and the immunologic apparatus. In man, special attention should be given to the influence of immune responses linked to histocompatibility antigens, since these responses are important in determining cancer susceptibility in the mouse. Information from such studies should assist in the discovery of individuals at high risk who might then be subject to improved measures of cancer control.

REFERENCES

1. Kersey, J., Spector, B., and Good, R.A. Immunodeficiency and cancer. *In* Weinhouse, S., and Klein, G., eds. *Advances in Cancer Research,* Academic Press, New York, 1973, pp. 211–230.

2. Gatti, R.A., and Good, R.A. Occurrence of malignancy in immunodeficiency diseases. *Cancer 28:*89–98, 1971.

3. McKhann, C.F. Primary malignancy in patients undergoing immunosuppression for renal transplantation. *Transplantation 8:*209–212, 1969.

4. Schneck, S.A., and Penn, I. De-novo brain tumours in renal transplant recipients. *Lancet 1:*983–986, 1971.

5. Kersey, J., Spector, B., and Good, R.A. Primary immunodeficiency diseases and cancer: The Immunodeficiency-Cancer Registry. *Int. J. Cancer 12:*333–347, 1973.

6. Walder, B.K., Robertson, M.R., and Jeremy, D. Skin cancer and immunosuppression. *Lancet 2:*1232–1283, 1971.

7. Hoover, R., and Fraumeni, J.F., Jr. Risk of cancer in renal transplant recipients. *Lancet 2:*55–67, 1973.

8. Waldmann, T.A., Strober, W., and Blaese, R.M. Immunodeficiency disease and malignancy: Various immunologic deficiencies of man and the role of immune processes in the control of malignant disease. *Ann. Intern. Med. 77:*605–628, 1972.

9. Good, R.A., Biggar, W.D., and Park, B. Immunodeficiency in man. *In* Amos, B., ed. *Progress in Immunology,* Academic Press, New York, 1971, p. 700.

10. Sedgwick, R.P., and Boder, E. Ataxia-telangiectasia. *In* Vinken, P.J., and Bruyn, G.W., eds. *Handbook of Clinical Neurology,* North Holland Publishing Co., Amsterdam, 1972, pp. 267–339.

11. Kersey, J., Spector, B.D., and Good, R.A. Cancer in children with primary immunodeficiency disorders. *J. Pediatrics 84:*263–264, 1974.

12. Spector, B.D., Kersey, J., and Good, R.A. Unpublished data.

13. Jackson, J.F. Ataxia-telangiactasia. *In* Lynch, H.T., ed., *Skin, Heredity, and Malignant Neoplasms,* Medical Exam. Publ. Co., Inc., Flushing, New York, 1972, pp. 94-103.

14. Epstein, W.L., Fudenberg, H.H., Reed, W.B., et al. Immunologic studies in ataxia-telangiectasia. I. Delayed hypersensitivity and serum immune globulin levels in probands and first-degree relatives. *Int. Arch. Allergy 30:*15-29, 1966.

15. Haerer, A.F., Jackson, J.F., and Evers, C.G. Ataxia-telangiectasia with gastric adenocarcinoma. *J.A.M.A. 210:*1884-1897, 1969.

16. Sholman, L., and Swift, M.A. Pancreatic carcinoma and diabetes mellitus in families of ataxia-telangiectasia probands (Abstract). *Am. J. Hum. Genet. 24:*48a, 1973.

17. Fraumeni, J.F., Jr., Vogel, C.K., and DeVita, V.T. Familial chronic lymphocytic leukemia. *Ann. Intern. Med. 71:*279-284, 1969.

18. Fraumeni, J.F., Jr., Wertelecki, W., Blattner, W.A., et al. Varied manifestations of a familial lymphoproliferative disorder. *Am. J. Med.* In press.

19. Anderson, R., et al. Unpublished data.

20. Vandeputte, M., Denys, J., Leyten, R., et al. The oncogenic activity of polyoma virus in thymectomized rats. *Life Sci. 2:*475-478, 1963.

21. Defendi, V., Roosa, R.A., and Koprowski, H. Effects of thymectomy at birth on response of tissue, cells and viral antigens. *In* Good, R.A. and Gabrielson, A.E. eds. *The Thymus in Immunobiology,* Hoeber and Harper, New York, 1964, pp. 504-520.

22. Allison, A.C. and Taylor, R.B. Observations on thymectomy and carcinogenesis. *Cancer Res. 27:*703-707, 1967.

23. Allison, A.C., Berman, L.D., and Levy, R.H. Increased tumor induction by adenovirus type 12 in thymectomized mice treated with anti-lymphocyte serum. *Nature (Lond.) 295:*185-187, 1967.

24. Allison, A.C., and Law, L.W. Effects of antilymphocyte serum on virus oncogenesis. *Proc. Soc. Exp. Biol. Med. 127:*207-212, 1968.

25. McEndy, D.P., Boon, M.C., and Furth, J. On the role of thymus, spleen, and gonads in the development of leukemia in high-leukemia stock of mice. *Cancer Res. 4:* 377-384, 1944.

26. Gross, L. Development and serial cell-free passage of a highly potent strain of mouse leukemic virus. *Proc. Soc. Exp. Biol. Med. 94:*767-771, 1957.

27. Kaplan, H.S., Hirsch, B.B., and Brown, M.B. Indirect induction of lymphomas in irradiated mice. IV. Genetic evidence of the origin of the tumor cells from the thymic grafts. *Cancer Res. 16:*434-436, 1956.

28. Siegler, R., and Rich, M.A. Unilateral histogenesis of AKR thymic lymphoma. *Cancer Res. 23:*1669-1678, 1963.

29. Goodman, S.B., and Block, M.H. The histogenesis of Gross's viral induced mouse leukemia. *Cancer Res. 23:*1634-1640, 1963.

30. Peterson, R.D.A., Hendrickson, R., and Good, R.A. Reduced antibody forming capacity during the incubation period of passage A leukemia in C3H mice. *Proc. Soc. Exp. Biol. Med. 114:*517-520, 1963.

31. Dent, P.B., Peterson, R.D.A., and Good, R.A. A defect in cellular immunity during the indubation period of passage A leukemia in C3H mice. *Proc. Soc. Exp. Biol. Med. 119:* 869-871, 1965.

32. Peterson, R.D.A., Burmester, B.R., Friedrickson, D.N., et al. Effect of bursectomy and thymectomy on the development of visceral lymphomatosis in the chicken. *J. Natl. Cancer Inst. 32:*1343-1354, 1964.

33. Cooper, M.D., Payne, L.N., Dent, P.B., et al. The role of the bursa in avian lymphoid leukosis (Abstract). *Fed. Proc. 25:*10, 1966.

34. Radzichovaskaja, R. Effect of thymectomy on Rous virus tumor growth induced in chickens. *Proc. Soc. Exp. Biol. Med. 126:*13–15, 1967.

35. McArthur, W.P., Carswell, E.A., and Thorsbecke, G.J. Growth of Rous sarcomas in bursectomized chickens. *J. Natl. Cancer Inst. 49:*907–909, 1972.

36. Malmgren, R., Benison, B.E., and McKinley, T.W. Reduced antibody titers in mice treated with carcinogenic and cancer chemotherapeutic agents. *Proc. Soc. Exp. Biol. Med. 79:*484–488, 1952.

37. Prehn, R.T. Function of depressed immunologic reactivity during carcinogenesis. *J. Natl. Cancer Inst. 31:*791–805, 1963.

38. Stutman, O. Carcinogen-induced immune depression: Absence in mice resistant to chemical oncogenesis. *Science 166:*620–621, 1969.

39. Mäkelä, O. Influence of immunological reactions on carcinogenesis. *In* Doll, R., and Vodopija, I., eds. *Host Environment Interactions in the Etiology of Cancer in Man.* I.A.R.C. Scientific Publications No. 7, I.A.R.C., Lyon, 1973, pp. 285–290.

40. Rygaard, J., and Povlsen, C.O. The mouse mutant nude does not develop spontaneous tumors. An argument against immunological surveillance. *Acta Pathol. Microbiol. Scand. 82B:*99–106, 1974.

41. Stutman, O. Tumor development after 3-methylcholanthrene in immunologically deficient athymic-nude mice. *Science 183:*534–536, 1974.

42. Allison, A.C., Monga, J.N., and Hammond, V. Increased susceptibility to viral oncogenesis of congenitally thymus-derived nude mice. *Nature (Lond.) 252:*746–747, 1974.

43. Hecht, F., McCaw, B.K., and Koler, R.D. Ataxia-telangiectasia: Clonal growth of translocation lymphocytes. *N. Engl. J. Med. 289:*286–291, 1973.

44. Hirsch, M.S., Phillips, S.M., Solnik, C., et al. Activation of leukemia viruses by graft-versus-host and mixed lymphocyte reactions in vitro. *Proc. Natl. Acad. Sci. USA 69:*1069–1072, 1972.

45. Schwartz, R.S. Immunoregulation, oncogenic viruses, and malignant lymphomas. *Lancet 1:*1266–1269, 1972.

46. Takemoto, K.K., Rabson, A.S., Mullarkey, M.F., et al. Isolation of papovirus from brain tumor and urine of a patient with Wiskott-Aldrich syndrome. *J. Natl. Cancer Inst. 53:*1205–1207, 1974.

47. Thomas, L. *In* Lawrence, H.S., ed. *Cellular and Humoral Aspects of the Hypersensitivity States.* Hoeber, New York, 1959, pp. 529–532.

DISCUSSION

Dr. Li raised the possibility that chronic antigenic stimulation predisposes to lymphoproliferative malignancy in renal transplant patients, and **Dr. Kersey** concurred referring to experimental studies on the progression of graft versus host disease to lymphoma.

Dr. Higginson challenged the causal association of immunodeficiency and malignancy, suggesting that these conditions are epiphenomena. In reply, **Dr. Kersey** discussed a family with ataxia-telangiectasia (A-T) and gastric carcinoma, in which the diseases were concurrent in some family members but segregated independently in others. A family member with gastric carcinoma alone would presumably be a carrier of the recessively inherited gene for A-T.

Dr. Hoover, referring to unpublished data from the registry of primary immune deficiency syndromes with cancer, noted a definite excess of stomach cancer when lymphoproliferative neoplasms are removed from the analysis. The possibility of immunologic determinants of stomach cancer was supported by **Dr. Fraumeni,** who reported a family with multiple cases of gastric carcinoma in which a high frequency of cell-mediated immune deficiency and antiparietal cell antibodies were found. **Dr. Fraumeni** and **Dr. Henderson** also summarized studies on other families with an excess of lymphoproliferative malignancy and evidence of subclinical immune deficiency. **Dr. Kersey** then reported a multiple-case family with acute lymphocytic leukemia over two generations, in which preliminary study suggests linkage between subclinical immune deficiency (depressed T-cell numbers) and the HL-A-2-5 pattern.

Dr. Bahn reiterated that the tumor primarily associated with renal transplantation is lymphoma, and **Dr. Kersey** emphasized that this lymphoma is generally the reticulum cell sarcoma type, frequently confined to the central nervous system. The tumors are not found exclusively in the frontal lobe where, according to **Dr. Rawson,** lymphomas of the nervous system have previously been localized.

Dr. Henderson questioned the role of viruses in the pathogenesis of lymphomas associated with immune deficiency. **Dr. Kersey** stated that Takemoto and Blaese at the National Institutes of Health have isolated SV 40-like agents from the tumors of patients with the Wiskott-Aldrich syndrome. Whether this virus is etiologic or merely a passenger agent is not yet clear, but it points to the need for further collaboration between immunologists and virologists in delineating the pathogenesis of these tumors.

William A. Blattner

4

ACQUIRED DISEASES

A. C. Templeton, M.D.

Pathology Department
St. Vincent Hospital
Worcester, Massachusetts

A statistically valid association between acquired disease and cancer may be explained as follows:

1) The disease may predispose to cancer.
2) The cancer may predispose to the disease.
3) The disease may increase the chance of diagnosis of cancer but not cause an increase in incidence.
4) Some third factor may cause both the disease and cancer which are not otherwise related.
5) The treatment of the disease may cause cancer.
6) The disease and cancer are in reality phases of the same process.

This chapter will emphasize those clinically apparent symptom-producing disease states which may result in an increased risk of cancer. Inapparent infections or asymptomatic lesions which may be the early stages in tumor formation are covered in other chapters. Table 1 lists the conditions discussed and the tumors with which they are associated.

INFECTIOUS STATES

Viral, bacterial, plasmodial, and metazoan infections have all been implicated in cancer development, but in most cases the precise interrelationships have not been elucidated.

TABLE 1
Acquired diseases which have been implicated as
predisposing to cancer

1. *Infectious states*	*Reference*	*Cancer*
a. Viral		
Herpes group organisms		
Herpes simplex virus		
type 2	1,2	cervix, penis
Epstein-Barr virus	3,4	lymphoma
Hepatitis B	5,6	liver
Mumps orchitis	7	testes
b. Bacterial		
Fistula		
Osteomyelitis	8,9	skin, soft tissue
Urethra	11	skin
Phagedenic ulcers	11	skin
Syphilis	12	tongue
Tuberculosis	13	lung
c. Plasmodial		
Malaria	14,15	lymphoma
d. Parasitic		
Schistosomiasis	16-20	
S. hematobium		bladder
S. mansoni	21	lymphoma
Clonorchis sinensis	22	biliary tract
Intestinal parasites	23,24	lymphoma
2. *Noninfectious inflammatory states*		
Gastritis	25-31	stomach
Crohn's disease	32-34	intestine
Ulcerative colitis	35,36	colon, bile ducts
Adult celiac disease	37	intestine, lymphoma
Cirrhosis	38-41	liver
Pulmonary fibrosis	42-44	lung
(pneumoconiosis, hematite lung, scleroderma, sarcoid, etc.)		
Hashimoto's disease	45	lymphoma of thyroid
Sjögren's syndrome	46	lymphoma
Pancreatitis	47,48	pancreas

TABLE 1 (Continued)

3. *Endocrine states*	*Reference*	*Cancer*
Diabetes	48,49	pancreas
Thyrotoxicosis	50,51	breast
Cystic mastopathy	52-54	breast
Prostatic hyperplasia	55,56	prostate
Stein-Leventhal syndrome	57	uterus
4. *Nutritional disorders*		
Iron excess	41,60	liver
Iron deficiency	61,62	pharynx, esophagus
Iodine deficiency	63	thyroid
Vitamin A deficiency	64	colon, other
Vitamin B deficiency	61,66	liver
Alcoholism	67-70	esophagus, oropharynx, larynx, liver, pancreas
Obesity	71-73	breast, uterus
5. *Trauma*		
Calculi		
Urinary stones	74	renal pelvis
Gallstones	75	gallbladder
Burns (thermal, caustic)	8,11	skin
	76	esophagus
6. *Postoperative states*		
Immune interference		
Appendectomy	77-79	(?)
Tonsillectomy	80	Hodgkin's disease
Thymectomy	81,82	(?)
Transplantation	83	lymphoma
Radical mastectomy	84	lymphangiosarcoma
7. *Benign proliferations*		
Polyps (adenomatous)	85,86	colon
Nevi	87,88	melanoma
Hydatidiform mole	89	choriocarcinoma
Enchondroma	90	chondrosarcoma
Paget's disease of bone	91	bone

TABLE 1 (Continued)

8. *Other disorders*	*Reference*	*Cancer*
Myeloproliferative states	92	leukemia
Pernicious anemia	25	leukemia, stomach
Heroin addiction	93	Hodgkin's disease
Pharyngeal pouch	94	pharynx
Bladder diverticulum	95	bladder

Viral Diseases

Herpesvirus infections have been linked with many cancers. The incidence of cancer of the cervix is increased in patients with herpes genitalis due to herpes simplex virus type 2, but whether the relation is causal or due to some common third factor is, as yet, uncertain [1,2]. From a practical point of view, however, patients who have had an attack of genital herpes can be regarded as being at excess risk. Herpes simplex virus type 2 infection has also been linked with penile carcinoma, but the same problems of proving a causal relation apply. The Epstein-Barr virus (EBV) has been associated with Burkitt's lymphoma and nasopharyngeal carcinoma, but the infections are clinically inapparent. Infectious mononucleosis caused by EBV is followed sometimes by cancer, but the risk does not seem high [3,4].

Australia hepatitis B antigen is a cause of hepatitis which may progress to cirrhosis. In Uganda, 40 percent of patients with hepatocellular carcinoma had positive tests for Australia antigen whether cirrhosis was present or not [5,6]. In other parts of the world, the proportion is much lower. Causality remains to be proven, but it appears that patients with hepatitis virus B infections who are unable to suppress the long-term production of antigen are prone to cancer.

Mumps orchitis has been suggested as a precursor of testicular tumors [7], but an analytical study will be necessary to determine any relationship.

Bacterial Diseases

Bacterial diseases predisposing to cancer are typically chronic infections with extensive fibrosis and persistent regenerative stress. In these conditions, it is difficult to separate the effects of bacterial products, scarring itself, regenerating cells, and treatment given. Certain skin tumors are related to osteomyelitis fistulas, varicose ulcers, or tropical ulcers [8,9]. In general, the longer the ulcer has been present, the greater the risk of tumor. Most common are squamous carcinomas of low-grade malignancy, but rapidly metastasizing fibrosarcomas have been described. The risk of developing such tumors is particularly high with tropical phagedenic ulcers, perhaps because the resident flora are capable of manufacturing carcinogens. Staphylococci are only rarely associated with such tumors, but gram-negative organisms are almost always present [10]. Fistulas of the urethra and rectum and vesicovaginal fistulas may all predispose to squamous carcinomas; these situations are rare in Western countries, but are serious public health problems in developing countries [11].

Syphilitic glossitis may predispose to lingual cancer. In one series, 40 percent of patients with cancer of the tongue had a positive serology [12] but, in this and other series, suitable controls were not surveyed. Tuberculosis and other scar-producing pulmonary infections have been implicated in the pathogenesis of adenocarcinoma of the lung [13]. The association is based on pathological studies, and epidemiologic evidence is slim.

Plasmodial Disease

Malaria has been implicated as a risk factor in Burkitt's lymphoma because of the strong geographic correlation between these two diseases [14]. The role of the malarial infection may be to induce a period of immune suppression so that viral infection is modified. Alternatively, the long-term particulate stress may increase immunocyte turnover. The risk of other forms of lymphoma also seems to be modified by malarial infection, but not to the same extent as Burkitt's tumor [15].

Parasitic Infections

Schistosomiasis *(Schistosoma haematobium)* has been associated, both clinically and geographically, with bladder cancer in Egypt [16]. In laboratory studies, the eggs are capable of inducing proliferation of transitional epithelium [17]. Schistosomiasis was found also in 71 percent of bladder cancer patients in the Gold Coast as compared with 1.4 percent of the population in general [18]. The carcinogenic mechanism may be related to increased levels of urinary glucuronidase in patients with significant egg loads. Schistosomiasis is associated primarily with squamous carcinomas, although these tumors occur also in the absence of infection [19,20]. Thus, urinary schistosomiasis is clearly associated with bladder cancer in certain countries, but the relative risk is difficult to estimate, probably in the order of four- or fivefold. By contrast, *S. mansoni* infection of the bowel does not predispose to colorectal cancer, although the tumors developing in patients with schistosomiasis have a rather distinctive appearance [11]. In a case series from Brazil [21], *S. mansoni* has been linked to follicular lymphoma of the spleen.

Clonorchis sinensis infection is responsible for the high rates of intrahepatic bile duct cancer in the Far East [22]. Parasitic infections of various types have been correlated geographically with certain subtypes of Hodgkin's disease and with Mediterranean lymphoma [23,24], but causal relationships remain to be proven.

NONINFECTIOUS INFLAMMATORY CONDITIONS

Gastritis and intestinal metaplasia are regularly found in association with stomach cancer. Patients with atrophic gastritis and pernicious anemia have a risk of developing stomach cancer four or five times normal [25] and 10 percent of patients with pernicious anemia develop gastric cancer before they die [26]. Chronic gastritis may be divided into two forms. One is diffuse, complete, and associated with gastric antibodies and pernicious anemia. The second form is patchy and is neither associated with antibodies nor pernicious anemia [27]. Most gastric cancers are associated with the second type, and the association is particularly strong with well-differentiated tumors of the pyloric antrum [28,29]. The relationships between gastric ulcer and cancer are much less certain and have been debated for years. A recent study in England on patients undergoing partial gastrectomy showed a greater risk of stomach cancer in patients who had a gastric ulcer than in patients who had a duodenal lesion [30]. In contrast, a study in the United States showed no excess risk in patients with gastric ulcer whether treated medically or surgically [31].

Patients with Crohn's disease (regional enterocolitis) have an elevated risk of adenocarcinoma of the small intestine based on clinical series, although only 28 cases of this association have been reported [32,33]. One study [33] showed an equivocal rise in the incidence of colorectal cancer, but a recent series from the Mayo Clinic [34] revealed a risk 20 times greater than in controls. In ulcerative colitis, the incidence of colorectal cancer is about 10 times greater than in the general population. The risk is related to the extent of the colitis, its duration, and the age at onset [35]. An excess of biliary cancer has also been reported in ulcerative colitis on the basis of case studies [36]. In addition, adult celiac disease (nontropical sprue) carries an increased risk of intestinal lymphoma and probably carcinoma [37].

Fifty to ninety percent of hepatocellular carcinoma occurs in association with cirrhosis. In Uganda and the United States about 15 percent of cirrhotics have hepatocellular cancer present at autopsy [38,39], but a figure of 44 percent was reported from South Africa [40]. The risk of developing cancer varies with different types of cirrhosis. Micronodular (nutritional) forms carry the smallest risk, and the postnecrotic macronodular pattern, the highest. The risk probably increases if Australia antigen is detected [6]. Hemochromatosis also predisposes to liver cancer, but the risk is sharply reduced by phlebotomy [41].

Inflammatory damage to the lung may be followed by scar formation with surrounding atypical proliferation of cells called tumorlets [13]. The significance of such lesions in the genesis of lung cancer is debated. Case studies have documented tumors developing in the neighborhood of bullet wounds and tuberculous lesions [42], and an excess of lung cancer has been linked with diffuse lung fibrosis such as certain forms of pneumoconiosis and scleroderma (progressive systemic sclerosis) [43]. In a recent study [44], patients with sarcoidosis were reported to have a three-fold increased risk of lung cancer and an eleven-fold excess of lymphoma, perhaps related to the reduced immune capacity associated with this disease [44].

Autoimmune disorders such as Hashimoto's disease [45] and Sjögren's syndrome [46] are associated with the development of lymphomas, primarily in the organs affected by the underlying disorder. In addition, pancreatitis is often found at autopsy in patients with pancreatic cancer, but if pancreatitis does predispose to cancer, the association is quite weak [47].

ENDOCRINE STATES

In surveys of cancer mortality in diabetes, a significant excess risk of pancreatic cancer has been consistently noted [48, 49], being twofold in females and 1.5-fold in males. The association may be weaker if cases are omitted where the cancer might have antedated the diabetes [48]. The incidence of some tumors, particularly lung cancer, is lower than usual, possibly because many diabetic patients are Jewish [49].

The relation of thyroid disease to cancer is complex and poorly understood. Compared with normal controls, patients with thyroid disease have a higher mortality from breast cancer [50], though the incidence seems unchanged. Patients with untreated myxedema are reportedly prone to pituitary tumors [51].

Alterations in sex hormone production may result in clinically detectable diseases associated with cancer. Retrospective studies have shown about a four-fold increase in the risk of breast cancer among women with benign cystic mastopathy [52]. Intraductal dysplasia is the component most strongly associated with cancer development [53]. Since only 5 percent of women with cancer have had a previous biopsy, this information is of limited value as a predictor of risk and studies of whole breast sections have shown these changes to be very common in the aging breast [54].

The relation of prostatic hyperplasia to clinical cancer of the prostate is disputed due to difficulties in defining hyperplasia and latent tumors. One study showed no association, while another found a threefold to fourfold increase in risk [55,56]. Studies of mastopathy and prostatic hyperplasia are complicated by the fact that diagnosis necessitates removal of tissue for histology, a process that may itself influence the likelihood of cancer formation.

Young women with the Stein-Leventhal syndrome are prone to various endo-metrial lesions, including well-differentiated adenocarcinomas. These reactions may be reversible following curettage and restitution of ovulation. The endo-metrial tumors rarely metastasize and are readily curable [57]. Ovarian function also influences breast cancer risk; the incidence of this disease has been correlated with the urinary estrogen fractions in population surveys [58], and is clearly reduced following oophorectomy [59].

NUTRITIONAL DISORDERS

Theoretically, adaptation of cellular function by nutritional abnormalities, such as vitamin and protein deficiency or carbohydrate excess, might alter tumor incidence. However, hard data on these relationships in humans are difficult to come by.

Thirty percent of patients with hemochromatosis and cirrhosis had hepato-cellular carcinoma at the time of death [60]. This risk is substantially reduced by phlebotomy as a means of removing iron [41]. Iron deficiency has been implicated in the Plummer-Vinson (Paterson-Kelly) syndrome which pre-disposes to postcricoid carcinoma in Swedish women [61]. The role of other factors such as vitamin lack and autoimmune reactions in such cases is unclear [62]. African women suffer from severe iron deficiency, but sideropenic webs have not been described and postcricoid cancer is very rare [11].

A geographical correlation has been described in areas with iodine de-ficiency and high rates for follicular cancer of the thyroid [63]. The association is difficult to quantify because of histologic problems in distinguishing hyper-plasia from well-differentiated cancer. In addition, mortality statistics in dif-ferent countries do not distinguish between follicular and papillary tumors. Papillary tumors are frequently induced by radiation and are not associated with iodine deficiency.

Vitamin A deficiency increases the effectiveness of carcinogens involving the colon [64] and lung in animal systems [64], and may alter the behavior of human tumors such as those arising in the conjunctiva [65] and bladder. Vitamin B deficiency has been suggested as an etiologic factor in human pharyn-geal [61] and hepatocellular [66] cancers.

Alcoholism predisposes to cancers of the mouth, pharynx, esophagus, larynx, and possibly the pancreas and liver [67-70]. The precise mechanisms are un-clear, but interactions with smoking have been demonstrated. Esophageal cancer may be related to the nitrosamine content of some beverages [67]. For most tumors, a deficiency state associated with alcoholism probably plays a critical role. The alcohol-related liver cancers are hepatocellular carcinomas associated with cirrhosis, although the risk of cancer in alcoholic cirrhosis is lower than with other types of cirrhosis.

Obesity has been reported to be a risk factor in cancers of the breast and endometrium, particularly among elderly patients [71-73]. The relationships, which may reflect dietary constituents, are not sufficiently strong to be useful for screening purposes.

TRAUMA

The place of trauma in the genesis of cancer is hotly debated, particularly when litigation is contemplated. Trauma may promote a tumor in a previously initiated site in experimental animals; in humans, chronic irritation is undoubtedly carcinogenic in some situations. For example, longstanding urinary stones may predispose to cancer of the renal pelvis [74]. Gallstones are an important risk factor in carcinoma of the gallbladder [75], although the contributions of trauma and other factors are difficult to distinguish. Thermal trauma may account for the increased risk of lip cancer in pipe smokers.

Scars following burns, bites, infections, corrosive damage, and vaccinations have all been implicated in the genesis of cancers, particularly of the skin [8, 65], lung [13,42], and esophagus [76]. Single episodes of trauma have been associated with the development of osteosarcoma, testicular tumors, and breast cancer. Although such trauma usually leads to the recognition of a preexisting tumor, it is possible that in rare instances cancer is induced in this manner. Trauma may precipitate malignant change in previously benign lesions, such as nevi on the sole of the foot [65] or osteochondromas.

POSTOPERATIVE STATES

Operations in which immunocompetent cells are removed have been suggested as a risk factor in cancer. Tonsillectomy, splenectomy, appendectomy and thymectomy have come under suspicion, but evidence of a significant cancer hazard is slim. Appendectomy was linked to cancer in two retrospective series [77,78], but a prospective survey found no association [79]. Tonsillectomy has been related to Hodgkin's disease [80] but other reports have been negative. Thymectomy in adults does not predispose to cancer [81], but may protect against the increased risk of breast cancer reported with myasthenia gravis [82]. Recipients of renal transplants have an increased risk of cancer, particularly reticulum cell sarcoma of the brain [83]. Whether the cancer risk is due to splenectomy, antimitotic drugs, steroids, anti-lymphocyte serum, or the implantation of foreign tissue itself is unknown.

A few patients with breast cancer develop the Stewart-Treves syndrome following radical mastectomy [84]. In this syndrome lymphangiosarcoma arises in the post-mastectomy lymphedematous arm. Lymphedema in other situations (filariasis, Milroy's disease) is only rarely followed by such tumors.

BENIGN PROLIFERATIONS

Villous papilloma of the colon is frequently (48 percent of biopsies) complicated by cancer, whether the papilloma is sessile or pedunculated [85]. The proportion of tubular adenomas (adenomatous polyps) which develop cancer is much lower (less than 1 percent); however, these lesions are so common that the number of cancers developing in them is still significant. The proportion of colorectal cancers associated with preexisting polyps is unknown, but the importance of polyps is suggested by the reduction of cancer risk in groups undergoing regular colonoscopy with removal of all adenomatous polyps [86].

The proportion of malignant melanomas developing in preexisting benign nevi is also unclear, with estimates between 100 percent [87] and 25 percent [88]. Nevi of the palms and soles are probably at greatest risk.

Women with hydatidiform mole have a risk of developing choriocarcinoma at least 1,000 times higher than women with a normal pregnancy. The incidence of both conditions is much higher in the Far East than in Western nations [89].

Many benign skeletal lesions may undergo malignant change. Chondrosarcoma develops in about 25 percent of patients with multiple enchondromas and in about 3 percent of treated solitary enchondromas. Osteochondroma only rarely (less than 1 percent) is complicated by malignant tumors [90]. In extensive Paget's disease of bone, the risk of osteosarcoma is increased about thirty-fold, and this association accounts for the majority of osteosarcomas seen in middle life. Nevertheless, only 1 percent of patients with Paget's disease develop sarcoma [91].

OTHER CONDITIONS

Myeloproliferative disorders and sideroblastic anemias are probably early phases of acute leukemia rather than separate diseases predisposing to cancer. Nevertheless, diagnosis offers an opportunity to treat leukemia before it is fully expressed [92]. Patients with pernicious anemia have an increased risk of myelocytic leukemia, with estimates of the relative risk varying from a 50 percent to a 350 percent increase [25].

Clinical observations have suggested that heroin addiction may predispose to Hodgkin's disease [93], but the many variables related to addiction should be considered as possible risk factors.

Pharyngeal diverticula are associated with tumors within the pouch itself [94], whereas the tumors with bladder diverticula seem to develop either in the pouch or elsewhere in the bladder [95].

CONCLUSIONS

Patients with symptomatic diseases which predispose to cancer are an important group because such people have already come to their doctor. This fact circumvents the problem of persuading people to come for screening tests. Some of the risks are well known, and, in follow-up of patients with ulcerative colitis and pernicious anemia, anticipation of colon and stomach cancers, respectively, is already part of standard medical practice. In many other situations, calculation of relative risk is hindered by lack of information on the incidence of the underlying disease in the population. Thus, the prevalence of diabetes may change from 1 to 16 percent of the population depending on the diagnostic definitions applied. The true incidence of appendicitis, pancreatitis, prostatic hyperplasia, and cystic mastopathy is all largely guessed at. Case-control studies enable some estimate of risk to be made, but the selection of suitable controls is often difficult. Once an excess risk has been established, careful follow-up of a group of patients should ensue. The purposes of such studies are to test etiologic hypotheses and to determine the efficacy of intervention in preventing cancer. For example, the effect of removing adenomatous polyps of the colon in a defined population on the incidence of colorectal cancer could be measured. Such a study would have both etiologic and preventive significance. Retrospective surveys are usually hampered by the lack of homogeneous definitions of disease, and etiologic hypotheses can seldom be proved by this means, though guidance as to preventive measures may be obtained. Prospective studies on a circumscribed sedentary community should be instituted to define these risks more closely. This type of study requires long-term follow-up, and a prepaid health program would provide a good group to work with. The most fruitful studies are likely to be done in relatively small groups with high-quality information. Large population surveys have already indicated trends and have delineated areas of interest. Study of tightly defined groups followed over periods of time is now required to delineate these risks more precisely.

REFERENCES

1. Nahmias, A.H., and Roizman, B. Infection with herpes simplex viruses 1 and 2. *N. Engl. J. Med. 289:*667–674, 719–725, 781–789, 1973.
2. Nahmias, A.H., Naib, Z., and Jossey, W.E. Genital herpes and cervix cancer—can a causal relation be proven? *In* Biggs, P.M., de The, G., Payne, L.N., eds. *Oncogenesis and Herpes Viruses* I.A.R.C., Lyon, 1973, pp. 403–407.
3. Connelly, R.R., and Cristine, B.W. A cohort study of cancer following infectious mononucleosis. *Cancer Res. 34:*1172–1178, 1974.
4. Miller, R.W., and Beebe, G.W. Infectious mononucleosis and the empirical risk of cancer. *J. Natl. Canc. Inst. 50:*315–321, 1973.

5. Vogel, C.L., Anthony, P.P., Mody, N., et al. Hepatitis associated antigen in Ugandan patients with hepatocellular carcinoma. *Lancet 11:*621–624, 1970.

6. Vogel, C.L., Anthony, P.P., Sadikali, F., et al. Hepatitis associated antigen and antibody in hepatocellular carcinoma. *J. Natl. Cancer Inst. 48:*1583–1588, 1972.

7. Gilbert, J.B. Tumors of testis following mumps orchitis. *J. Urol. 51:*296–300, 1944.

8. Cruikshank, A.H., McConnell, E.M., and Miller, D.G. Malignancy in scars tropical ulcers and sinuses. *J. Clin. Pathol. (Lond.) 16:*573–580, 1963.

9. Shepherd, J.J. Tribal variation in cutaneous tumors of the leg. *E. Afr. Med. J. 44:* 600–602, 1966.

10. Manale, B.L., and Brower, T.D.: The significance of bacterial flora in carcinoma in chronic osteomyelitis. *Surg. Gynecol. Obst. 136:*63–64, 1973.

11. Templeton, A.C., ed. *Tumors in a Tropical Country*. Recent Results in Cancer Research, vol. 41. Springer-Verlag, Heidelberg, 1973.

12. Murray, J.F. Endemic syphilis or yaws. A review of the literature from South Africa. *S. Afr. Med. J. 31:*821–824, 1957.

13. Spencer, H. *Pathology of the Lung*, 2nd ed., Pergamon, London, 1970, p. 826.

14. Kafuko, G.W., and Burkitt, D.P. Burkitt's lymphoma and malaria. *Int. J. Cancer 6:* 1–9, 1970.

15. Serck-Hanssen, A., and Purohit, G.P. Histiocytic medullary reticulosis. *Brit. J. Cancer 32:*506–516, 1968.

16. Hashem, M. The aetiology and pathogenesis of the bilharzial bladder cancer. *J. Egypt. Med. Assoc. 44:*857–966, 1961.

17. Kuntz, R.E., Cheever, A.W., and Myers, B.J.: Proliferative epithelial lesions of the urinary bladder of non-human primates infected with schistosoma hematobium. *J. Natl. Cancer Inst. 68:*223–235, 1972.

18. Edington, G.M. Malignant disease in the Gold Coast. *Brit. J. Cancer 10:*595–605, 1956.

19. Anthony, P.P. Malignant tumors of the kidney, bladder and urethra. *In* Templeton, A.C., ed. *Tumors in a Tropical Country,* Springer-Verlag, Heidelberg, 1973.

20. Dunham, L., Bailar, J.C., and Laqueur, G.L. Histologically diagnosed cancers in 693 Indians of the U.S., 1950-65. *J. Natl. Cancer Inst. 50:*1119–1128, 1973.

21. Andrade, Z., and Abreu, W.N. Follicular lymphoma of the spleen in patients with hepatosplenic *Schistosomiasis Mansoni*. *Am. J. Trop. Med. Hyg. 20:*237–243, 1971.

22. Gibson, R.B. *Parasites, liver disease and liver cancer*. I.A.R.C. Scientific Publications No. 1, Lyon, 1971.

23. Ramat, B., and Many, A. Primary intestinal lymphoma. Clinical manifestations and possible effect of environmental factors. *In* Grundman, E. and Tulinius, H., eds. *Current Problems in the Epidemiology of Cancer and Lymphomas.* Springer-Verlag, Heidelberg, 1972.

24. Correa, P., and O'Conor, G.T. Epidemiological patterns of Hodgkin's disease. *Int. J. Cancer 8:*192–201, 1971..

25. Blackburn, E.K., Callender, S.T., Dacie, J.V., et al. Pernicious anemia and leukemia. *Int. J. Cancer 3:*163–170, 1968.

26. Zamcheck, N., Grable, E., Ley, A.B., et al. Occurrence of gastric cancer among patients with pernicious anemia at the Boston City Hospital. *N. Engl. J. Med. 252:*1103–1110, 1955.

27. Strickland, R.G., and McKay, I.R. A reappraisal of the nature and significance of chronic atrophic gastritis. *Am. J. Dig. Dis. 18:*426–440, 1973.

28. MacDonald, W.C. Clinical and pathologic features of adenocarcinoma of the gastric cardia. *Cancer 29:*724–732, 1972.

29. Munoz, N., and Matko, I. Histological types of gastric cancer and its relationship with intestinal metaplasia. *In* Grundman, E. and Tulinius, H., eds. *Current Problems in the Epidemiology of Cancer and Lymphoma.* Springer-Verlag, Heidelberg, 1972.

30. Nicholls, J.C. Carcinoma of the stomach following partial gastrectomy for benign gastroduodenal lesions. *Br. J. Surg. 61:*244-249, 1974.

31. Hirohata, T. Mortality from gastric cancer and other causes after medical or surgical treatment for gastric ulcer. *J. Natl. Cancer Inst. 41:*895-908, 1968.

32. Saeed, W., Kim, S., and Burch, B.H.: Development of carcinoma in regional enteritis. *Arch. Surg. 108:*376-379, 1974.

33. Darke, S.G., Parks, A.G., Gronogo, T.L., et al. Adenocarcinoma and Crohn's disease. *Br. J. Surg. 60:*169-175, 1973.

34. Weedon, D.D., Shorter, R.G., Ilstrup, D.M., et al. Crohn's disease and cancer. *N. Engl. J. Med. 289:*1099-1103, 1973.

35. Devraede, G.J., Taylor, W.F., Saver, W.G., et al. Cancer risk and life expectancy of children with ulcerative colitis. *N. Engl. J. Med. 285:*17-21, 1971.

36. Ross, A.P., and Broasch, J.W. Ulcerative colitis and carcinoma of the proximal bile ducts. *Gut 14:*94-97, 1973.

37. Pemberton, J. Adult celiac disease, reticulosis and carcinoma. *Am. J. Dig. Dis. 17:*851-853, 1972.

38. Steiner, P.E. Carcinoma of the liver in the United States. *Acta Uni. Int. Contra Cancrum 13:*628-645, 1957.

39. Shaper, A.G. Cirrhosis and primary liver cell carcinoma in Uganda. *J. Trop. Geogr. Med. 22:*161-166, 1970.

40. Becker, B.J.P., and Chatgidakis, C.B. Primary carcinoma of the liver in Johannesburg. *Acta Uni. Int. Contra Cancrum 17:*650-653, 1961.

41. Hines, C., Davis, W.D., and Ferranti, W.A. Hepatoma developing in hemochromatosis in spite of adequate treatment by multiple phlebotomies. *Am. J. Dig. Dis. 16:*349-355, 1971.

42. Spencer, H., and Raeburn, C.: Pulmonary (bronchiolar) adenomatosis. *J. Pathol. Bacteriol. 71:*145-154, 1956.

43. Hagganti, M.T., and Holti, G. Systemic sclerosis with pulmonary fibrosis and oat cell carcinoma. *Acta Derm. Venereol. 53:*369-373, 1973.

44. Brincker, H., and Wilbeck, E. The incidence of malignant tumors in patients with respiratory sarcoidosis. *Br. J. Cancer 29:*247-251, 1974.

45. Cox, M. Malignant lymphoma of the thyroid. *J. Clin. Pathol. 17:*591-601, 1964.

46. Anderson, C.G., and Talal, N. The spectrum of benign to malignant lymphoproliferation in Sjögren's syndrome. *Clin. Exp. Immunol. 10:*199-221, 1972.

47. Wynder, E.L., Mabuchi, K., Maruchi, N., et al. Epidemiology of cancer of the pancreas. *J. Natl. Cancer Inst. 50:*645-668, 1973.

48. Bell, E.T. Carcinoma of the pancreas: 1. Clinical and pathologic study of 609 necropsied cases, 2. The relation of carcinoma of the pancreas to diabetes mellitus. *Am. J. Pathol. 33:*499-523, 1957.

49. Kessler, I.I. Cancer mortality among diabetics. *J. Natl. Cancer Inst. 46:*673-686, 1971.

50. Editorial. The thyroid and breast cancer. *Br. Med. J. I:*472, 1974.

51. Boyce, R., and Beadles, C.F. Enlargement of the hypophysis cerebri in myxoedema; with remarks upon hypertrophy of the hypophysis, associated with changes in the thyroid body. *J. Pathol. Bacteriol. 1:*223, 1892.

52. Davis, H.H., Simons, M., David, J.B. Cystic disease of the breast—relationship to cancer. *Cancer 17:*957-978, 1964.

53. Black, M.M., Barclay, T.H., Cutler, S.J., et al. Association of atypical characteristics of benign breast lesions with subsequent risk of breast cancer. *Cancer 29:*338-343, 1972.

54. Wellings, S.R., and Jensen, H.M. On the origin and progression of ductal cancer in the human breast. *J. Natl. Cancer Inst. 50:*1111-1118, 1973.

55. Armenian, H.K., Lilienfeld, A.M., Diamond, E.L., et al. Relationship between benign prostatic hyperplasia and cancer of the prostate. *Lancet 2:*115-117, 1974.

56. Greenwald, P., Kirmos, V., Tolan, A.K., et al. Cancer of the prostate among men with benign prostatic hyperplasia. *J. Natl. Cancer Inst. 53:*335-340, 1974.

57. Fechner, R.E., and Kaufman, R.H. Endometrial adenocarcinoma in Stein-Leventhal syndrome. *Cancer 34:*444-452, 1974.

58. MacMahon, B., Cole, P., and Brown, J. Etiology of human breast cancer. A review. *J. Natl. Cancer Inst. 50:*21-42, 1973.

59. Feinleib, M. Breast cancer and artificial menopause—a cohort study. *J. Natl. Cancer Inst. 41:*315-329, 1968.

60. Berk, J.E., and Lieber, M.M. Primary carcinoma of the liver in hemochromatosis. *Am. J. Med. Sci. 202:*708-714, 1941.

61. Wynder, E.L., Hultberg, S., Jacobsson, F., et al. Environmental factors in cancer of the upper alimentary tract. *Cancer 10:*470-487, 1957.

62. Chisholm, M. The association between webs, iron and post-cricoid carcinoma. *Postgrad. Med. J. 50:*215-219, 1974.

63. Wahner, H.W., Cuello, C., Correa, P., et al. Thyroid cancer in an endemic goiter area, Cali, Colombia. *Am. J. Med. 40:*58-66, 1966.

64. Newberne, P.M., and Rogers, A.E. Rat colon carcinomas associated with aflatoxin and marginal vitamin A. *J. Natl. Cancer Inst. 50:*439-448, 1973.

65. Davies, J.N.P., Tank, R., Meyer, R., et al. Cancer of the integumentary tissues in Uganda Africans. The basis for prevention. *J. Natl. Cancer Inst. 41:*31-51, 1968.

66. Wilk, M., and Wynder, E.L. Uber die Wirkung polycyclischer, aromatischer Kohlenvasserstoffe auf isoliente mitochondrien de Mausleber. *Z. Natur. 21B:*161-166, 1966.

67. Cook, P. Cancer of the esophagus in Africa. *Br. J. Cancer 25:*853-880, 1971.

68. Schwartz, D., Lellough, J., Flamant, R., et al. Alcohol and cancer. Results of a retrospective investigation. *Rev. Fr. Etiol. Clin. Biol. 7:*590-604, 1962.

69. Hakulinen, T., Lehtimaki, L., Lehtonen, M., et al. Cancer morbidity among two male cohorts with increased alcohol consumption. *J. Natl. Cancer Inst. 52:*1711-1714, 1974.

70. Burch, G.E., and Ansoni, A. Chronic alcoholism and carcinoma of the pancreas. *Arch. Intern. Med. 122:*273-275, 1968.

71. De Waard, F., and Baanders-van Halewijn, E.A. A prospective study in general practice on breast-cancer risk in postmenopausal women. *Int. J. Cancer 14:*153-160, 1974.

72. Hems, G. Epidemiological characteristics of breast cancer in middle and late age. *Br. J. Cancer 24:*226-233, 1970.

73. Wynder, E.L., Escher, G., and Mantel, N. An epidemiological investigation of cancer of the endometrium. *Cancer 19:*489-520, 1966.

74. Maclean, J.T., and Fowler, V.B. Pathology of tumors of the renal pelvis and ureter. *J. Urol. 75:*384-423, 1965.

75. Hart, J., Modan, B., and Shani, M. Cholelithiasis in the etiology of gallbladder neoplasms. *Lancet 1:*1151-1153, 1971.

76. Imre, G., and Kapp, M. Arguments against long-term conservative treatment of esophageal strictures due to corrosive lesions. *Thorax 27:*594-597, 1972.

77. Bierman, H.R. Human appendix and neoplasia. *Cancer 21:*109-118, 1968.

78. McVay, J.R., Jr. The appendix in relation to neoplastic disease. *Cancer 17:*929–937, 1964.

79. Moertel, C.G., Nobrega, F.T., Elveback, L.R., et al. A prospective study of appendectomy and predisposition to cancer. *Surg. Gynecol. Obst. 138:*549–556, 1974.

80. Vianna, N.J., Greenwald, P., and Davies, J.N.P. Tonsillectomy and Hodgkin's disease. The lymphoid tissue barrier. *Lancet 1:*431–432, 1971.

81. Vessey, M.P., and Doll, R. Thymectomy and cancer. A follow-up study. *Br. J. Cancer 26:*53–58, 1972.

82. Papatestas, A.E., Osserman, K.E., and Kark, A.E. The relationship between thymus and oncogenesis. *Br. J. Cancer 25:*635–645, 1971.

83. Penn, I., and Starzl, T.E. Malignant tumors arising de novo in immunosuppressed organ transplant recipients. *Transplantation (Baltimore) 14:*407–417, 1972.

84. Stewart, F.W., Treves, N. Lymphangiosarcoma in post-mastectomy lymphedema. *Cancer 1:*64–81, 1968.

85. Kurzon, M., Ortega, R., and Rwylin, A.M. The significance of papillary features in polyps of the large intestine. *Am. J. Clin. Pathol. 62:*447–454, 1974.

86. Gilbertsen, V.A. Proctosigmoidoscopy and polypectomy in reducing the incidence of rectal cancer. *Cancer* (suppl.) to *34:*936–939, 1974.

87. Allen, A.C., and Spitz, S. Malignant melanoma. *Cancer 6:*1–45, 1953.

88. Becker, S.W. Dermatological investigation of melanin pigmentation in the biology of melanoma. *Ann. N.Y. Acad. Sci. 4:*82–100, 1948.

89. Holland, J.F., and Hreshchyhyn, M.M. *Choriocarcinoma.* U.I.C.C. Monogr. Series 3, Springer-Verlag, Berlin, 1967.

90. Dorfman, H. Malignant transformations of benign bone lesions. *In Proceedings of the Seventh National Cancer Conference*, pp. 901–913, Lippincott, New York, 1973.

91. MacKenzie, A., Court-Brown, W.M., Doll, R., et al. Mortality from primary tumors of bone in England and Wales. *Br. Med. J. 1:*1782–1790, 1961.

92. Fisher, W.B., Armentrout, S.A., Weisman, R., et al. Preleukemia. A myelodysplastic syndrome often terminating in acute leukemia. *Arch. Intern. Med. 132:*226–232, 1973.

93. Dworsky, R.L., and Henderson, B.E. Hodgkin's disease clustering in families and communities. *Cancer Res. 34:*1161–1163, 1974.

94. Turner, M.J. Carcinoma as a complication of pharyngeal pouch. *Br. J. Radiol. 36:* 206–209, 1963.

95. Melicow, M.M. Tumors of the urinary bladder. A clinico-pathological analysis of over 2,500 specimens and biopsies. *J. Urol. 74:*498–521, 1955.

DISCUSSION

Dr. Lipkin emphasized the importance of familial factors in many so-called acquired diseases. Thus, Crohn's disease and ulcerative colitis, both alleged to be "acquired" diseases, sometimes occur in familial aggregation. The role of genetic susceptibility in these diseases should be clarified. However, the concept that "family groupings" reflect "genetic factors" was challenged. Dr. Davies stated that if lightning struck a particular family and killed all the members, one should not ascribe genetic causation in their demise.

Dr. Koss stressed the need for detailed histologic diagnoses, which may enable the detection of important epidemiologic correlations. In response, Dr.

Schneiderman questioned the epidemiologic value of meticulous attention to pathologic documentation and demonstrated the usefulness of "dirty data" in making valuable etiologic hypotheses. He felt that one must be realistic and make some compromises in data collection and classification, so that adequate numbers of cases are available for epidemiologic investigation. This point of view, according to **Dr. Templeton**, is not inconsistent with the need for careful pathologic documentation in developing etiologic hypotheses for many tumors, although such documentation might be more loosely handled in cancer control studies. **Dr. Blattner** cited the need for applying newer laboratory methodology in the pathologic classification of tumors. In particular, immunologic markers for B- and T-lymphocytes provide an opportunity for refined classification of leukemias and lymphomas that might generate important etiologic insights. **Dr. Higginson** also reiterated the value of careful histopathologic correlation; in the case of mesothelioma, precise classification was essential to identify the etiologic factors in certain occupational groups. He advised geographic studies of cancer risk (particularly in areas where complete autopsies are possible) to enable correlations with environmental exposures.

Henry T. Lynch

5

PRECANCEROUS LESIONS

Leopold G. Koss, M.D.

Department of Pathology
Montefiore Hospital and Medical Center
Albert Einstein College of Medicine
Bronx, New York

INTRODUCTION

During the last 25 years, major strides have been made in the definition, recognition, and understanding of patterns of behavior of precancerous lesions. However, current knowledge is largely confined to organs with an epithelium accessible to clinical sampling, and pertains to precursor lesions of many but not all carcinomas. Nevertheless, in our understanding of the natural history of human cancer, the importance of this group of diseases cannot be underestimated. Little is known about precancerous lesions of tissues of mesenchymal derivation, encompassing sarcomas and diseases of blood-forming organs.

MEANS OF DETECTION AND DIAGNOSIS

Most precancerous lesions are not identifiable as such by clinical examination. In general, these lesions either form no visible or palpable abnormalities or, if such abnormalities occur, they cannot be differentiated from benign processes. Therefore, the diagnosis of precancerous lesions is essentially a microscopic one, based on a sample that is either obtained for unrelated reasons or as a result of a deliberate search for precursors of invasive cancer.

Cytologic techniques have proved their value in the search for precancerous lesions of the uterine cervix, endometrium, vagina, bronchus, larynx, buccal cavity, stomach and esophagus, and the urinary bladder. Occasionally, cytologic examination of other organs, such as the cornea and conjunctiva of the eye, skin, large bowel, pancreas, and prostate, has given interesting results in experienced hands [1]. Considerable experience based on knowledge of tissue morphology is required for accurate interpretation of the cytologic sample.

The *biopsy* is an essential tool in the localization of lesions identified by cytology. Furthermore, because of limitations inherent in the cytologic sample, the biopsy may reveal a lesion that is at variance with the cytologic diagnosis. On the other hand, biopsy is not necessarily more accurate than cytology because it reflects the status of a small area. Therefore, contrary to some opinions, a cytologic diagnosis is often more accurate than a histologic diagnosis. The biopsy may also serve as a primary means of detecting precancerous lesions, which is particularly significant in organs not readily amenable to cytologic sampling such as the breast. Most precancerous lesions of the breast are discovered on incidental biopsies with or without mammography.

In investigations of the breast and gastrointestinal tract, *roentgenology* has proved particularly useful. Because of the frequent association of early breast cancer with calcification, mammography may be helpful in selecting patients for surgical exploration [2]. Similarly, differences in gastric and esophageal motility may yield helpful diagnostic hints [3]. In the colon, certain potentially precancerous lesions such as polyps may be uncovered.

There is no evidence at the present level of technology that *thermography* is useful in the detection of precancerous lesions [4].

The *immunologic technique* area of endeavor is very promising, but at this time there is no evidence that precancerous lesions may be identified by immunologic testing of patients.

Definition

Precancerous epithelial lesions are morphologic abnormalities with microscopic characteristics of cancer confined to the epithelium of origin, i.e., showing no evidence of invasive growth. Such lesions are obligate antecedents of invasive carcinoma, i.e., invasive carcinoma always originates from a precancerous lesion. Such lesions, if not treated or otherwise molested, will progress to invasive cancer within a time span and in a proportion of cases that may vary from organ to organ. The rate of invasive cancer following these lesions must exceed, in a statistically significant fashion, the rate expected in a normal population. Alternately, if such lesions are removed or destroyed, cancer will not develop from this particular site or organ. There is no conclusive information as to whether such lesions can regress spontaneously.

Principles of Recognition

Microscopic recognition of cancer depends on certain features that encompass nuclear and mitotic abnormalities and abnormal patterns of growth.

Classification of cancer is based on three essential features:
1) Histologic differentiation, such as squamous or glandular
2) Patterns of growth, i.e., noninfiltrating or infiltrating, exophytic or ulcerated
3) Degree of cytologic abnormality (grading), based on degree and percentage of nuclear abnormalities and the type and location of mitotic abnormalities.

There is no obvious reason why precancerous lesions should not be identified and classified according to the same set of principles. Yet, many pathologists are reluctant to accept for precancerous lesions these simple, common sense criteria, partly because the biologic characteristics of the precancerous lesions are at a considerable variance with invasive carcinoma.

Biologic Characteristics of Precancerous Lesions

In notably the uterine cervix, endometrium, bladder, breast, and skin, several biologic features of precancerous lesions have been recognized [1]. The progression of precancerous lesions to invasive cancer is an unpredictable process that cannot be prognosticated from morphologic appearance [2]. The time lapse between the identification of precancerous lesions and the development of invasive cancer may be extremely variable, from a few months to many years, and it varies from organ to organ. In some organs such as the uterine cervix and the breast, the average duration of the process is estimated at 10 years or more. In other organs, such as the urinary bladder or the stomach, this time lapse appears to be much shorter [3]. Virtually nothing is known about the biologic events that govern the capricious behavior of precancerous lesions.

Despite ignorance in this area, numerous attempts have been made to establish prognostic criteria based on morphology. These criteria often depart from the principles of identification and classification of cancer discussed above and, furthermore, are not reproducible among various, or even the same, observers. This problem applies particularly to the uterine cervix.

PRECANCEROUS LESIONS OF VARIOUS ORGANS

Uterine Cervix

As a consequence of cytologic screenings and numerous clinical studies, precancerous lesions of the uterine cervix are well known today. Cancer of the uterine cervix and its precancerous states occur excessively among women with high levels of sexual exposure, especially when exposure is initiated in adolescence. The role of a transmissible agent such as herpes simplex virus type 2 in the genesis of cancer of the cervix is under active investigation [5,6].

Epidermoid Carcinoma

Natural history. The initial changes usually occur in the form of nuclear enlargement confined to epithelial cells in the squamous epithelium, adjacent to the endocervial epithelium (so-called squamocolumnar junction, or the transformation zone of the colposcopist). From here the lesions may spread onto the squamous epithelium of the portio, the endocervical epithelium, or both. With the passage of time, the severity of the intraepithelial change may increase. In a small percentage of cases, perhaps 5 percent, primary origin in the epithelium of the endocervical canal may be anticipated.

Dysplasia and carcinoma in situ. As discussed, attempts to establish morphologic prognostic criteria of the precancerous lesions unfortunately have been unrealistically based, not on the degree of epithelial changes (i.e., proportion and placement of abnormal cells), but on the appearance of the surface of the altered epithelium. Carcinoma in situ was defined in these attempts as a lesion composed throughout of cancer cells without surface differentiation and with ominous prognosis. "Dysplasia" was vaguely defined [7] as "all other disturbances of differentiation of the squamous epithelial lining of surface and glands." Matters were complicated further by the dysplasias being subdivided into mild, moderate, and severe. The separation of carcinoma in situ from dysplasia implied the existence of two essentially similar processes of carcinogenesis, one benign and one malignant.

In my judgment, the criteria of separation of most forms of dysplasia, particularly the moderate and severe, from carcinoma in situ are unrealistic and misleading. There is only one, not two, neoplastic process in the uterine cervix [8, 9], as reflected in surveys of the experienced pathologists who could not agree among themselves on the classification of any given lesion and could not confirm their own diagnoses on review of the same material. It has been succinctly stated [10] that "one man's dysplasia is another man's carcinoma in situ." The precancerous lesions of the uterine cervix form a spectrum of morphologic abnormalities of capricious behavior and unpredictable prognosis for which the term "intraepithelial neoplasia," as suggested by Richart [11], appears suitable. Grading of intraepithelial neoplasia (e.g., I to III, or IV) would convey the degree of morphologic abnormality without detracting from the essential nature of these lesions.

There is excellent biologic and follow-up evidence to support the unified concept of precancerous lesions of the uterine cervix. Studies of nucleic acid content of cells [12], cytogenetics [13, 14], tissue culture [15], and ultrastructure [16] show great similarities between dysplasia and carcinoma in situ. In carefully conducted follow-up surveys [17-19], no essential differences of behavior could be elicited on the strength of the morphologic assessment.

Clinical significance. The difficulty in assessing fully the prognostic significance of the intraepithelial neoplasia lies in the very process of discovery and diagnosis. The lesion detected cytologically and further localized and identified by biopsy is no longer in its natural state. Even small biopsies have a major impact on the distribution and behavior of intraepithelial lesions [17]. Few follow-up surveys fulfill rigid criteria of clinical surveillance. Our own studies [17] disclosed that, after biopsies, carcinoma in situ disappears in about 40 percent of cases, and so do lesser lesions (mild and moderate dysplasia, grouped as "borderline lesions"). On the other hand, the borderline lesions progressed to carcinoma in situ in about 40 percent of cases. In studies on dysplasia Richart [19], using cytology and colposcopy to the exclusion of biopsies, failed to reveal any significant rate of regression. Progression, however, while predictable for histologic classes of lesions, was unpredictable for any given lesion, although some produced invasive cancer. Stern and Neely [20] demonstrated that patients with dysplasia had a 1,600 times greater chance of developing carcinoma in situ than women with a normal cervix.

The significance of these lesions also was demonstrated by Marshall [21] on a group of 20,000 women in the closed, stable population of a Seattle health plan; eradication of carcinoma in situ led to disappearance of invasive carcinoma of the cervix. So far, demonstration of this sequence in large population groups [22, 23] has been only partly successful for two main reasons: 1) the difficulty of reaching women in low socioeconomic levels who are most affected by cervical cancer, and 2) neglect of lesions known as dysplasia. Despite these failures, the incidence of invasive carcinoma of the cervix has declined in a number of communities [22-24].

Adenocarcinoma

Because adenocarcinoma of the cervix is relatively rare (not more than 5 percent of all cervical cancers), recognition of precancerous states as a public health measure is not as important as for epidermoid carcinoma. Nevertheless, cervical adenocarcinoma in situ is well known [1]; the cancerous changes are confined to the endocervical glands without evidence of invasion of the stroma. Many of these lesions are associated with epidermoid carcinoma in situ.

Clinical significance. Because of the rarity of these lesions and usual treatment by surgery, no follow-up studies are known. Endocervical adenocarcinoma in situ may be associated with invasive carcinoma; therefore, it can be considered as a precursor lesion of invasive cancer.

Vagina

Carcinoma in situ of the squamous type and related lesions of the vagina may be primary [25] or secondary to previously treated carcinoma of the uterine cervix [26]. Methods for detection and histologic identification of these lesions are similar to those used for the uterine cervix. Well-differentiated lesions of squamous epithelium of the type usually observed on the portio of the uterine cervix prevail in the vagina. Because of the low frequency of these lesions, statistical evidence having to do with the progression of vaginal carcinoma in situ has not been obtained to date. However, the behavior of vaginal carcinoma is quite different from that of cancer of the uterine cervix. Even superficially invasive vaginal cancers tend to produce early metastases [1], whereas this is rarely true of similar lesions of the uterine cervix. Therefore, it appears paramount to localize and identify these conditions at the earliest possible state. This is often associated with major clinical difficulties in the localization of these lesions.

There are two aspects of vaginal carcinoma that deserve special mention: 1) vaginal carcinoma originating in adenosis of the vagina, and 2) vaginal and cervical carcinoma in situ occurring after radiotherapy for cancer of the uterine cervix.

Adenosis of the vagina was identified recently in offspring of women who received diethylstilbestrol during pregnancy [27]. This condition may also occur without exposure to drugs [28]. Teenage girls with adenosis are prone to develop vaginal adenocarcinoma similar in histologic appearance to adenocarcinoma of the endocervix. Adenosis may be incidentally discovered by cytologic smears, but more commonly it is identified by biopsy in specialized centers.

Postradiation carcinoma in situ of the vagina and cervix is of the epidermoid type and may occur 1 or more years after apparently successful treatment of cancer of the cervix [29]. This disease has an ominous prognosis because of its association with invasive carcinoma elsewhere in the pelvis or its progression to invasive cancer in a rather short time. The same disease has been identified by others [30] as "postirradiation dysplasia," but the term seems inappropriate for a lesion with such a grave prognosis.

Endometrium

Carcinoma of the endometrium has a very different epidemiologic profile than carcinoma of the cervix. It is essentially a disease associated with a disturbance or arrest of endometrial shedding [1]. The underlying reason may be a disturbance of ovulation, a hormone-producing tumor of the ovary, or other factors that interfere with endometrial cycling. The consequence of focal or generalized arrest of endometrial shedding is endometrial hyperplasia. Whether one can prognosticate the outcome of hyperplasia has provoked much discussion [31, 32]. In my judgment, it is not possible.

One form of endometrial hyperplasia, called "endometrial carcinoma in situ" or "adenomatous hyperplasia," was shown in retrospective and prospective studies to progress to endometrial carcinoma in a substantial percentage of cases [31, 33]. Although other forms of hyperplasia, such as cystic or proliferative hyperplasia, have not had the benefit of similar studies, anecdotal evidence and personal experience suggest that they also can progress to endometrial cancer.

Because endometrial hyperplasia and carcinoma usually produce menstrual abnormalities or bleeding, the discovery of these lesions is generally based on histologic evidence obtained by curettage. However, in at least some cases, the lesions are asymptomatic. In such instances, cytologic techniques may lead to identification of lesions [34, 35].

Breast

Precancerous lesions confined to the ductal system of the breast have been identified for many years [36]. Ductal carcinoma in situ or intraductal carcinoma may be incidentally discovered in frozen sections for benign breast lesions. Paget's disease of the nipple may also be associated with ductal carcinoma in situ [37]. Some controversy pertains to the assessment of intraductal carcinoma; in most lesions, invasion of the parenchyma of the breast occurs early or at least at the time of the discovery. Therefore, many observers believe that intraductal carcinoma should be treated at par with invasive cancer of the breast [38].

Lobular Carcinoma in Situ

Unlike intraductal carcinoma, the entity known as lobular carcinoma in situ was thrust only recently into the foreground of diagnostic problems. Although described briefly in the 1940's by Ewing [39] and by Foote and Stewart [40], it did not become generally known until the 1960's [41]. The lesion is difficult to identify: enlarged terminal acini (lobules) are filled with loosely arranged atypical cells. The process often spreads to adjacent minor ducts. Follow-up studies of lobular carcinoma in situ disclosed that a significant percentage of patients with this lesion develop homolateral breast cancer after 2 to 20 years. More importantly, perhaps, contralateral breast cancer also develops in a significant percentage of these patients [41]. This fact is in keeping with Stewart's statement [42] that "the most frequent precancerous lesion of the breast is a cancer of the opposite breast." It was estimated that the risk of developing homolateral breast cancer for women with lobular carcinoma in situ is approximately 70 percent in 24 years, whereas the chance of developing carcinoma of the opposite breast is about 40 percent [41]. Because of the very long time span before the true nature of the lobular carcinoma in situ can be assessed, the significance of this disease has been questioned [43, 44]. Some observers prefer the term "atypical lobular hyperplasia" to lobular carcinoma in situ and thus avoid the necessity for a mastectomy. The unpredictability of behavior and the very long-term follow-up studies required to assess fully the significance of such lesions must again be stressed. However, lobular carcinoma in situ undoubtedly fulfills the histologic and clinical criteria for a precancerous lesion. Lack of familiarity with this lesion by many practicing pathologists and surgeons is now the principal source of difficulty.

Mammography may be occasionally helpful in the diagnosis of these lesions because of the presence of tiny calcifications [45]. Similar calcifications, however, may also occur in benign breast lesions.

Diagnosis of early breast cancer by X-ray studies of breast biopsies was first promoted at the Memorial Hospital for Cancer [46]. By this method, small inconspicuous cancers can be uncovered that escape the initial observer. However, small cancers of the breast should not be confused with early cancers. Even very small cancers of the breast can produce metastases, as long as they are invasive. On the other hand, there are no known instances of metastatic cancer from lobular carcinoma in situ.

Recent epidemiologic studies have disclosed a familial tendency among women with bilateral carcinoma of the breast. Further, in such families breast cancer may develop early [47]. Often, the early cancer is lobular carcinoma in situ, which occurs on the average in women 10 years younger than those with invasive cancer. Lobular carcinoma of the breast and epidermoid carcinoma in situ of the uterine cervix are remarkably similar in that the outcome of the lesion in individual cases is totally unpredictable and progression to invasive carcinoma usually takes many years.

Lung

Epidermoid Carcinoma

Cigarette smoking is the key epidemiologic factor in bronchogenic epidermoid carcinoma and its keratinizing (squamous) variant. Short of major public health measures that will reduce or alter cigarette consumption, there is no hope for preventing this disease.

The existence of epidermoid carcinoma in situ of the bronchus was amply documented in autopsy material by Auerbach et al. [48]. This postmortem evidence was confirmed by cytologic studies [49-51] of asymptomatic smokers with negative X-ray findings who were examined cytologically, either because of trivial symptoms or as a part of major surveys. By use of bronchoscopic techniques [52], the lesions initially identified by cytology can be localized and treated. Long-term follow-up will be required to determine whether carcinoma of the bronchus can be successfully prevented by the search for such precancerous lesions. The matter is complicated by several factors. First, Auerbach et al. [48] documented that carcinoma in situ of the bronchus is often a multifocal lesion. It may be anticipated, therefore, that even if one such lesion is successfully treated, others may occur during the patient's lifespan. Second, it was shown that carcinoma in situ of the bronchus is also a result of manifold progressive changes within the bronchial epithelium such as squamous metaplasia, atypical squamous metaplasia, and carcinoma in situ [53]. Without long-term prospective studies, we cannot determine today which of these changes are reversible, and thus innocuous in nature, and which are irreversible, and thus capable of progression to invasive cancer. The problem is like that of the uterine cervix in which prognostication of the natural history of any precancerous lesions is fraught with difficulty.

The dilemma is compounded by the fact that carcinoma of the bronchus can produce distant metastases with only minimal infiltration at the site of the primary tumor. Therefore, one is somewhat pessimistic about our ability to successfully prevent lung cancer by treatment of precancerous changes.

Adenocarcinoma

The risk of pulmonary adenocarcinoma does not appear to be significantly influenced by cigarette smoking. Histologic evidence from surgical and post-mortem material strongly suggests that at least some forms of bronchogenic adenocarcinoma are associated with precursor abnormalities in terminal bronchioles and perhaps within the alveoli [54]. Such lesions can be observed occasionally in the form of cytologic abnormalities in sputum [1, 55], but this identification apparently has not led to successful localization or resection of early bronchogenic adenocarcinoma.

Larynx

Carcinoma in situ of the larynx is a well-known lesion that may be discovered through biopsy or cytologic technique [1, 56]. The number of such lesions recorded is too small for a statistical evaluation of the rate and speed of progression to invasive cancer.

Oral Cavity

The early stages of squamous and epidermoid cancer of the oral cavity are not readily recognizable by dentists or other observers who have a chance to discover them in the early stages [57]. Clinical evidence suggests that the non-keratinizing carcinoma in situ forms red velvety patches in the epithelium of the oral cavity. They are often mistaken for inflammation. On the other hand, the heavily keratinizing carcinoma of the oral cavity forms white patches that are usually considered as benign leukoplakia.

While cytologic detection techniques appear rather useless for the assessment of white patches (which should be biopsied for diagnosis), considerable success has been recorded [57, 58] for the cytologic diagnosis of the red velvety patches of nonkeratinizing carcinoma in situ. A cytologic scrape of the lesion may reveal the true nature of the disease and may lead to prompt and effective treatment. This method is equally successful in the follow-up of patients with previously treated carcinoma of the oral cavity [59]. The recurrent cancer may also manifest itself in a rather innocuous fashion and may be promptly discovered by cytology.

Urinary Bladder

Since the beginning of this century, evidence has accumulated that exposure to chemicals is a major factor in the origins of bladder cancer. Aromatic amines are the principal offender, but other compounds may play a role [60].

The notion that carcinoma of the urinary bladder is preceded and accompanied by precancerous changes is relatively recent. While such observations were occasionally made in the early 1950's [61], current knowledge is based on a systematic survey [62] of patients exposed to para-aminodiphenyl. During this survey, certain patients had cytologic abnormalities in their urinary sediment that did not correspond to any visible tumors of the urinary bladder. It was assumed [62], and subsequently documented [63], that such patients had a nonpapillary carcinoma in situ that could not be detected cystoscopically. Subsequently, numerous examples of nonpapillary carcinoma in situ of the urinary bladder were discovered in populations not known to be exposed to carcinogens [1,64-65]. Today, approximately 100 instances of nonpapillary carcinoma in situ are on record [67]. The rate of recurrent cancer and progression to invasive carcinoma of the bladder is approximately 80 percent over a period of 5 years. Thus, nonpapillary carcinoma in situ of the bladder has an ominous prognosis in contrast to the capricious and usually slow progression of carcinoma in situ of the cervix and lobular carcinoma in situ of the breast.

Nonpapillary carcinoma in situ also has been observed simultaneously with papillary lesions of the bladder and, in some instances, after treatment of such lesions [67]. Hence, the thought has evolved that the prognosis of papillary and nonpapillary carcinoma of the urinary bladder depends not only on the grade and stage of the primary tumor, but also on the status of the epithelium of the bladder elsewhere.

Indeed, our studies [68] and those of Schade and Swinney [69] show that patients with epithelial abnormalities outside of the area of the primary tumor have a serious prognosis. Hence, the assessment of risk should include cytologic study of the urinary sediment and multiple biopsies of bladder epithelium even in situations where there is no clinical evidence of widespread disease.

Evidence is accumulating that papillary neoplasia, such as papillomas and papillary carcinomas, do not originate de novo in the normal urothelium [67]. Rather, these lesions appear to be secondary to an increase in the number of epithelial layers (hyperplasia). Hence, a new role has to be attributed to epithelial hyperplasia, especially if accompanied by nuclear abnormalities.

Gastrointestinal Tract

Esophagus

A recent cytologic survey from China [70] documented that dysplasia and carcinoma in situ are precursor lesions of esophageal cancer. In the Western World, a few cases of esophageal carcinoma in situ are on record [1, 71, 72], usually discovered incidentally by biopsies or cytologic techniques. Because of the rarity of these lesions, no comments can be made as to their clinical significance. However, following the Chinese example, a systematic search for carcinoma in situ should be instituted in certain areas of the world, such as parts of South Africa and northern Iran where carcinoma of the esophagus is very common.

Stomach

Great progress has been made in the identification of early gastric cancer, through systematic search for this disease in Japan where carcinoma of the stomach is very prevalent and where conspicuous efforts toward early detection have been made [73]. Cytologic techniques [74, 75], fibrogastroscopy [76], gastric camera, or a combination, have led to the discovery of numerous cases of early gastric cancer. There is some objection to the term "carcinoma in situ" when applied to the stomach, since lymph node metastases may be observed with very superficial carcinomas apparently still confined to the mucosa [73]. Although this is a rare event, the term "intramucosal carcinoma" has been suggested and appears acceptable. The prognosis of patients who were surgically treated for intramucosal carcinoma of the stomach is remarkably good; whereas survival rates for advanced gastric cancer are very low, survival rates for intramucosal carcinoma of the stomach are nearly 100 percent for 10 years.

There is good evidence [73, 74] that gastric carcinoma follows certain abnormalities of gastric epithelium such as atrophic gastritis and intestinal metaplasia. How these changes relate to the dietary habits that have been implicated in gastric cancer is not yet known.

Colon

In some hands, notably those of Raskin et al. [77, 78], colonic cytology has proved remarkably accurate in identifying colon cancer in nearly 100 percent of patients. The techniques used are extremely meticulous, time-consuming, and require the attention of a devoted and skilled staff; therefore, they have not been generally accepted. Simplification of Raskin's methods have been attempted [79, 80]; however, the benefit derived from these new methods is not yet evident. Nevertheless, carcinoma in situ of the colon does exist either as a flat sessile lesion or as a focal abnormality in adenomatous polyps. Whether all polyps should be considered precancerous is debatable [81]. It is, of course, known that in polyposis of the colon, the danger of colonic carcinoma is very high. It is probably safe to state, that when a polypoid lesion of the colon is found, every attempt should be made to examine it histologically.

Skin

Precancerous lesions of the skin such as Bowen's disease, actinic keratosis, arsenical keratosis, or Queyrat's erythroplasia of the glans penis are well known [82]. It is generally accepted that only a small percentage of precancerous skin lesions will progress to invasive cancer. Usually invasive carcinoma is of the basal cell type [82], whereas in a small percentage of cases it is of the squamous cell type [83]. Patients with Bowen's disease are known to produce only a small fraction of invasive cancers when compared with the number of preinvasive lesions. More importantly, Bowen's disease may be associated with systemic cancer in a significant percentage of cases [84].

Extramammary Paget's disease may affect any part of the skin where epidermis and certain types of sweat glands coexist. Thus, Paget's disease has been observed in the vulva, perineum, anus, and conjunctiva [85, 86]. In most instances where documentation was adequate, Paget's disease has been associated with an underlying carcinoma of sweat glands. There are, however, instances where the documentation of an underlying carcinoma may be extremely difficult. In a series of such cases, we observed [85] in situ carcinoma of sweat glands as a probable source of cancer cells growing in the epidermis. In Paget's disease of the vulva, cell attachments apparently develop between Paget's cells and adjacent normal cells, indicating a symbiosis between these two cell types [87].

Other Organs

Pancreas

The pancreas has not been sufficiently investigated to warrant any firm statement about precancerous lesions. Occasionally, carcinoma of the pancreatic ducts has been uncovered by cytologic methods before any clinical evidence of tumor [88]. It is debatable whether this type of investigation of the pancreas lends itself to general use, but in view of the rising incidence of this disease, an attempt may prove worthwhile.

Liver

Very little is known about early stages of hepatic cancer. Should such knowledge become available, therapy of this disease may prove elusive. However, in certain parts of the world, notably China and Africa, liver cancer is extremely common, and further efforts are needed to identify morphologically precancerous states.

Eye and Other Organs

Carcinoma in situ of the conjunctiva has been described cytologically and histologically [89]. Precancerous lesions have been identified in other organs, but they are so rare that any statement about their significance is not warranted.

COMMENT

Morphologically identifiable precancerous lesions of various organs have certain features in common as well as those that are characteristic for each individual organ. Nearly all organs have in common the relative unpredictability of behavior of precancerous lesions. This feature is particularly striking for carcinoma in situ of the uterine cervix and the skin, and for lobular carcinoma in situ of the breast. In these three organs, it has not hitherto been possible to separate the lesions that will progress to invasive carcinoma from lesions that will remain stationary or possibly regress. Perhaps the most important area of our future endeavors should be the analysis of epidemiologic factors that may account for such disparities of behavior.

More predictable is the behavior of carcinomas in situ of the bladder, stomach, and probably bronchus. The time span involved between the identification of the precancerous lesions and progression to invasive cancer also varies from organ to organ. For the cervix, the endometrium, and the breast, 10 or more years appear to be required. For the bladder and the lung, apparently a much shorter time is needed. We do not know why this is so. It may be related to the anatomic setting in which carcinomas in situ occur or to the immunologic setting of the patient. In any event, this matter clearly deserves further investigation.

A deliberate, concentrated national effort toward detection of precancerous lesions may have a beneficial effect on the rate of invasive cancer of organs such as the cervix, endometrium, lung, urinary bladder, and gastrointestinal tract. These studies must comprise a major epidemiologic component.

REFERENCES

1. Koss, L.G. *Diagnostic Cytology and its Histopathologic Bases,* 2nd ed. J.B. Lippincott Co., Philadelphia, 1968.

2. Koehl, R.H., Snyder, R.E., Hutter, R.V.P., et al. The incidence and significance of calcifications within operative breast specimens. *Am. J. Clin. Pathol. 53:*3-14, 1970.

3. McNeer, G., and Peck, G.T. *Neoplasms of the Stomach.* J.B. Lippincott Co., Philadelphia, 1967.

4. Strax, P. New techniques in mass screening for breast cancer. *Cancer 28:*5163-5168, 1971.

5. Kessler, I.I. Perspectives on the epidemiology of cervical cancer with special reference to herpesvirus hypothesis. *Cancer Res. 34:*1091-1110, 1974.

6. Nahamias, J.A., Naib, Z.M., and Josey, W.E. Epidemiological studies relating genital herpetic infection to cervical carcinoma. *Cancer Res. 34:*1111-1117, 1974.

7. International agreement on histological terminology for the lesions of the uterine cervix. *Acta Cytol. 6:*235, 1962.

8. Koss, L.G. Concept of genesis and development of carcinoma of the cervix. *Obstet. Gynecol. Surv. 24:*850–860, 1969.

9. Johnson, L.D., Nickerson, R.J., Easterday, C.L., et al. Epidemiologic evidence for the spectrum of change from dysplasia through carcinoma in situ to invasive cancer. *Cancer 22:*901-914, 1968.

10. Hulme, G.W., and Eisenberg, H.S. Carcinoma in situ of the cervix in Connecticut. *Am. J. Obstet. Gynecol. 102:*415–425, 1968.

11. Richart, R.M. Natural history of cervical intraepithelial neoplasia. *Clin. Obstet. Gynecol. 10:*748-784, 1967.

12. Wagner, D., Sprenger, E., and Blank, M.H. DNA–content of dysplastic cells of the uterine cervix. *Acta Cytol. 16:*517-522, 1972.

13. Granberg, I. Chromosomes in preinvasive, microinvasive, and invasive cervical carcinoma. *Hereditas 68:*165-218, 1971.

14. Spriggs, A.I., Bowey, C.E., and Cowdell, R.H. Chromosomes of precancerous lesions of the uterine cervix. New data and a review. *Cancer 27:*1239-1254, 1971.

15. Wilbanks, G.A. Tissue culture in early cervical neoplasia. *Obstet. Gynecol. Surv. 24:*804-837, 1969.

16. Shingleton, H.M., and Wilbanks, G.D. Fine structure of human cervical intraepithelial neoplasia in vivo and in vitro. *Cancer 33:*981-989, 1974.

17. Koss, L.G., Stewart, F.W., Foote, F.W., et al. Some histological aspects of behavior of epidermoid carcinoma in situ and related lesions of the uterine cervix. A long-term prospective study. *Cancer 16:*1160-1211, 1963.

18. Hall, J.E., and Walton, L. Dysplasia of cervix. A prospective study of 206 cases. *Am. J. Obstet. Gynecol. 100:*662-671, 1968.

19. Richart, R.M., and Barron, B.A. A follow-up study of patients with cervical dysplasia. *Am. J. Obstet. Gynecol. 105:*386-393, 1969.

20. Stern, E., and Neely, P.M. Dysplasia of the uterine cervix–incidence of regression, recurrence and cancer. *Cancer 17:*508-512, 1964.

21. Marshall, E.E. Effect of cytologic screening on the incidence of invasive carcinoma of the cervix in a semi-closed community. *Cancer 18:*153-156, 1965.

22. Boyes, D.A. The British Columbia screening program. *Obstet. Gynecol. Surv. 24:*1005-1011, 1969.

23. Dickinson, L., Mussey, M.E., Soule, E.H., et al. Evaluation of the effectiveness of cytologic screening for cervical cancer. I. Incidence and mortality trends in relation to screening. *Mayo Clin. Proc. 47:*533-544, 1972.

24. Handy, V.H., and Wieben, E. Detection of cancer of the cervix: A public health approach. *Obstet. Gynecol. 25:*348-355, 1965.

25. Moran, J.P., and Robinson, H.J. Primary carcinoma in situ of the vagina. Report of 2 cases. *Obstet Gynecol. 20:*405, 1962.

26. Boyes, D.A., Worth, A.J., and Fidler, H.K. The results of treatment of 4389 cases of pre-clinical cervical squamous carcinoma. *J. Obstet. Gynaecol. Br. Commonw. 77:*769-780, 1970.

27. Herbst, A.L., Robboy, S.L., Scully, R.E., et al. Clear-cell adenocarcinoma of the genital tract in young females. Analysis of 170 registry cases. *Am. J. Obstet. Gynecol. 119:*713-724, 1974.

28. Kurman, R.J., and Scully, R.E. The incidence and histogenesis of vaginal adenosis. An autopsy study. *Hum. Pathol. 5:*265-276, 1974.

29. Koss, L.G., Melamed, M.R., and Daniel, W.W. In situ epidermoid carcinoma of cervix and vagina following radiotherapy for cervix cancer. *Cancer 14:*353, 1961.

30. Wentz, W.B., and Reagan, J.W. Clinical significance of postirradiation dysplasia of the uterine cervix. *Am. J. Obstet. Gynecol. 106:*812–817, 1970.

31. Gusberg, S.B., and Kaplan, A.L. Precursors of corpus cancer. V. Adenomatous hyperplasia as stage 0 carcinoma of endometrium. *Am. J. Obstet. Gynecol. 87:*662–676, 1963.

32. Way, S. Aetiology of carcinoma of body of uterus. Ingleby lecture for 1953. *J. Obstet. Gynaecol. Br. Emp. 61:*46–58, 1954.

33. Hertig, A.T., Sommers, S.C., and Bengloff, H. Genesis of endometrial carcinoma. III. Carcinoma in situ. *Cancer 2:*964–971, 1949.

34. Koss, L.G., and Durfee, G.R. Cytologic diagnosis of endometrial carcinoma. Result of ten years of experience. *Acta Cytol. 6:*519–531, 1962.

35. Reagan, J.W., and Ng, A.B.P. *The Cells of Uterine Adenocarcinoma,* 2nd ed. Williams and Wilkins, Baltimore, 1973.

36. McDivitt, R.W., Stewart, F.W., and Berg, J.W. Tumors of the breast. *In Atlas of Tumor Pathology,* 2nd series, fascicle 2. Armed Forces Institute of Pathology, Washington, D.C., 1968.

37. Ashikari, R., Park, K., Huvos, A.G., et al. Paget's disease of the breast. *Cancer 26:*680–685, 1970.

38. Ashikari, R., Hajdu, S.I., and Robbins, G.F. Intraductal carcinoma of the breast (1960–1969). *Cancer 28:*1182–1187, 1971.

39. Ewing, J. *Neoplastic Diseases. A Treatise on Tumors,* 4th ed. W.B. Saunders, Philadelphia, 1940.

40. Foote, F.W., Jr., and Stewart, F.W. Lobular carcinoma in situ: A rare form of mammary cancer. *Am. J. Pathol. 17:*491–495, 1941.

41. McDivitt, R.W., Hutter, R.V.P., Foote, F.W., Jr., et al. In situ lobular carcinoma— A prospective follow-up study indicating cumulative patient risks. *J.A.M.A. 201:*82–86, 1967.

42. Stewart, F.W. Tumors of the breast. *In Atlas of Tumor Pathology,* Section 9, fascicle 30. Armed Forces Institute of Pathology, Washington, D.C., 1950.

43. Haagensen, C.D. *Diseases of the Breast,* 2nd ed. W.B. Saunders, Philadelphia, 1971; pp. 503–527.

44. Wheeler, J.E., Enterline, H.T., Roseman, J.M., et al. Lobular carcinoma in situ of the breast. Long-term follow-up. *Cancer 34:*554–563, 1974.

45. Hutter, R.V.P., Snyder, R.E., Lucas, J.C., et al. Clinical and pathologic correlation with mammographic findings in lobular carcinoma in situ. *Cancer 23:*826–829, 1969.

46. Snyder, R.E., and Rosen, P. Radiography of breast specimens. *Cancer 28:*1608–1611, 1971.

47. Anderson, D.E. Some characteristics of familial breast cancer. *Cancer 28:*1500–1504, 1971.

48. Auerbach, O., Stout, A.P., Hammond, E.C., et al. Changes in bronchial epithelium in relation to cigarette smoking and in relation to lung cancer. *N. Engl. J. Med. 265:*253–267, 1961.

49. Melamed, M.R., Koss, L.G., and Cliffton, E.E. Roentgenologically occult lung cancer, diagnosed by cytology. Report of 12 cases. *Cancer 16:*1537–1551, 1963.

50. Holman, C.W., and Okinaka, A. Occult carcinoma of the lung. *J. Thorac. Cardiovasc. Surg. 47:*466–471, 1964.

51. Woolner, L.B., David, E., Fontana, R.S., et al. In situ and early invasive broncho-genic carcinoma: Report of 28 cases with postoperative survival data. *J. Thorac. Cardiovasc. Surg. 60:*275–290, 1970.

52. Marsh, B.R., Frost, J.K., Erozan, Y.S., et al. Occult bronchogenic carcinoma. Endoscopic localization and television documentation. *Cancer 30:*1348–1352, 1972.

53. Nasiell, M. The Epithelial Picture in the Bronchial Mucosa in Chronic Inflammatory and Neoplastic Lung Disease and Its Relation to Smoking. A Comparative Histologic and Sputum-Cytologic Study. Tryckeribolaget Ivar Haeggstrom AB, Stockholm, 1968.

54. Meyer, E.C., and Liebow, A.A. Relationship of interstitial pneumonia honeycombing and atypical epithelial proliferation to cancer of the lung. Cancer 18:322-351, 1965.

55. Kern, W.H. Cytology of hyperplastic and neoplastic lesions of terminal bronchioles and alveoli. Acta Cytol. 9:372-379, 1965.

56. Frable, W.J., and Frable, M.A. Cytologic diagnosis of carcinoma of the larynx by direct smear. Acta Cytol. 12:318-324, 1968.

57. Sandler, H.C. Cytological screening for early mouth cancer. Interim report of the Veterans Administration Cooperative Study of Oral Exfoliative Cytology. Cancer 15:1119, 1962.

58. Stahl, S.S., Koss, L.G., Brown, R.C., Jr., et al. Oral cytologic screening in a large metropolitan area. J. Am. Dent. Assoc. 75:1385, 1967.

59. Hutter, R.V.P., and Gerold, F.P. Cytodiagnosis of clinically inapparent oral cancer in patients considered to be high risks. A preliminary report. Am. J. Surg. 112:541-546, 1966.

60. Hueper, W.C. Occupational and Environmental Cancers of the Urinary System. Yale Univ. Press, New Haven, 1969.

61. Crabbe, J.G.S. Cytological methods of control for bladder tumours of occupational origin. In Wallace, D.M., ed. Tumours of the Bladder. Livingstone, Edinburgh, 1959, pp. 56-76.

62. Koss, L.G., Melamed, M.R., Ricci, A., et al. Carcinogenesis in the human urinary bladder. Observations after exposure to para-aminodiphenyl. N. Engl. J. Med. 272:767-770, 1965.

63. Koss, L.G., Melamed, M.R., and Kelly, R.E. Further cytologic and histologic studies of bladder lesions in workers exposed to para-aminodiphenyl: Progress report. J. Natl. Cancer Inst. 43:233-243, 1969.

64. Voutsa, N.G., and Melamed, M.R. Cytology of in situ carcinoma of the human urinary bladder. Cancer 16:1307-1316, 1963.

65. Melamed, M.R., Voutsa, N.G., and Grabstald, H. Natural history and clinical behavior of in situ carcinoma of the human urinary bladder. Cancer 17:1533-1545, 1964.

66. Utz, D.C., Hanash, K.A., and Farrow, G.M. The plight of the patient with carcinoma in situ of the bladder. J. Urol. 103:160-164, 1970.

67. Koss, L.G. Tumors of the urinary bladder. In Atlas of Tumor Pathology, 2nd series, fascicle 11. Armed Forces Institute of Pathology. Washington, D.C. In press.

68. Koss, L.G., Tiamson, E.M., and Robbins, M.A. Mapping cancerous and precancerous bladder changes. A study of the urothelium in ten surgically removed bladders. J.A.M.A. 227:281-286, 1974.

69. Schade, R.O.K., and Swinney, J. Precancerous changes in bladder epithelium. Lancet 2:943-946, 1968.

70. Co-ordinating Group for Research on Esophageal Carcinoma, Chinese Academy of Medical Sciences and Honan Province. Studies on the relationship of dysplasia to carcinoma of the esophagus. In Abstracts of Proceedings of the 4th International Cancer Congress. Vol. 3, 1974, p. 472.

71. Imbriglia, J.E., and Lopusniak, M.S. Cytologic examination of sediment from the esophagus in a case of intra-epidermal carcinoma of the esophagus. Gastroenterology 13: 457-463, 1949.

72. Ushigama, S., Spjut, H.J., and Noon, G.P. Extensive dysplasia and carcinoma in situ of esophageal epithelium. Cancer 20:1023-1029, 1967.

73. Kurokawa, T., Kajitani, T., and Oota, K. Carcinoma of the Stomach in Early Phase. Nakayama-Shoten Co., Tokyo, 1967.

74. Schade, R.O.K. *Gastric Cytology, Principles, Methods and Results.* Edward Arnold, London, 1960.

75. Raskin, H.F., Kirsner, J.B., Palmer, W.L., et al. Gastrointestinal cancer; definitive diagnosis by exfoliative cytology. *Arch. Intern. Med. 101:*731-740, 1958.

76. Kasugai, T. Evaluation of gastric lavage cytology under direct vision by the fiber-gastroscope, employing Hank's solution as a washing solution. *Acta Cytol. 12:*345-351, 1968.

77. Raskin, H.R., Palmer, W.L., and Kirsner, J.B. Exfoliative cytology in diagnosis of cancer of the colon. *Dis. Colon Rectum 2:*46-57, 1959.

78. Raskin, H.F., and Pleticka, S. Exfoliative cytology of the colon. Fifteen years of lost opportunity. *Cancer 28:*127-130, 1971.

79. Cameron, A.B., and Thabet, R.J. Recovery of malignant cells from enema returns in carcinoma of colon. *Surg. Forum 10:*30-33, 1959.

80. Katz, S., Sherlock, P., and Winawer, S.J. Rectocolonic exfoliative cytology. A new approach. *Am. J. Dig. Dis. 17:*1109-1116, 1972.

81. Horn, R.C. Malignant potential of polypoid lesions of the colon and rectum. *Cancer 28:*146-152, 1971.

82. Allen, A.C. *The Skin. A Clinicopathological Treatise,* 2nd ed. Grune & Stratton, New York, 1967.

83. Hugo, N.E., and Conway, H. Bowen's disease, its malignant potential and relationship to systemic cancer. *Plast. Reconstr. Surg. 39:*190-194, 1967.

84. Graham, J.H., and Helwig, E.B. Bowen's disease and its relationship to systemic cancer. *Arch. Dermatol. 83:*738-758, 1961.

85. Koss, L.G., Ladinsky, S., and Brockunier, A. Paget's disease of the vulva. *Obstet. Gynecol. 31:*513-525, 1968.

86. Yates, D.R., and Koss, L.G. Paget's disease of the esophageal epithelium. Report of first case. *Arch. Pathol. 86:*447-452, 1968.

87. Koss. L.G., and Brockunier, A., Jr. Ultrastructural aspects of Paget's disease of the vulva. *Arch. Pathol. 87:*592-600, 1969.

88. Raskin, H.F., Wenger, J., Sklar, M., et al. Diagnosis of cancer of pancreas, biliary tract, and duodenum by combined cytologic and secretory methods. I. Exfoliative cytology and description of rapid method of duodenal intubation. *Gastroenterology 34:* 996-1008, 1958.

89. Dykstra, B.A., and Dykstra, P.C. Cytologic diagnosis of carcinoma in situ (Bowen's disease) of the conjunctiva of the eye. (abstract). *In Proceedings of 15th Annual Meeting of the American Society of Cytology.* Denver, Colo., October, 1967.

DISCUSSION

Dr. Berg commented that contradictory observations sometimes are made following initial reports of a precancerous lesion. He referred to a recent report that the risk of invasive breast cancer was not markedly elevated following diagnosis of an in situ lesion, in contrast to previous studies. The situation would be clarified by prospective studies that provide estimates of cancer risk following precancerous lesions. Dr. Koss replied that diagnostic procedures such as biopsy alter the biology of precancerous lesions, so that investigators often are faced with a choice between: 1) studies on lesions that undergo a change in behavior by diagnosis, or 2) cytologic observations, with the danger that early lesions become invasive during the study.

Dr. A. B. Miller inquired whether host factors interfere with the progression of precancerous lesions, and **Dr. Koss** replied that such lesions behave in a "capricious manner" by mechanisms that are not clearly understood. **Dr. Cole** asked whether the definition of precancerous lesions might be broadened to permit the possibility of regression. **Dr. Koss** knew of no convincing evidence for this process.

Dr. Kersey observed lymphocyte infiltration in some of the slides shown by Dr. Koss and suggested that such cells around a focus of invasion might reflect a host response to tumor antigenicity resulting in control of the development and progression of precancerous lesions.

Dr. Cohen asked whether it ever had been shown that a virus infection produced a tumor via a precancerous lesion. **Dr. Koss** answered that the in vitro studies on viral-induced tumors have not been shown to apply to humans. He knew of no instance in man in which a change from normal tissue to malignant neoplasia did not involve the intermediate stage of a precancerous lesion.

Alan S. Morrison

6

MULTIPLE PRIMARY NEOPLASMS

Bruce S. Schoenberg, M.D., M.P.H.

*Department of Neurology and Department of Medical
Statistics and Epidemiology
Mayo Medical School
Rochester, Minnesota*

Investigations of multiple primary malignancies have been especially reward-
ing in providing information to those concerned with the prevention, diagnosis,
treatment, and etiology of cancer. The earliest studies were isolated case reports
documenting the phenomenon and providing criteria for distinguishing metastatic disease from a new, independent, primary neoplasm. They were followed
by case series, yielding estimates of the frequency of occurrence of multiple
primaries. Unfortunately, the series reflected individual experiences of particular
physicians or medical institutions. Data based on such selected groups did not
always accurately indicate the epidemiologic patterns of multiple primary cancer
in the general population. A number of case-control comparisons were then
carried out, based on the assumption that the cases being examined were representative of all such cases and that the controls were representative of the general population. However, the validity of this assumption was often unknown.
The establishment of tumor registries and good follow-up procedures greatly
aided the identification of sufficient individuals with multiple primary malignancies to make better investigations possible. The most sophisticated studies
in this category were based on data from well-defined population groups.

A population-based tumor registry is ideal for such an analysis, particularly
if it has a large well-defined group under observation for 10 or more years. Such
data can be analyzed to determine whether an individual with a malignancy in
a particular organ or tissue has an increased, decreased, or unchanged risk of
developing a second primary malignancy in the same or another organ or tissue.

If the patient with one cancer had a decreased chance of developing a new malignancy, the presence of the first tumor may have protected the individual; studies of the mechanism of such protection might be useful. If, on the other hand, one cancer places the patient at higher risk for a second primary malignancy, the same oncogenic factors may be operating in the pathogenesis of both neoplasms. Such analyses are useful in identifying the high-risk cancer patient, and these individuals deserve further study for possible etiologic factors.

METHODOLOGY

This paper will concentrate on the findings of three types of published investigations:
1) Case reports or series with supporting evidence (genetic, epidemiologic, etc.) that the observed associations of particular multiple primary neoplasms are real;
2) Ad hoc studies of a group of patients with a particular tumor to determine their multiple primary cancer experience, frequently involving a priori hypotheses as to what associations will be found;
3) Large-scale surveys of the multiple primary cancer experience obtained from an analysis of data reported to a central registry, rarely involving a priori hypotheses as to what associations will be found.

It should be emphasized that a few case reports of two or more neoplasms occurring within the same individual do not constitute proof of a significant biologic association. The two tumors must be shown to occur together more frequently than expected on the basis of chance. The optimal methodology for such an analysis is one that makes it possible to compare the *observed* and *expected* number of second primary malignancies. A person-years approach, as detailed recently [1], is the most convenient method to use. The overall survival experience for patients with a first primary malignancy is converted to person-years of exposure, i.e., person-years of exposure to the risk of developing a new primary cancer. This technique is based on the assumption that five persons observed for 1 year have a similar experience to one person observed for 5 years. Age-, sex-, and site-specific incidence rates are then applied to the appropriate person-years of exposure to obtain the expected number of second primary cancers at any particular site. Such a procedure adjusts for the age and sex distribution and survival experience of patients with a first primary cancer. The incidence rates used in an analysis of this type should be derived from the same population yielding the first primary malignancies. Otherwise, differences between the observed and expected number of second primaries might be attributable to differences in the characteristics (other than age and sex, which are taken into account in the calculations) between: 1) the population yielding the incidence rates and 2) the population to which these rates are applied. A population-based tumor registry fulfills this condition.

Since the probability of developing a second primary cancer is very small, the number of second primary cancers can be expected to follow a Poisson distribution. The statistical significance of the results (ratio of observed-to-expected second primaries) can be tested with a table of significance factors for the ratio of a Poisson variable to its expectation [2].

RESULTS

In examining results, one must constantly consider certain possibilities for bias. For example, metastatic disease may be mistaken for an independent primary malignancy. The problem of misclassification is likely to be greater when two tumors occur in close anatomical or temporal proximity. Therefore, histologic confirmation of the tumors as independent primary neoplasms is important. The group who already developed one cancer may be more closely followed medically than the population without a malignancy, so that subsequent cancers are likely to be discovered more often and earlier in patients who have had a cancer. One must use clinical judgment in evaluating the results by considering the possible effects of treatment and problems in differential diagnosis.

An example of an association caused largely by artifact is the excess of prostatic cancer in males with first primary cancer at a variety of different sites. This relationship reflects: 1) the common diagnosis of occult primary prostatic cancer at autopsy and 2) the fact that autopsies are more common in patients who have died of cancer than in the general population of deaths. Finally, multiple comparisons have been made in the large-scale surveys of multiple primary malignancies, and some statistically significant results would be expected on the basis of chance. It becomes imperative, therefore, to distinguish biologic from statistical significance. Before accepting a statistically significant association as real, one must search for supporting evidence from other sources. A common etiologic mechanism more likely is involved for site-group combinations exhibiting a two-way association (cancer at site 2 occurs more frequently than expected in patients with cancer at site 1, *and* vice versa) than a one-way association.

To determine whether the cancer patient is at increased risk for a second primary malignancy, one can analyze the experience of a population-based central registry. In Connecticut [3], results for nonsimultaneously diagnosed tumors indicate that individuals with one malignant neoplasm have 1.29 times the risk of developing a new independent primary tumor when compared to individuals who never had cancer ($P<0.01$). However, the increased risk of multiple primary tumors is highly selective on a site-specific basis. Table 1 presents Connecticut registry data indicating the risk of a subsequent primary malig-

TABLE 1

Risk of nonsimultaneously diagnosed second primary malignancy by
site in patients with first primary malignancy

Site of second primary malignancy	Observed	Expected	$\dfrac{\text{Observed}}{\text{Expected}}$
Lip	43	30.46	1.41[a]
Tongue	71	28.08	2.53[b]
Salivary gland	16	11.02	1.45
Mouth	79	37.64	2.10[b]
Pharynx	65	36.02	1.80[b]
Esophagus	75	62.62	1.20
Stomach	227	305.98	0.74[b]
Small intestine	23	13.47	1.71[b]
Colon	655	496.44	1.32[b]
Rectum	304	256.46	1.19[b]
Liver, gallbladder and biliary passages	85	98.79	0.86
Pancreas	116	130.56	0.89
Nose and sinuses	11	7.38	1.49
Larynx	51	43.98	1.16
Lung and bronchus	331	278.00	1.19[b]
Other respiratory organs	9	5.04	1.78
Breast	944	492.64	1.92[b]
Cervix uteri	112	127.85	0.88
Corpus uteri	157	104.99	1.50[b]
Uterus, unspecified	49	56.66	0.86
Ovary	172	97.19	1.77[b]
Other female genital organs	39	20.82	1.87[b]
Prostate	459	342.80	1.34[b]
Testis	12	3.59	3.34[b]
Other male genital organs	5	6.55	0.76
Kidney and ureter	119	69.10	1.72[b]
Bladder	239	189.25	1.26[b]
Melanoma of skin	45	26.01	1.73[b]
Eye	15	7.15	2.10[a]
Brain and nervous system	21	33.90	0.62[a]
Thyroid	30	20.32	1.48
Bone	11	10.06	1.09
Soft tissue	48	24.08	1.99[b]
Lymphoma and myeloma	98	99.95	0.98
Leukemia	118	100.85	1.17
Other sites	168	211.34	0.79[b]
Total	5,022	3,887.05	1.29[b]

[a] $0.01 < P < 0.05$.
[b] $P < 0.01$.

nancy by anatomical site of the second primary in patients with a first primary cancer. For example, the cancer patient is at increased risk for developing subsequent malignant neoplasms of the lip and tongue, but not at increased risk for lymphoma, myeloma, and leukemia. Just as the risk of second primaries varies with the anatomical site of the second primary, the risk is also highly dependent upon the anatomical location of the first primary cancer. As shown [3], individuals with a first cancer of the lip are at high risk for cancer of the tongue, but brain tumor patients are not. Instead of presenting a detailed analysis of all the studies of multiple primaries, certain tumor complexes were grouped according to possible etiologic explanations (Table 2).

The first category in Table 2 includes site-group combinations linked by possible common environmental or genetic factors. A number of ad hoc studies and systematic reviews of tumor registry experience demonstrate that patients with colon cancer are at high risk for developing new, independent, colon malignancies [3-5], and that women with breast cancer are prone to cancer of the opposite breast [3, 6]. This excess risk within the same organ or in paired organs might be explained by exposure of similar tissue to the same carcinogenic factors. The exact nature of the factors involved remains unknown, although hormonal, dietary, and genetic profiles of these patients are being evaluated.

Patients with cancer of the upper respiratory and gastrointestinal tracts tend to develop a second neoplasm within this same anatomical location [3, 7]. Cigarette smoking, responsible for single tumors at these sites, also enhances the risk of multiple primary cancers of the mouth, pharynx, larynx, esophagus, and lung [8-12]. There is disagreement, however, as to whether cessation of smoking after the first primary cancer lowers the risk of developing a second independent malignancy. Since lung cancer and bladder cancer are strongly correlated with cigarette consumption [13, 14], one might expect to find a relationship between these tumors. In the Connecticut tabulations [3], only a one-way association was found—an excess of second primary lung cancer among bladder cancer patients. The most likely explanation for the lack of a two-way association is that patients with lung cancer do not live long enough for bladder cancer to develop.

In a cohort of individuals with scrotal carcinoma attributed to industrial exposure to mineral oil, three patients subsequently developed primary lung cancer [15]. A follow-up survey [16] of the survival experience of all scrotal-cancer patients reported to a central tumor registry in the same geographic area revealed an excess of second primaries of the upper digestive and respiratory system. Occupational exposure to mineral oil mist was suggested as the etiologic factor responsible for this association.

A group at high risk for one cancer may also be prone to other cancers because of common demographic factors (which may, of course, reflect common biological factors). Investigators using registry data and employing the person-

TABLE 2

Examples of site-group pairs with excess of observed/expected second primary malignancies

Explanation of results | Complexes of multiple primary neoplasms

I Common etiologic factors

A. Same or paired organs

Multicentric colorectal carcinoma
Bilateral breast carcinoma

B. Chemical carcinogens

1. Tobacco

Carcinomas of upper respiratory and gastrointestinal tracts
Carcinomas of lung and bladder

2. Mineral oil

Carcinomas of scrotum and lung

C. Endocrine and nutritional

Carcinomas of breast, uterine corpus, ovary, and colon
Meningioma and carcinoma of breast(?)

D. Genetic

Carcinomas of colon and uterine corpus
Retinoblastoma and lower extremity osteosarcoma
Multiple endocrine adenomatosis: tumors of anterior pituitary, parathyroid, pancreatic islet cells, and, less frequently, neoplasms of the
thyroid, adrenal cortex, and carcinoid tumors of the intestine and
bronchus
von Hippel-Lindau disease: hemangiomas of the retina and cerebellum
with an excessive frequency of hypernephroma, pheochromocytoma,
and ependymoma

108

TABLE 2 (Continued)

Explanation of results

    D.   Genetic (continued)   Complexes of multiple primary neoplasms

                                        von Recklinghausen's disease: multiple neurofibromas, glioma, meningioma, acoustic neuroma, and pheochromocytoma

                                        Pheochromocytoma, medullary thyroid carcinoma, multiple neuromas, and parathyroid tumors

                                        Turcot's syndrome: polyposis of colon and brain tumors

                                        Gardner's syndrome: polyposis of colon with osteomas, fibromas, lipomas, and epidermal cysts

II.   Treatment

    A.   Radiation   Rectal cancer following cancer of the uterine corpus or cervix

                                          Osteosarcoma, soft-tissue sarcoma, or skin cancer of the orbit following retinoblastoma

    B.   Chemotherapy   Other neoplasms following Hodgkin's disease

                                          Acute myeloblastic or acute myelomonoblastic leukemia following multiple myeloma

    C.   Surgery   Lymphangiosarcoma following breast cancer

III. Immune defects   Thymoma and other primary neoplasms

                                          Chronic lymphatic leukemia and skin cancer

TABLE 2 (Continued)

Explanation of results | Complexes of multiple primary neoplasms

IV. Unknown etiologic significance

A. Confirmed by other studies | Breast and salivary gland cancers

B. Unconfirmed by other studies | Prostate or testis cancers with leukemia

110

years approach adjust for age and sex in computing the number of expected second primary cancers. Therefore, these characteristics cannot be used to explain the reported associations.

Two registry studies [3, 17] document an association between cancers of the breast, uterine corpus, ovary, and colon in women. Numerous studies [18-22] show that patients with breast cancer are more frequently unmarried, or if married, have lower pregnancy rates than comparable controls. Similarly, endometrial cancer patients have a high frequency of infertility [23-26]. A study of the role of marital status in cancer mortality [27] revealed that nuns have a higher risk of malignant neoplasms affecting the large intestine, breast, uterine corpus, and ovary than the general female population. Finally, a study of female patients with colon cancer [28] revealed a higher proportion of infertility among these patients than among comparable controls. Here we have a single factor, infertility or reduced fertility, that may be a function of some other factor(s), but is associated with an increased risk of cancer of the female breast, colon, ovary, and uterine corpus.

In a paper correlating international cancer death rates, Wynder et al. [29] compared mortality rates for cancer of the breast and colon in women for 21 countries and found a positive correlation. They hypothesized that dietary habits have a direct effect on increasing the risk of colon cancer in women and an indirect effect, mediated through hormonal mechanisms, on increasing the risk of breast cancer.

An association between breast cancer and meningioma in women was discovered from the Connecticut Tumor Registry data [30]. Although yet to be substantiated by other investigations, this result raises interesting etiologic possibilities when considered in conjunction with other epidemiologic features of meningiomas. First, meningiomas are the only common intracranial neoplasm with a higher incidence in females [31]; second, the abrupt appearance or enlargement of this tumor during pregnancy has been reported [32]. Thus, the association between breast cancer and meningioma may be related to hormonal factors.

Genetic investigations of cancer and studies of multiple primary malignancies complement one another. The same constellation of tumors occurring among members of the same family can also be found in a single individual. As Anderson noted [33], hereditary cancers are often found 1) at several locations within one organ, 2) bilaterally in paired organs, or 3) at multiple sites within a specific tissue type, wherever this tissue exists in the body.

The study by Lynch et al. [34] of six cancer-prone families revealed a frequency of multiple primary neoplasms much above the figures reported from large series of cancer patients. These families were distinguished primarily by the frequent occurrence of endometrial and colon carcinoma. Other investigators [35, 36] reported similar families that point to genetic determinants, although environmental factors cannot be excluded with certainty.

A nationwide investigation [37] of 1,623 children hospitalized with retino-blastoma revealed 30 with a second primary cancer. In 11 such cases, the second tumor could not be attributed to radiotherapy for the retinoblastoma. Of the 11 cases, 3 of the second primaries were osteosarcomas and 3 were brain tumors. A second study [38] dealing with 1,130 retinoblastoma patients reported seven additional bone tumors in areas far removed from the radiation field. The excess of second primary tumors, mainly osteosarcomas, has been limited to patients with bilateral disease. Since a familial pattern is usually apparent in cases of bilateral retinoblastoma (and only in a small percentage of cases with unilateral tumor), a genetic mechanism is probably involved in the development of both the retinoblastoma and osteosarcoma.

Mendelian inheritance has been described in several syndromes involving specific histologic types of multiple primary neoplasms. Patients with multiple endocrine adenomatosis have neoplasms often arising from the anterior pituitary, parathyroid, and pancreatic islet cells. Less frequently, they may develop carci-noids of the intestine and bronchus, and tumors of the thyroid and adrenal cortex [39]. Patients with von Hippel-Lindau disease have hemangiomas of the retina and cerebellum and are at increased risk for developing hypernephroma, pheochromocytoma, and ependymoma [40]. Von Recklinghausen's disease (mul-tiple neurofibromatosis) carries an increased risk of other neurogenic tumors such as glioma, meningioma, acoustic neuroma, and pheochromocytoma [41]. Pheochromocytoma and medullary thyroid carcinoma (Sipple syndrome) occur together in the same individual or in different members of the same family and are sometimes associated with mucosal neuromas and parathyroid tumors [42]. The familial pattern seen in these syndromes is consistent with autosomal domi-nant inheritance.

Familial polyposis of the colon may be associated with brain tumors in the Turcot syndrome [43, 44] or with osteomas, fibromas, lipomas, and epidermal cysts in the constellation of Gardner's syndrome [45]. Some doubt the exis-tence of Turcot's syndrome as a distinct clinical entity since the brain tumors have been of diverse histologic types [43].

Only rarely are such familial syndromes detected by large-scale site-specific analysis of tumor registry data. The association between tumors of specific histologic types may be diluted by the large number of other tumors included in the same site classification. However, once a particular syndrome involving multiple primary neoplasms has been discovered, tumor registry data are very useful in identifying other examples of the syndrome.

One factor that may predispose to cancer is treatment, i.e., treatment for a first cancer may induce a second cancer. Tabulations from a Connecticut survey [1] indicate that patients with a first cancer of the uterine cervix or corpus are at increased risk for developing rectal carcinoma. The carcinogenic potential of radiation, often used in treating genital cancer, should be considered

[46, 47], particularly since radiation for cancer of the uterine corpus or cervix may induce cancer in a nearby structure such as the rectum [48-51]. To explore this hypothesis more fully, the excess risk of rectal cancer after a uterine malignancy was analyzed [3] by time interval between the first and second cancers. The excess risk of rectal cancer was limited to the period 5 or more years following uterine cancer, which is consistent with possible radiation induction of the rectal carcinoma. The observed and expected numbers of second primary rectal cancers were calculated separately for those uterine-cancer patients who were treated with radiation, and for those who were treated by other means. The excess risk was limited to the group that had received radiation. Another example of radiation-induced cancer is the excess occurrence of osteosarcomas, soft-tissue tumors, and skin cancers within the radiation field of children treated for retinoblastoma [37].

A study [52] of subsequent primary malignancies in 425 patients treated for Hodgkin's disease revealed a relative risk for second primaries of 3.8 in those given intensive radiotherapy without intensive chemotherapy. Those treated with chemotherapy alone had a relative risk of 4.3; because of the small number of cases, this difference was not statistically significant. In patients receiving intensive radiotherapy and intensive chemotherapy the relative risk increased to 29, suggesting that chemotherapeutic agents and radiation may have multiplicative effects in oncogenesis. The carcinogenic potential of chemotherapeutic agents has further support from a series of 26 patients with multiple myeloma treated with alkylating agents who subsequently developed acute leukemia, primarily of the myelocytic or myelomonocytic types [53]. No increase in leukemia among myeloma patients was noted before these antineoplastic agents came into general use. The drugs may produce this excess risk by any one of three possible means: 1) a direct carcinogenic effect, 2) suppression of the immune system, or 3) an increase in survival, thereby providing a prolonged time interval for subsequent primary neoplasms to develop as a result of any oncogenic mechanism.

An analysis of the Connecticut multiple primary malignancy experience [3] indicates an excess of soft-tissue tumors following breast cancer. These neoplasms were primarily lymphangiosarcomas of the upper extremities, a known sequela of radical mastectomy with obstructive lymphedema. Thus, various modalities employed in treating cancer may in themselves increase the patient's risk of developing a new primary neoplasm.

Kidney transplant patients receiving immunosuppressive therapy have an elevated risk of cancer, particularly lymphoreticular neoplasms and skin cancer [54]. Moreover, patients with immunodeficiency syndromes have a high frequency of leukemia and lymphoreticular tumors [55]. The question arises as to whether these patients have an intrinsic abnormality of the reticuloendothelial system that leads to malignant transformation, or whether the high occurrence of malignancies is the result of immunosuppression. Such observations have prompted much interest in the occurrence of second primary cancers in patients with a first primary malignancy of organs involved in the immune response.

Souadjian et al. [56] discovered that 21 percent of 146 thymoma patients followed for 20 years developed a nonthymic malignancy. This exceeded the risk of second primary neoplasms found among a group of patients with parathyroid tumors serving as controls. Berg [57] reported an excess of skin cancer developing in patients with lymphoma and leukemia, particularly chronic lymphatic leukemia or chronic myelogenous leukemia. Using tabulations from the Charity Hospital Tumor Registry, Newell et al. [58] also found an excess of skin cancer among white patients with Hodgkin's disease or leukemia, but felt these observations might be due to artifacts of reporting. Moriarty [59] reported that patients with chronic lymphatic leukemia are prone to skin cancer, and suggested that the excess of skin cancer was the result of immunologic incompetence.

Multiple tumors in organs apparently unrelated either functionally or anatomically are not readily explained, but may be valuable in providing clues to etiology. Such associations may allow us to relate a tumor whose epidemiologic pattern is unknown to one whose epidemiologic pattern has been well delineated. The relationship between cancer of the breast and salivary gland was discovered by Berg et al. [60] and was substantiated by data from the Connecticut Tumor Registry [3]. However, the etiology of this relationship remains obscure. Finally, data from the Connecticut Tumor Registry [3] reveal an association of unknown etiologic significance between leukemia and cancer of both the prostate and testis. This relationship was described in case reports [61, 62], but has yet to be documented in other case-control comparisons.

IMPLICATIONS FOR CANCER CONTROL AND ETIOLOGY

Studies of multiple primary malignancies derived from the experience of a population-based tumor registry are of immediate value in cancer control programs. Findings of such studies highlight particular organs or tissues most likely to develop a second primary cancer, and are useful to the clinician concerned with detecting the second malignancy at the earliest possible stage. They also help clarify the carcinogenic potential of various treatment modalities currently employed in the care of the cancer patient. When applied to questions of etiology, such studies provide corroboration for other epidemiologic investigations into the pathogenesis and causes of cancer. They also serve to complement the findings of genetic investigations. Discovering hitherto unsuspected relationships between tumors may permit one to apply what is currently known about one tumor to understand the etiology of an associated neoplasm. Finally, studies of multiple primary cancers should assist in the identification of particular segments of the population for further study to elucidate the factors and mechanisms involved in oncogenesis.

SUGGESTIONS FOR THE FUTURE

The findings of studies of multiple primary neoplasms do not provide definitive answers, but rather are useful in formulating and testing hypotheses. One must be cautious to distinguish: 1) real from artifactual relationships and 2) biological from statistical significance. Other studies are needed to corroborate and evaluate the findings concerning multiple primaries. Detailed reviews of case histories and pathological specimens should be undertaken to test the relationships suggested. As we are able to follow larger population groups of cancer patients over longer periods, it will be possible to define the risk of subsequent primary cancer with more precision, not only in terms of sex, tumor site, and time interval between tumors as currently done [3], but also in terms of the histologic type of the associated neoplasms. Thus, the association between intracranial tumors and breast cancer was clarified by narrowing the broad group of intracranial neoplasms to meningiomas. Such an analysis requires nearly complete microscopic confirmation of both the first and subsequent primary tumor.

Finally, just as this present volume is devoted to defining the *high-risk* cancer patient, it would probably be quite useful to examine the characteristics of the *low-risk* cancer patient. Analysis of existing tabulations [3] of patients at low risk for multiple primary malignancy may be fruitful in discovering the mechanisms involved in the reduction of risk. Such findings would be most applicable to efforts aimed at the primary prevention of malignant neoplasms.

REFERENCES

1. Schoenberg, B.S., and Christine, B.W. The association of neoplasms of the colon and rectum with primary malignancies of other sites. *Am. J. Proctol. 25:*41–60, 1974.

2. Bailar, J.C., III, and Ederer, F. Significance factors for the ratio of a Poisson variable to its expectation. *Biometrics 20:*639–643, 1964.

3. Schoenberg, B.S. *Multiple Primary Malignancies: The Connecticut Experience.* Springer-Verlag, New York. In press.

4. Dencker, H., Liedberg, G., and Tibblin, S. Multiple malignant tumours of the colon and rectum. *Acta Chir. Scand. 135:*260–262, 1969.

5. Devitt, J.E., Roth-Moyo, L.A., and Brown, F.N. The significance of multiple adenocarcinomas of the colon and rectum. *Ann. Surg. 169:*364–367, 1969.

6. Robbins, G.F., and Berg, J.W. Bilateral primary breast cancers: A prospective clinicopathological study. *Cancer 17:*1501–1527, 1964.

7. Berg, J.W., Schottenfeld, D., and Ritter, F. Incidence of multiple primary cancers. III. Cancers of the respiratory and upper digestive system as multiple primary cancers. *J. Natl. Cancer Inst. 44:*263–274, 1970.

8. Higginson, J., and Muir, C.S. Epidemiology. *In* Holland, J.F., and Frei, E., III, eds. *Cancer Medicine.* Lea & Febiger, Philadelphia, 1973, pp. 258-275.

9. Castigliano, S.G. Influence of continued smoking on the incidence of second primary cancers involving mouth, pharynx, and larynx. *J. Am. Dent. Assoc. 77:*580-585, 1968.

10. Wynder, E.L., Dodo, H., Bloch, D., et al. Epidemiologic investigation of multiple primary cancer of the upper alimentary and respiratory tracts. I. A retrospective study. *Cancer 24:*730-739, 1969.

11. Moore, C. Cigarette smoking and cancer of the mouth, pharynx, and larynx. *J.A.M.A. 218:*553-558, 1971.

12. Schottenfeld, D., Gantt, R.C., and Wynder, E.L. The role of alcohol and tobacco in multiple primary cancers of the upper digestive system, larynx, and lung: A prospective study. *Prev. Med. 3:*277-293, 1974.

13. Lilienfeld, A.M., Levin, M.L., and Moore, G.E. The association of smoking with cancer of the urinary bladder in humans. *Arch. Int. Med. 98:*129-135, 1956.

14. Doll, R., and Hill, A.B. Mortality in relation to smoking: Ten years' observations of British doctors. *Br. Med. J. 1:*1399-1410, 1964.

15. Editorial. Hazard of mineral-oil mist? *Lancet 2:*967-968, 1960.

16. Holmes, J.G., Kipling, M.D., and Waterhouse, J.A.H. Subsequent malignancies in men with scrotal epithelioma. *Lancet 2:*214-215, 1970.

17. Schottenfeld, D., Berg, J.W., and Vitsky, B. Incidence of multiple primary cancers. II. Index cancers arising in the stomach and lower digestive system. *J. Natl. Cancer Inst. 43:*77-86, 1969.

18. Heiberg, B., and Heiberg, P. Some investigations into the occurrence of carcinoma of the breast with special reference to the ovarian function. *Acta Chir. Scand. 83:*479-496, 1940.

19. Harnett, W.L. A statistical report on 2529 cases of cancer of the breast. *Br. J. Cancer 2:*212-239, 1948.

20. Gilliam, A.G. Fertility and cancer of the breast and of the uterine cervix: Comparisons between rates of pregnancy in women with cancer at these and other sites. *J. Natl. Cancer Inst. 12:*287-304, 1951

21. Wynder, E.L., Bross, I.J., and Hirayama, T. A study of the epidemiology of cancer of the breast. *Cancer 13:*559-601, 1960.

22. Lilienfeld, A.M. The epidemiology of breast cancer. *Cancer Res. 23:*1503-1513, 1963.

23. Sommers, S.C., Hertig, A.T., and Bengloff, H. Genesis of endometrial carcinoma. II. Cases 19 to 35 years old. *Cancer 2:*957-963, 1949.

24. Speert, H. Carcinoma of the endometrium in young women. *Surg. Gynecol. Obst. 88:*332-336, 1949.

25. Dockerty, M.B., Lovelady, S.B., and Foust, G.T., Jr. Carcinoma of the corpus uteri in young women. *Am. J. Obstet. Gynecol. 61:*966-981, 1955.

26. Corscaden, J.A. *Gynecologic Cancer,* 3rd ed. Williams & Wilkins Co., Baltimore, 1962, p. 333.

27. Fraumeni, J.F., Jr., Lloyd, J.W., Smith, E.M., et al. Cancer mortality among nuns: Role of marital status in etiology of neoplastic disease in women. *J. Natl. Cancer Inst. 42:*455-468, 1969.

28. Acheson, R.M., Chapple, M., and Eisenberg, H. Infertility as a risk factor for carcinoma of the colon in women. (Submitted for publication).

29. Wynder, E.L., Hyams, L., and Shigematsu, T. Correlations of international cancer rates; an epidemiological exercise. *Cancer 20:*113-126, 1967.

30. Schoenberg, B.S. The unique association between meningiomas and breast cancer (abstract). *Neurology 24:*356, 1974.

31. Schoenberg, B.S., and Christine, B.W. Neoplasms of the brain and cranial meninges: A study of incidence, epidemiological trends, and survival (abstract). *Neurology 20:*399, 1970.

32. Michelsen, J., and New, P.F.I. Brain tumour and pregnancy. *J. Neurol. Neurosur. Psychiatry 32:*305-307, 1969.

33. Anderson, D.E. Familial susceptibility. This volume, 1975.

34. Lynch, H.T., Krush, A.J., and Larsen, A.L. Heredity and multiple primary malignant neoplasms: Six cancer families. *Am. J. Med. Sci. 254:*322-329, 1967.

35. Savage, D. A family history of uterine and gastrointestinal cancer. *Br. Med. J. 2:*341-343, 1956.

36. Hauser, I.J., and Weller, C.V. A further report on the cancer family of Warthin. *Am. J. Cancer 27:*434-449, 1936.

37. Jensen, R.D., and Miller, R.W. Retinoblastoma: Epidemiologic characteristics. *N. Engl. J. Med. 285:*307-311, 1971.

38. Kitchin, F.D., and Ellsworth, R.M. Pleiotropic effects of the gene for retinoblastoma. *J. Med. Genet. 11:*244-246, 1974.

39. Johnson, G.J., Summerskill, W.H.J., Anderson, V.E., et al. Clinical and genetic investigation of a large kindred with multiple endocrine adenomatosis. *N. Engl. J. Med. 277:*1379-1385, 1967.

40. Fraumeni, J.F., Jr. Genetic factors. *In* Holland, J.F., and Frei, E., III, eds. *Cancer Medicine.* Lea & Febiger, Philadelphia, 1973, pp. 7-15.

41. Rubinstein, L.J. Tumors of the central nervous system. *In Atlas of Tumor Pathology,* 2nd series, fascicle 6. Armed Forces Institute of Pathology, Washington, D.C., 1972, pp. 302-303.

42. Schimke, R.N., Hartmann, W.H., Prout, T.E., et al. Syndrome of bilateral pheochromocytoma, medullary thyroid carcinoma, and multiple neuromas. *N. Engl. J. Med. 279:*1-7, 1968.

43. Turcot, J., Despres, J.P., and St. Pierre, F. Malignant tumors of the central nervous system associated with familial polyposis of the colon: Report of two cases. *Dis. Colon Rectum 2:*465-468, 1959.

44. Baughman, F.A., Jr., List, C.F., Williams, J.R., et al. The glioma-polyposis syndrome. *N. Engl. J. Med. 281:*1345-1346, 1969.

45. Gardner, E.J., and Richards, R.C. Multiple cutaneous and subcutaneous lesions occurring simultaneously with hereditary polyposis and osteomatosis. *Am. J. Hum. Genet. 5:*139-147, 1953.

46. Novak, E.R., and Woodruff, J.D. Postirradiation malignancies of the pelvic organs. *Am. J. Obstet. Gynecol. 77:*667-675, 1959.

47. Willson, J.R., Beecham, C.T., and Carrington, E.R. *Obstetrics and Gynecology,* 2nd ed. C.V. Mosby Co., St. Louis, 1963, pp. 631-633.

48. Slaughter, D.P., and Southwick, H.W. Mucosal carcinoma as a result of irradiation. *Arch. Surg. 74:*420-429, 1957.

49. Smith, J.C. Carcinoma of the rectum following irradiation of carcinoma of the cervix. *Proc. R. Soc. Med. 55:*701-702, 1962.

50. MacMahon, C.E., and Rowe, J.W. Rectal reaction following radiation therapy of cervical carcinoma: Particular reference to subsequent occurrence of rectal carcinoma. *Ann. Surg. 173:*264-269, 1971.

51. Qizilbash, A.H. Radiation-induced carcinoma of the rectum: A late complication of pelvic irradiation. *Arch. Pathol. 98:*118-121, 1974.

52. Arseneau, J.C., Sponzo, R.W., Levin, D.L., et al. Nonlymphomatous malignant tumors complicating Hodgkin's disease: Possible association with intensive therapy. *N. Engl. J. Med. 287:*1119-1122, 1972.

53. Karchmer, R.K., Amare, M., Larson, W.E., et al. Alkylating agents as leukemogens in multiple myeloma. *Cancer 33:*1103–1107, 1974.

54. Penn, I., and Starzl, T.E. A summary of the status of *de novo* cancer in transplant recipients. *Transplant. Proc. 4:*719, 1972.

55. Kersey, J.H., Spector, B.D., and Good, R.A. Primary immunodeficiency diseases and cancer: The immunodeficiency-cancer registry. *Int. J. Cancer 12:*333–347, 1973.

56. Souadjian, J.V., Silverstein, M.N., and Titus, J. Thymoma and cancer. *Cancer 22:* 1221–1225, 1968.

57. Berg, J.W. The incidence of multiple primary cancers. I. Development of further cancers in patients with lymphomas, leukemias, and myeloma. *J. Natl. Cancer Inst. 38:*741–752, 1967.

58. Newell, G.R., Krementz, E.T., Roberts, J.D., et al. Multiple primary neoplasms in blacks compared to whites. I. Further cancers in patients with Hodgkin's disease, leukemia, and myeloma. *J. Natl. Cancer Inst. 52:*635–638, 1974.

59. Moriarty, M. Skin carcinoma and chronic lymphatic leukemia—An association. *J. Irish Med. Assoc. 67:*177–180, 1974.

60. Berg, J.W., Hutter, R.V.P., and Foote, F.W., Jr. The unique association between salivary gland cancer and breast cancer. *J.A.M.A. 204:*771–774, 1968.

61. Lynch, H.T., Larsen, A.L., Magnuson, C.W., et al. Prostate carcinoma and multiple primary malignancies. *Cancer 19:*1891–1897, 1966.

62. Guerrier, K.R., and Persky, L. Combined leukemia, carcinoma, and hyperplasia of the prostate. *Arch. Surg. 98:*365–366, 1969.

DISCUSSION

Dr. Houten emphasized the importance of the time interval between the occurrence of first and second primary tumors and wondered whether studies have been made of second-cancer risk while the first tumor was still active in the patient. **Dr. Schoenberg** stated that this important issue has not been evaluated. **Dr. Bahn** urged further studies of the latent period in multiple primary cancers—paying special attention to the role of treatment in inducing second cancers.

Dr. Henderson reported on the occurrence of 12 testicular cancers, as opposed to an expected 3.5, in a series of patients with multiple primary cancers. He suggested that an etiologic explanation should be sought. **Dr. Cohen** called for studies to assess the possibility that oncogenic viruses are responsible for certain combinations of miltiple primary cancers.

Dr. E. C. Hammond pointed out that a high fatality rate from the first cancer limits development of a second cancer. For example, when lung cancer victims are carefully examined at autopsy, microscopic evidence of carcinoma of the larynx is found in excess. Thus, patients dying of lung cancer are at increased risk for a second primary, but death occurs before the second primary becomes clinically apparent.

Discussing the relationship between osteogenic sarcoma and retinoblastoma, **Dr. Knudson** noted that children treated by radiation for retinoblastoma are very prone to osteogenic sarcoma in the radiation field. Since persons with retinoblastoma are predisposed also to osteogenic sarcomas outside the radiation field, the exceptional risk of radiogenic sarcomas in these children appears due in part to constitutional factors. This finding is evidence for the role of host susceptibility to a mutagenic agent.

Henry T. Lynch

7

OVERVIEW: HOST FACTORS

Robert W. Miller, M.D.

Epidemiology Branch, National Cancer Institute
Bethesda, Maryland

It is important to learn not only what causes cancer, but also who is most susceptible and why. We know that relatively crude observations at the bedside have led to new understanding of the fundamental biology of cancer. Clues have been developed that could not have come from animal experimentation. At this point, the laboratory has an important role in elucidating the mechanisms involved and in studying interactions of host factors and environmental agents.

HIGH RISK OF WILMS' TUMOR

No one could have suspected, apart from observations in man, that Wilms' tumor occurs in a constellation of four growth excesses: 1) malignant neoplasia, 2) hamartomas (benign developmental neoplasms), 3) congenital hemihypertrophy, and 4) the visceral cytomegaly syndrome [1]. What accounts for this link among various manifestations of growth abnormality in the same person or among close relatives? Tissue culture studies may tell us, and they are finally getting underway in several laboratories.

HIGH RISK OF LEUKEMIA

Leukemia is associated with a very different constellation of disorders. The groups at high risk of this neoplasm have in common a chromosomal abnormality,

121

visible by old cytogenetic techniques in Down's syndrome, Fanconi's aplastic anemia, Bloom's syndrome [2,3] and chronic myelocytic leukemia [4]. Chromosomal abnormalities are now increasingly being found in acute myelocytic leukemia through the use of new banding techniques [5,6]. Thus, from rare conditions, we appear to be developing a generalization concerning leukemogenesis, namely, that the myelocytic form of the neoplasm is caused or accompanied by cytogenetic abnormality.

RETINOBLASTOMA AND CHROMOSOMAL DELETION

Chromosome abnormalities are also involved in certain forms of retinoblastoma in association with congenital malformations (D-deletion syndrome) [7]. New high-powered microscopic techniques in combination with new banding procedures for staining chromosomes have revealed the segment of chromosome 13 that is involved in the development of retinoblastoma in the D-deletion syndrome, and the neighboring segment that is involved in the associated malformations [8].

HIGH RISK OF LYMPHOMA

Dr. Kersey showed (Chapter 3) that in lymphoma, as contrasted with leukemia, the groups at high risk have in common an inborn immunological abnormality. Again, the observations began at the bedside—with a single case of congenital X-linked agammaglobulinemia reported in 1952 by Colonel Ogden Bruton [9]. In 1965, Dr. Good's group at Minnesota [10] pieced together evidence from eight cases of lymphoma with ataxia-telangiectasia, three cases with Wiskott-Aldrich syndrome, and three cases with congenital agammaglobulinemia to formulate an hypothesis about immunodeficiency states predisposing to lymphoma. The main thrust of the hypothesis remains intact as additional cases have been added during the past 9 years [11].

RELATION TO ENVIRONMENTAL EFFECTS

Many will ask what these rarities have to do with environmentally induced leukemia or lymphoma. The same relationships appear to exist with regard to environmental exposures as to inborn abnormalities. In leukemia, exposure to radiation or to benzene produces long-lasting chromosomal breaks that may well be involved in leukemogenesis observed after such exposures [2]. Environmentally induced immunosuppression, in the form of drugs given for renal transplantation, produces lymphoreticular neoplasia [12] and thus shares an effect in common with inborn immunodeficiency disorders [10,11].

HIGH RISK OF GONADOBLASTOMA

One Venn diagram can simplify 20 pages of narrative in explaining relationships among diseases. Dr. Mulvihill (Chapter 1) has thus summarized a two-part serial recently published by Schellhas [13,14] showing, from a comprehensive literature search, that gonadoblastoma occurs: 1) only in patients with gonadal dysgenesis, and 2) only when a Y-chromosome component is present in conjunction with the Turner phenotype or otherwise.

MULTIPLE PRIMARIES AND FAMILIES AT HIGH RISK OF CANCER

Dr. Anderson reported (Chapter 2) that pedigree analysis is a most effective means of studying familial cancer, a conclusion in accord with our own experience. He emphasized familial aggregation of cancers of a single cell type. Other cancers of certain dissimilar cell types may also aggregate in what appears to be family cancer syndromes, i.e., families in which certain, and at times rare, tumors occur among close relatives (e.g., osteosarcoma, adrenocortical carcinoma, rhabdomyosarcoma, glioma, and breast cancer) [15-17]. These tumors occur in various combinations, not only among close relatives, but also as double primaries—discussed in Chapter 6 by Dr. Schoenberg. The same combinations of cancers that occur excessively as second primaries appear to occur excessively among close relatives (Figure 1). These occurrences in individuals and their families may tell us something about the common origins of certain of these tumors and about their prevention or early detection.

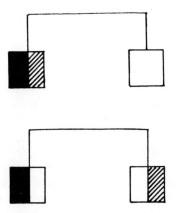

FIGURE 1.   Schematic representation showing the same double primary cancer in a person (above) as occurs individually among sibs (below).

Another type of familial aggregation was not brought out clearly, namely, that in which specific cancers and specific noncancerous diseases occur among close relatives. Dr. Meadows et al. [18], for example, found that in a sibship of three children with Wilms' tumor, the mother had congenital hemihypertrophy. Dr. Fraumeni has made a fine art as well as good science studying families with cancer in the same depth that individuals with rare diseases have previously been evaluated. By so doing, he found immunological disorders among relatives of patients with lymphomas, sometimes with clinical disease, e.g., idiopathic thrombocytopenic purpura and Hodgkin's disease [19]. In cancer-prone families, healthy members sometimes show the same laboratory aberrations that are found in the cancer-affected members, an observation that suggests these aberrations portend a high risk of cancer [20]. In these instances, one can offer not only genetic counseling, but also occupational counseling. The person with immunological abnormality and a family history of lymphoma might be advised, for example, not to work in a virus laboratory [21].

HIGH RISK FROM ACQUIRED DISEASES

Dr. Templeton's subject, acquired disorders that predispose to cancer (Chapter 4), is almost too broad to be absorbed. It is no doubt just as important to define acquired diseases that predispose to cancer as it is to find other factors that do the same, not only for the sake of the patient, but also for the sake of learning about the mechanism. One preexistent disorder that Dr. Templeton did not mention concerns bone infarcts, a sequel to decompression sickness seen among caisson workers. The specific tumor occurring at the site of these infarcts, as among those not resulting from caisson disease, is malignant fibrous histiocytoma [22]. The rarity of this tumor suggests that its concurrence with old infarcts is caused by something other than chance.

REGRESSION OF IN SITU TUMORS?

Dr. Koss reviewed in situ lesions (Chapter 5), and noted that he knew of none in which spontaneous regression could be studied. Actually there is one— below the age-range of Dr. Koss's interests—in pediatrics. Neuroblastoma in situ (microscopic neuroblastoma) was reported in 1963 by Beckwith and Perrin [23] to occur excessively in the adrenals of infants under 3 months old who came to autopsy for noncancerous diseases. The frequency of in situ neuroblastoma among these infants was 40 times more common than is clinical neuroblastoma. No in situ neuroblastoma was seen at autopsy in infants over 3 months. Apparently the lesions regress or mature to normal tissue. Turkel and Itabashi [24] subsequently found that all fetuses in a substantial series have at least one such lesion, the peak frequency being at 17 to 20 weeks gestational age.

In a recent publication [25], two infants with an unusual form of widely disseminated neuroblastoma (Type IV S) were reported to have experienced total regression of the tumor without therapy. The tumor occurred in the skin and other organs, but not in bone except for the marrow. Because neuroblastoma of this type is said to respond well to treatment, the authors elected to observe the children closely for a short interval before giving medication. The tumors soon began to regress and had disappeared entirely by the time the children reached 1 year of age. One wonders if this category of neuroblastoma is an exaggerated form of neuroblastoma in situ, visible in the infant and subject to study to determine what magic accounts for regression. The results could lead to new concepts of prevention or therapy.

WHO SHOULD BE SCREENED FOR HERITABLE CANCERS?

Which adults should be screened for detection of genetically induced cancers has been questioned. Opportunities for large-scale screening on the basis of high risk may come, but such opportunities are not yet here. Dr. Anderson indicated that only about 3 percent of breast cancer is hereditary. He also showed how the population can be narrowed to those at very high risk of breast cancer; e.g., women 20 to 49 years of age with a first-degree relative who had bilateral breast cancer [26]. This approach may serve as a model in determining who should be screened for other cancers. At present, identifying host factors that carry a high risk for cancer appears to be of greater value for studies of causation, which can lead to prevention, than for screening and early detection.

RECOMMENDATIONS

In developing several worthwhile recommendations, one might ask who is at high risk of discovering host factors that predispose to cancer. I claim it is the bedside etiologist—the person who thinks as much or more about etiology than he does about diagnosis or therapy. This category of physician is in extremely short supply, so my recommendations begin with alleviating this shortage and progress to communication improvements:

1) Screen to identify persons with an aptitude to think etiologically at the bedside—students in medical schools, colleges, or high schools.

2) Establish positions for bedside etiologists on the faculties in certain clinical departments (pediatrics, medicine, pathology) and at cancer centers—to search for new clues in the history of the patient, his family, or community. On ward rounds, etiologists would focus their attention on factors that may have contributed to the patient's illness.

3) Develop simple checklists of etiologic information that should be obtained at cancer centers for each patient admitted. The questions asked must be tailored to the type of tumor, as illustrated from discussions at the conference concerning leukemia, lymphoma, Wilms' tumor, and other neoplasms.

4) Develop new means to disseminate information fast. At present, reports of etiologic interest are scattered throughout the medical literature. We have developed a Childhood Cancer Etiology Newsletter that spreads information rapidly, generates new thinking, and increases requests for advice.

5) To improve the interaction among epidemiologists, clinicians, and laboratory investigators, small brainstorming sessions should be held regularly to discuss new information.

REFERENCES

1. Miller, R.W. Etiology of childhood cancer. *In* Sutow, W.W., Vietti, T.J., Fernbach, D.J., eds. *Clinical Pediatric Oncology.* C.V. Mosby Co., St. Louis, 1973, pp. 9–10.

2. Miller, R.W. Persons at exceptionally high risk of leukemia. *Cancer Res. 27:*2420–2423, 1967.

3. German, J. Genes which increase chromosomal instability in somatic cells and predispose to cancer. *Prog. Med. Genet. 8:*61–101, 1972.

4. Mastrangelo, R., Zuelzer, W.W., and Thompson, R.I. The significance of the Ph¹ chromosome in acute myeloblastic leukemia: Serial cytogenetic studies in a critical case. *Pediatrics 40:*834–841, 1967.

5. Sakurai, M., Oshimura, M., Katati, S., et al. 8–21 translocation and missing sex chromosomes in acute leukaemia. *Lancet 2:*227–228, 1974.

6. Rowley, J.D. Nonrandom chromosomal abnormalities in hematologic disorders of man. *Proc. Natl. Acad. Sci. USA.* In press, 1975.

7. O'Grady, R.B., Rothstein, T.B., and Romano, P.E. D-group deletion syndromes and retinoblastoma. *Am. J. Ophthalmol. 77:*40–45, 1974.

8. Orye, E., Delbeke, M.J., and van den Abeele, B. Retinoblastoma and long arm deletion of chromosome 13. Attempts to define the deleted segment. *Clin. Genet. 5:*457–464, 1974.

9. Bruton, O.C. Agammaglobulinemia. *Pediatrics 9:*722–728, 1952.

10. Peterson, R.D.A., Cooper, M.D., and Good, R.A. Disorders of the thymus and other lymphoid tissues. *Prog. Med. Genet. 4:*1–31, 1965.

11. Kersey, J.H., Spector, B.D., and Good, R.A. Primary immunodeficiency diseases and cancer: The Immunodeficiency-Cancer Registry. *Int. J. Cancer 12:*333–347, 1973.

12. Hoover, R., and Fraumeni, J.F., Jr. Risk of cancer in renal-transplant recipients. *Lancet 2:*55–57, 1973.

13. Schellhas, H.F. Malignant potential of the dysgenetic gonad. Part I. *Obstet. Gynecol. 44:*298–309, 1974.

14. Schellhas, H.F. Malignant potential of the dysgenetic gonad. Part II. *Obstet. Gynecol. 44:*455–462, 1974.

15. Li, F.P., and Fraumeni, J.F., Jr. Rhabdomyosarcoma in children: Epidemiologic study and identification of a familial cancer syndrome. *J. Natl. Cancer Inst. 43:*1365–1373, 1969.

16. Li, F.P., and Fraumeni, J.F., Jr. Soft tissue sarcomas, breast cancer, and other neoplasms. A familial syndrome? *Ann. Intern. Med. 71:*747–752, 1969.

17. Miller, R.W. Deaths from childhood leukemia and solid tumors among twins and other sibs in the United States, 1960-67. *J. Natl. Cancer Inst. 46:*203–209, 1971.

18. Meadows, A.T., Lichtenfeld, J.L., and Koop, C.E. Wilms's tumor in three children of a woman with congenital hemihypertrophy. *N. Engl. J. Med. 291:*23–24, 1974.

19. Creagan, E.T., and Fraumeni, J.F., Jr. Familial Hodgkin's disease .*Lancet 2:*547, 1972.

20. Fraumeni, J.F., Jr., Wertelecki, W., Blattner, W.A., et al. Varied manifestations of a familial lymphoproliferative disorder. *Am. J. Med.* In press, 1975.

21. Allison, A.C. Immunosuppression and cancer. *In* Hellman, A., Oxman, M.N., and Pollack, R., eds. *Biohazards in Biological Research.* Cold Spring Harbor, N.Y., 1973, p. 287.

22. Mirra, J.M., Bullough, P.G., Marcove, R.C., et al. Malignant fibrous histiocytoma and osteosarcoma in association with bone infarcts. Report of 4 cases, 2 in caisson workers. *J. Bone J. Surg. 56-A:*932–940, 1974.

23. Beckwith, J.B., and Perrin, E.V. In situ neuroblastomas: Contribution to the natural history of neural crest tumors. *Am. J. Pathol. 43:*1089–1104, 1963.

24. Turkel, S.B., and Itabashi, H.H. The natural history of neuroblastic cells in the fetal adrenal gland. *Am. J. Pathol. 76:*225–244, 1974.

25. Schwartz, A.D., Dadash-Zadeh, M., Lee, H., et al. Spontaneous regression of disseminated neuroblastoma. *J. Pediatr. 85:*760–763, 1974.

26. Anderson, D.E. A genetic study of human breast cancer. *J. Natl. Cancer Inst. 48:* 1029–1034, 1972.

DISCUSSION

Dr. **Cole** emphasized that the concept of regressibility is essential in defining precancerous lesions and in distinguishing these from cancerous lesions. In the natural history of precancerous lesions, the incidence of tumors is much lower than would be expected, thus regression must be taking place. Identifying the factors which influence regression is a promising avenue for study.

He also pointed out the applications of different risk measures in assessing high-risk groups. If one is interested in etiologic studies, estimates of relative risk are useful. However, estimates of absolute or attributable risk find application in cancer control and screening.

Dr. **Bahn** asked about the application of screening programs to high-risk groups. **Dr. R. W. Miller** replied that screening may help identify environmental as well as genetic factors in cancer etiology. Common mechanisms such as chromosome breaks on a heritable or environmental basis have a common outcome, e.g., leukemia. Therefore, screening high-risk patients, such as members of high-risk families, for etiologic factors may elucidate new mechanisms in oncogenesis. Dr. **Rawson** interjected that epidemiologic observations may give critical leads for laboratory study. Dr. **Miller** agreed, but pointed out that man is frequently unique with no counterpart animal models suitable for etiologic study (e.g., Fanconi's anemia and Down's syndrome). To some extent this limits laboratory identification of etiologic mechanisms.

Dr. Wynder indicated that as the new cancer centers are set up around the country, a requirement for minimal historical data should be established as a base for etiologic studies. The therapy orientation of cancer centers now often overshadows studies of etiology. In fact, full-time nurse epidemiologists or "physician etiologists" should be hired for the centers to monitor for etiologic clues. **Dr. Miller** pointed out that a checklist of epidemiologically significant information might facilitate this monitoring.

Dr. Cohen questioned whether coordinated efforts are being made to keep track of long-term survivors with childhood cancer to assess the risk of second primary cancers. **Dr. Miller** knew of no nationwide program, but discussed an ongoing multi-hospital survey in the follow-up of childhood Wilms' tumor. In surveys of patients with polycythemia vera, multiple myeloma, and Hodgkin's disease, leukemia has been reported in excess. Such relationships may have the following explanations: 1) cure of the primary malignancy may allow, as part of the natural history of the disease, an underlying tumor diathesis to emerge, or 2) treatment of the first neoplasm may be carcinogenic. Both mechanisms seem to function in the case of sarcomas following retinoblastoma.

William A. Blattner

ENVIRONMENTAL FACTORS

8

TOBACCO

E. Cuyler Hammond, Sc. D.

American Cancer Society
New York, New York

A great many things said about cancer are debatable because of lack of solid evidence, conflicting evidence from different investigations, or different interpretations of the evidence. This is not so with respect to the impact of tobacco use on the risk of cancer at several sites. It would be hard to find another subject so thoroughly and extensively investigated during the last 25 years [1-3]. The degree of consistency of findings is truly remarkable considering the different methods employed and considering the fact that many of the studies were conducted by scientists who had been highly skeptical of the findings of their predecessors. The subject of tobacco-related cancer is so familiar that a detailed review would be pointless. Therefore, I will present selected issues, briefly discuss some areas of uncertainty, and then turn to suggestions for future work.

HISTORICAL ASPECTS

Over 100 years ago, there was evidence linking betel nut chewing to mouth cancer, and good reason to suspect that tobacco included in the wad was the major culprit [4]. This use of tobacco is still a major cause of cancer in some parts of Asia. The effects of chewing tobacco and snuff have not been so extensively studied, but probably contribute little to the risk of cancer simply because these exposures are now uncommon in most parts of the world [5].

Many years ago Bouisson conducted a beautiful set of studies clearly demonstrating that smoking—particularly the smoking of short-stem clay pipes called

131

"mouth burners"—was the major cause of lip cancer in France. Apparently, his findings were generally accepted but aroused little interest and were almost forgotten. Indeed, the whole subject of tobacco and cancer was largely neglected until a rapid and continuing increase occurred during this century in lung cancer death rates [1]. Oschner [6] noted that virtually all of his lung cancer patients were cigarette smokers and suggested that the tremendous rise in cigarette consumption—which began during World War I—was responsible for the increase in disease. The rest of the story is well known to all.

CANCER RISK AMONG CIGARETTE SMOKERS

The relationship between cigarette smoking and cancer may be illustrated by a prospective epidemiological study of over one million men and women who were enrolled between October 1, 1959, and March, 1960, and traced through September 30, 1965 [7, 8]. The findings are consistent with dozens of other studies conducted by many different investigators in many different countries. Mortality ratios for cancer were computed by dividing the age-standardized death rate of cigarette smokers by the age-standardized death rate of those who never smoked regularly (Table 1). Cigarette smoking increases the risk of lung cancer to a greater degree than any other cancer site. In addition, cigarette smoking (as well as pipe and cigar smoking) multiplies the risk of cancer of the buccal cavity (lip, mouth, and tongue) and pharynx by a factor of about three to ten depending upon the type and amount of smoking. It is hard to estimate the mortality ratio with any precision because the rate in nonsmoking men in the United States is very low. As shown in several studies, heavy drinking of alcoholic beverages increases the risk of mouth and throat cancer even further in smokers [9].

Furthermore, cigarette smoking greatly increases the risk of cancers of the larynx and esophagus. Again the rarity of these cancers in non-smoking American men makes it difficult to estimate the exact degree of risk in terms of mortality ratios. Smoking also multiplies the risk of bladder cancer, particularly among men under the age of 65. This finding has been confirmed by many studies and appears beyond dispute.

The increased risk of cancer of the pancreas in cigarette smokers is supported by histologic evidence. Atypical changes have been observed in the nuclei of pancreatic duct cells among smokers coming to autopsy, with the extent of such changes increasing with the amount of smoking [10]. The relation of smoking to cancer at other sites is less definitely established. In several studies, for example, deaths ascribed to liver cancer have occurred more frequently in cigarette smokers than nonsmokers [1]. However, in many cases, there is considerable doubt as to whether the liver was the primary site of cancer. The association may be due to lung cancer with liver metastases being mistakenly reported as primary liver cancer. This subject is worth further investigation.

TABLE 1
Cancer mortality ratios among men with history of cigarette smoking
compared with men who never smoked regularly;
American Cancer Society Survey [7]

	Age 45-64	Age 65-79
Total Cancer	2.14	1.76
Lung	7.84	11.59
Buccal cavity, pharynx	9.90	2.93
Larynx	6.09	8.99
Esophagus	4.17	1.74
Bladder	2.00	2.96
Kidney	1.42	1.57
Prostate	1.04	1.01
Pancreas	2.69	2.17
Liver, biliary passages	2.84	1.34
Stomach	1.42	1.26
Colon, rectum	1.01	1.17
Leukemia	1.40	1.68
Lymphoma	1.38	0.80
Other specified sites	1.64	1.14
Unspecified sites	2.23	1.78

DOSE-RESPONSE RELATIONSHIPS

It is well known that lung cancer death rates increase with the amount of cigarette smoking (Table 2). This finding has been confirmed by many studies [1-3]. It is less well known that lung cancer death rates increase with depth of inhalation of cigarette smoke and are far higher among people who started cigarette smoking in their early teens than among people who took up the habit later in life.

Tables 1 and 2 illustrate the cancer risk from cigarette smoking in men. In women the patterns are essentially the same, but with one big difference, namely the relationship between smoking and cancer risk (expressed in terms of mortality ratios) is far less pronounced. This difference is largely, but not entirely, explained by the fact that among cigarette smokers in the United States who are now over the age of 50, women as a group took up the habit at a later age then men, tend to inhale the smoke less deeply, and smoke fewer cigarettes per day. It is also true that when filter-tip cigarettes began to displace nonfilter cigarettes, they were more popular among female than male smokers.

TABLE 2

Lung cancer mortality ratios among men aged 35-84 years,
according to current number of cigarettes smoked per day,
degree of inhalation, and age began smoking;
American Cancer Society survey [8].

Current no. cigarettes/day	Ratio
1-9	4.62
10-19	8.62
20-39	14.69
40+	18.77
Degree of inhalation	
None	8.00
Slight	8.92
Moderate	13.08
Deep	17.00
Age began smoking	
25+	4.08
20-24	10.08
15-19	14.69
<15	16.77
Never smoked regularly	1.00

PIPE AND CIGAR SMOKING

As a group, men with a lifetime history of only pipe or cigar smoking have a lung cancer death rate which is significantly higher than that of men who never smoked but considerably lower than that of men who smoked even a few cigarettes per day (Table 3). Upon further examination, it turns out that most pipe and cigar smokers do not inhale the smoke while most cigarette smokers, even light smokers, do inhale. It appears that those few pipe and cigar smokers who inhale are at as great or greater risk of lung cancer than cigarette smokers.

PREVENTABILITY OF LUNG CANCER

A very large number of men, now over the age of 50, have been smoking cigarettes ever since there were teenagers. Must we tell them that what they have done cannot be undone? Probably so in relation to emphysema; apparently not

TABLE 3

Lung cancer mortality ratios among men aged 35-84 years,
according to type of smoking (lifetime history);
American Cancer Society survey [8].

	Ratio
Never smoked regularly	1.00
Pipe only	2.23
Pipe and cigar	1.23
Cigar only	2.15
Cigarette and other	8.23
Cigarette only	10.08

in relation to lung cancer (Table 4). These data and other studies [1-3] indicate that lung cancer death rates are lower among ex-cigarette smokers than those who continue the habit, and are lower among those who have not smoked for many years than those who have not smoked for a few years. Histologic findings in bronchial epithelium are consistent with these epidemiological observations [11].

In this situation the evidence appears to be indisputable, but the interpretation is open to at least a shadow of a doubt. The obvious interpretation is that when a long-term cigarette smoker gives up the habit his risk of lung cancer gradually diminishes and eventually approaches the very low risk for people who have never smoked. The shadow of a doubt is based upon evidence that those with the lowest lifetime pulmonary exposure to cigarette smoke are the most likely to give up the habit permanently. This introduces a bias. Whether the bias is sufficiently great to account for the observations must be investigated before we can be absolutely certain of the interpretation. The problem may be resolved by tracing subjects for a long period of time and periodically obtaining information on their smoking habits. This is one of the reasons which impelled us to extend our prospective study for an additional seven years.

FUTURE STUDIES

Further research on the subject of cigarette smoking and cancer should be aimed at answering two seemingly very simple questions: 1) Does reduction in the tar and/or nicotine content of cigarettes significantly reduce the risk of cancer incurred by smoking cigarettes? 2) If so, is there an accompanying decrease or increase in the risk of death from other serious diseases, especially coronary heart disease?

For many years, there has been an almost steady decline in the per capita consumption of pipe tobacco, cigar tobacco, chewing tobacco and snuff. More

TABLE 4

Age-standardized death rates for lung cancer among men aged 50-69
who were ex-cigarette smokers, by former number of cigarettes smoked
per day, and years since last smoking; comparison with death rates
for men who were current cigarette smokers, and men who
never smoked regularly; American Cancer Society survey [8].

	Death rates	
Ex-cigarette smokers (yrs. since last smoking)	Smoked 1–19 cigarettes/day	Smoked 20+ cigarettes/day
Under 1 year	114	283
1–4 years	53	162
5–9 years	20	104
10+ years	7	29
Total ex-smokers	28	101
Current cigarette smokers	120	271
Never smoked regularly	16	16

recently, the per capita consumption of cigarette tobacco decreased due to the
use of less tobacco per cigarette. This trend can be ascribed to the fact that filter-
tip cigarettes generally contain less tobacco than nonfilter cigarettes. While the
pounds of cigarette tobacco per capita decreased, the numbers of cigarettes per
capita decreased briefly on several occasions and then increased again. These
fluctuations, taken alone, are about as meaningful as reporting the numbers of
bottles of alcoholic beverages consumed per year without mentioning changes
in the average amount of alcohol per bottle.

Nevertheless, during the last 20 years or so, there has been a dramatic decline
in the average amount of tar and nicotine delivered in the smoke from cigarettes
consumed in the United States [12]. As a result, the per capita consumption of
cigarette tar and nicotine has greatly decreased. This trend should, within a
decade or so, lead to a reduction in lung cancer death rates—that is, *if* tar and
nicotine in cigarette smoke are mainly responsible for the cancer producing
effects, and *if* reduced exposure to these ingredients can lower the risk of cancer
among people who were heavily exposed for many years.

There is some preliminary evidence from our ongoing prospective study that
both of the two conditions may be true. Male cigarette smokers were classified
according to the tar and nicotine content of the cigarettes smoked at the time
of enrollment, and the figures were standardized according to the number of
cigarettes smoked per day. Men who smoked cigarettes with the lowest amount

of tar and nicotine had the lowest lung cancer death rates. Retrospective studies have revealed similar findings [13, 14].

This relationship suggests that reduction in tar and nicotine in cigarette smoke lowers the risk of lung cancer, but there is at least a shadow of doubt—resulting from a suspicion of biasing factors similar to those discussed in relation to the effects of giving up smoking.

There is a further problem. Death rates from coronary heart disease were no lower—indeed, they were a trifle higher—in men who smoked low tar-nicotine cigarettes than in men who smoked high tar-nicotine cigarettes. This finding may be due to biasing factors, which need to be evaluated in future studies. The issue is of prime importance; if reduction in tar and nicotine greatly reduces the risk of cancer—without aggravating the risk of coronary heart disease—then the means are at hand to achieve a splendid breakthrough in cancer control.

REFERENCES

1. U.S. Department of Health, Education, and Welfare. *Smoking and Health. Report of the Advisory Committee to the Surgeon General of the Public Health Serivce.* U.S. Govt. Print. Off., Washington, D.C., 1964.

2. U.S. Department of Health, Education, and Welfare. *The Health Consequences of Smoking - 1974.* U.S. Govt. Print. Off., Washington, D.C., 1974.

3. World Health Organization. *Smoking and Its Effects on Health. Report of a WHO Expert Committee.* WHO Technical Report Series No. 568. WHO, Geneva, 1975.

4. Orr, I. M. Oral cancer in betel nut chewers in Travancore; its aetiology, pathology, and treatment. *Lancet 2:*575-580, 1933.

5. Wynder, E. L., Bross, I. J., and Feldman, R. M. A study of the etiological factors in cancer of the mouth. *Cancer 10:*1300-1323, 1957.

6. Ochsner, A., and DeBakey, M. Symposium on cancer: Primary pulmonary malignancy. *Surg. Gynecol. Obstet. 68:*435-451, 1939.

7. Hammond, E. C. Smoking in relation to the death rates of one million men and women. *Natl. Cancer Inst. Monogr. 19:*127-204, 1966.

8. Hammond, E. C. Smoking habits and air pollution in relation to lung cancer. *In* Lee, H. K., ed. *Environmental Factors in Respiratory Disease,* Academic Press, New York, 1972.

9. Rothman, K. J. Alcohol. This volume, 1975.

10. Auerbach, O. Unpublished data.

11. Auerbach, O., Stout, A. P., Hammond, E. C., et al. Changes in bronchial epithelium in relation to cigarette smoking and in relation to lung cancer. *N. Engl. J. Med. 265:*253-267, 1961.

12. Wynder, E. L., and Hoffmann, D. The tenth anniversary of the Surgeon General's Report on Smoking and Health: Have we made any progress? *J. Natl. Cancer Inst. 54:* 533-534, 1975.

13. Wynder, E. L., Mabuchi, E. L., and Beattie, E. J. The epidemiology of lung cancer. Recent trends. *J.A.M.A. 213:*2221-2228, 1970.

14. Bross, J. D., and Gibson, R. Risk of lung cancer in smokers who switch to filter cigarettes. *Am. J. Public Health 58:*1396-1403, 1968.

DISCUSSION

The discussion centered on tobacco usage as a risk factor in population subgroups, such as racial minorities in the United States. For American Indians and Asian-Americans, the data are scanty. Lung cancer appears to be increasing in lower socioeconomic groups, due perhaps to the concomitant increase in advertising and sale of cigarettes among the poor. However, bladder cancer is less common among blacks than among whites, due perhaps to the absence of Negroes in certain industries until recently and to the different patterns of tobacco usage, as illustrated by studies in Veterans Administration hospitals.

Dr. Wynder stated that some 40 percent of all male cancer deaths is attributed to cigarette smoking. These deaths result from cancers of the lung, larynx, oral cavity, pharynx, esophagus, and bladder. In addition, a large percentage of deaths from coronary artery disease and emphysema, particularly among white men, is attributable to cigarette smoking.

Finally, **Dr. Goldsmith** indicated the need to obtain smoking data on migrants moving from farm to rural areas and from rural to urban areas. Cancer trends among population subgroups who have stopped smoking should also be investigated. However, there is no need to prove repeatedly that tobacco usage in any form (smoked, dipped, or chewed) is bad for one's health, since the hazard has been adequately shown.

Andrew Z. Keller

9

ALCOHOL

Kenneth J. Rothman, Dr. P.H.

Department of Epidemiology
Harvard School of Public Health
Boston, Massachusetts

INTRODUCTION

Ethyl alcohol has been part of the human diet for thousands of years. Evidence suggests it was consumed by prehistoric man and probably has been a ubiquitous feature of human society since Neolithic times. Alcohol consumption remains prevalent today throughout the world. Most Americans drink at least occasionally, and a significant proportion consume alcohol to the extent that it interferes with an orderly and healthy existence.

Alcohol has many and varied metabolic and pharmacologic effects. While there is little reason to implicate alcohol as a carcinogen on a priori grounds, neither is it unthinkable that such a pharmacologically active substance could initiate or promote carcinogenesis. Alcohol is generally imbibed as naturally fermented fruit juice or grain extract or, in distilled form, in a variety of vehicles. Such beverages often contain contaminants, some of which may have carcinogenic activity. The usual compounds present are congeners to ethanol, aliphatic molecules with six or fewer carbons in most distilled spirits, and one or more oxygen atoms, generally in hydroxyl form [1]. As a class, these compounds are irritants to skin and mucous membranes, and in large doses have strong pharmacologic actions characterized as "paint remover effect" (including nausea, vomiting, confusion, and central nervous system depression). Congeners occur in different concentrations in various alcoholic beverages, being plentiful, for example, in bourbon and nearly absent in vodka. Compounds other than ethanol congeners are thought to be in some alcoholic beverages. For example, it is suspected that nitrosamines, which are established carcinogens [2], or precursors of nitrosamines are in the maize beer consumed in areas of Africa where esophageal cancer is common [3].

Because alcohol is consumed in intimate association with other biologically active compounds, it is difficult to distinguish its effect on cancer risk from that of the congeners or other contaminants. Experimental work with animals should be helpful in this regard, but the evidence to date is sparse. The work of Stënback [4] and Kuratsune et al. [5] suggests that alcohol increases cancer risk, but not acting alone; rather, it acts as a cocarcinogen, enhancing the carcinogenic effect of other agents.

The effect on humans drinking alcohol is also confounded by factors that are by habit associated with alcohol consumption and may influence cancer risk. The most important of these factors is tobacco consumption, which is a strong risk factor for several sites of cancer and highly correlated with alcohol consumption in most populations. Accurate assessment of the carcinogenicity of alcohol is impossible without removal of the confounding effect introduced by the generally greater tobacco consumption of alcohol drinkers. The failure or inability to control for the effect of tobacco limits the utility of several follow-up studies of alcoholics [6-9], which otherwise would prove highly informative about the effects of prolonged heavy consumption of alcohol in humans. Also it may be difficult to separate other facets of the life of alcohol drinkers affecting their cancer risk from the effect of alcohol. For example, alcohol consumption usually displaces calories that may be accompanied by essential nutrients; malnourishment conceivably could alter cancer risk and thus confound the potential effect of alcohol.

Despite these difficulties, the balance of evidence strongly supports the view that alcohol consumption increases the risk of cancer in humans. This evidence accrues mainly from case-control studies of cancer of specific sites in which the major confounder, tobacco consumption, was controlled [10-15]. Additional evidence comes from cohort studies by analysis of proportional mortality [6, 8]. These analyses demonstrate an excess of cancers in the mouth, pharynx, and larynx relative to the lung, presumably attributable, at least in part, to alcohol. For these sites, there is scant evidence that is not consistent with an association between alcohol consumption and cancer risk.

CANCER OF SPECIFIC SITES

Mouth and Pharynx

Alcohol and tobacco are both well established as strong risk factors for cancer of the mouth and pharynx [10-12]. Together these two agents are estimated to account for approximately three-fourths of cancers of the oral cavity in males in the United States [16], presuming their relationship to risk of oral cancer is causal. Cohort studies examining cause of death [6–8] and cancer morbidity [9] among alcoholics support the idea that alcoholics have a higher risk than non-alcoholics of developing and dying from cancer of the mouth or pharynx. Further evidence supporting the causal connection between consumption of alcoholic beverages and cancer risk comes from the clear dose-response relationship present for each of several levels of tobacco consumption, including nonsmoking (Table 1). Heavy drinkers experience a risk 2 to 6 times higher than nondrinkers, the effect depending on and increasing with the amount of tobacco smoked. The combined effect of heavy smoking and drinking results in a risk more than 15 times as great as that for those who neither smoke nor drink, whereas heavy smoking alone results in no more than a two- to threefold increase in risk.

Table 1 indicates that alcohol is a risk factor for cancer of the oral cavity even without smoking; however, the effect of alcohol seems considerably greater when accompanied by smoking, which suggests a synergistic effect compatible with evidence from animal studies that alcohol acts as a cocarcinogen. The synergistic effect of alcohol and tobacco on the risk of oral cancer, with an index analogous in interpretation to the risk ratio [17], was estimated from these data to be 2.6 (1.0 would denote no synergy), which suggests the effect of alcohol in increasing the risk of oral cancer depends strongly on tobacco consumption.

TABLE 1

Risk ratios for oral cancer according to level of exposure to alcohol and smoking[a, b]

Alcohol per day (oz.)	Cigarette equivalents per day			
	0	Less than 20	20–39	40 or more
None	1.00	1.52	1.43	2.43
< 0.4	1.40	1.67	3.18	3.25
0.4–1.5	1.60	4.36	4.46	8.21
> 1.5	2.33	4.13	9.59	15.5

[a]Risks are expressed relative to a risk of 1.00 for persons who neither smoked nor drank.
[b]Source: Rothman and Keller [16].

The relatively small increase in risk experienced by alcohol drinkers who do not smoke could represent an interaction of alcohol with nontobacco carcinogens. Alternatively, the increase in risk seen in nonsmokers might reflect a small but direct primary carcinogenic effect of alcoholic beverages.

Larynx

Laryngeal cancer occurs much more frequently in alcoholics than nonalcoholics [6-8]. Although this increase may be partly attributable to heavy smoking among alcoholics, the relative frequency of laryngeal and lung cancers in alcoholics differs dramatically from the proportions generally seen in nonalcoholic heavy smokers. This fact suggests that drinking alcohol accounts for at least part of the excess of laryngeal cancer observed among alcoholics. In a case-control study of 347 cases and matched controls, Wynder, Bross, and Day [13] examined the association between alcohol consumption and risk for laryngeal cancer, while controlling for the effect of smoking. Alcohol consumption, particularly heavy whiskey consumption, elevated the risk for laryngeal cancer more than 10 times compared to abstinence or moderate drinking. These data support the idea that, although smoking may initiate laryngeal cancer, alcohol serves as a promoter rather than a primary carcinogen.

Esophagus

Esophageal cancer occurs with a wide range of frequency in different geographic areas; it is rare in the United States but common in certain other areas, particularly in a broad belt across central Asia [18]. In Western countries, there seems to be an association between esophageal cancer risk and alcohol consumption, as documented in correlation studies in France [19] and the United States [20]. The U.S. study shows a steep increase in esophageal cancer mortality rates with increasing amounts of distilled spirits sold per capita. Kamionkowski and Fleshler [21], in a case-control study of 50 patients with esophageal cancer and 106 controls (with cancer of the colon), estimated that the risk for esophageal cancer is 17 times greater for alcoholics than for nonalcoholics. More pertinent evidence for the role of alcohol consumption comes from case-control studies that examined the association of alcohol consumption with risk for cancer of the esophagus while controlling for smoking history. Restricting comparison to moderate smokers, Wynder and Bross [14] estimated that heavy drinkers experience a risk more than 25 times that of nondrinkers. In Puerto Rico, where incidence rates for cancer of the esophagus are high, Martinez [15], with 400 cases and 1,200 controls, also found a strong association with alcohol consumption after adjusting for tobacco use.

Because the geographic variation of esophageal cancer is exceptional, the exact nature of the relationship with alcohol consumption is particularly interesting, since alcohol consumption is nearly ubiquitous and varies geographically less than esophageal cancer rates. In some areas, such as the Ghurjev district of the Kazakhstan Province of the U.S.S.R., esophageal cancer is the most commonly diagnosed cancer, with an incidence rate exceeding 500 cases per 100,000 males per year [22]. Near the Caspian Sea, a thirtyfold gradient in disease incidence in females exists along a small strip of several hundred kilometers [23]. Such variation cannot easily be attributed to the amount of alcohol consumed [24, 25], which suggests that other factors besides alcohol consumption have an important function. This suggestion is consistent with the idea that the carcinogenic agent elevating the risk in alcohol drinkers is not alcohol but a contaminant.

The high rate of esophageal cancer among certain African groups has been ascribed to the locally brewed maize beer [26], which is thought to be contaminated with nitrosamines or substances that are converted into nitrosamines in the stomach [3]. Similarly, the high rate in Puerto Rico has been blamed on the impure, illicitly distilled rum commonly consumed throughout the island [15]. In France, where alcohol consumption is generally high, esophageal cancer rates vary considerably between regions, thus seeming to be related to the type of alcohol spirits produced and, presumably, consumed [19].

Stomach

Whereas fluids pass quickly through the esophagus coming only briefly into contact with the epithelium, they remain in intimate and prolonged contact with the mucosa of the stomach. Thus, it might be reasoned that consumption of alcoholic beverages, strongly associated with cancer of the esophagus, would also be associated with risk of stomach cancer. A slight association with cancer of the cardiac portion of the stomach has been observed [27], but the association is weak and is absent for cancers of the noncardiac portion of the stomach. The best evidence against a role for alcohol in cancer of the stomach comes from the cohort studies of alcoholics: no excess of stomach cancers was observed. In three studies, the observed-to-expected ratios for cancer of the stomach among alcoholics were 1.0 [8], 0.8 [6], and 0.8 [9]. Nevertheless, the distinctive clinical and epidemiologic features of cancer of the gastric cardia, in addition to its reported association with alcohol consumption, argue that at least some cases of stomach cancer may be linked to alcohol consumption.

Liver

Primary cancer of the liver reportedly occurs with great frequency (10 to 30 percent) among alcoholics with cirrhosis [28-30]. The risk is so high relative to that in nondrinkers—in whom hepatoma occurs rarely, at least in Western countries—it seems unlikely that the association would be spurious.

These observations seem inconsistent with the low rates of hepatoma reported in Western countries, considering that about 10 percent of alcoholics develop advanced cirrhosis [6]. However, hepatoma may be more common, at least in Europe, than has been assumed [31].

Strangely, cohort studies of mortality among alcoholics do not show an excess of cancers of the liver. In the largest series of deaths among alcoholics [8], 4 cancers of the liver (and biliary passages) were found, with 4.2 expected. This result, however, is somewhat difficult to interpret because the expected number was derived from proportional cancer mortality figures. In another study of alcoholics [6], there were 68 deaths from liver cirrhosis, with no hepatomas. The conflict between the strong association suggested from the high attack rate of hepatoma in people with alcoholic cirrhosis and the absence of such an association in the cohort studies of alcoholics needs resolution. Since selection bias may be a problem in the cirrhosis series, the evidence should be regarded with caution. Even a skeptic, however, would be prudent to acknowledge the strong possibility for a causal role of alcohol in the development of hepatoma.

Rectum

A correlation analysis [32] of age-adjusted mortality data and beer consumption by state revealed a high correlation between death from rectal cancer and beer consumption, after controlling for cigarette consumption and urbanization; similar results were obtained using international mortality data. There was little association between rectal cancer mortality and spirit consumption. As the authors point out, the association between beer and rectal cancer should be considered only tentative until it can be established in studies with individuals. If the association indeed proves valid and causal, it strengthens the belief that it is not alcohol but other ingredients that are the primary determinants for cancer related to alcohol consumption.

Other Sites

Alcohol has been proposed as a risk factor for cancer of several other sites, notably the prostate and pancreas. Evidence for these associations is sparse and conflicting [33]. Mortality studies among alcoholics suggest that if alcohol is an etiologic factor in cancer of these sites, the increase in risk is relatively small.

OVERALL INCREASE IN CANCER RISK FROM ALCOHOL

Of the 173,665 cancer deaths in 1968 among males in the United States, 159,111 of the cancers occurred in sites for which no evidence suggests a causal association with consumption of alcoholic beverages [34]. Even if as much as 75 percent of the remaining deaths were attributed to alcohol consumption (and this percentage is probably too high), then only about 11,000 cancer deaths would be attributed to alcohol consumption. This figure represents about a 7 percent increase in cancer deaths over what would have occurred in the absence of alcohol consumption. The comparable figure in females is a 2 percent increase in cancer deaths. Thus, alcohol is potentially related to only a small fraction of cancer deaths in the United States.

These figures give an idea of the impact of alcohol on cancer mortality in the United States, but they do not answer the primary question an individual might pose: What are the comparative risks of developing (any) cancer for drinkers and nondrinkers of alcohol (or preferably, the risk function)? The comparative risks for specific sites outlined in this chapter, although instructive in evaluation of the scientific aspects of the carcinogenicity of alcohol consumption, does not completely answer this question.

An estimate of the probability at age 15 of subsequently developing cancer in the United States is 0.26 [35]. To estimate the probability of developing cancer after age 15 for nondrinkers, subtract the probabilities (or appropriate fractional parts) for developing cancers related to alcohol consumption. With such calculations the probability of developing cancer for nondrinkers is roughly 0.24 to 0.25, about 6 percent less than the average value for a 15-year-old male.

It is more difficult to estimate the probability of developing cancer for alcohol drinkers in order to evaluate the increment in overall cancer risk. It can be approximated with knowledge of the proportion of people who are "drinkers," although it is difficult to decide what figure would be appropriate. If two-thirds of the adult population were assumed to drink little enough to experience a negligible increase in cancer risk, the average probability of 0.26 would result if the remaining one-third experienced a probability of 0.29, which represents about a 20 percent increase in cancer risk over nondrinkers and "moderate" drinkers. If instead the increased risk were considered to be concentrated in the 20 percent of the adult population that drinks most heavily, then the probability of developing cancer among these heavy drinkers would be 0.32, a substantial increase of 30 percent in cancer risk for this group.

The preceding are only rough estimates derived from oversimplified assumptions. The actual increase in cancer risk from alcohol would of course be a complex function dependent upon many factors, such as amount of alcoholic beverages consumed, type of beverage, smoking habits, and a variety of host factors. Nevertheless, these rough estimates of increased risk are in the same range as those observed in cohort studies of cancer mortality among alcoholics [6, 9].

PROSPECTS FOR CONTROL

The evidence clearly suggests that consumption of alcoholic beverages causes an increase in cancer risk for certain sites. The increased risk is dose related and, at least for cancer of the oral cavity, also depends to a large extent on tobacco consumption. Thus, an effective campaign against smoking would also decrease the carcinogenic effect of alcohol.

The preponderance of evidence supports the view that alcohol does not usually initiate cancer but acts as a cocarcinogen, magnifying the carcinogenic activity of other cancer-inducing agents such as tobacco. An important consequence of this hypothesis, were it to prove correct, would be that alcohol-related cancers could be prevented by eliminating carcinogens that are unrelated to alcohol consumption (i.e., except by habit, such as smoking) or that are undesirable contaminants of alcoholic beverages.

Primary prevention of alcohol-related cancer also could be achieved through campaigns directed at limiting alcohol intake. It appears unlikely that alcohol use will be proscribed again in the United States. Furthermore, the increased risk for cancer experienced by heavy users of alcohol is probably of less public health importance than other sometimes more devastating health and social consequences. These problems are enough of a concern to motivate, in their own right, programs aimed at preventing or reversing chronic, excessive, alcohol consumption. Although increased risk for cancer should in principle provide an added impetus to such control programs, it seems likely that this hazard would be overshadowed by the more direct consequences of excessive drinking.

Alcoholics, particularly those who smoke heavily, experience a greatly increased risk of cancer that is concentrated in a few anatomic sites. Early detection and treatment, particularly for mouth and pharynx cancer where detection is relatively simple, would be a natural way to seek to control cancer in such a high-risk group. Screening programs for mouth and pharynx cancer are being implemented in some areas, primarily as an adjunct to routine dental examination by dentists. However, the efficacy of such programs in reducing morbidity or mortality is not yet demonstrated. Furthermore, alcoholics are less likely to visit dentists than nonalcoholics and are unlikely to benefit from existing programs.

To the extent that alcoholics can be approached as a group (through reform organizations or other channels), it would seem advisable to implement trial screening programs to evaluate the potential benefit of early cancer detection and treatment. The feasibility of such programs has been demonstrated by Kissin et al. [36], who detected 10 head and neck cancers in 3,007 alcoholics who volunteered for a simple screening examination. Undoubtedly many alcoholics would not be reached through such programs, but educational programs about screening (which seem to achieve more success than primary prevention programs) might be useful in publicizing and thereby extending the potential efficacy of any contemplated screening program.

SUGGESTIONS FOR RESEARCH

Much of the available evidence indicates that alcohol elevates cancer risk by acting synergistically as a cocarcinogen with other primary carcinogens. Since this mode of action carries considerably different implications than would a primary carcinogen, priority in research should be given to clarifying this interaction. To this end, further work with animals would be desirable along the lines of the experiments of Stënback [4] and Kuratsune et al. [5], in which the carcinogenicity of alcohol acting alone and in combination with other agents was examined.

In humans, studies should focus on establishing whether different vehicles or types of alcoholic beverages are related to different sites of cancer [10, 13, 19, 32]. There is reason to suspect that consumption of vodka, which is essentially diluted pure ethanol [1], might be less carcinogenic than spirits with more congeners or contaminants, such as bourbon or Scotch whiskey. Research in this area would help elucidate the mechanism of action by which alcoholic beverages increase cancer risk.

REFERENCES

1. Murphree, H. Effects of alcoholic beverages containing large and small amounts of congeners. *In* Sardesai, V.M., ed. *Biochemical and Clinical Aspects of Metabolism* (Chap. 25). Charles C. Thomas, Springfield, Ill., 1969.

2. Lijinsky, W., and Epstein S.S. Nitrosamines as environmental carcinogens. *Nature (Lond.) 225:*21–23, 1970

3. Editorial: Esophageal carcinoma in Africa. *Lancet i:* 622, 1972.

4. Stënback, F. The tumorigenic effect of ethanol. *Acta Pathol. Microbiol. Scand. 77:* 325–326, 1969.

5. Kuratsune, M., Kohchi, S., Horie, A., et al. Test of alcoholic beverages and ethanol solutions for carcinogenicity and tumor-promoting activity. *Gann 62:*395–405, 1971.

6. Schmidt, W., and de Lint, J. Causes of death of alcoholics. *Q. J. Stud. Alcohol 33:* 171–185, 1972.

7. Pell, S., and D'Alonzo, C.A. A five-year mortality study of alcoholics. *J. Occup. Med. 15:*120–125, 1973.

8. Monson, R.R., and Lyons, J.L. Proportional mortality among alcoholics. *Cancer.* In press, 1975.

9. Hakulinen, T., Lehtimaki, L., Lektonen, M., et al. Cancer morbidity among two male cohorts with increased alcohol consumption in Finland. *J. Natl. Cancer Inst. 52:*1711–1714, 1974.

10. Wynder, E.L., Bross, I.J., and Feldman, R. A study of etiological factors in cancer of the mouth. *Cancer 10:*1300–1323, 1957.

11. Vincent, R.G., and Marchetta, F. The relationship of the use of tobacco and alcohol to cancer of the oral cavity, pharynx or larynx. *Am. J. Surg. 106:*501–505, 1963.

12. Keller, A.Z., and Terris, M. The association of alcohol and tobacco with cancer of the mouth and pharynx. *Am. J. Public Health 55:*1578–1585, 1965.

13. Wynder, E.L., Bross, I.J., and Day, E. Epidemiological approach to the etiology of cancer of the larynx. *J.A.M.A. 160:*1384-1391, 1956.

14. Wynder, E.L., and Bross, I.J. A study of etiological factors in cancer of the esophagus. *Cancer 14:*389-413, 1961.

15. Martinez, I. Factors associated with cancer of the esophagus, mouth and pharynx in Puerto Rico. *J. Natl. Cancer Inst. 42:*1069-1094, 1969.

16. Rothman, K.J., and Keller, A.Z. The effect of joint exposure to alcohol and tobacco on risk of cancer of the mouth and pharynx. *J. Chron. Dis. 25:*711-716, 1972.

17. Rothman, K.J. Synergy and antagonism in cause-effect relationships. *Am. J. Epidemiol. 99:*385-388, 1974.

18. Kmet, J., and Mahboubi, E. Esophageal cancer in the Caspian littoral of Iran: Initial studies. *Science 175:*846-853, 1972.

19. Tuyns, A.J. Cancer of the esophagus; further evidence of the relation to drinking habits in France. *Int. J. Cancer 5:*152-156, 1970.

20. Schoenberg, B.S., Bailar, J.C., III, and Fraumeni, J.F., Jr. Certain mortality patterns of esophageal cancer in the United States, 1930-67. *J. Natl. Cancer Inst. 46:*63-73, 1971.

21. Kamionkowski, M.D., and Fleshler, B. The role of alcohol intake in esophageal carcinoma. *Am. J. Med. Sci. 249:*696-700, 1965.

22. Doll, R. The geographical distribution of cancer. *Br. J. Cancer 23:*1-8, 1969.

23. Mahboubi, E., Kmet, J., Cook, P.J., et al. Oesophageal cancer study in the Caspian littoral of Iran: The Caspian Center Registry. *Br. J. Cancer 28:*197-214, 1973.

24. Mahboubi, E. Epidemiologic study of esophageal cancer in Iran. *Int. Surg. 56:*68-71, 1971.

25. deJong, U.W., Breslow, N., Goh Ewe Hong, J., et al. Aetiological factors in oesophageal cancer in Singapore Chinese. *Int. J. Cancer 13:*291-303, 1974.

26. Cook, P. Cancer of the oesophagus in Africa. *Br. J. Cancer 25:*853-880, 1971.

27. MacDonald, W.C. Clinical and pathologic features of adenocarcinoma of the gastric cardia. *Cancer 29:*724-732, 1973.

28. Parker, R.G.F. The incidence of primary hepatic carcinoma in cirrhosis. *Proc. R. Soc. Med. 50:*145-147, 1957.

29. Leevy, C.M., Gellene, R., and Ning, M. Primary liver cancer in cirrhosis of the alcoholic. *Ann. N. Y. Acad. Sci. 114:*1026-1040, 1964.

30. Lee, F.I. Cirrhosis and hepatoma in alcoholics. *Gut 7:*77-85, 1966.

31. International Agency for Research on Cancer: *Alcohol and Cancer Report.* Interim report. I.A.R.C., Lyons, December 1973.

32. Breslow, N.E., and Enstrom, J.E. Geographic correlations between cancer mortality rates and alcohol-tobacco consumption in the United States. *J. Natl. Cancer Inst. 53:*631-639, 1974.

33. Lowenfels, A.B. Alcohol and cancer. *N.Y. State J. Med. 74:*56-59, 1974.

34. Murray, J.L., and Axtell, L.M. Impact of cancer: years of life lost due to cancer mortality. *J. Natl. Cancer Inst. 52:*3-7, 1974.

35. Ferber, B., Handy, V.H., Gerhardt, P.R., et al. *Cancer in New York State Exclusive of New York City, 1941-1960.* Bureau of Cancer Control, New York State Department of Health, 1962.

36. Kissin, B., Kaley, M.M., Su, W.H., et al. Head and neck cancer in alcoholics; the relationship to drinking, smoking and dietary patterns. *J.A.M.A. 224:*1174-1175, 1973.

DISCUSSION

Dr. **Rothman** concluded his paper by recommending two central areas for future research: 1) study of the mode of action of alcohol as a carcinogen or cocarcinogen, and 2) further experimental work in animals. The discussion pursued these two themes. **Dr. Higginson** emphasized that it is alcoholic *beverages,* not alcohol per se, that may be related to certain cancers. He pointed out that the solvent action of ethanol has never been adequately investigated. Wines, for example, are known to contain some 1,500 substances, and the possible carcinogenic or cocarcinogenic effect of alcoholic beverages may reflect the combination of the solvent action of ethanol and the various compounds dissolved. **Dr. Rothman** agreed that the etiologic agents may be the impurities and compounds in wines, rather than the ethanol or tannic acid content. In France, there is some evidence that the geographic distribution of esophageal cancer corresponds with the regional differences in wine produced and, presumably, consumed.

Pursuing this point, **Dr. Henderson** inquired whether the high rates of esophageal cancer among black populations might be related to patterns of consumption of alcoholic beverages containing various impurities and/or carcinogens. **Dr. Rothman** said that the high incidence of esophageal cancer in Puerto Rico may reflect consumption of locally brewed impure rum. Similarly, a high incidence of esophageal cancer is reported in some areas of France where homemade apple cider is consumed.

Dr. Saffiotti pointed out that it is not clear whether alcohol functions as a carcinogen, or cocarcinogen, or through an indirect mechanism (e.g., alteration of the bacterial flora of the gastrointestinal tract). Secondly, evaluation of the carcinogenic or cocarcinogenic effect of alcohol will be difficult if the active ingredients are the impurities, because the competing toxic effect of ethanol may prevent the application of sufficient dosage of this compound. **Dr. Hirohata** stressed the difficulties in extrapolating results from animal studies to human populations. His group has successfully fed alcohol (Vat 69 and Johnny Walker Scotch) to rats and mice and has available some quantitative information, but estimation of the absolute and relative risk factors in man requires a population study.

Dr. Wynder discussed the problems encountered in trying to disentangle the effects of alcohol and tobacco in relation to cancer. He referred especially to pancreatic cancer, where the role of alcoholic beverage consumption and smoking is still not clear. The few available studies that control for the effect of tobacco report contradictory results. In his own material from Memorial Hospital, where the data were standardized for tobacco usage, no association was found between alcohol consumption and cancer of the pancreas.

Concluding the discussion, both **Dr. Wynder** and **Dr. Rothman** stated that, despite our fragmentary knowledge of the specific etiologic agent, it is clear that two-thirds of cancers associated with consumption of alcoholic beverages and smoking could be prevented by eliminating the smoking factor. Similarly, in patients with one primary lesion, steps could be taken by the clinician to prevent development of a second malignancy.

Josef Vana

10

RADIATION

Seymour Jablon

Follow-Up Agency
National Academy of Sciences
Washington, D.C.

INTRODUCTION

In 1972, the United Nations Scientific Committee on the Effects of Atomic Radiation (UNSCEAR) stated: "It is generally accepted that cancer is the major long-term somatic effect of radiation on human beings" [1]. The first definite evidence that a form of cancer, leukemia, was associated in man with chronic exposure to ionizing radiation was published in 1944, when March [2] reported that radiologists were 10 times as likely as other physicians to die of leukemia. He obtained his data by scanning the obituary notices in the *Journal of the American Medical Association* for the period 1929-1943. Ulrich [3], using a similar methodology, obtained a comparable result for 1935-1944; finally March [4], in 1950, covered the 20-year period 1929-1948 and reported that 4.7 percent of all deaths among radiologists were attributable to leukemia, as contrasted with 0.5 percent for other physicians.

The suspicion that ionizing radiation might cause leukemia had been raised by experimental results (many of which are cited by March), the earliest dating back to 1906 [5]. In 1944, Henshaw and Hawkins [6] also noted that the incidence of leukemia in physicians as a class was 1.7 times that in the general population; they related this increased risk to use of and exposure to X-rays by many physicians.

The difficulties in obtaining exact information regarding the leukemogenic or, more generally, carcinogenic effects of ionizing radiation are great: Even after very large doses, the probability that cancer will occur is but a few percent, latent periods extend at least as long as 3 decades, and accurate information regarding doses received is often lacking. Nevertheless, the importance of the problem is so great that investigators have studied virtually every large irradiated group that could be identified.

Interest in the problem of radiation carcinogenesis has its roots in two rather different considerations. First, to establish standards for population or occupational exposures to radiation requires a balancing of benefits against risks. Such an exercise is, at best, difficult, but becomes impossible lacking numeric estimates of the cancer risk attendant upon particular levels of exposure. The second consideration is deeper. When we completely understand the process of radiation carcinogenesis, we shall be a long way toward understanding carcinogenesis in general.

Radiation leukemogenesis differs from other radiation carcinogenesis in two important ways: First, as will be discussed, the minimum latent period for leukemia is no more than 2 years as against at least 5 for other cancers; and second, leukemia is a rare enough disease that cases which are, with high probability, radiation-induced can be identified in heavily exposed groups and their characteristics studied. For other radiation-induced tumors this identification is impossible, except for some of those resulting from ingested radionuclides.

The kinds of ionizing radiation that will be discussed include photons (X-rays and gamma rays), uncharged particles (neutrons), and charged particles (electrons, or beta particles and helium nuclei, or alpha particles).

Radiation dose is measured in rads, 1 rad being the quantity of radiation that deposits 100 ergs per gram of tissue. An important quality of radiation is linear energy transfer (LET) which measures the rate at which energy is deposited along the photon or particle path. Typical values of LET, measured in keV per micron, are 100 for 5 MeV alpha particles, 20 for 2.5 MeV neutrons, and 0.30 for 1.33 $MeV^{60}Co$ gamma rays. Thus, the distribution of energy along gamma-ray tracks is some 60 times sparser than along neutron tracks. Energy deposition from neutron or alpha particle irradiation is markedly nonuniform in tissue of some size, as in a man's trunk, much more so than that from X-rays.

Radiations of different kinds have quite different effects in biological systems for equal energy deposition (dose). It is customary in radiobiology, therefore, to characterize radiation by its relative biological effectiveness (RBE) using X-rays or gamma rays as a standard. For example, to say that a given kind of radiation has an RBE of 5 means that 100 rads would produce the same effect as 500 rads of X-rays. However, because for many biological effects the response to X-rays is not a linear function of the dose, the RBE is not a function merely of the two kinds of radiation being compared, but varies with the dose and also with the particular effect being studied.

RADIOGENIC LEUKEMIA

Whole-Body Irradiation

The groups exposed to whole-body irradiation include physicians, especially radiologists and other specialists who commonly use X-ray equipment; X-ray technologists; and the populations of Hiroshima and Nagasaki who received radiation, chiefly gamma rays and neutrons, coming from the atomic explosions.

Several authors reported the excessive occurrence of leukemia among physicians, especially radiologists [2-4,6,7]. The relative risk for American radiologists in comparison with other physicians is reported as between 4.3 [7] and 9.2 [4]. These estimates apply to radiologists who survived beyond age 50, who therefore entered practice at a time when risks from radiation exposure were not appreciated and who were exposed over many decades. It is difficult to estimate the doses received by radiologists in the early years, hence the data are of limited value for purposes of numerical risk estimations. Nevertheless, the reports [8], establish clearly that chronic, repeated exposures to relatively small doses of radiation of the order of 0.4 to 2 rads per week can increase the risk of leukemia severalfold.

Court Brown and Doll [9], however, found no evidence of an increased incidence of leukemia among British radiologists who entered the specialty after 1920, and only a small increase among those who entered before that time. They conjectured that the reason for the discrepancy was the smaller doses received by radiologists in Britain, who exercised greater precautions than those in the United States.

Miller and Jablon [10] studied men who served as X-ray technicians in the United States Army during World War II and found only a very small (statistically nonsignificant) excess of deaths attributed to leukemia over an 18-year follow-up period. Presumably, the doses received by these men were insufficient to produce an observable leukemia effect.

Among the most useful epidemiologic data are those derived from the experience of the Japanese atomic-bomb survivors [11]. Nearly 24,000 had radiation doses estimated at 10 rads or more, and the fact that the exposures occurred at a fixed moment in time enables determination of the distribution of latent periods between exposure and onset of disease or death.

Leukemia was first identified in 1948 among the survivors who had received large doses [12]; thus, the minimum latent period was a little over 2 years. Incidence reached a peak in 1951-1952, after which it declined slowly. As late as 1970-1972, however, the leukemia death rate was still significantly elevated among survivors who had received doses of 100 rads or more [13]. Among the survivors, two-thirds of the leukemias were acute; the remainder were chronic myeloid. Chronic lymphatic leukemia (CLL) did not increase.

Partial-Body Irradiation

Preeminent among the studies of leukemia after partial-body irradiation is that of Court Brown and Doll [14,15], who followed more than 14,000 British spondylitis patients for periods ranging from 5 to 25 years. Follow-up information was obtained from death certificates. The observed number of deaths from leukemia was nearly 10 times expectation (52 vs 5.48) and from aplastic anemia nearly 30 times (15 vs 0.51). However, after reviewing pathological material of the 15 cases diagnosed as aplastic anemia, the authors state that 8 were likely to be misdiagnosed cases of leukemia, 4 were probable cases of aplastic anemia, and for the remainder neither diagnosis could be justified by the available clinical material. The latent periods observed were like those seen in the Japanese survivors—mortality from leukemia reached a peak in the interval 3 to 5 years after irradiation, then declined slowly. There was but a single leukemia death more than 15 years after exposure, but few subjects had been observed for as long as 20 years.

Among the British spondylitis cases, as among the Japanese atomic-bomb survivors, CLL was not increased; over 80 percent were acute leukemias, and most of the remainder, chronic myeloid.

Other, smaller therapy series showing an increased leukemia risk include women treated for menorrhagia [16,17], children irradiated for supposedly enlarged thymus glands [18], and children treated for tinea capitis [19]. However, in some studies, patients treated with radiation for cervical cancer had no subsequent increased risk of leukemia [20,21]. Hutchison's report [20] is especially noteworthy, since it is based on more than 20,000 patients. A possible explanation of the negative results in these instances is that very large radiation doses given to sharply circumscribed regions of the body may effectively sterilize the cells within the zone of irradiation.

Internal Emitters

Reports of studies of leukemia after the administration of ^{131}I or ^{32}P have conflicted. Pochin [22] and Brincker et al. [23] found a significant excess among patients treated with ^{131}I for thyroid carcinoma, as did Modan and Lilienfeld [24] in polycythemia vera patients treated with ^{32}P. A large increase in the risk of leukemia was also reported among patients injected with Thorotrast [25,26]. On the other hand, large-scale studies of patients treated with ^{131}I for hyperthyroidism [27-29] showed no significant increase in leukemia from the rate in patients not so treated; however, the radiation doses were much smaller among these patients than among those treated for carcinoma.

Risk Estimates

Table 1 summarizes the risks for leukemia in relation to radiation dose, adapted from the BEIR report [30]. Only those studies are cited for which explicit risk estimates could be made. It is plain that there is good overall agreement among the various studies as to the risks per rad of leukemia and that children are more sensitive than adults. For children, there are about three

TABLE 1
Risk estimates for leukemia [30]

Population	Reference no.	No. of subjects	Dose in rads[a] Range	Dose in rads[a] Mean	Relative risk (O/E)[b]	Cases induced per million PYR
Age at exposure: under 10 years						
A-bomb survivors	33	4,507	10-600	69	19/2.93 = 6.5	2.6
Thymus X-ray recipients	18	1,451	<60-600+	65	6/0.96 = 6.2	3.0
Tinea capitis patients	19	2,043	200-400	30	4/0.9 = 4.4	3.4
Age at exposure: 10 years or more						
A-bomb survivors	33	19,472	10-600	86	62/16.8 = 3.7	1.5
Menorrhagia patients	16	2,068	550-1,050	136	6/1.3 = 4.6	1.2
Spondylitis patients	15	14,554	250-2,750	372	52/5.48 = 9.5	0.9

[a] Range is given for external dose; mean dose is mean dose to marrow, except for atomic-bomb survivors, for whom it is mean external dose. Risk estimates are based on mean dose.
[b] O/E = observed-to-expected ratio.

cases of leukemia induced per million person-year-rads (PYR) over a 20-to-25-year follow-up period, whereas for adults the corresponding figure appears to be 1 to 1.5.

As Table 1 shows, all risk estimates are derived from experience after relatively large doses. No data are available or are ever likely to be regarding the effect of very small doses, since the required population sizes are enormous for assessing the leukemogenic potential for man of, say, 100 millirad. Therefore, the risk estimates quoted involve the *assumption* that the risk per rad is independent of dose level and dose rate. However, it is known that in many experimental situations, although a linear dose response function is found over a wide range of doses for high LET radiation, for low LET radiation the response is more nearly represented by a second degree function and is decreased at a low dose rate. It has been suggested [31,32], in fact, that the leukemogenic response to gamma rays follows a square law and, presumably, involves a double-stranded DNA break as an essential element in the initiation of the leukemogenic process [32].

RADIOGENIC CANCERS OTHER THAN LEUKEMIA

External Irradiation

Among the Japanese atomic-bomb survivors, excessive mortality from cancer excluding leukemia was observed beginning about 1960, some 15 years after exposure, among persons whose doses were estimated at more than 100 rads [33]. Although relative risk was greatest among children exposed below age 10 [34], absolute risks were greater in adults, being 1.2 deaths per million PYR in children, but 4.7 per million PYR in adults [30]. The cancers that occurred among exposed children included widely metastasizing thyroid tumors, brain tumors, salivary gland tumors, and cancers of the gastrointestinal system [34]. Among adults, the excess cancer mortality was principally accounted for by respiratory cancers, breast cancer, cancer of the gastrointestinal system, excluding the stomach [33], and lymphosarcoma [35]. Interestingly, no excesses were seen with respect to gastric cancer or cancer of the uterus, both of which are of high incidence in Japan. In addition to the fatal cancers, carcinoma of the thyroid gland was found greatly increased among Japanese survivors who received physical examinations under the Adult Health Study program of the Atomic Bomb Casualty Commission [36]. The increases occurred primarily among persons who received radiation doses exceeding 200 rads when they were under age 40.

Similarly, among the British spondylitis patients, mortality from cancers of heavily irradiated sites was apparently increased some 6 years after the first course of radiotherapy [15]. In these patients, excesses were especially notable for cancers of the pharynx, pancreas, bronchi, and lymphatic and hemopoietic system, other than leukemia. The only notable point of discrepancy is that among the spondylitics, gastric cancer was significantly increased (relative risk, 1.7) but not among the Japanese survivors.

Among children irradiated for supposedly enlarged thymus glands, in addition to the increase in leukemia previously mentioned, very large excesses were found for thyroid carcinoma and tumors of the salivary glands [18].

An increased risk of breast cancer has been reported among women exposed to fairly large doses of radiation. Among the atomic-bomb survivors, the increases in relative risk were most notable among those 10 to 19 years of age at exposure [33,37], whose doses were estimated at 50 rads or more. Similarly, increases in breast cancer were found among women treated with X-ray for post-partum mastitis [38] and among women who received multiple fluoroscopies while being treated with artificial pneumothorax for pulmonary tuberculosis [39].

Although, as mentioned above, radiation therapy for carcinoma of the cervix has not resulted in any apparent increase in leukemia, an increased risk of malignancy of the uterine corpus has been reported [40], the cases occurring 5 to 18 years after the X-ray therapy.

Specific cancer risks in relation to radiation dose, adapted from the BEIR report [30], are shown in Table 2. Although the risk estimates derived from different surveys do not always agree, it is perhaps surprising that the variation is no larger than it is. The greatest variation is in the risk for breast cancer, where the largest estimate is 6 times the smallest. However, as mentioned above, breast cancer risks are strongly related to age at irradiation, so variation among different series is to be expected. Moreover, the risk for breast cancer *incidence* would be perhaps twice the risk for breast cancer *mortality*, and would be marked by a shorter latent period.

Internal Emitters

The principal groups of persons who have had substantial exposure to internal alpha-particle emitters are the radium dial painters; patients treated with radium, chiefly in Germany; patients in whom thorium dioxide (Thorotrast) was used as a contrast medium for roentgenographic purposes; and certain groups of miners exposed to high atmospheric levels of radon. Alpha particles, as mentioned previously, have very high LET. Accordingly, their energy is released within a short range in tissue so that cells in the immediate vicinity of the emitter receive extraordinarily large radiation doses, while cells at some distance receive little or none. The tissues at risk are, therefore, those proximate to the sites of deposition of the radionuclides.

Radium-226 and thorium-232 have very long half-lives; hence, following their ingestion and lodgment, the subject receives continuous radiation. Radon-

TABLE 2

Risk estimates for cancer excluding leukemia following external radiation [30]

Population	Reference No.	No. of subjects	Dose in rads Range	Dose in rads Mean	Relative risk (O/E)	Cases induced per million PYR
All cancer excluding leukemia (mortality)						
Atomic-bomb survivors, under 10 years	33	4,507	10-600	69	6/2.1 = 2.9	1.2
Atomic-bomb survivors, age 10 or more	33	19,472	10-600	86	615/544 = 1.13	4.7
Spondylitis patients[a]	15	14,554	250-2,750	400[b]	631/285 = 2.2	4.6
Thyroid cancer (incidence)						
Atomic-bomb survivors, under 10 years	34	811	10-600	143	6/1.6 = 3.8	1.9
Thymus X-ray recipients, under 10 years	18	2,878	5-1,200	229	19/0.14 = 136	2.5
Breast cancer (mortality)						
Atomic-bomb survivors, age 10 or more	33	11,968	10-600	81	26/12.9 = 2.0	1.4
Fluoroscopy recipients	39	243	50-7,000	1,215	10.5	8.4
Mastitis patients	38	606	50-450	200	11/4.23 = 2.6	6.0
Lung cancer (mortality)						
A-bomb survivors	33	19,472	10-600	86	71/56.8 = 1.25	0.93
Spondylitis patients	15	14,554	250-2,750	400	96/54.2 = 1.8	1.2

158

222 has a short half-life, but its radioactive daughters (isotopes of polonium, lead, and bismuth) have half-lives ranging up to 21 years. These daughter products, attached to small airborne particles, are inhaled and deposited in the bronchial tree.

Radium has chemical activity similar to calcium and, like calcium, tends to be incorporated into bone. One isotope, radium-224, which was used in the therapy of ankylosing spondylitis and of tuberculosis, has a half-life of less than 4 days; unlike radium-226, therefore, most energy is released while the radium is at the bone surface, rather than after incorporation into the matrix.

Data on follow-up studies of the radium cases are cited in the 1972 UNSCEAR report [1]. Among 780 former radium dial painters, 71 presumably induced tumors have been identified, 51 of them bone sarcomas, and 20 carcinomas of the paranasal sinuses and mastoid. All these tumors developed among the 238 persons whose accumulated doses exceeded 700 rads; 30 percent of those with doses over 700 rads developed them.

Among 925 juveniles treated with radium-224 (half-life, 3.6 days), mostly for bone tuberculosis, 43 bone sarcomas were identified during a 25-year follow-up period. The lowest dose for which a sarcoma was seen exceeded 300 rads, but few patients had received smaller doses.

A series of 2,428 persons who received Thorotrast in Portugal between 1930 and 1955 was studied by da Silva Horta and others [26]. Although only 1,178 were completely traced through 1970, the occurrence of cancers in this sub-group is very great. There were 12 deaths from leukemia, at least 5 times the number expected at population rates. A more notable finding was the unusually high rate of liver cancer, most frequently hemangioendothelioma, although cholangiocarcinomas and hepatomas also occurred. Of 23 histologically confirmed liver cancers, 15 were hemangioendotheliomas, 6 cholangiocarcinomas, and 2 hepatomas. Because of the incomplete follow-up and great difficulty in obtaining adequate dosimetry for these Thorotrast patients, it is almost impossible to compute estimates of cancer risk per rad. Similarly, van Kaick and his colleagues [25] studied causes of death among 1,050 Thorotrast patients in Germany and found in addition to the increase in leukemia previously mentioned 94 deaths attributed to liver cancer, more than 20 times the proportion in 800 control deaths. Most of the liver cancer deaths occurred 15 to 30 years after Thorotrast injection, with the peak at 25 to 30 years.

Miners who work in radon-containing air are known to be at high risk of lung cancer. Among these groups [1] are miners in Czechoslovakia and Saxony, fluorspar miners in Canada, and iron-ore miners in Britain. Assessment of radon dosage is very difficult for miners, and it is only for the uranium miners in Colorado that the Working Level Month (WLM) could be devised as at least a rough index to exposure. Lung cancer mortality increased with increasing cumulative WLM, reaching nearly 24 times expectation in the group with greatest exposure. Most of the excess lung cancer cases were accounted for by small-cell and undifferentiated tumors.

Most of the miners studied were cigarette smokers; the separate roles of smoking and radon exposure in the causation of the lung cancers cannot be described explicitly nor can it be determined whether the two effects act independently or whether there is synergism. Clearly, however, even after standardization for smoking, radon exposure is strongly related to lung cancer.

Finally, among 53 residents of Rongelap (Marshall Islands) exposed in 1954 to fallout from a weapons test, 3 (5.7 percent) developed carcinomas of the thyroid gland in addition to nearly one-third who had benign adenomatous nodules. The doses to the thyroid of ingested radioiodine are estimated to have ranged from 160 to 1,400 rads.

PRENATAL IRRADIATION

Stewart et al. [41] reported that children, irradiated as fetuses during diagnostic X-rays given their mothers, had a nearly twofold excess risk of dying from leukemia or other cancer before the age of 10. Following this report, Stewart and her colleagues studied a vastly increased number of cases and addressed various collateral questions. This work led to investigations by several others who sought to confirm her findings. In 1962 MacMahon [42] found a relative risk of 1.52 for death from all cancers within 10 years of birth among children irradiated in utero. Graham et al. [43] and other investigators also confirmed this work with respect to leukemia.

Nevertheless, the question has remained whether the prenatal X-ray was the *cause* of the subsequent cancer, or merely associated with its occurrence through the operation of various possible forms of bias. Stewart and Kneale [44] estimated from the Oxford Survey data that the carcinogenic effect of X-ray on the fetus, during the first 10 years of postnatal life, was 57 deaths per million PYR. An effect of this magnitude implies that among the fetuses exposed to radiation from the atomic bombs in Japan, about 37 deaths from cancer should have occurred during 1945-1955 among the 1,292 exposed children. In fact, however, there was only 1 such death, and the number to be expected at Japanese national death rates was 0.75 [45].

Diamond et al. [46] did a prospective study involving more than 55,000 children, almost equally divided between white and black; one-third of the children received X-rays and two-thirds were controls. The results were surprising. Among the black children, X-ray seemed to carry no risk, whether of death from leukemia, from other cancers, or from other causes. Among white children treated with X-ray, there was a relative risk of 2.9 for death from leukemia, but 0.87 for other cancers. For leukemia and other cancers combined, the risk was 1.50, virtually identical with that found by MacMahon [42]. But, most remarkably, the relative risk for death from all causes *except* cancer was 1.9 among the white children, and from accidents, in particular, was 2.0!

Further, the finding of Graham et al. [43], that the relative risk of death from leukemia was 1.56 for X-ray of the mother *during* the pregnancy and 1.55 for X-ray *prior to* the relevant conception has raised further serious question whether the association of prenatal X-ray with childhood cancer is, in fact, causal, or a reflection of unknown biases.

NONIONIZING RADIATION

Ultraviolet Radiation

Ultraviolet radiation differs from most ionizing radiation in two important ways beyond not causing ionizations: it has low penetrating ability in biologic materials; and its absorption in biologic material is markedly nonrandom, occurring principally in conjugated systems such as nucleic acids and proteins [47]. Thus, ultraviolet radiation is highly damaging to DNA, principally to DNA contained in epidermal cells.

It is not surprising, therefore, that exposure to ultraviolet radiation appears to be associated with the occurrence of skin cancer. Emmett, in an extensive review of the literature [48], cites a strong association between cumulative exposure to the sun and squamous cell carcinoma of the skin; a somewhat weaker association with basal cell epithelioma; and a much less clearcut association with malignant melanoma, except for the particular type designated "lentigo maligna melanoma." On the other hand, an ad hoc committee of the National Academy of Sciences recently asserted [49] that for a Caucasian population living at 40° latitude (Philadelphia) no less than 40 percent of the melanomas and 80 percent of the squamous and basal cell carcinomas are caused by ultraviolet light.

It is difficult to establish precise risk estimates for ultraviolet light induction of skin cancer. Both basal and squamous cell carcinomas are relatively benign lesions with low mortality, and published data probably understate their true incidence by a wide margin. However, melanoma mortality rates among white males are about 75 percent larger in the band of states from Louisiana to South Carolina than in the band from Washington to Minnesota; for other skin cancer, the corresponding ratio is about 2.5 [50].

Microwave Radiation

Microwave radiation, such as emitted by radar equipment or microwave ovens, transmits energy to biological systems as heat [51]. Although the effects are not completely understood, it appears that the thermal effects are the most important. No ionizations are produced by microwaves. Although a number of deleterious effects of microwaves on mammalian systems have been identified, there are no data to suggest that cancer induction is included among them [52].

INDICATIONS FOR FUTURE WORK

Although much work on assessing radiation cancer risks has been done, present knowledge is not adequate to satisfy society's needs. For example, data are beginning to become available regarding the value of screening programs that include mammography in reducing case fatality rates for breast cancer. Are breast cancers induced in well women by radiation received during the screening examination? If so, how many, and how does this number compare with the number of lives saved? These questions cannot be answered now with any accuracy, and it is necessary to exploit the few series that can provide the needed answers. Although there are many groups of irradiated persons, radiation doses must be known and follow-up be reasonably complete and of long duration—30 years or more—to obtain adequate risk estimates. Only a few studies of irradiated groups meet these criteria, and they must be prosecuted vigorously.

A second opportunity exists in the careful study of the carcinogenic effects of different kinds of radiation. Alpha particles, neutrons, and photons vary greatly as to the distribution of their energy within the cell on a microscale. It is possible to exploit these differences to learn about the probable sizes of targets involved in the intracellular cancerogenic event induced by radiation. Such studies have already begun with respect to leukemogenesis, and further work of this kind should be actively pursued. Progress in this area probably will require close collaboration and interaction between epidemiologists and laboratory scientists. Finding mechanisms that will foster the needed interdisciplinary cross-fertilizations is an important task for research administrators.

REFERENCES

1. United Nations Scientific Committee on the Effects of Atomic Radiation. *Ionizing Radiation: Levels and Effects. Effects.* Volume II. United Nations, New York, 1972.
2. March, H.C. Leukemia in radiologists. *Radiology 43:*275–278, 1944.
3. Ulrich, H. The incidence of leukemia in radiologists. *N. Engl. J. Med. 234:*45–46, 1946.
4. March, H.C. Leukemia in radiologists in a 20-year period. *Am. J. Med. Sci. 220:*282–286, 1950.
5. Ziegler, K. Experimentelle und Klinische Untersuchungen uber die Histogenese der Myeloischen Leukamie, Gustave Fischer, Jena, 1906.
6. Henshaw, P.S., and Hawkins, J.W. Incidence of leukemia in physicians. *J. Natl. Cancer Inst. 4:*339–346, 1944.

7. Seltser, R., and Sartwell, P.E. The influence of occupational exposure to radiation on the mortality of American radiologists and other medical specialists. *Am. J. Epidemiol. 81:*2–22, 1965.

8. Warren, S. Longevity and causes of death from irradiation in physicians. *J. A.M. A 162:*464–468, 1956.

9. Court Brown, W.M., and Doll, R. Expectation of life and mortality from cancer among British radiologists. *Br. Med. J. 2:*181–187, 1958.

10. Miller, R.W., and Jablon, S. A search for late radiation effects among men who served as X-ray technologists in the U.S. Army during World War II. *Radiology 96:*269–274, 1970.

11. Ishimaru, T., Hoshino, T., Ichimaru, M., et al. Leukemia in atomic bomb survivors. Hiroshima and Nagasaki, 1 October 1950-30 September 1966. *Radiat. Res. 45:*216–233, 1971.

12. Brill, A.B., Tomonaga, M., and Heyssel, R.M. Leukemia in man following exposure to ionizing radiation: summary of findings in Hiroshima and Nagasaki, and comparison with other human experience. *Ann. Intern. Med. 56:*590–609, 1962.

13. Moriyama, I.M., and Kato, H. *JNIH-ABCC Life Span Study Report 7: Mortality Experience of A-Bomb Survivors, 1970-72, 1950-72.* Atomic Bomb Casualty Commission Technical Report 15-73, Hiroshima, Japan, 1973.

14. Court Brown, W.M., and Doll, R. *Leukemia and Aplastic Anemia in Patients Irradiated for Ankylosing Spondylitis.* Her Majesty's Stat. Off., London, 1957.

15. Court Brown, W.M., and Doll, R. Mortality from cancer and other causes after radiotherapy for ankylosing spondylitis. *Br. Med. J. 2:*1327–1332, 1965.

16. Alderson, M.R., and Jackson, S.M.: Long-term follow-up of patients with menorrhagia treated by irradiation. *Br. J. Radiol. 44:*295-298, 1971.

17. Doll, R., and Smith, P.G. The long-term effects of X-irradiation in patients treated for metropathia hemorrhagica, *Br. J. Radiol. 41:*362–368, 1968.

18. Hempelmann, L.H., Pifer, J.W., Burke, G.J., et al. Neoplasms in persons treated with X-rays in infancy for thymic enlargement: A report on the third follow-up survey. *J. Natl. Cancer Inst. 38:*317–341, 1967.

19. Albert, E.R., and Omran, A.R. Follow-up study of patients treated by X-ray epilation for tinea capitis. *Arch. Environ. Health 17:*899–950, 1968.

20. Hutchison, G.B. Leukemia in patients with cancer of the cervix uteri treated with radiation. A report covering the first five years of an international study. *J. Natl. Cancer Inst. 40:*951–982, 1968.

21. Zippin, C., Bailar, J.C., III, Kohn, H.I., et al. Radiation therapy for cervical cancer: Late effects on life span and on leukemia incidence. *Cancer 28:*937-942, 1971.

22. Pochin, E.E.: Long-term hazards of radioiodine treatment of thyroid carcinoma. *In* Hedinger, C., ed. *Thyroid Cancer,* UICC Monograph Series, Vol. 12, Springer-Verlag Berlin, 1969, pp. 293–304.

23. Brincker, H., Hansen, H.S., and Andersen, A.P. Induction of leukaemia by ^{131}I treatment of thyroid carcinoma. *Br. J. Cancer 28:*232–237, 1973.

24. Modan, B., and Lilienfeld, A.M. Polycythemia vera and leukemia—the role of radiation treatment. *Medicine 44:*305–344, 1965.

25. van Kaick, G., Muth, H., Lorenz, D., et al. *In* Mays, C.W., ed. *Proceedings of The International Symposium on Biological Effects of* [224]*Ra and Thorotrast.* Health Physics, In press, 1975.

26. Abbatt, J.D. Human leukemic risk data derived from Portuguese Thorotrast experience. *In Radionuclide Carcinogenesis, Proceedings of the 12th Annual Hanford Biology Symposium.* United States Atomic Energy Commission, 1973.

27. Saenger, E.L., Thomas, G.E., and Tompkins, E.A. Incidence of leukemia following treatment of hyperthyroidism. *J.A.M.A. 205:*855–862, 1968.

28. Pochin, E.E. Leukemia following radioiodine treatment of thyrotoxicosis. *Br. Med. J. 2:*1545–1550, 1960.

29. Werner, S.C., Gittelsohn, A.M., and Brill, A.B. Leukemia following radioiodine therapy of hyperthyroidism. *J.A.M.A. 177:*646–648, 1961.

30. Advisory Committee on the Biological Effects of Ionizing Radiations, National Academy of Sciences-National Research Council: *The Effects on Populations of Exposure to Low Levels of Ionizing Radiation.* U.S. Govt. Print. Off., Washington, D.C., 1972.

31. Mays, C.W., Lloyd, R.D., and Marshall, J.H. Malignancy risk to humans from total body X-ray irradiation. *In Proceedings Third International Congress of the International Radiation Protection Association,* 1973.

32. Jablon, S. Leukemia, lymphoma and radiation. *In Proceedings 11th-International Cancer Congress.* Excerpta Medica Int. Congr. Ser. No. 351, Vol. 3, pp. 239–243, 1975.

33. Jablon, S., and Kato, H. Studies of the mortality of A-bomb survivors. 5. Radiation dose and mortality, 1950–1970. *Radiat. Res. 50:*649–698, 1972.

34. Jablon, S., Tachikawa, K., Belsky, J.L., et al. Cancer in Japanese exposed as children to atomic bombs. *Lancet 1:*927–932, 1971.

35. Nishiyama, H., Anderson, R.E., Ishimaru, T., et al. The incidence of malignant lymphoma and multiple myeloma in Hiroshima and Nagasaki atomic bomb survivors, 1945–1965. *Cancer 32:*1301–1309, 1973.

36. Wood, J.W., Tamagaki, H., Neriishi, S., et al. Thyroid carcinoma in atomic bomb survivors, Hiroshima-Nagasaki. *Am. J. Epidemiol. 89:*4–14, 1969.

37. Wanebo, C.K., Johnson, K.G., Sato, K., et al. Breast cancer after exposure to the atomic bombing of Hiroshima and Nagasaki. *N. Engl. J. Med. 279:*667–671, 1968.

38. Mettler, F.A., Hempelmann, L.H., Dutton, A.M., et al. Breast neoplasms in women treated with X-rays for acute post-partum mastitis. *J. Natl. Cancer Inst. 43:*803–811, 1969.

39. Myrden, J.A., and Hiltz, J.E. Breast cancer following multiple fluoroscopies during artificial pneumothorax treatment of pulmonary tuberculosis. *Can. Med. Assoc. J. 100:*1032–1034, 1969.

40. Fehr, P.E., and Prem, K.A. Malignancy of the uterine corpus following irradiation therapy for squamous cell carcinoma of the cervix. *Am. J. Obstet. Gynecol. 119:*685–692, 1974.

41. Stewart, A., Webb, J., and Hewitt, D. A survey of childhood malignancies. *Br. Med. J. 1:*1495–1508, 1958.

42. MacMahon, B.: Prenatal X-ray exposure and childhood cancers. *J. Natl. Cancer Inst. 28:*1173–1191, 1962.

43. Graham, S., Levin, M.L., Lilienfeld, A.M., et al.: Preconception, intrauterine, and postnatal irradiation as related to leukemia. *Natl. Cancer Inst. Monogr. 19:*347–371, 1966.

44. Stewart, A., and Kneale, G.W. Radiation dose effects in relation to obstetric X-rays and childhood cancers. *Lancet 1:*1185–1188, 1970.

45. Jablon, S., and Kato, H. Childhood cancer in relation to prenatal exposure to atomic bomb radiation. *Lancet 2:*1000–1003, 1970.

46. Diamond, E.L., Schmerler, H., and Lilienfeld, A.M.: The relationship of intrauterine radiation to subsequent mortality and development of leukemia in children. *Am. J. Epidemiol. 97:*283–313, 1973.

47. Jagger, J. Ultraviolet effects. *In* Dalrymple, G.V., Gaulden, M.E., Kollmorgen, G.M., and Vogel, H.H. Jr., eds. *Medical Radiation Biology.* W.B. Saunders, Philadelphia, 1973.

48. Emmett, E.A. Ultraviolet radiation as a cause of skin tumors. *CRC Crit. Rev. Toxicol. 2:*211–255, 1973.

49. Environmental Studies Board, Ad Hoc Panel on the Biological Impacts of Ultra-
violet Radiation. *Biological Impacts of Increased Intensities of Solar Ultraviolet Radiation.*
National Academy of Sciences, Washington, D.C., 1973.
50. Burbank, F. Patterns in cancer mortality in the United States: 1950-1967.
*Natl. Cancer Inst. Monogr. 33:*1971.
51. Michaelson, S.M. Biological effects of microwave exposure. *In* Cleary, S.F., ed.
Biological Effects and Health Implications of Microwave Radiation DRH/DBE 70-2.
Symposium Proceedings. U.S. Department of Health, Education, and Welfare, Washington,
D.C., 1970.
52. Healer, J.: Review of studies of people occupationally exposed to radio frequency
radiation. *In* Cleary, S.F., ed. *Biological Effects and Health Implications of Microwave
Radiation DRH/DBE 70-2.* Symposium Proceedings. U.S. Department of Health, Education,
and Welfare, Washington, D.C., 1970.

DISCUSSION

Dr. R. W. Miller asked for clarification of statements on the rates of
energy deposition in tissue, particularly in relation to the effects on DNA. **Mr.
Jablon** replied that the leukemogenic response to neutrons appears to be
linear, whereas the response to photons (gamma rays) apparently follows a
square law. Furthermore, in vitro studies have shown that neutrons result in
double-stranded breaks in DNA; photons result in single-stranded breaks. Thus,
neutrons might act by a single DNA "hit" (i.e., one hit affecting two closely
spaced targets), whereas two separate hits usually would be required for photons
to have the same effect. **Dr. Miller** stated that, compared to the rates in
Nagasaki, the higher rates of leukemia at low-dose exposures in Hiroshima, where
the amount of neutron irradiation was relatively high, were consistent with such
a mechanism. **Mr. Jablon** agreed with this interpretation.

Dr. Houten commented that data from the Tri-State Leukemia Survey
indicated the amount of radiation accompanying a single abdominal X-ray film
resulted in an increased incidence of leukemia. A markedly elevated risk was observed in subsets of the surveyed population, for example, in children with asthma
who also had received prenatal irradiation. He also emphasized the possibility of
an effect from irradiation prior to conception. **Mr. Jablon** replied that no
elevation in leukemia rates was observed in the group of Japanese exposed pre-
natally during gestation to much higher levels of irradiation from the atomic
bomb.

Alan S. Morrison

11

OCCUPATION

Philip Cole, M.D., and Marlene B. Goldman

Department of Epidemiology
Harvard School of Public Health
Boston, Massachusetts

HISTORICAL PERSPECTIVES

The first systematic review of occupational hazards was Ramazzini's *De Morbis Artificum Diatriba,* published in 1700 [1]. It records the excess risk of breast cancer experienced by nuns; however, Ramazzini correctly suggested that this risk reflected celibacy and not the occupational endeavors of nuns. The first direct connection between an occupational exposure and risk of a specific cancer was that of chimney sweeping and cancer of the scrotum, pointed out by Pott in 1775 [2]. He recognized this association because he saw several affected chimney sweeps but little or none of the disease in persons with other occupations. We infer that the disease was exceedingly rare in general, and that the risk ratio for chimney sweeps was quite high. We can make no inference about the absolute risk of cancer of the scrotum among chimney sweeps; the disease may have been rare or common among them.

About 1880, Härting and Hesse [3] showed that "mountain disease" of Schneeberg and Joachimsthal was a lung neoplasm. This condition, a fatal chronic pulmonary disease, was recognized as an entity in the Middle Ages because of its frequent occurrence among young miners despite its rarity in the general population [4]. In 1895, the German surgeon, Rehn [5], published

The authors are indebted to Miss Rita Ouellet for assistance and to the American Cancer Society who supported Dr. Cole in his work by an award (PRA No. 115).

his perceptions on bladder cancer among dye workers. The observations suggesting a hazard to Rehn were different from those that led Pott, and Härting and Hesse to their conclusions. Bladder cancer was well recognized although uncommon in Rehn's day; however, he diagnosed three cases of bladder cancer over a relatively brief period among the workers at a small factory. Rehn's association was based not on an exceedingly high risk ratio (later observations suggest a risk ratio of 30 or so) but, rather, on the absolute high frequency of the disease among exposed persons.

During the past several decades, instances of occupational carcinogenesis have continued to be recognized both on the basis of an extremely high risk ratio (usually owing to the rarity of the disease in the general population) and a high incidence rate among exposed persons (e.g., lung cancer among uranium miners). The twentieth century has seen the development of the epidemiologic method, which has permitted the recognition of only moderate increases in risk, say threefold, even for cancers that are not rare in the general population. For example, a recent retrospective cohort study [6] of mortality among rubber workers suggests that they have a risk ratio of 3 of dying from leukemia, compared to the general male population.

It seems likely that existing epidemiologic methods will allow the identification of groups at high risk of cancer because of their occupational experience. These methods are imperfect, however, and limitations in study design and types of data should be borne in mind when occupational carcinogenesis is studied. Retrospective cohort studies, the type most often done in the study of occupational carcinogenesis, have two major disadvantages to overcome: the long time-lapse between the introduction of a carcinogen into the work environment and its recognition as such, and the reliance on mortality rather than incidence data. Both difficulties can be reduced by prospective cohort studies with continuous surveillance of the health of workers. Such studies, admittedly, would be feasible only for certain large, stable, occupational groups. They do offer the valuable opportunity, however, to discover all the major adverse health effects associated with a particular exposure.

Another approach to supplement the retrospective cohort study is the population-based case-control study. Very few have been done but they can be quite useful, both for quantifying recognized hazards and for identifying new ones. They probably should be undertaken only for diseases suspected to be caused in large part by occupational exposures and in populations where more than 2 or 3 percent of the individuals have sustained the exposure of interest.

OCCUPATION AS AN EPIDEMIOLOGIC VARIABLE

In the United States, among those of working age, about 75 percent of men and 40 percent of women are gainfully employed [7]. For most men and many women, employment is a major part of life's experience. Yet, despite their obvious significance, occupational exposures have not been of much concern to the general public. This indifference, and the great diversity of occupational exposures, make them particularly resistant to epidemiologic study.

There are many specific problems making occupation difficult to study. Many workers are unaware of the conditions surrounding them or the substances they handle. The latter difficulty often results because a particular agent is known by a trivial chemical or trade name. Many persons change occupations from time to time, and may forget or lose interest in the experiences of former occupations. Further difficulties result because many occupational titles have no specific exposure connotation—a single title may refer to occupations involving exposure to very different substances; equally problematic, a particular exposure may be sustained in occupations with dissimilar titles or duties. The value of occupational titles as an index of exposure is further reduced by their upward social drift, particularly on death certificates. These difficulties are vexing in case-control studies, which are dependent on memory, and in any study that uses titles rather than descriptions of duties or exposures to categorize occupations. Such studies, especially when negative, are not persuasive.

Two more difficulties affect virtually all studies of occupational carcinogenesis. Most cancers probably have an "incubation" period of 20 years or more. In industrialized countries, technologic advances and changing needs are such that many industries evolve rapidly. As they do, new jobs and exposures come into being and others cease to exist. Thus, a given study might uncover a carcinogenic exposure that has already ceased. At the same time, the more recent replacement exposure cannot be evaluated because the requisite incubation period has not elapsed. Finally, a problem results because occupation is so closely related to social class. Indeed, in many studies occupational "level"—not exposure—is used to designate an individual's social class. Social class, in turn, is a correlate of risk for many cancers, including some for which the association is quite strong. The possible confounding by social class and other characteristics (e.g., race) of an employed group should be evaluated before it is inferred that a causal association exists between the occupational exposure and a cancer. For example, soft-coal miners were reported [8] at increased risk of cancer of the stomach, but when the effects of social class were evaluated [9], the association was much reduced.

To balance the discussion of occupation as an epidemiologic variable, we should mention some characteristics that make it suitable for study. For certain types of occupations, such as skilled trades and professions, exposures are reasonably easy to delineate and are experienced for a working lifetime. Less often, unskilled workers in some industries hold a single position for decades. In such cases, if investigations or control programs are conducted in collaboration with management or a trade union, highly valid long-term exposure information may be available.

OBJECTIVES OF OCCUPATIONAL STUDIES

Studies of occupational carcinogenesis usually report only whether an apparent association between an occupation suspected of being hazardous and a particular malignancy is statistically significant. When possible, the identity of the responsible agent is also given. Often, considerably more valuable information is available. For example, many studies give no idea of the magnitude (risk ratio, relative risk) of the increased cancer risk. Usually, the attributable risk or etiologic fraction [10, 11] is missing. The etiologic fraction among the exposed (EF_e) is the proportion of cases of the cancer in question among the workers that results from the exposure under study. The total etiologic fraction (EF_t) is the proportion of the disease in question, among the referent population, that results from the exposure. It would be reasonable to consider the referent population to be either all employees on the site where the investigation was conducted or the residents of the geographic area from which the workers come. The EF_t, using all workers as the referent, should prove a useful measure for comparing results between studies. The magnitude of the excess risk alone (as measured, say, by the risk ratio) will differ between similar studies, depending on the criteria used to characterize an "exposed" worker. However, the EF_t is much less susceptible to this difficulty because as the criteria for exposure are relaxed, with concomitant reduction in the risk ratio, the proportion of the referent population that is exposed increases and the EF_t remains constant.

Another potentially interesting item, since it could have profound implications for prevention, is the relationship of excess risk to age-at-starting exposure. In one study [12], all the excess risk of bladder cancer among men with occupational exposures was confined to those whose exposure began prior to age 25. If this finding were confirmed, it would have considerable significance. Studies of occupational carcinogenesis are needed to determine the relationship of excess risk to age at first exposure. At least two issues appear involved: First, younger persons might be more susceptible to cancer induction; and second, only persons who are first exposed while young may work long enough to sustain carcinogenic exposures. (The latter explanation did not apply in the bladder cancer study cited.) In either case, the implication is that only persons, say, 40 and over should be placed in possibly carcinogenic work environments. Yet, on the basis of existing knowledge, we cannot make this recommendation. Several studies [13, 14] suggested that elderly persons are actually more susceptible than the young to cancer induction. These relationships should be worked out in detail so that their preventive implications can be exploited. It may be that both the young and the old are susceptible, but that the middle-aged are relatively resistant to carcinogenesis.

Closely tied to the age-at-starting issue is duration of exposure. Several studies [12, 15] suggested that relatively short occupational exposures (e.g., 6 months to a year) appreciably increase cancer risk. However, it seems there is also a relationship of increased excess risk with increasing duration of exposure. Again, preventive strategies might follow from an understanding of these temporal factors.

An additional temporal factor is the duration of the interval between beginning exposure and the manifestation of disease. Concepts of carcinogenesis and cancer growth do not serve us well here, nor do the lessons learned from infectious disease epidemiology. Detailed knowledge of this interval, its components (induction, incubation periods), length, variability, and determinants would contribute to the understanding of human carcinogenesis. It might also have control implications for screening schedules.

Largely ignored have been the determinants of cancer in addition to the occupational exposure. One exception is the important finding [16] that, apparently, asbestos will produce lung cancer only in smokers. Other agent-agent and host-agent interactions should be sought. The implications would seem to be both of a general scientific and preventive nature.

OCCUPATIONAL CARCINOGENESIS–AGENT CLASSIFICATION

Table 1 is a classification of agents used in the occupational environment and recognized as having caused cancers in man. For each agent, the target organ is given and the risk ratio and incubation periods are estimated. These estimates are the writers' interpretation of information in the references cited. Associations based on risk ratios <2 have not been included except in instances where, for one reason or another, the association is of special interest, or the risk ratio, although not estimated, is likely to be high. A detailed description of epidemiologic and other evidence substantiating the carcinogenicity of several substances listed in Table 1 has been presented elsewhere by Fraumeni [17].

Organic agents, especially the aromatic hydrocarbons, have been the most thoroughly studied occupational carcinogens. The magnitude of the excess risk and temporal aspects of chemical carcinogenesis have been worked out best for this group of compounds. For example, Case et al. [15] studied these issues extensively with respect to β-naphthylamine, benzidine, and bladder cancer. They estimated that workers in the dyestuffs industry had about 30 times the risk of the general population of dying from bladder cancer (risk ratios of 87 and 14 for β-naphthylamine and benzidine, respectively) and that the incubation period of the disease was about 19 years.

Several heavy metals, fibers, and dusts (Table 1) have also been implicated in occupational carcinogenesis, but not as persuasively as the aromatic hydrocarbons. The observation with respect to wood and cancer of the nasal sinuses

TABLE 1
Classification of Occupational Carcinogens

A. Organic agents
1. Aromatic hydrocarbons

Agents	Affected organ(s)	Incubation period (years)	Risk ratio	Occupation	References
Coal soot Coal tar Other products of coal combustion	Lung, larynx, skin, scrotum, urinary bladder	9–23	2–6	Gashouse workers, stokers, and producers; asphalt, coal tar, and pitch workers; coke-oven workers; miners; still cleaners; chimney sweeps	4, 19–28
Petroleum Petroleum coke Wax Creosote Anthracene Paraffin Shale Mineral oils	Nasal cavity, larynx, lung, skin, scrotum	12–30	2–4	Contact with lubricating, cooling, paraffin or wax fuel oils, or coke; rubber fillers; retortmen; textile weavers; diesel jet testers	4, 17, 23–25, 29–33
Benzene	Bone marrow (leukemia)	6–14	2–3	Explosives, benzene, or rubber cement workers; distillers; dye users; painters; shoemakers	34–37

TABLE 1 (Continued)

A. Organic agents (continued)

1. Aromatic hydrocarbons (continued)

Agents	Affected organ(s)	Incubation period (years)	Risk ratio	Occupation	References
Auramine Benzidine α-naphthylamine β-naphthylamine Magenta 4-aminodiphenyl 4-nitrodiphenyl	Urinary bladder	13–30	2–90	Dyestuffs manufacturers and users; rubber workers (pressmen, filtermen, laborers); textile dyers; paint manufacturers	5, 38–51
2. Alkylating agents					
Mustard gas	Larynx, lung trachea, bronchi	10–25	2–36	Mustard gas workers	52, 53
3. Others					
Isopropyl oil	Nasal cavity	10+	21	Producers	4, 21, 23, 24, 54, 55
Vinyl chloride	Liver (angiosarcoma), brain	20–30	200 (liver) 4 (brain)	Plastic workers	56–59

173

TABLE 1 (Continued)

A. Organic agents (continued)

  3. Others (continued)

Agents	Affected organ(s)	Incubation period (years)	Risk ratio	Occupation	References
Bis(chloromethyl) ether Chloromethyl methyl ether	Lung (oat cell carcinoma)	5+	7–45	Chemical workers	17, 60–62

B. Inorganic agents

  1. Metals

Agents	Affected organ(s)	Incubation period (years)	Risk ratio	Occupation	References
Arsenic	Skin, lung, liver	10+	3–8	Miners; smelters; insecticide makers and sprayers; tanners; chemical workers; oil refiners; vintners	4, 17, 24, 30, 63–68
Chromium	Nasal cavity and sinuses, lung, larynx	15–25	3–40	Producers, processors, and users; acetylene and aniline workers; bleachers; glass, pottery and linoleum workers; battery makers	4, 17, 21, 24, 69–72

174

TABLE 1 (Continued)

B. Inorganic agents (continued)

1. Metals (continued)

Agents	Affected organ(s)	Incubation period (years)	Risk ratio	Occupation	References
Iron oxide	Lung, larynx	—	2–5	Iron ore (hematite) miners; metal grinders and polishers; silver finishers; iron foundry workers	4, 17, 21, 23, 24, 26, 30, 73–77
Nickel	Nasal sinuses, lung	3–30	5–10 (lung) 100+ (nasal sinuses)	Nickel smelters, mixers, and roasters; electrolysis workers	4, 17, 21, 14, 78–81
2. Fibers					
Asbestos	Lung, pleural and peritoneal mesothelioma	4–50	1.5–12	Miners; millers; textile, insulation, and shipyard workers	4, 17, 82–85
3. Dusts					
Wood	Nasal cavity and sinuses	30–40	—	Woodworkers	86–88
Leather	Nasal cavity and sinuses, urinary bladder	40–50	50 (nasal sinuses) 2.5 (bladder)	Leather and shoe workers	12, 89

175

TABLE 1 (Continued)

C. Physical agents

1. Nonionizing radiation

Agents	Affected organ(s)	Incubation period (years)	Risk ratio	Occupation	References
Ultraviolet rays	Skin	varies with skin pigment and texture	—	Farmers; sailors	90, 91

2. Ionizing radiation

X-rays	Skin, bone marrow (leukemia)	10–25	3–9	Radiologists; medical personnel	92, 93
Uranium Radon Radium Mesothorium	Skin, lung, bone, bone marrow (leukemia)	10–15	3–10	Radiologists; miners; radium dial painters; radium chemists	94–96

3. Other

Hypoxia	Bone	—	—	Caisson workers	97

is especially perplexing but appears valid. The observations on hypoxia and trauma as possible causes of bone sarcoma are tenuous but of considerable interest, if correct.

In reviewing Table 1, it is important to keep in mind that many sites where occupational cancers arise are only rarely involved with spontaneous cancers—at least in Western countries. Such sites include nose, sinuses, liver, and scrotum. Thus, even if workers are placed at a fivefold risk, it may not be true that their risk is high in an absolute sense. While this fact may have little or no implication for the need to control the exposure, it does suggest that efforts to reduce morbidity or mortality by screening will have to be evaluated carefully.

Table 2 is excerpted from Table 1 with the observations arranged so that the classification is by site rather than by carcinogenic agent. In addition, the criteria for inclusion in Table 2 are more stringent in that the associations listed between disease sites and agents may be considered established. The occupations listed are those where the agents in question are used; it is not necessarily true that every occupational group is known to have experienced the related cancer in excess.

CONTROL OF OCCUPATIONAL CARCINOGENESIS

Existing epidemiologic methods are adequate for demonstrating carcinogenic hazards in the work environment even when the excess risk is rather small and the disease in question is relatively common in the general population. However, this capacity for recognition depends on the actual occurrence of disease and, by itself, has no preventive or control value. Ideally, we should prevent occupational cancers from occurring. Failing that, we should strive to eliminate a fatal outcome in cases that do occur. Technical and epidemiologic approaches are likely to be useful both in the areas of prevention and mortality reduction.

Technical progress to prevent occupational cancer is now advancing rapidly. The major approaches are process modification (usually to totally closed systems), material substitution, and personal protective measures. They, however, are exposure-specific and will not be discussed here. More fundamental is the plan to use lower organisms or laboratory animals to screen compounds of potential industrial value before they arrive in the workplace. The advantages of such screening are likely to be great, but the costs are staggering; and, as pointed out by Hueper and Conway [18], negative results are not to be interpreted as exonerating an agent.

Epidemiologic approaches to the prevention of occupational cancer have not been developed. Presumably, such approaches will be based on a knowledge of temporal aspects of occupational carcinogenesis and personal characteristics, such as age and sex, according to which sensitivity to carcinogens vary. In addition, epidemiology has a role to play in prevention as part of the design

TABLE 2

Occupations Conveying an Increased Risk of Developing Cancer, by Site

Site	Agents	Occupations
Liver	Arsenic, vinyl chloride	Tanners; smelters; vintners; plastic workers
Nasal cavity and sinuses	Chromium, isopropyl oil, nickel, wood and leather dusts	Glass, pottery, and linoleum workers; battery makers; nickel smelters, mixers, and roasters; electrolysis workers; wood, leather, and shoe workers
Lung	Arsenic, asbestos, chromium, coal products, dusts, iron oxide, mustard gas, nickel, petroleum, ionizing radiation, bis(chloromethyl) ether	Vintners; miners; asbestos users; textile users; insulation workers; tanners; smelters; glass and pottery workers; coal tar and pitch workers; iron foundry workers; electrolysis workers; retortmen; radiologists; radium dial painters; chemical workers
Bladder	Coal products, aromatic amines	Asphalt, coal tar, and pitch workers; gas stokers; still cleaners; dyestuffs users; rubber workers; textile dyers; paint manufacturers; leather and shoe workers
Bone	Ionizing radiation	Radium dial painters
Bone marrow	Benzene, ionizing radiation	Benzene, explosives, and rubber cement workers; distillers; dye users; painters; radiologists; radium dial painters

and evaluation of surveillance mechanisms and etiologic studies. However, all public health approaches to the prevention of occupational cancer are to complement, not replace or make less stringent, the industrial hygiene practices that should be in effect.

With respect to mortality reduction among persons who develop occupational cancer, both technical and epidemiologic methods again seem likely to be useful. Technical advances are required in the area of screening for the development of tests that are highly sensitive and, especially, highly specific. Of course, technical advances will be made in most of the areas of diagnosis and treatment. Epidemiologic approaches to mortality reduction will be in the form of improving the design and evaluation of proposed early disease detection programs. Such programs may prove quite useful. Nonetheless, the impact of screening on cancer morbidity and mortality is uncertain; at present, they are not programs on which we can rely.

REFERENCES

1. Ramazzini, B. *De Morbis Artificum Diatriba (Diseases of Workers)*. Translated by W.C. Wright. Hafner, New York, 1964.

2. Pott, P. *Chirurgical Observations*. Hawes, Clarke, & Collings, London, 1775.

3. Härting, F.H., and Hesse, W. Der Lungenkrebs, die Bergkrankheit in den Schneebergen Gruben. *Vjschr. Med. Gerich. 30*:296–309; *31*:102–132, 313–337, 1879.

4. Hueper, W.C. *Occupational & Environmental Cancers of the Respiratory System*. Springer-Verlag, New York, 1966.

5. Rehn, L. Blasengeschwülste bei Fuchsin-Arbeitern. *Arch. Klin. Chirurgie 50:* 588–600, 1895.

6. McMichael, A.J., Spirtas, R., and Kupper, L.L. An epidemiologic study of mortality within a cohort of rubber workers. *J. Occup. Med. 16:* 458–464, 1974.

7. U.S. Bureau of the Census. *Census of Population: 1970. Detailed Characteristics. Final Report PC(1)–D1. U.S. Summary*. U.S. Govt. Print. Off., Washington, D.C., 1973.

8. Matolo, N.M., Klauber, M.R., Gorishek, W.M., et al. High incidence of gastric carcinoma in a coal mining region. *Cancer 29:* 733–737, 1972.

9. Creagan, E.T., Hoover, R.N., and Fraumeni, J.F., Jr. Mortality from stomach cancer in coal mining regions. *Arch. Environ. Health 28:* 28–30, 1974.

10. Cole, P., and MacMahon, B. Attributable risk percent in case-control studies. *Br. J. Prev. Soc. Med. 25:* 242–244, 1971.

11. Miettinen, O.S. Proportion of disease caused or prevented by a given exposure, trait or intervention. *Am. J. Epidemiol. 99:* 325–332, 1974.

12. Cole, P., Hoover, R., and Friedell, G.H. Occupation and cancer of the lower urinary tract. *Cancer 29:* 1250–1260, 1972.

13. Hoover, R., and Cole, P. Temporal aspects of occupational bladder carcinogenesis. *N. Engl. J. Med. 288:* 1040–1043, 1973.

14. Doll, R. Susceptibility to carcinogenesis at different ages. *Gerontol. Clin. (Basel) 4:* 211–221, 1962.

15. Case, R.A.M., Hosker, M.E., McDonald, D.B., et al. Tumours of the urinary bladder in workmen engaged in the manufacture and use of certain dyestuff intermediates in the British chemical industry. Part I. *Br. J. Ind. Med. 11:* 75–104, 1954.

16. Selikoff, I.J., Hammond, E.C., and Churg, J. Asbestos exposure, smoking and neoplasia. *J.A.M.A. 204:* 106-112, 1968.

17. Fraumeni, J.F., Jr. Chemicals in the induction of respiratory tract tumors. *In Proceedings of the 11th International Cancer Congress.* Excerpta Medica Int. Congr. Ser. No. 351, Vol. 3, 1975, pp. 327-335.

18. Hueper, W.C., and Conway, W.D. *Chemical Carcinogenesis and Cancers.* Charles C. Thomas, Springfield, Ill., 1964.

19. Doll, R. The causes of death among gas-workers with special reference to cancer of the lung. *Br. J. Ind. Med. 9:* 180-185, 1952.

20. Doll, R. Etiology of lung cancer. *Adv. Cancer Res. 3:* 1-50, 1955.

21. Doll, R. Occupational lung cancer: A review. *Br. J. Ind. Med. 16:* 181-190, 1959.

22. Doll, R., Vessey, M.P., Beasley, R.W., et al. Mortality of gas-workers–final report of a prospective study. *Br. J. Ind. Med. 29:* 394-406, 1972.

23. Hueper, W.C. *Occupational Tumors and Allied Diseases.* Charles C. Thomas, Springfield, Ill., 1942.

24. Hueper, W.C. *A Quest Into the Environmental Causes of Cancer of the Lung.* Pub Health Monogr 36, Public Health Service. U.S. Govt. Print. Off., Washington, D.C., 1956.

25. Kennaway, N.M., and Kennaway, E.L. A study of the incidence of cancer of the lung and larynx. *J. Hyg.* (Camb.) *36:* 236-267, 1936.

26. Kennaway, N.M., and Kennaway, E.L. A further study of the incidence of cancer of the lung and larynx. *Br. J. Cancer 1:* 260-298, 1947.

27. Lloyd, J.W. Long-term mortality study of steelworkers. V. Respiratory cancer in coke plant workers. *J. Occup. Med. 13:* 53-68, 1971.

28. Kawai, M., Amamoto, H., and Harada, K. Epidemiologic study of occupational lung cancer. *Arch. Environ. Health 14:* 859-864, 1967.

29. Bell, B. Paraffin epithelioma of the scrotum. *Edinb. Med. J. 22:* 135, 1876.

30. Dontenwill, W. Occupational atmospheric carcinogens (other than fibers). *In* Clark, R.L., Cumley, R.W., McCay, J.E., and Copeland, M.M., eds. *Oncology 1970.* Vol. 5. Yearbook Medical Publishers, Chicago, 1971, pp. 63-74.

31. Fischer, H.G.M., Priestly, W., Eby, L.T., et al. Symposium on cancer control program for high-boiling catalytically cracked oils; properties of high-boiling petroleum products; physical and chemical properties as related to carcinogenic activity. *A.M.A. Arch. Ind. Hyg. 4:* 315-324, 1951.

32. Henry, S.A. *Cancer of the Scrotum in Relation to Occupation.* Oxford Univ. Press, London, 1946.

33. Huguenin, R., Fauvet, J., and Bourdin, J.S. Rôle éventuel des nébulisations de certaines huiles industrielles dans l'étiologie du cancer bronchopulmonaire. *Bull. Soc. Med. Paris 65:* 1020-1022, 1949.

34. Aksoy, M., Dinçol, K., Akgün, T., et al. Haematological effects of chronic benzene poisoning in 217 workers. *Br. J. Ind. Med. 28:* 296-302, 1971.

35. Aksoy, M., Dinçol, K., Erdem, S., et al. Acute leukemia due to chronic exposure to benzene. *Am. J. Med. 52:* 160-166, 1972.

36. Ishimaru, T., Okada, H., Tomiyasu, T., et al. Occupational factors in the epidemiology of leukemia in Hiroshima and Nagasaki. *Am. J. Epidemiol. 93:* 157-165, 1971.

37. Thorpe, J.J. Epidemiologic survey of leukemia in persons potentially exposed to benzene. *J. Occup. Med. 16:* 375-382, 1974.

38. Bonser, G.M., Faulds, J.S., and Stewart, M.J. Occupational cancer of the urinary bladder in dyestuffs operatives and of the lung in asbestos textile workers and iron-ore miners. *Am. J. Clin. Pathol. 25:* 126-134, 1955.

39. Case, R.A.M. The expected frequency of bladder tumour in works populations. *Br. J. Ind. Med. 10:* 114-120, 1953.

40. Case, R.A.M., and Hosker, M.E. Tumour of the urinary bladder as an occupational disease in the rubber industry in England and Wales. *Br. J. Prev. Soc. Med. 8:* 39–50, 1954.

41. Case, R.A.M., Hosker, M.E., McDonald, D.B., et al. Tumours of the urinary bladder in workmen engaged in the manufacture and use of certain dyestuff intermediates in the British chemical industry. *Br. J. Ind. Med. 11:* 75–104, 1954.

42. Case, R.A.M. Tumours of the urinary tract as an occupational disease in several industries. *Ann. R. Coll. Surg. Engl. 39:* 213–235, 1966.

43. Clayson, D.B. *Chemical Carcinogenesis.* Little, Brown and Co., Boston, 1962.

44. Cole, P., Hoover, R., and Friedell, G.H. Occupation and cancer of the lower urinary tract. *Cancer 29:* 1250–1260, 1972.

45. Goldblatt, M.W. Occupational cancer of the bladder. *Br. Med. Bull. 4:* 405–417, 1947.

46. Koss, L.G., Melamed, M.R., Ricci, A., et al. Carcinogenesis in the human urinary bladder. Observations after exposure to para-aminodiphenyl. *N. Engl. J. Med. 272:* 767–770, 1965.

47. Koss, L.G., Melamed, M.R., and Kelly, R.E. Further cytologic and histologic studies of bladder lesions in workers exposed to para-aminodiphenyl: progress report. *J. Natl. Cancer Inst. 43:* 233–243, 1969.

48. Melick, W.F., Escue, H.M., Naryka, J.J., et al. The first reported cases of human bladder tumors due to a new carcinogen–xenylamine. *J. Urol. 74:* 760–766, 1955.

49. Owen, R. Occupational cancer of the renal tract: recent developments in epidemiology and legislation in Great Britain. *J. Natl. Cancer Inst. 43:* 253–254, 1969.

50. Veys, C.A. Two epidemiological inquiries into the incidence of bladder tumors in industrial workers. *J. Natl. Cancer Inst. 43:* 219–226, 1969.

51. Wendel, R.G., Hoegg, U.R., and Zavon, M.R. Benzidine: a bladder carcinogen. *J. Urol. 111:* 607–610, 1974.

52. Beebe, G.W. Lung cancer in World War I veterans: possible relation to mustard-gas injury and 1918 influenza epidemic. *J. Natl. Cancer Inst. 25:* 1231–1252, 1960.

53. Wada, S., Miyanishi, M., Nishimoto, Y., et al. Mustard gas as a cause of respiratory neoplasia in man. *Lancet 1:* 1161–1163, 1968.

54. Eckardt, R.E. *Industrial Carcinogens.* Grune & Stratton, New York, 1959.

55. Weil, C.S., Smyth, H.F., Jr., and Nale, T.W. Quest for a suspected industrial carcinogen. *A.M.A. Arch. Ind. Hyg. 5:* 535–547, 1952.

56. Creech, J., Johnson, M.N., and Block, B. *Morbid. Mortal. Wkly. Rep. 23,* No. 49, 1974.

57. Creech, J.L., and Johnson, M.N. Angiosarcoma of liver in the manufacture of polyvinyl chloride. *J. Occup. Med. 16:* 150–151, 1974.

58. Monson, R.R., Peters, J.M., and Johnson, M.N. Proportional mortality among vinylchloride workers. *Lancet 2:* 397–398, 1974.

59. Tabershaw, I.R., and Gaffey, W.R. Mortality study of workers in the manufacture of vinyl chloride and its polymers. *J. Occup. Med. 16:* 509–518, 1974.

60. Laskin, S., Kuschner, M., Drew, R.T., et al. Tumors of the respiratory tract induced by inhalation of bis (chloromethyl) ether. *Arch. Environ. Health 23:* 135–136, 1971.

61. Figueroa, W.G., Raszkowski, R., and Weiss, W. Lung cancer in chloromethyl methyl ether workers. *N. Engl. J. Med. 288:* 1096–1097, 1973.

62. Brown, S.M., and Selvin, S. Lung cancer in chloromethyl methyl ether workers. *N. Engl. J. Med. 289:* 693–694, 1973.

63. Hueper, W.C. Environmental factors in the production of human cancer. *In* Raven, R.W., ed. *Cancer.* Butterworths, London, 1957.

64. Kuratsune, M., Tokudome, S., Shirakusa, T., et al. Occupational lung cancer among copper smelters. *Int. J. Cancer 13:* 552–558, 1974.

65. Lee, A.M., and Fraumeni, J.F., Jr. Arsenic and respiratory cancer in man: An occupational study. *J. Natl. Cancer Inst. 42:* 1045–1052, 1969.

66. Neubauer, O. Arsenical cancer: A review. *Br. J. Cancer 1:* 192–251, 1947.

67. Regelson, W., Kim, U., Ospina, J., et al. Hemangioendothelial sarcoma of liver from chronic arsenic intoxication by Fowler's solution. *Cancer 21:* 514–522, 1968.

68. Yeh, S. Skin cancer in chronic arsenicism. *Hum. Pathol. 4:* 469–485, 1973.

69. Baetjer, A.M. Pulmonary carcinoma in chromate workers. *A.M.A. Arch. Ind. Hyg. 2:* 487–516, 1950.

70. Bidstrup, P.L., and Case, R.A.M. Carcinoma of the lung in workmen in the bichromates-producing industry in Great Britain. *Br. J. Ind. Med. 13:* 260–264, 1956.

71. Enterline, P.E. Respiratory cancer among chromate workers. *J. Occup. Med. 16:* 523–526, 1974.

72. Machle, W., and Gregorius, F. Cancer of the respiratory system in the United States chromate-producing industry. *Public Health Rep. 63:* 1114–1127, 1948.

73. Bonser, G.M., Faulds, J.S., and Stewart, M.J. Occupational cancer of the urinary bladder in dyestuffs operatives and of the lung in asbestos textile workers and iron-ore miners. *Am. J. Clin. Pathol. 25:* 126–134, 1955.

74. Boyd, J.T., Doll, R., Faulds, J.S., et al. Cancer of the lung in iron ore (haematite) miners. *Br. J. Ind. Med. 27:* 97–105, 1970.

75. Faulds, J.S. Haematite pneumoconiosis in Cumberland miners. *J. Clin. Pathol. (Lond.) 10:* 187–199, 1957.

76. Faulds, J.S., and Stewart, M.J. Carcinoma of the lung in haematite miners. *J. Pathol. 72:* 353–366, 1956.

77. McLaughlin, A.I.G., and Harding, H.E. Pneumoconiosis and other causes of death in iron and steel foundry workers. *A.M.A. Arch. Ind. Health 14:* 350–378, 1956.

78. Doll, R. Cancer of the lung and nose in nickel workers. *Br. J. Ind. Med. 15:* 217–223, 1958.

79. Doll, R., Morgan, L.G., and Speizer, F.E. Cancers of the lung and nasal sinuses in nickel workers. *Br. J. Cancer 24:* 623–632, 1970.

80. Morgan, J.G. Some observations on the incidence of respiratory cancer in nickel workers. *Br. J. Ind. Med. 15:* 224–234, 1958.

81. Pedersen, E., Høgetveit, A., and Andersen, A. Cancer of respiratory organs among workers at a nickel refinery in Norway. *Int. J. Cancer 12:* 32–41, 1973.

82. Doll, R. Mortality from lung cancer in asbestos workers. *Br. J. Ind. Med. 12:* 81–86, 1955.

83. Enticknap, J.B., and Smither, W.J. Peritoneal tumours in asbestosis. *Br. J. Ind. Med. 21:* 20–31, 1964.

84. Selikoff, I.J., Churg, J., and Hammond, E.C. Asbestos exposure and neoplasia. *J.A.M.A. 188:* 22–26, 1964.

85. Wagner, J.C., Sleggs, C.A., and Marchand, P. Diffuse pleural mesothelioma and asbestos exposure in the North Western Cape Province. *Br. J. Ind. Med. 17:* 260–271, 1960.

86. Acheson, E.D., Cowdell, R.H., Hadfield, E., et al. Nasal cancer in woodworkers in the furniture industry. *Br. Med. J. 2:* 587–596, 1968.

87. Hadfield, E.H. A study of adenocarcinoma of the paranasal sinuses in woodworkers in the furniture industry. *Ann. R. Coll. Surg. Engl. 46:* 301–319, 1970.

88. Mosbech, J., and Acheson, E.D. Nasal cancer in furniture-makers in Denmark. *Dan. Med. Bull. 18:* 34–35, 1971.

89. Acheson, E.D., Cowdell, R.H., and Jolles, B. Nasal cancer in the Northamptonshire boot and shoe industry. *Br. Med. J. 1:* 385–393, 1970.

90. Silverstone, H. Skin cancer in Queensland, Australia. *In Report of the Airlie House Conference on Sunlight and Skin Cancer.* National Institutes of Health, Bethesda, Md., 1964.

91. Urbach, F. Geographic pathology of skin cancer. *In The Biologic Effects of Ultraviolet Radiation.* Pergamon Press, Oxford, 1969.

92. Court-Brown, W.M., and Doll, R. Expectation of life and mortality from cancer among British radiologists. *Br. Med. J. 2:* 181–187, 1958.

93. Seltser, R., and Sartwell, P.E. The influence of occupational exposure to radiation on the mortality of American radiologists and other medical specialists. *Am. J. Epidemiol. 81:* 2–22, 1965.

94. Saccomanno, G., Archer, V.E., Auerbach, O., et al. Histologic types of lung cancer among uranium miners. *Cancer 27:* 515–523, 1971.

95. Wagoner, J.K., Archer, V.E., Carroll, B.E., et al. Cancer mortality patterns among U.S. uranium miners and millers, 1950 through 1962. *J. Natl. Cancer Inst. 32:* 787–801, 1964.

96. Wagoner, J.K., Archer, V.E., Lundin, F.E., et al. Radiation as the cause of lung cancer among uranium miners. *N. Engl. J. Med. 173:* 181–188, 1965.

97. Mirra, J.M., Bullough, P.G., Marcove, R.C., et al. Malignant fibrous histiocytoma and osteosarcoma in association with bone infarcts. *J. Bone Joint Surg. (Am.) Vol. 56A:* 932–940, 1974.

DISCUSSION

Dr. Koss disagreed with statements that we know little about the natural history of occupational cancers, or that we need to assess the value of screening occupationally exposed persons. In men exposed to para-aminodiphenyl, cytologic screening was successful in detecting several cases of bladder cancer without the necessity of cystoscopy. He also indicated that cytologic screening in uranium miners for the early effects of respiratory exposure to radon daughter products has been satisfactory.

Dr. Cole rejoined that the data cited by Dr. Koss did not indicate risk associated with the exposure. He stressed that case identification by screening does not prove the usefulness of the screening process; the effectiveness should be judged by reduction in mortality and morbidity, and not merely by the number of cases found. In this sense he felt that the impact of screening programs in occupational cancer needs to be examined.

Dr. Bahn discussed the need for controlled trials of screening, and asked whether it was desirable to carry them out in occupational groups. The reply was that unless the rate is as high as 3 to 4 cases per thousand, screening has not been of value despite a high risk ratio. For example, there is a fivefold excess relative risk of nasal-sinus cancer in some occupational groups, but screening would not be useful because the absolute risk is so small.

Dr. Selikoff stressed that when cancer occurs in young employed persons, a very careful occupational exposure history should be taken. These patients may be the earliest cases associated with a previously unsuspected environmental carcinogen. Secondly, other toxic effects are often a clue to carcinogenic potential. For example, hepatotoxicity of vinyl chloride should have raised suspicions of a risk of liver cancer. In addition, current studies of cancer in work populations exposed three decades ago may be futile because the types of exposure may have changed over time. Instead, it may be more productive to maintain continuous study of occupational groups. Examples are the ongoing surveys of 225,000 members of the Painters Union and 125,000 members of the Printing Pressmen Union. The observations should focus not only on cancer but on other toxic effects as well.

Dr. Selikoff proposed that several types of exposures should be assigned priority for study: 1) exposures involving large numbers of workers, 2) exposures that began several decades ago and continue at present, 3) exposures involving both the general community and occupational groups, and 4) exposures to new materials, particularly those producing other toxic reactions.

In conclusion, **Dr. Cole** stated that occupationally related cancers provide a major opportunity for prevention through interruption of exposure.

John R. Goldsmith

12

DRUGS

Robert Hoover, M.D., and Joseph F. Fraumeni, Jr., M.D.

Epidemiology Branch, National Cancer Institute
Bethesda, Maryland

Western societies are often called "medicated" or "over-medicated," because of their massive use of prescription and over-the-counter drugs. Intrinsically, these substances are biologically and chemically active, so that unintended reactions are relatively common. Acute side effects have always been of great concern to those marketing, consuming, or regulating drugs; for that reason, they are usually well documented through toxicity studies and clinical trials. Long-term side effects, including cancer, are much more difficult to evaluate and remain largely unknown. This chapter summarizes the epidemiologic evidence for drug-induced cancer in man. The limited number of agents implicated to date signifies not that other drugs are innocuous, but that the need for study is urgent.

Drug-cancer relationships in laboratory animals and man may be classified as follows:

1) Drug exposures associated with cancer in man.
2) Drug exposures carcinogenic in laboratory animals that with investigation have thus far demonstrated no carcinogenicity for man.
3) Drug exposures carcinogenic in laboratory animals that have not been evaluated in man.
4) Drug exposures either not carcinogenic in laboratory animals or whose carcinogenicity is unknown.

This presentation emphasizes the first two categories. Although the last two categories include the vast majority of pharmacologic compounds produced, a review of laboratory research with these agents is beyond the scope of this report. However, some criteria are presented for selecting which drugs should be evaluated in man.

DRUGS ASSOCIATED WITH HUMAN CANCER

Agents related to cancer in man, recently reviewed by Fraumeni and Miller [1], are listed in Table 1. Some agents were removed from clinical use when their carcinogenic potential was recognized, but others are still used because estimates of risk-benefit ratios warrant their administration in certain diseases. However, as different conditions are added to the therapeutic indications for a drug, new assessments of risk-benefit ratios must be made.

Radioisotopes exert carcinogenic effects by release of ionizing radiation at deposition sites in the body. For example, radioactive phosphorus increases the risk of acute myelocytic leukemia (AML) in patients with polycythemia vera [2]. Radium and mesothorium, bone-seeking isotopes once used for bone tuberculosis and other illnesses, produce a high rate of osteogenic sarcoma and carcinoma in mucous membranes near bone, particularly the paranasal sinuses [3,4]. The same effect results from occupational exposures among radium-dial painters and radium chemists. Radioiodine used in high doses for thyroid cancer probably increases the risk of leukemia [5], but no effect is evident when lower amounts are used for hyperthyroidism [6]. Thorotrast, deposited in the reticuloendothelial system after use in radiographic studies, is a cause of hepatic hemangioendothelioma and AML [7].

Immunosuppressive agents (antimetabolites, corticosteroids, antilymphocyte serum) are suspected of being contributing factors to the high cancer risk experienced by recipients of renal transplants. The mechanism undoubtedly involves some alteration of immunologic processes rather than chemical induction of malignant change. In a recent follow-up study [8] of over 6,000 recipients of renal transplants, the risk of lymphoma was about 35 times normal—derived almost entirely from a risk of reticulum cell sarcoma that was 350 times higher than expected. Skin and lip cancers occurred up to four times more often than expected, whereas the risk of other cancers was 2½ times more frequent, due largely to soft tissue sarcoma and hepatobiliary carcinoma. Recent data [9] suggest that the risk is increased also for adenocarcinomas of the lung. Since persons with heritable immunodeficiency syndromes are susceptible to lymphoma and possibly other cancers [10], immunosuppressive drugs most likely are involved in posttransplant carcinogenesis. Despite case reports of cancer developing in patients with other conditions treated with these drugs, no study has as yet determined whether there is any excess of malignancy. Perhaps the predisposition to neoplasia in transplant recipients results from an interaction between immunosuppression and immunostimulation by antigens from the grafted kidney. The mechanism will be

TABLE 1
Cancers Related to Drug Exposures in Man

DRUG	RELATED CANCER
Radioisotopes	
Phosphorus (P^{32})	Acute leukemia
Radium, mesothorium	Osteosarcoma, sinus carcinoma
Thorotrast	Hemangioendothelioma of liver
Immunosuppressive drugs (for renal transplantation)	
Antilymphocyte serum	Reticulum cell sarcoma
Antimetabolites	Soft tissue sarcoma, other cancers (skin, liver)
Cytotoxic drugs	
Chlornaphazine	Bladder cancer
Melphalan, cyclophosphamide	Acute myelomonocytic leukemia
Hormones	
Synthetic estrogens	
Prenatal	Vaginal and cervical adeno-carcinoma (clear-cell type)
Postnatal	Endometrial carcinoma (adenosquamous type)
Androgenic-anabolic steroids (for aplastic anemia)	Hepatocellular carcinoma
Others	
Arsenic	Skin cancer
Phenacetin-containing drugs	Renal pelvis carcinoma
Coal-tar ointments	Skin cancer
Diphenylhydantoin?	Lymphoma
Chloramphenicol?	Leukemia
Amphetamines?	Hodgkin's disease
Reserpine?	Breast cancer

important to establish. Although the cancer risk associated with immunosuppressive drugs is considered acceptable for renal transplantation, similar risks for less serious disorders might be unacceptable.

Cytotoxic agents used in cancer chemotherapy are often carcinogenic in laboratory animals, and some may induce cancer in man [11]. Chlornaphazine was withdrawn from use in 1964 when high doses for treating polycythemia vera and Hodgkin's disease (HD) were found to cause bladder tumors [12]. This drug is a derivative of β-naphthylamine, previously known to be a bladder carcinogen in industrial workers. Certain alkylating agents also seem to elevate the risk of acute leukemia, especially the myelocytic and myelomonocytic types. Most striking is the increase in leukemia among patients with multiple myeloma treated with melphalan or cyclophosphamide [13], although one cannot yet exclude the possibility that improved survival permits the development of a hematopoietic neoplasm related to the origin or natural history of myeloma.

Another effect of cytotoxic drugs was suggested by a recent follow-up study [14] of HD, which showed that intensive chemotherapy enhanced the risk of second cancers originating at heavily irradiated sites.

Synthetic estrogens, particularly diethylstilbestrol (DES), triggered much recent concern about the carcinogenic effects of drugs. First evidence for a human transplacental carcinogen came in 1971, when a link was reported between DES and a cluster of vaginal adenocarcinoma in Boston among eight women between 14 and 22 years of age [15]. At present, prenatal exposure to synthetic estrogens has been linked to clear cell carcinomas of the vagina and cervix in over 100 patients 7 to 29 years of age [16]. However, based on a recent follow-up study [17], the rate for the cancers after in utero exposure to estrogens has been estimated thus far to be no greater than 4 per 1,000 and probably considerably less [16]. Synthetic estrogens given after birth may also induce cancer. In a study of 24 patients receiving DES for at least 5 years for gonadal dysgenesis, endometrial carcinoma developed in two and possibly three cases [18]. Along with three cases in the literature, the tumors were diagnosed between 28-35 years of age, and most were of an unusual mixed or adenosquamous type.

Androgenic-anabolic steroids have been implicated by several reports of patients developing hepatocellular carcinoma after long-term treatment of aplastic anemia, mainly the Fanconi type, with oxymetholone or methyltestosterone derivatives [19]. Further evaluation is needed, particularly in groups receiving these medications for other reasons.

Inorganic arsenicals have not been shown carcinogenic in experimental animals, but when taken internally they are a cause of skin cancer in man [20, 21]. The skin cancers following arsenical use are characteristically multiple, involve unexposed parts of the body and unusual locations (e.g., palms of the hand), and are associated with arsenical pigmentation and hyperkeratosis. Instances of lung cancer and liver hemangioendothelioma have been attributed to medicinal arsenic. These occurrences may not be in excess of expectation [21, 22], but would be compatible with what is known about cancer risks in occupational studies of arsenic exposure [22, 23].

Phenacetin in analgesic mixtures, when given in large doses, can cause chronic pyelonephritis and papillary necrosis. Reports from various countries [24-26] indicate that patients with "analgesic nephropathy" are at high risk of developing transitional cell tumors of the renal pelvis.

Coal tar and creosote preparations that contain polycyclic aromatic hydrocarbons have been reported to cause skin cancer in laboratory animals, in exposed workers, and in patients using these preparations [27].

Diphenylhydantoin (Dilantin) is one of four drugs under suspicion, along with chloramphenicol, amphetamines, and reserpine. There is some evidence of carcinogenicity in humans, but epidemiologic testing is inadequate. Dilantin occasionally induces lymphoid reactions that regress on cessation of therapy, but transformation to malignant lymphoma has occurred in several patients [28]. The nature of this association remains to be defined, but recent evidence [29, 30] in man and laboratory animals suggests that Dilantin may predispose to lymphoma by its capacity to concurrently depress and stimulate immune responses. Three separate studies [31-33] make it obvious that if there is an excess risk, it is almost certainly of small magnitude and perhaps acceptable, given the drug's efficacy in the treatment of epilepsy.

Chloramphenicol and other bone marrow-depressing drugs have been implicated by case studies in the development of leukemia [34, 35]. A causal relationship would be consistent with the potential of leukemogens (radiation, benzene, alkylating agents) to produce aplastic anemia [35, 36]. The production of chromosomal defects by chloramphenicol supports the possibility of a leukemia hazard, since such defects are seen in various conditions at high risk of leukemia [35, 36].

Amphetamine intake, mainly for weight reduction, was linked to a sixfold excess risk of Hodgkin's disease according to a recent case-control study [37]. With the problems involved in obtaining a reliable drug history, and with a subsequent negative study [38], this relationship needs further investigation.

Reserpine is indicated in three recent surveys [39-41] as a risk factor in breast cancer and possibly other tumors in persons treated for hypertension. Reserpine may be linked to breast cancer by its known capacity to stimulate prolactin release in humans [42]. But further studies are needed to evaluate the role of hypertension, social class, obesity, and other variables that may influence the association.

Often a drug with carcinogenic potential cannot be replaced by an equally effective, safe agent, so that some sort of risk-benefit decision must be made. To effectively make such a decision, the risk of cancer should not only be quantified, but also characterized with respect to dose-response, latent period, susceptibility factors, and the effect of cocarcinogens. In only a few cases, however, has the magnitude of excess risk been estimated in absolute or relative terms. Only very rarely are the "finer points" of an association delineated.

DRUGS CARCINOGENIC IN LABORATORY ANIMALS BUT SHOWING NO EFFECT IN MAN

Exactly which drugs are placed in this category depends on how rigorous an epidemiologic evaluation is expected. Adequate analytic studies of reasonable numbers of exposed persons followed over time have been conducted on only two drugs: *isoniazid* [43] and the *female steroidal sex hormones (including contraceptives)* [44-48]. This short list attests to the difficulties in evaluating cancer risk in man and unraveling the various components of risk (e.g., age, latent period, and cocarcinogen exposures) which also complicate the laboratory assessment of carcinogenicity.

The long latent period between exposure to a carcinogen and manifestation of the cancer is perhaps the single most important obstacle to adequate evaluation. This is illustrated by the apparent relation of alkylating agents to acute leukemia. In 26 reported cases of leukemia complicating multiple myeloma, the average latent period was about 4½ years [13]. Since the primary indication for this therapy is a usually fatal malignancy, the identification of risk was dependent on following up a large number of relatively long-term survivors.

If the latent period and other risk variables are not taken into account, the recognition and interpretation of relationships may be obscured. These variables may also interact with each other, as illustrated by the capacity of DES to cause genital tract adenocarcinomas. In this situation, the neoplasms are caused by a specifically timed prenatal exposure (probably first trimester), a latent period usually over 10 years, and possibly a concomitant surge of endogenous estrogens during puberty (acting as a promoting factor).

Because of the problems involved in evaluating drugs in man, any negative findings must be considered with caution. With *oral contraceptives,* three recent well-designed and executed analytic studies [46-48] to assess the risk of breast cancer showed either no association or perhaps slight protection. However, oral contraceptives have been available only since 1960 and in widespread use since 1965. Thus, the "latent period" that has now elapsed between exposure and the evaluation for disease is limited to 10 to 15 years for even the earliest of users.

Adequate assessment of a drug-cancer relationship requires knowledge of the epidemiology of the cancer in question. This information helps in distinguishing a drug effect from the natural history of the underlying disease and in identifying groups of people that might be particularly susceptible to a drug. It is known, for example, that a woman who has her first child before 18 years of age has one-third the risk of breast cancer of a woman having her first child after the age of 35 [49]. Perhaps younger women are also more susceptible to the effects of steroidal hormones.

In a recent survey [50] of Boston-area women of predominantly middle and upper social class, those entering the breast cancer age range had not used oral contraceptives in early reproductive life, because the drugs were not available. The exposure being studied in these women, therefore, may not be as relevant as exposure at a younger, more susceptible age. These difficulties, coupled with recent reports that oral contraceptive users are prone to liver tumors [51] and in situ cervical cancer [52], point to the need for continued monitoring.

OTHER DRUG EXPOSURES

The last two categories of drug exposures concern agents not yet evaluated in man. Experimentalists are better equipped to evaluate laboratory evidence of carcinogenicity. However, in assessing priorities for epidemiologic study of these drugs, it would seem prudent to weigh: 1) relative carcinogenicity in the laboratory, along with 2) the magnitude of population exposure, and 3) various parameters of this exposure (e.g., age, length of treatment, reason for treatment). Mentioned here are only a few drugs that would qualify for epidemiologic study at the earliest opportunity.

Various agents in *cancer chemotherapy* show carcinogenic potential in the laboratory. They have enabled some young people with cancer to survive long periods [53, 54] and are used in combination much earlier in the natural history of various malignancies. Furthermore, the agents are employed increasingly in nonmalignant conditions [55, 56], so that a major effort is now required to assess the long-term risks.

Laboratory research has raised concern about a group of drugs classed as *tertiary amines.* Included in this group are a number of widely prescribed drugs such as oxytetracycline and chlorpromazine. Experimentally, these agents, in the presence of a large amount of nitrite and an appropriately acidic medium, form highly carcinogenic nitrosamines [57]. In man also, the drugs may produce nitrosamines after interacting with dietary nitrites in an acid stomach. Widespread population exposure over many years and chronic use by some people dictate the need for epidemiologic evaluation. Study of chlorpromazine and other phenothiazines may be justified by an entirely different rationale. These agents are potent stimulators of prolactin release in females [42]. Since prolactin may be a risk factor in breast cancer, the risk of this neoplasm should be estimated among a group of women treated with heavy doses.

Iron dextran should be investigated because of its carcinogenicity in animals, widespread use, and case reports of malignancies at the site of injection [58, 59].

It has been claimed in the public press that women receiving *Depo-Provera* for contraception have a risk of in situ cervical cancer higher than that of the general population as determined by the Third National Cancer Survey. The results are in doubt since the exposed (and not the comparison) group comes from a highly screened population. However, the magnitude of the risk reported and the carcinogenicity of progestogens in the laboratory [60] indicate the need for further studies.

ESTIMATES OF POPULATION EXPOSURE TO DRUGS

In determining which drugs to evaluate by epidemiologic study, it would be useful to know the magnitude and characteristics of exposure to various drugs in the population. Marketing and prescription surveys have provided marginally useful data. For example, 500 drugs account for approximately 85 percent of all prescriptions [61]. However, estimates are needed of population exposure to drugs by type, duration of use, and therapeutic indication. Data specific for age, race, sex, social class, and possibly other risk factors would be desirable. This type of information was collected at least once by the National Health Survey [62], but publication of the survey was economically oriented and did not identify particular drugs or conditions. The best available information is probably that collected by a commercial drug information service [63]. Prescription data are given according to age, sex, and therapeutic indication; but there are serious limitations to this resource, and a more useful information system should be developed [64]. In addition, special surveys should be conducted of detailed characteristics of consumption of very commonly used drugs. The patterns of drug usage in "special risk" populations, such as pregnant women, also should be studied.

These surveys would help not only in selecting drugs for evaluation, but also in quantifying the population risk and designing control programs when an association has been established. This information would be critical to risk-benefit decisions.

IMPLICATIONS AND RECOMMENDATIONS

Cancer Etiology

Identification of drug-associated cancers helps not only by indicating medicinal hazards, but also by providing information on possible occupational, dietary, or other environmental dangers from the same agents (e.g., inorganic arsenic, coal-tar derivatives, DES). In this manner, the role of nitrosamines in human carcinogenesis could be clarified by a study of users of the tertiary amine drugs. In addition, drug-cancer associations may provide insight into carcinogenic mechanisms. Immunologic determinants, for example, have been clarified by the study of cancer in immunosuppressed transplant recipients.

Despite widespread population exposure to drugs that physiologically might be expected to increase the risk of malignancy, only limited knowledge of drug-induced cancer has been accumulated. For one reason the source of productive clues has been primarily clinical observations. The alert clinician usually detects an environmental hazard through clusters of unusual, rather than common, events. The initial observation is often a cluster of patients with a rare tumor type, such as clear cell adenocarcinomas, or adenosquamous carcinomas of the genital tract (DES), liver hemangioendotheliomas (arsenic, Thorotrast), or myelomonocytic leukemia (alkylating agents). More common tumors may be recognized by unusual sites of presentation (e.g., brain lymphomas in transplant recipients, palms of the hands for arsenical skin cancer), or by associations with known toxic manifestations (e.g., arsenical dermatosis, analgesic nephropathy).

Recognition of drug relationships may also be enhanced by short latent periods (excess lymphoma risk within 1 year of renal transplantation). Thus, it is unlikely that a clinician would be able to link a drug to a common neoplasm occurring 10 to 50 years after exposure. This may be the situation for reserpine, which is under suspicion not on the basis of clinical observations, but from a systematic survey of cancer risk following drug exposures.

The clinical approach, obviously productive in the past, should be encouraged. Practitioners providing etiologic clues should be able to consult the National Cancer Institute, the International Agency for Research on Cancer, and other agencies. Promising leads should be pursued by epidemiologic study. However, with the increasing exposure of our society to a large battery of pharmacological agents, many taken by healthy individuals, some mechanism is needed to determine which drugs to evaluate systematically in man, rather than waiting for a risk large enough to become clinically obvious.

With the advances in comparative physiology and laboratory carcinogenicity testing, some decisions can be made on an interdisciplinary basis. Perhaps a first step would be a meeting of laboratory scientists, epidemiologists, and clinical pharmacologists to decide on drug exposures needing human evaluation. Priorities may be ranked on the strength and relevance of laboratory results, magnitude of population exposure, duration of drug use, special characteristics of consumers, and the ease or difficulty with which appropriate groups could be identified for evaluation. High priority should be given to studies of patient groups exposed to drugs known to be carcinogenic in other groups (e.g., DES for the menopause, androgens for male infertility).

Another recommendation is to incorporate drug histories into case-control studies of cancer and to conduct cohort studies concerned with any outcome. The format of the drug histories could vary, but might as a minimum be a checklist of suspected drugs. Drug surveillance programs, such as the one at Boston University [38, 39], are concerned with these studies and show great potential for identifying long-term, as well as short-term, effects. These systems should continue to be used to generate and test hypotheses. To date, however, they have evaluated only those drugs taken recently (within 3 months of hospitalization for the Boston program). Perhaps the programs can be expanded in the future to include earlier drug histories.

Record-linkage systems, while much discussed, have contributed little to our understanding of the long-term effects of drugs. Theoretically, they seem to be ideal mechanisms to use for drug evaluation. Linking prescription information with subsequent hospital and diagnostic data for groups of people within prepaid health plans should be a relatively easy and inexpensive way of screening drugs for associations needing more intensive evaluation. With the likelihood of some form of national health insurance imminent, the opportunity for this type of study should be increased. The reasons for the failure of such record-linking efforts in the past need to be explored to determine if this is a feasible mechanism for drug screening.

Finally, a change in government policy might greatly facilitate studies of drug-induced cancer. The drug industry should be assigned some responsibility for evaluating long-term effects of drugs in man, just as it is now responsible for demonstrating safety regarding acute or toxic effects. A promising drug should not necessarily be withheld from general consumption until long-term follow-up studies have been done. A drug company, however, might be required to construct a surveillance mechanism in order to conduct a follow-up study, if warranted, on the first 50,000 to 100,000 individuals who received significant amounts of a new drug. This information would be furnished on demand to the FDA for appropriate evaluation up to 60 years after the introduction of a drug. Although the financial feasibility of this recommendation needs to be explored, it should not be inordinately expensive, particularly in terms of total drug sales; therefore, it should not substantially increase the cost of drugs. In fact, the money saved by not having to initiate such studies from scratch some 20 years after significant exposure could be great.

Cancer Control

Although the human data on drug-induced cancer is sparse, some steps can be taken in the areas of prevention, early diagnosis, and treatment. Control activities would benefit from the surveys previously outlined that could provide adequate data on drug-consumption patterns in this country. For instance, in the early 1960's DES was still being given to a surprisingly large number of pregnant women years after its efficacy in preventing spontaneous abortion had been disproved [65]. Even with the recent publicity about carcinogenic hazards to the fetus, within the past year prescriptions for DES were still being written for pregnant women [63]. Other illustrations of drug abuse (e.g., anabolic steroids given to athletes, chloramphenicol for upper respiratory infections) should prompt action in the form of professional education or drug regulation.

Two types of screening programs are possible. First is a coordinated local or national program of periodic screening for patient groups exposed to known carcinogenic drugs who are no longer being seen for the condition that led to such therapy (e.g., women exposed in utero to DES, long-term survivors of malignancies). A second type of screening is continuous monitoring by physicians of patients being seen for the conditions that led to their drug exposure (e.g., renal transplant recipients, reserpine-treated hypertensive women). This approach should not be restricted to only those patient groups with proved carcinogenic exposures, but should also include those taking "suspect" drugs. However, the effectiveness of this continued monitoring for cancer depends on the physician's awareness of the possible risk involved. While for some physician groups this awareness may be high, for others it will require an intensive program of professional education.

Last year, dermatologists wrote 99,000 prescriptions for methotrexate for severe psoriasis, and urologists wrote 125,000 prescriptions for androgens for such conditions as the male climacteric and sterility [63]. These groups, and others like them, who may not be aware of the potential hazards of these drugs, should receive the emphasis in campaigns for professional awareness. Similarly, it is not clear how many of the over 300 groups performing renal transplants are aware of the high risk of skin cancer in transplant recipients and the unusually malignant course of this neoplasm if not treated early [66].

Finally, while it is important to discourage the inappropriate use of carcinogenic drugs and to encourage screening and early treatment of exposed patients, it is also imperative to identify the biochemical mechanism of drug carcinogenesis through experimental research. In this way, new drugs may be developed that are equally effective but not carcinogenic, and agents may be added to therapeutic regimens that would block the carcinogenic action [67].

REFERENCES

1. Fraumeni, J.F., Jr., and Miller, R.W. Drug-induced cancer. *J. Natl. Cancer Inst.* *48:*1267-1270, 1972.

2. Modan, B., and Lilienfeld, A.M. Leukaemogenic effect of ionizing-irradiation treatment in polycythaemia. *Lancet 2:*439-441, 1964.

3. Hasterlik, R. J., and Finkel, A.J. Diseases of bones and joints associated with intoxication by radioactive substances, principally radium. *Med. Clin. North Am.* *49:*285-296, 1965.

4. Spiess, H. 224Ra-induced tumors in children and adults. *In Delayed Effects of Bone Seeking Radionuclides.* Symposium Proceedings, Univ. of Utah Press, Salt Lake City, Utah, 1969, pp. 227-247.

5. Brinker, H., Hansen, H.S., and Anderson, A.P. Induction of leukaemia by ^{131}I treatment of thyroid carcinoma. *Br. J. Cancer 28:*232-237, 1973.

6. Saenger, E.L., Thomas, G.E., and Tompkins, E.A. Incidence of leukemia following treatment of hyperthyroidism. *J.A.M.A. 205:*147, 1969.

7. da Silva Horta, J., Cayolla da Motta, L., Abbatt, J.D., et al. Malignancy and other late effects following administration of thorotrast. *Lancet 2:*201-205, 1965.

8. Hoover, R., and Fraumeni, J.F., Jr. Risk of cancer in renal transplant recipients. *Lancet 2:*55-57, 1973.

9. Hoover, R. Unpublished data.

10. Kersey, J.H., Spector, B.D., and Good, R.A. Primary immunodeficiency diseases and cancer: The immunodeficiency-cancer registry. *Int. J. Cancer 12:*333-347, 1973.

11. Ryser, H.J-P. Chemical carcinogenesis. *N. Engl. J. Med. 285:*721-734, 1971.

12. Thiede, T., Chievitz, E., and Christensen, B.C. Chlornaphazine as a bladder carcinogen. *Acta Med. Scand. 175:*721-725, 1964.

13. Karchmer, R.K., Amare, M., Larsen, W.E., et al. Alkylating agents as leukemogens in multiple myeloma. *Cancer 33:*1103-1107, 1974.

14. Arseneau, J.C., Sponzo, R.W., Levin, D.L., et al. Nonlymphomatous malignant tumors complicating Hodgkin's disease. *N. Engl. J. Med. 287:*1119-1122, 1972.

15. Herbst, A.L., Ulfelder, H., and Poskanzer, D.C. Adenocarcinoma of the vagina: Association of maternal stilbestrol therapy with tumor appearance in young women. *N. Engl. J. Med. 284:*878-881, 1971.

16. Herbst, A.L., Robboy, S.J., Scully, R.E., et al. Clear-cell adenocarcinoma of the vagina and cervix in girls: Analysis of 170 registry cases. *Am. J. Obstet. Gynecol. 119:* 713-724, 1974.

17. Lanier, A.P., Noller, K.L., Decker, D.G., et al. Cancer and stilbestrol. *Mayo Clin. Proc. 48:*793-799, 1973.

18. Cutler, B.S., Forbes, A.P., Ingersol, F.M., et al. Endometrial carcinoma after stilbestrol therapy in gonadal dysgenesis. *N. Engl. J. Med. 287:*628-631, 1972.

19. Mulvihill, J.J., Ridolfi, R.L., Schultz, F.R., et al. Hepatic adenoma in Fanconi anemia treated with oxymetholone. *J. Pediatr. 87:* 122-124, 1975.

20. Neubauer, O. Arsenical cancer: A review. *Br. J. Cancer:1:* 192-251, 1947.

21. *IARC Monograph on the Evaluation of the Carcinogenic Risk of Chemicals to Man: Some Inorganic and Organometallic Compounds.* Vol. 2. I.A.R.C., Lyon, 1973, pp. 48-73.

22. Lee, A.M., and Fraumeni, J.F., Jr. Arsenic and respiratory cancer in man: An occupational study. *J. Natl. Cancer Inst. 42:*1045-1052, 1969.

23. Ott, M.G, Holder, B.B., and Gordon, H.L. Respiratory cancer and occupational exposure to arsenicals. *Arch. Environ. Health 29:*250-255, 1974.

24. Bengtsson, U., Angervall, L., Ekman, H., et al. Transitional cell tumors of the renal pelvis in analgesic abusers. *Scand. J. Urol. Nephrol. 2:*145-150, 1968.

25. Taylor, J.S. Carcinoma of the urinary tract and analgesic abuse. *Med. J. Aust. 1:* 407-409, 1972.

26. Johansson, S., Angervall, L., Bengtsson, U., et al. Uroepithelial tumors of the renal pelvis associated with abuse of phenacetin-containing analgesics. *Cancer 33:*743-753, 1974.

27. Rook, A.J., Gresham, G.A., and Davis, R.A. Squamous epithelioma possibly induced by the therapeutic application of tar. *Br. J. Cancer 10:*17-23, 1956.

28. Gams, R.A., Neal, J.A., and Conrad, F.G. Hydantoin-induced pseudo-pseudolymphoma. *Ann. Intern. Med. 69:*557-568, 1968.

29. Kruger, G., Harris, D., and Sussman, E. Effect of Dilantin in mice. II. Lymphoreticular tissue atypia and neoplasia after chronic exposure. *Z. Krebsforsch. 78:*290-302, 1972.

30. Grob, P.J., and Herold, G.E. Immunological abnormalities and hydantoins. *Br. Med. J. 2:*561-563, 1972.

31. Anthony, J.J. Malignant lymphoma associated with hydantoin drugs. *Arch. Neurol.* 22:450-454, 1970.
32. Clemmesen, J., Fuglsang-Frederiksen, V., and Plum, C.M. Are anticonvulsants oncogenic? *Lancet 1:*705-707, 1974.
33. Li, F.P., Willard, D.R., and Goodman, R. Malignant lymphoma after diphenylhydantoin (Dilantin) therapy. *Cancer.* In press.
34. Fraumeni, J.F., Jr. Bone marrow depression induced by chloramphenicol or phenylbutazone. Leukemia and other sequelae. *J.A.M.A. 201:*828-834, 1967.
35. Fraumeni, J.F., Jr. Clinical epidemiology of leukemia. *Semin. Hematol. 6:*250-260, 1969.
36. Fraumeni, J.F., Jr., and Miller, R.W. Epidemiology of human leukemia: Recent observations. *J. Natl. Cancer Inst. 38:*593-605, 1967.
37. Newell, G.R., Rawlings, W., Kinnear, B.K., et al. Case-control study of Hodgkin's disease. I. Results of the interview questionnaire. *J. Natl. Cancer Inst. 51:*1437-1441, 1973.
38. Boston Collaborative Drug Surveillance Program. Amphetamines and malignant lymphoma. *J.A.M.A. 229:*1462-1463, 1974.
39. Boston Collaborative Drug Surveillance Program. Reserpine and breast cancer. *Lancet 2:*669-671, 1974.
40. Armstrong, B., Stevens, N., and Doll, R. Retrospective study of the association between use of Rauwolfia derivatives and breast cancer in English women. *Lancet 2:*672-675, 1974.
41. Heinonen, O.P., Shapiro, S., Tuominen, L., et al. Reserpine use in relation to breast cancer. *Lancet 2:*675-677, 1974.
42. Turkington, R.W. Prolactin secretion in patients treated with various drugs. *Arch. Intern. Med. 130:*349-354, 1972.
43. Hammond, E.C., Selikoff, I.J., and Robitzek, E.H. Isoniazid therapy in relation to later occurrence of cancer in adults and in infants. *Br. Med. J. 2:*792-795, 1967.
44. Burch, J.C., and Byrd, B.F. Effects of long-term administration of estrogens on the occurrence of mammary cancer in women. *Ann. Surg. 174:*414-418, 1971.
45. Wynder, E.L., and Schneiderman, M.A. Exogenous hormones - boon or culprit? *J. Natl. Cancer Inst. 51:*729-731, 1973.
46. Vessey, M.P., Doll, R., and Sutton, P.M. Investigation of the possible relationship between oral contraceptives and benign and malignant breast disease. *Cancer, 28:*1395-1399, 1971.
47. Arthes, F.G., Sartwell, P.E., and Lewison, E.F. The pill, estrogens and the breast. Epidemiologic aspects. *Cancer 28:*1391-1394, 1971.
48. Henderson, B.E., Powell, D., Rosario, I., et al. An epidemiologic study of breast cancer. *J. Natl. Cancer Inst. 53:*609-614, 1974.
49. MacMahon, B., Cole, P., Lin, T.M., et al. Age at first birth and breast cancer risk. *Bull. W.H.O. 43:*209-221, 1970.
50. Hoover, R., and Cole, P. Oral contraceptive use in metropolitan Boston. In preparation.
51. Mayes, E.T., Christopherson, W.M., and Barrows, G.H. Focal nodular hyperplasia of the liver. *Am. J. Clin. Pathol. 61:*735-746, 1974.
52. Ory, H.W., Conger, S.B., Naib, Z., et al. The relationship between oral contraceptive use and cervical carcinoma in situ. Annual Meeting of the American Public Health Association, San Francisco, November 1973.
53. Everson, R.B., Fraumeni, J.F., Jr., and Myers, M.H. Improved survival in Wilms' tumour. *Lancet 1:*1290-1291, 1974.
54. Holland, J.F. Hopes for tomorrow versus realities of today; therapy and prognosis of acute lymphocytic leukemia of childhood. *Pediatrics 45:*191-193, 1970.

55. Turk, J.L. The use of cyclophosphamide in non-neoplastic disease. *Proc. Roy. Soc. Med. 66:*805-810, 1973.

56. Harris, C.C. Malignancy during methotrexate and steroid therapy for psoriasis. *Arch. Dermatol. 103:*501-504, 1971.

57. Lijinsky, W. Reaction of drugs with nitrous acid as a source of carcinogenic nitrosamines. *Cancer Res. 34:*255-258, 1974.

58. Robinson, C.E.G., Bell, D.N., and Sturdy, J.H. Possible association of malignant neoplasm with iron-dextran injection. *Br. Med. J. 11:*648-650, 1960.

59. MacKinnon, A.E., and Bancewicz, J. Sarcoma after injection of intramuscular iron. *Br. Med. J. 2:*277-279, 1973.

60. Nelson, L.W., Carlton, W.W., and Weikel, J.H. Canine mammary neoplasms and progestogens. *J.A.M.A. 219:*1601-1606, 1972.

61. Maronde, R.F., Burks, D., Lee, P.V., et al. Physician prescribing practices. *Am. J. Hosp. Pharm. 26:*566-573, 1969.

62. National Center for Health Statistics. *Cost and Acquisition of Prescribed and Nonprescribed Medicines, United States, July 1964-June 1965.* Series 10, No. 33, U.S. Govt. Print. Off., Washington, D.C., 1966.

63. Lea, Inc. *National Disease and Therapeutic Index.* Ambler, Pa., 1974.

64. Rucker, T.D. Drug use: Data, sources, and limitations. *J.A.M.A. 230:*888-890,1974.

65. The Boston Collaborative Drug Surveillance Program. Diethylstilbestrol in pregnancy. *Cancer 31:*573-577, 1973.

66. Koranda, F.C., Dehmel, E.M., Kahn, G., et al. Cutaneous complications in immunosuppressive transplant recipients. *J.A.M.A. 229:*419-424, 1974.

67. Apple, M.A. Active intervention to prevent cancer in vivo with prophylactic drugs. *J. Clin. Pharm. 15:*29-35, 1975.

DISCUSSION

The relationship of birth-control pills and hepatoma was considered by some participants to be a serious public health threat. **Dr. Shubik** supported Richard Doll's opinion that birth-control pills are definitely related to the development of hepatoma in treated women. Furthermore, **Dr. Henderson** stated that 19 of 21 cases of liver adenoma studied by Edmundson in Los Angeles were associated with oral contraceptives.

With respect to the nitrosation problem in the gastrointestinal tract, **Dr. Shubik** felt this might be avoided by the addition of ascorbic acid to drugs susceptible to nitrosation. This has been done for tetracycline and should be used routinely. **Dr. Shubik** also reported that Flagyl, Meridozol, phenobarbital, and griseofulvin have produced tumors in animals and need to be studied in man. Studies of veterans who received griseofulvin while in Vietnam may yield valuable information. Perhaps the use of Flagyl and Meridozol should be restricted to life-threatening situations.

Dr. Davies commented that we must not lose sight of the vehicles used in drug compounding, since these vehicles may have carcinogenic or other toxic effects. An example might be the toxicity associated with vinyl chloride used in aerosol propellants. **Dr. Mulvihill** emphasized the potential importance of genetic factors in evaluating responses to drugs. Screening for known genetic traits, such as α-1-antitrypsin deficiency, may identify persons who would respond abnormally to drugs or who should not work with certain substances.

Dr. Henderson pointed out that case-control studies of Hodgkin's disease (with respect to amphetamines) and breast cancer (with respect to menopausal estrogens) have produced conflicting results, due apparently to the difficulty in obtaining appropriate controls. Dr. Hoover concluded the discussion by agreeing with Dr. Shubik that the relation of birth-control pills to hepatoma is a major problem to be solved. He hoped that the National Health Insurance currently under consideration might improve the opportunities for record linkage and discovery of adverse drug effects.

Glyn G. Caldwell

13

DIET

John W. Berg, M.D.

Cancer Epidemiology Research Center
University of Iowa
Iowa City, Iowa

INTRODUCTION

Food comes late in the discussion of environmental carcinogens, not because we think it an unimportant source of risk, but because of the paucity of well-documented carcinogenic situations. Most cancers in the United States are culture-linked, and many are associated with particular dietary patterns. Also, there is no shortage of carcinogens in our diets. The difficulty is that these aspects are not fitted together: cancers are linked with dietary patterns but not with specific carcinogens, while the association of a particular dietary carcinogen to any kind of cancer is tenuous, to say the least. This review can only elaborate on the impasse. It will focus on candidate dietary carcinogens. Specific cancers will be considered primarily in relation to specific dietary factors.

Part of our difficulty is that we generally are working in situations of low host susceptibility, low biologic activity, or very low dosage. In this country, bowel cancer is our most common major cancer, and current evidence suggests lifelong exposure to a ubiquitous carcinogen. Yet the lifetime risk of developing a clinically apparent bowel cancer is about 5 percent. In such situations, even direct single-factor associations are difficult to establish. For dietary factors, the impression at this time is that the associations are not simple but depend

Supported by Public Health Service Contract NOI CP43200 with the National Cancer Institute.

strongly on combinations of noxious agents, cofactors, and natural or acquired metabolic peculiarities of the host.

The bright side of complex risk situations is that once understood they should offer more options for control and more chances of finding a workable program of prevention. However, accurate descriptions of dietary risk factors must emphasize the weakness of most cases against them, yet stress the overall likelihood that definite connections between specific dietary chemicals and cancers exist and will be demonstrated given sufficiently sophisticated epidemiology. The reader must decide whether these cancer problems have resisted solution because we do not have the technical tools or because too few people have applied appropriate techniques.

The other subjective decision is: When is there enough evidence to act upon one of the discussed hypotheses and remove the risk factor from food? Since we view this question as a sociopolitical one, it will not be considered here. Rather, suggestions for action will involve the gathering of further evidence.

The references cited will be to general reviews where possible, since they offer the most efficient lead to evaluative work by others and to more complete bibliographies.

CARCINOGENS IN THE DIET

Aflatoxins

Aflatoxins are naturally occurring substances that came to prominence as carcinogens because they produced liver cancers in fish in natural feeding situations and in rats under laboratory conditions. There is strong evidence associating them with the high rate of liver cancer found in many populations, although they have not been linked with cancer in this country.

Aflatoxins are lactones and derivatives produced by strains of *Aspergillus flavus* growing on peanuts, grains, and other foods [1, 2]. These fungi grow well only under conditions of sustained high humidity. Aflatoxins are the most potent carcinogens known for rats [1]. They are about 10 times as potent on a weight basis as dimethylnitrosamine (DMN), which in turn is an order of magnitude more potent than the polycyclic hydrocarbons.

Normal practices of food and grain storage in this country make aflatoxin contamination of local food unlikely. Imports from tropical countries, where the climate is right for *Aspergillus* growth, are the danger sources. The major human food item at risk is peanuts, and they are monitored by the Department of Agriculture and Food and Drug Administration (FDA) for aflatoxin levels [3]. Since 1967, Brazil nuts have been inspected also.

The most direct evidence that aflatoxins can be carcinogenic for man comes from the Netherlands [4]. A small cohort of Dutch workers extracting oils from peanuts contaminated with aflatoxins was studied. Their rate of cancer (multiple kinds) and liver disease taken together was more than 3 times that in matched controls. There was just 1 liver cancer among the 11 malignancies, although in international studies only liver cancer has been linked to aflatoxin ingestion.

In parts of Africa and the Far East, local grain stores are heavily contaminated with aflatoxin. Oettlé [5] was among the first to emphasize the concentration of liver cancer in regions of high humidity where *Aspergillus* growth is favored. Recent reports from countries such as Thailand [6], the Ivory Coast [7], Swaziland [8], Kenya [9], and the Philippines [10] emphasize the strong coincidence of aflatoxin and liver cancer regions.

In animal experiments, cofactors play a role. Some fatty acids promote the formation of hepatoxins by aflatoxin [11]. Diets deficient in lipotropes protect rats from aflatoxin liver cancer [12], as does diethylstilbestrol (DES) [13]. Vitamin A deficiency leads to the formation of intestinal cancer as well as liver cancer [14]. Presumably the situation in man is equally complex. In particular, the possible role of hepatitis viruses remains to be elucidated [15]. There is undoubtedly much more to be learned, but at this moment aflatoxin is the most probable important example of a human carcinogen reaching its victims through the food they eat.

Nitrosamines

Nitrosamines are powerful carcinogens for animals. They and their precursors can be found frequently in food. Thus, it is not surprising they are at or near the top of everyone's food hazard list.

Yet so many pieces of evidence connecting these compounds with human cancer are lacking that they currently can be considered only possible, not probable, human carcinogens. In particular, there is no probable link between them and any major amount of cancer in this country.

Nitrosamines are frightening because so many are strong carcinogens in animals at very low concentrations [16]. However, there are species and strain differences in susceptibility [17] that prevent automatic extrapolation from animal reactivity to human sensitivity. In fact, although nitrosamines first came to the attention of cancer researchers because of their toxicity to humans [16], there has been no direct association between these compounds and human cancer even in the industrial setting.

The other disturbing aspect of nitrosamines is the relative ease with which they can be formed from common precursors. A large number of secondary, tertiary, and quaternary amines will combine with nitrite to form nitrosamines. Reactions can take place under varying conditions of pH [18] and temperature so that nitrosamines may be formed in soil [19]; under conditions of food storage; during food preparation, such as the frying of bacon; or in the body [20, 21]. Bacteria may play a role either directly by catalyzing the amine-nitrite union or indirectly by reducing nitrate to nitrite [19,22]. Hence, the infected bladder and the achlorhydric stomach are considered particularly favorable sites for nitrosamine synthesis [22]. The necessary amines can be found in many foods, but they are also ingested in the pure form of many common medicines such as oxytetracycline, tolazamide, chlorpromazine, and quinacrine [23].

Balancing the argument of ubiquity is the low level of these compounds found in foods, usually near the threshold of accurate detection and identification. Significant biological levels have not, at this writing, been demonstrated in humans in contrast with the aflatoxin situation. While emphasizing the importance of test-tube reactions that could occur in vivo, the efficient blockage of nitrosamine formation by ascorbic acid must also be mentioned. The same individuals who put themselves at risk by eating bacon every morning may be protecting themselves by preceding the bacon with orange juice.

The Japanese offer the strongest epidemiologic correlation between nitrosamine-containing foods and cancer. Salted fish is an undoubted risk factor for stomach cancer and a major source of nitrosamines [24]. However, it is not clear how much overlap there is between the consumption of salted fish and smoked fish, with its high levels of polycyclic hydrocarbons. Nitrosamines have been reported in the diets of Africans and Iranians [25] in epidemic esophageal cancer areas, but involved such low levels that it is difficult to characterize the substances found or to determine why they should have such an impact on the populations in question.

The amine precursors are high in the nitrosamine-containing fish consumed by the Japanese. Nitrate in water supplies was linked in a general way with stomach cancer in Chile [26] and with liver, stomach, and esophageal cancer in the English borough of Worksop [22]. The overall cancer rate for the borough, however, was only 88 percent of that expected. In American data, the mortality from stomach cancer was higher in the 12 of 94 large cities with the least nitrate in the drinking water than in the 12 with the most (J. Berg, unpublished data). No study of cancer and diet in this country has associated nitrite-rich foods with increased cancer risk. As long as we have such a paucity of evidence, there will be a wide range of opinions on the danger of current levels of nitrate ingestion.

Polycyclic Aromatic Hydrocarbons

Polycyclic aromatic hydrocarbons have been the standard animal carcinogens and have received substantial attention as potential human carcinogens. Among the many such compounds, benzo[a]pyrene appears to be the most common in foods [27, 28]. It also was the first chemically pure carcinogen extracted from coal tar [29]. Dibenzanthracene is the second most common food contaminant of the group, and the first pure chemical proved carcinogenic. The third famous polycyclic compound, 3-methylcholanthrene, is less often found in food and may not be carcinogenic in primates [30]. Usually found as mixtures, there are many more of these compounds [27]; considering them as an epidemiologic group seems to be practical.

Industrial exposures and air pollution apparently are more important sources of polycyclics than foods in this country. As a first estimate, one can judge the level of these compounds in the diet by the intake of smoked foods. They include not only smoked fish [31] and hams, but also such foods as barbecued beef [32], cooking oils, and coffee [33].

Do foods containing polycyclics present any risk to the general population? Adequate studies have not been done, although they are technically feasible. The strongest correlation between dietary polycyclics and human cancer is that all populations consuming a great deal of smoked fish seem to be at high risk for stomach cancer [34]. The converse is not true: smoked foods cannot account for all high-risk stomach cancer. How much stomach cancer is from other sources of polycyclic hydrocarbons is another question and one that deserves more study. Polycyclics currently are considered the most carcinogenic component in polluted air [35], and air pollution has been associated with high stomach cancer rates [36]. Polycyclics settling from air onto food might even be a risk factor [33]. On the other hand, smokers surely swallow some of their inhaled tars, yet stomach cancer is only linked weakly to smoking [37].

Since bowel cancer is associated with beef intake [38], polycyclics produced in grilling may be a factor in that association. Again, the evidence called for seems available but is as yet uncollected. It will be argued that stomach and bowel cancers occur in different populations so that no simple correlation can exist between polycyclics and both sites. But we may be demanding too much when we ask for simple correlations. The site of carcinogenesis may be determined by different cofactors producing different pathways of metabolism or making one particular epithelium susceptible to the ingested carcinogen. The assessment here—that the evidence associating dietary polycyclics with human cancer still is weak—is a judgment of our efforts, not of the ultimate likelihood of risk from these common and powerful carcinogens.

Other Toxic Natural Food Constituents

In certain parts of the world, a cancer risk may be posed by natural plant foods. Some, such as cycasin, are generally toxic and will not be deliberately ingested. Others are less obviously noxious and provide a more subtle hazard. Among the toxins, cycasin is the most thoroughly studied [39]. If not leached from cycad meal, it can be metabolized to an active aglycone that is the same proximate carcinogen as is generated from DMN [40].

Of greater potential risk to humans are the carcinogens in bracken fern. This plant came to attention first by producing bladder cancer in cattle in Turkey [41]. Carcinogens also were in Japanese bracken, a common dietary item in

Japan [42]. The first specific carcinogen identified in bracken was shikimic acid (3, 4, 5-trihydroxy-1-cyclohexene-1-carboxylic acid), but still another more potent component needs to be identified [43]. Shikimic acid is widespread in plants [44]. Bracken is eaten in many other areas, but not all varieties have been tested for their carcinogenic potential. The high bowel cancer incidence in Scotland might be related to the ubiquity of bracken in forage areas, if not because of direct ingestion of fern by cattle, then by leaching of a carcinogenic agent from the plants and concentration in water or food. There is no experimental evidence for this hypothesis; however, since Scotland reports the world's highest bowel cancer mortality rate, it might merit investigation.

Safrole is a flavoring agent shown to be a carcinogen for animals [40]. No epidemiologic pattern of cancer has been related to its use and, in fact, no high-use population has been suggested for study.

Morton [45] has long held that the high incidence of esophageal cancer in Curacao and perhaps other regions as well resulted from the heavy consumption of medicinal teas made from a variety of plants. Carcinogenic activity now has been shown for several tannin-containing extracts of these plants [46], so the hypothesis remains viable. Other folk medicines contain pyrrolizidine alkaloids that are strong carcinogens [40]. Investigations are now underway to see if individuals in this country with a high intake of herbal products have a high cancer rate.

Cole et al. [47, 48] found an association between one of our most common beverages—coffee—and bladder cancer. Although not analyzed as thoroughly as the Curacao teas, coffee may contain some polycyclic hydrocarbons [33]. Caffeine itself is a potentiator for several carcinogens in animal systems [49], and it might do the same for humans. Although the epidemiologic evidence does not rule out mere mutual association of coffee and cancer to a third variable [50], the ubiquity of exposure to coffee should give high priority to investigations of the subject, especially biochemical and biological studies.

Food Additives

Besides the carcinogens naturally occurring in foods or formed during processing, one must consider those chemicals added to foods to enhance their appearance and flavor or to preserve them. Dyes used to color foods were the first group of compounds studied because of chemical similarities to other carcinogens. For instance, two compounds, FD&C Yellow Nos. 3 and 4, are derived by coupling aniline or orthotoluidine with 2-naphthylamine. Decoupling has been reported. Although not shown carcinogenic, the dyes are hepatotoxins and were removed from the approved list [51]. Decisions on safety do not appear to be consistent. Citrus Red No. 2, highly suspect as an animal carcinogen [51], is considered toxic in the WHO evaluation; however, it is still approved for use in the United States. On the other hand, FD&C Violet No. 1, long used as the stamping dye for meat inspection, was withdrawn on the basis of similar preliminary evidence [52].

One of the most important problems at the moment concerns artificial sweeteners—cyclamate and saccharin. Both compounds produce bladder cancer in mice by the pellet implantation method [53]. In addition, cyclamate produces bladder cancer when fed to rats [54, 55]. The active metabolite seems to be cyclohexylamine, which is formed by humans (in quite variable amounts) who ingest cyclamate [56]. Hence, while no cancers in humans have been specifically attributed to cyclamate, it has been banned as an additive. Saccharin has not been shown to be a complete carcinogen when fed to animals, but it does have cocarcinogenic properties [57]. Its active metabolites have not been identified; thus, human risks are less easily estimated.

Looking at epidemiologic patterns of human cancer does not add much to our judgments. Cyclamates came into common usage so recently that one would not expect to see their carcinogenic impact for some time. Saccharin, if a carcinogen, might be expected to have particularly high use in diabetics. The cancer incidence in diabetics is difficult to determine precisely [58, 59], but there is no suggestion of a special bladder cancer risk. Particularly relevant to the question would be data on the health of cyclamate workers. By anecdotal report, cyclamate airborne levels were high in parts of the production cycle. Study of individuals who worked under these conditions should provide direct evidence about the risks from this useful compound. The situation is the classic one in cancer epidemiology. Here we have a substantial theoretical risk of cancer for almost the entire U.S. population, compounds of substantial utility are involved, and although hundreds of man hours are spent on debating the philosophy of risk, no one will take the responsibility to seek out the facts about chemical-human interaction that would help us judge whether or not there is susceptibility.

Sato [60] and others suggested that salt is a risk factor for stomach cancer. Certainly the pickled vegetables and fish identified in Japanese dietary studies [61, 62] are highly salted foods. Most other investigators have not highlighted the salt intake of high-risk European groups. So often in a situation such as this one, it is not clear whether salt was overlooked, could not be measured, or was not correlated. In animals, salt produces acute gastric injury but chronic atrophic gastritis has not been described. These facts should not cause us to dismiss the possibility out of hand; rather they suggest that more experimental work and epidemiologic analyses are needed for evaluation.

Food Contaminants

Another large set of chemicals enters our food less directly. High rates of food yield come only when growth factors are added and natural hazards are eliminated. Hence, chemical fertilizers and pesticides are ubiquitous potential additives to plant foods, while antibiotics and growth stimulants find their way into meats and other animal products. Other contaminants are added during processing and even during packaging. Still others are transfers from other parts of the environment, such as when air pollutants settle on plants or pesticides applied to plants appear in drinking water. Usually the concentrations of these contaminants are low. Risks would be assumed to come first of all from those compounds that accumulate in the human body.

Conspicuous among compounds that accumulate are asbestos, DDT, and related compounds. DDT is one of several pesticides that can produce tumors in animals [63, 64]. Some groups of people were heavily exposed as long as 20 years ago, so its effects on human health should be well known. In fact, no adequate study on cancer risk in man has ever been done. Aldrin and dieldrin are somewhat newer compounds whose presence in food also has been considered a risk on the basis of animal experiments [63]. These compounds produce liver cancers in mice, but their effect on other species is debatable [65]. However, they have been banned and, ironically, may be replaced by arsenic [66], a proved carcinogen for humans, and heptachlor[67], an even more potent carcinogen in mice [63].

A special risk from asbestos or related compounds was suggested for individuals consuming polished rice [68]. The rice is polished by talc; despite washing, enough talc remains in the rice to be ingested and found in gastrointestinal tumors of rice eaters. Talc is also used in salami, peanuts, and chewing gum [52]. Asbestos often is found with talc, and asbestos workers uniformly have increased rates of stomach and bowel cancer. Talc particles are found in fully developed cancers, since the ulcerated surfaces of these cancers are fine portals for accumulating all sorts of material. A causal role would be more convincing if the particles were related to precancerous lesions. Most significant of all would be to identify specific tissue reactions to these particles in the lung, pleura, and peritoneum and to have these reactive areas associated with cancer development.

There is also a dietary burden of physically similar particles from another source. Plants growing in sandy soils may be expected to contain phytoliths: precipitated silicate casts of their vessels. They are in the same size range as asbestos fibers. Such foods as bamboo shoots are a rich source of these fibers (I. Selikoff, personal communication); hence, they are one more possible source of risk if ingested fibers are a significant factor in human cancer etiology.

Asbestos recently received publicity as a drinking-water contaminant, but the risk to humans is said to be nondemonstrable from death rates in the Duluth area where the exposure is a public issue [69]. The problem is far more widespread than it would be if contamination from single mine sources were the only source of asbestos in water and other beverages. Many water supplies contain some asbestos [70], and filtering is only partially effective in removing fibers. Since fibers have been found in rain water, it is postulated that urban air can be a source of contamination. Asbestos can be used for piping and is the usual material for filtering beer, wine, and soft drinks. In all cases, some fibers get into the final product. With so many sources of asbestos, it may be more efficient to examine total body burdens and relate them to cancer if possible than to estimate total intake from liquids, air pollution, and other sources.

Scientists have emphasized the need to obtain relevant facts on the dangers of food contaminants, but assembling these facts will only move the discussion into an ethical and philosophical framework. The best example is the problem of DES in beef [71]. DES is a known carcinogen for humans when high doses (about 2 grams) are given in the first trimester of pregnancy. Little argument took place about prohibiting the use of pellets of this material for fattening chickens, since the pellets could get into human foods. There is far less consensus about their use in beef, because even a heavy beef eater probably would consume no more than a few *micrograms* per year. Such a hormone level is below physiological levels of the natural estrogens for either men or women and well below the amount of "natural" estrogens consumed by someone adding wheat germ to his diet. Scientists seem to have provided most of the needed facts (except regarding thresholds) about this problem, and there seems no reason to think that DES in beef poses a *major* cancer risk. Whether there is *any* risk is likely to remain a matter of speculation; the cost-benefit analysis is essentially a political question.

Other possible food contaminants are so numerous that even listing them is beyond the scope of this review. In addition, surface water can contain and accumulate hundreds of organic and inorganic compounds including most known carcinogens [72], with the total effect being great enough to increase cancer rates in fish [73]. Currently used methods of purifying water for drinking do not eliminate the chemicals. It probably is epidemiologically hopeless to expect to link specific cancer risks to a specific contaminant; however, correlating high cancer risk with high general pollution levels may be forthcoming.

Trace Elements

Heavy metals are important industrial toxins and carcinogens as described in Chapter 11. Hence, they are *prima facie* potential dietary carcinogens. They enter the diet both in foods [74] and in drinking water. Soft water that is corrosive [75] may contain lead [76] and other metals in concentrations near those shown to reduce survival in animals [77].

Among several correlations between levels of carcinogenic trace metals in water supplies and increased cancer risk, one association seems unquestioned: A region of Taiwan has particularly high levels of arsenic in the well water, and the population of this area has a very high cancer rate. Skin cancer predominates, but lung cancer also seems increased [78].

Other suggested associations merit further investigation. The distribution of carcinogenic metals in water supplies in the United States matched the distribution of cancer mortality in a number of cases (Table 1). Often the same cancers were produced by these agents in laboratory animals [79]. For example, beryllium was associated with bone cancer, and lead with leukemia and bowel and kidney cancer. The opportunities for further investigation seem quite explicit, the only question being one of priority since the magnitude of the hypothesized effects does not suggest that these elements could be the primary environmental determinants of risk.

Trace elements may affect cancer risk in other ways than by direct carcinogenesis. Most cations are biologic competitors with other dietary constituents [80]. Future studies should be done with this in mind, since correlations may be found with deficiencies or excesses of elements not usually implicated in carcinogenesis.

A well-known example of carcinogenesis attributed to dietary imbalance in humans is the Plummer-Vinson iron deficiency syndrome [81, 82], associated in northern Scandinavia with a high risk of cancer developing in the affected pharyngeal and esophageal mucosa. A parallel suggestion is that African esophageal cancers flourish in an environment deficient in molybdenum (Mo) [83]. Low Mo in U.S. water supplies is correlated with excess esophageal cancer [84].

Selenium reduces tumor frequency in several experimental situations [85]. Cancer rates are lower in states and cities in the United States where higher selenium levels are found in plants, milk, or human blood [86]. The protection comes about because selenium is an effective antioxidant. Other antioxidants have the same anticarcinogenic effects [87], which appear to be very basic since even actinic carcinogenesis is affected [88]. The implications go far beyond selenium. Both vitamins C and E have antioxidant activities [89]. Most of us ingest biologically meaningful levels of the commercial antioxidants, butylated hydroxytoluene (BHT) and butylated hydroxyanisole (BHA). It has been postulated that these compounds have contributed to the drop in stomach cancer incidence in this country [90].

Other trace elements have been linked to cancer, although none of the studies has been developed to the point of removing contradictions or presenting a clear picture of altered human risk. Zinc is an inhibitor of 7,12-dimethylbenz[a]anthracene (DMBA) carcinogenesis in hamsters and rats [91, 92]; on the other hand, zinc deficiency inhibits tumor growth [93]. Stocks and Davies [94] associated soils having zinc excess or at least a high zinc-copper ratio with human stomach cancer, whereas others [95] say low zinc-high copper is the pattern consistent with cancer. Severe magnesium deficiency in rats produced an increased incidence of myelogenous leukemia [96] and lymphoma [97], while manganese deficiency depressed nickel subsulfide carcinogenesis in rats [98] and was correlated with high cancer rates in Finland [99]. Both substances, when present in drinking water, were associated with low cancer rates in a Dutch study [100].

TABLE 1
Statistically significant positive correlations
between metal concentrations and cancer death rates [79]

Metal	Cancer[a]	Probability of positive association
Arsenic	Larynx (161)	0.024
	Eye (192)	0.009
	Myeloid leukemia (204.1)	0.042
Beryllium	Breast (women) (170)	0.040
	Uterine cervix (171)	0.016
	Other uterus (172–174)	0.006
	Bone (196)	0.024
	All cancers (140–205)	0.016
Cadmium	Mouth and pharynx (140-149)	0.003
	Esophagus (150)	0.00004
	Large intestine (153, 154)	0.00001
	Larynx (161)	0.004
	Lung (162, 163)	0.001
	Breast (women) (170)	0.003
	Bladder (181)	0.009
	Myeloma (203)	0.008
	All lymphomas (200–203, 205)	0.016
	All cancers (140–205)	0.0005
Chromium	None	
Cobalt	None	
Iron	None	
Lead	Stomach (151)	0.0026
	Small intestine (152)	0.038
	Large intestine (153, 154)	0.009
	Ovary (175)	0.02
	Kidney (180)	0.008
	Myeloma (203)	0.042
	All lymphomas (200–203, 205)	0.0005
	All leukemia (204)	0.006
Nickel	Mouth and pharynx (140–149)	0.044
	Large intestine (153, 154)	0.031

[a] Numbers in parentheses indicate the code numbers used in the *International Classification of Diseases, Injuries, and Causes of Death (ICD)*.

The most instructive association of all is the one between iodine and thyroid cancer. Both iodine deficiency and excess appear carcinogenic. Iodine deficiency in Switzerland and Colombia leads to goiter and carcinoma of the follicular or anaplastic type. Iodine excess, found in Hawaii and Iceland for instance, has been linked to a high rate of papillary thyroid cancer [101]. Papillary thyroid cancer is less aggressive than other types, so iodine-deficient populations are more likely to show excess mortality from thyroid cancer. Apparently, any dietary imbalance, especially one affecting metabolically active tissue, may increase the risk of cancer.

The list linking high- and low-risk situations to trace element ingestion seems almost endless. In most instances, the implication is that the element modifies a primary risk situation. The biggest epidemiologic challenge is to determine major causes, but modification of risk deserves more attention since it is likely to be more feasible socially.

Vitamins

Vitamin A has been studied more than any other vitamin for its effects on carcinogenesis because of its importance to normal epithelial functioning. Added vitamin A decreases the carcinogenic effect of polycyclic hydrocarbons in several rodent systems, including hamster lung [102], cervix and forestomach [103], mouse skin [104], and prostate [105]. This effect may result in part from alterations in the metabolic pathways of the carcinogens [106]; in addition, it may involve biological antagonism to the metaplasia usually produced as an intermediate step to neoplasia. Vitamin A also has direct and indirect therapeutic properties against human skin cancers [107] and mouse leukemia in vitro [108]. It enhances bacillus Calmette-Guérin (BCG) immunotherapy as well [109]. Vitamin A deficiency in rats enhances salivary gland carcinogenesis [110] and increases bowel carcinogenesis [14, 111].

The salivary gland experiment was designed explicitly to investigate whether vitamin A deficiency is a factor in the high frequency of salivary gland cancer in Eskimos. Vitamin A deficiency also has been invoked as a likely contributor to the high level of nasopharyngeal cancer in Kenya [112] and as a possible cofactor in gastric carcinogenesis [113].

Other vitamins affect carcinogenesis. Bracken fern alone produced many bowel cancers but few bladder cancers in rats; when the rats were given additional thiamine, over half developed bladder cancers as well [114]. Riboflavin deficiency both inhibited [115] and enhanced [115, 116] experimental carcinogenesis, although no extrapolation to epidemiologic problems in human cancer has been suggested. Vitamin B_{12} deficiency slowed hepatic carcinogenesis [117], but pernicious anemia (a B_{12}-deficient condition) is a precancerous state with patients having an increased risk for stomach cancer and leukemia [118].

Apparently, vitamin C has not been tested in animal carcinogenesis. As an antioxidant, it should have a protective effect. Epidemiologically, it has been suggested that low vitamin C intake is characteristic of a region with a high rate of stomach cancer [119] and is more prevalent in stomach cancer patients than in controls [120]; this observation is consistent with studies [24, 121, 122] indicating a negative association between consumption of raw vegetables and stomach cancer.

Other Dietary Factors

Besides vitamins and trace elements, other dietary constituents modify carcinogenesis in experimental situations. Presumably, there are equivalent effects in humans, but these seem more likely to affect individual susceptibility or resistance to a carcinogen than to modify the risk of a whole population. This likelihood does not make them unimportant for study as they may help explain apparent epidemiologic inconsistencies. Further, they might lead to methods of risk reduction more socially acceptable than direct attacks on favorite, but carcinogenic, vices and addictions.

The most general effect observed experimentally is the reduction of tumor incidence by undernutrition [123]. The diets are much too drastic to be used on humans, and in any case the extrapolation to humans is doubtful. For example, the United States and India certainly represent extremes of general caloric intake for general populations, yet their age-specific cancer incidence rates are nearly identical. Experimental studies on underfeeding also have the problem that strictly defined diets may be borderline in some essential factor, and this situation, rather than caloric content per se, may influence the results. For example, mice on an artificial diet developed more tumors after radiation than did mice on an equicaloric natural diet [124]. The factor responsible was not identified.

Overfeeding has enhanced carcinogenesis in several experiments [125]. Most work has been done with rodents, but Anderson et al. [125] showed the same effects in cattle. Wynder has long felt that general overnutrition contributes to the high incidence of cancers of the breast, ovary, endometrium, and prostate in this country [126]. A general relationship between obesity and cancer has been reported, without indication of the types of cancer involved [127]. In another study, men 20 percent or more overweight had a 16 percent excess cancer mortality and women a 13 percent excess [128]. Endometrial cancer is the one cancer in this country consistently associated with obesity [129]. Breast cancer has been associated in other countries with both excess height and weight [130], but the association is not always found [131] and is too weak and confused with other variables [132] to be of practical screening use in this country.

Protein deficiency increases the tumorigenicity of DMN in a rat system but the effect seems partly due to reducing acute toxicity [133]. Moderate protein deficiency increases immune responses to tumors, whereas more marked malnutrition depresses these reactions [134]. As with calorie malnutrition, the extrapolation to the human situation is not yet demonstrated.

High levels of dietary fat increased the production of mammary cancer by DMBA in rats; the effect was greater during the promotional stage [135]. The effect of dietary fat must be associated with the concomitant level of dietary lipotropes. Marginal deficiency of these compounds enhanced the carcinogenicity of aflatoxin and some nitrosamines, whereas severe deficiency inhibited aflatoxin carcinogenesis [12, 136]. In other work [137], cyclopropenoid fatty acids increased aflatoxin carcinogenicity.

The property of tumor promotion may be the epidemiologic key in many important human situations. For example, bile and some of its fractions enhance bowel carcinogenesis [138, 139]. By increasing bile production and flow, high-fat diets could thus be an important factor in determining bowel cancer incidence. The hypothesis corresponds well with bowel cancer epidemiology that is currently under intense study. By contrast, although it is hypothesized that fiber may inhibit bowel carcinogenesis, the mechanism of this action and even the proper definition of "fiber" remains unknown [140].

A wide range of dietary constituents will influence individual susceptibility to carcinogens through their induction of different activity levels of microsomal enzymes, both in the body's detoxifying organs and in target cells [141]. For example, protein deficiency can increase the inactivation of some carcinogens and promote the activation of others [142, 143]. Some of the most active inducers of microsomal enzymes are flavones [144], found naturally in cabbage, turnips, broccoli, and other vegetables. Reviews on enzyme inducibility [141, 145-147] and publication of the papers from a symposium on related topics may be of interest [148]. Most, if not all, carcinogens are affected by manipulation of the microsomal system, including crude preparations of bracken fern [149] and urethan [150]. Inducers can be such varied compounds as steroids, phenobarbital, DDT, alcohol, and ozones. Inducibility is related to the genetic makeup of the cells as well as to their life history [151, 152].

The rapid development of knowledge about enzyme induction has produced almost too much information on possible dietary influences on carcinogenesis, since both activation and deactivation may be enhanced. We are well supplied with explanations for individual susceptibility or resistance, but unable to predict whether risks will be raised or lowered in particular situations. There seems to be an opportunity, however, for epidemiologic investigations. Alcohol, DDT, and phenobarbital are enzyme inducers, and all are markers of particular populations. Alcohol and DDT may be difficult to study because they are directly related to carcinogenesis. Epileptics, with their high doses of phenobarbital, are subject to other environmental modifications that affect cancer incidence [153]. Still, careful epidemiologic design should be able to unravel some of these complexities and produce generalizations about overall cancer risks in individuals with differing profiles of microsomal enzyme activity.

OVERVIEW AND RECOMMENDATIONS

A number of specific recommendations have been included in previous sections. One valuable means of delineating dietary carcinogens is to study the effects on man of suspected carcinogens in high-exposure groups, particularly industrial groups.

Secondly, there are reasonably strong hypotheses linking certain foodborne carcinogens to specific cancers: aflatoxin to liver cancer, nitrosamines and polycyclics to stomach cancer, tannins to esophageal cancer. These hypotheses should be tested and followed up in a similar manner to the studies of stomach cancer in Colombia described by Haenszel in Chapter 21.

To evaluate specific carcinogens responsible for other culture-linked cancers, such as pancreatic cancer in nonsmokers, the need is to identify populations suitable for case-control studies that could implicate the dietary factor or vehicle for the carcinogen. Then, if associations were found, as in the case of coffee and bladder cancer or beef and bowel cancer, studies of *mechanisms* should begin. Regardless of how seriously one takes the idea of coffee or beef as cancer causes, the association of common foods with common cancers should give follow-up studies top priority.

The difficulties preventing translation of a suspected dietary etiology into an effective lowering of risk are exemplified in the current status of the bowel cancer problem. From what we know about animal models, bowel cancer should be caused by an ingested carcinogen, most likely converted to an active compound by the bowel flora. Studies of diet, both retrospective and prospective, in middle class whites in this country have failed to identify a suspicious food. However, the same thing is true for coronary heart disease. The failure signifies relative uniformity of exposure, rather than no role for diet. Diets in different populations at low and high risk of bowel cancer differ in so many ways that there is no sharp focus. Knowing that a high-fat and high-animal-protein diet is characteristic of bowel cancer countries is of much less help than is the fat-coronary disease association because it does not suggest exposure to any known carcinogen.

Migrants provide the proper amount of dietary contrast as well as the evidence that bowel cancer is, in fact, environmental and probably dietary. The risk-associated foods—beef, string beans, and total starches [38]—still are fairly general and are not obvious special vehicles for any of the carcinogens discussed above. Beef fits better epidemiologically with bowel cancer than does any proposed alternative, including other fatty meat. Biologically, however, the epidemiologic specificity of beef makes no sense at all at present. We know of no constituent unique to beef or especially concentrated in beef that would cause bowel cancer. Animal fat generally fits better biochemically, since there are ways of metabolizing fat to carcinogens and promoters. Epidemiologically, the case against fat is weak because there are populations that have a high-fat intake but little bowel cancer, and there is no case-control study pointing to fat as a risk factor.

What is different and heartening about the bowel cancer problem is that it is being attacked by individuals, multidisciplinary teams, and multiteam working groups with broad outlooks as well as long-term commitments to the problem. They are restoring the balance of laboratory-field work needed in epidemiology. Their primary focus is man, and they are studying him biochemically and bacteriologically as well as by questionnaire. They are using animal models not only to mimic the human disease, but also for basic investigations of bacteriology, cell kinetics, bile metabolism, and the like [139, 154, 155]. In other words, at long last the strategy is to match the complexity of the investigations to the complexity of the problem. If the same approach is taken with other diet-related cancers, we should be able to replace our tentative and practically useless guesses about risk factors with enough understanding to lower current levels of risk.

For other cancers too there may be little profit from more and more descriptive epidemiology in general populations, despite the near certainty that food habits influence cancer patterns. It may be too simpleminded to look for dietary equivalents of cigarettes. With foods, instead of having obvious carcinogens, co-carcinogens, promoters, ciliatoxins, and so forth wrapped neatly in one package and causing cancer in a high proportion of the consumers, we may be dealing with more complex chains. Different environmental constituents may be furnishing different parts of the carcinogenic mixture at different times. A dominant role may be played by host susceptibility, conditioned by environmental factors acting at a different time than the carcinogen exposure. Thus, cancers of the stomach and esophagus are tied in different ways to deficiency states: esophageal cancer by various epidemiologic associations (e.g., to alcohol and to molybdenum or iron deficiency), and stomach cancer by its predilection for chronically inflamed and atrophic mucosa. Without preexisting deficiency, the actual carcinogens may be fairly harmless.

Contrariwise, cancers of the colon, breast, prostate, endometrium, and ovary all appear to be cancers of affluence. Bowel cancer probably is caused or promoted by metabolites of rich foods. While they could affect other tissues [156], the endocrine cancer risk might be set indirectly by general overnutrition causing overstimulation of the pituitary gland and target organs.

Cancers of the pancreas, hepatobiliary system, kidney, bladder, and possibly the lower rectum form a third group whose relation to food is less clear yet certainly worth pursuing from the standpoint of metabolic epidemiology; they comprise the excretion pathways for toxic materials, and as proved for cigarette smokers, they are vulnerable to the carcinogen they excrete.

To confirm or refute these possibilities and to utilize our knowledge for cancer prevention, we need to concentrate on metabolic epidemiology both in man and in animal models. Can we document different metabolic pathways in cancer patients or in cancer-prone epithelium? Do particular vitamin or other nutritional deficiencies produce esophageal or gastric epithelium that is especially vulnerable to carcinogens? Can the effects be aborted or established pathology reversed by remedying these deficiencies? Can the dangers of hormonal hyperactivity be minimized? Becoming more utopian, can we link cancer resistance so closely to a prudent diet and define this diet, even in childhood, so accurately that whole cultures can achieve as low risks for dietary cancers as they could, if they wished, for lung cancer?

REFERENCES

1. Kraybill, H.F. The toxicology and epidemiology of mycotoxins. *Trop. Geogr. Med. 21:* 1–18, 1969.

2. Wogan, G.N. Aflatoxin risks and control measures. *Fed. Proc. 27:* 932–938, 1968.

3. Duggan, R.E. Controlling aflatoxins. *FDA Papers.* pp. 13–18, April 1970.

4. Van Nieuwenhuize, J.P., Herber, R.F.M., de Bruin, A., et al. Aflatoxins: epidemiologic study on carcinogenicity at chronic low-level exposure in a factory population. *Tijdschr. Soc. Genesk. 51:* 754–760, 1973. *(Engl.* Abstr. in *Carcinogenesis Abstr. 11:* 906, 1974.)

5. Oettlé, A.G. Cancer in Africa, especially in regions south of the Sahara. *J. Natl. Cancer Inst. 33:* 383–439, 1964.

6. Shank, R.C., Bhamaropravati, N., Gordon, J.E., et al. Dietary aflatoxins and human liver cancer in two municipal populations of Thailand. *Food Cosmet. Toxicol.,* pp. 171–179, 1972.

7. Tuyns, A.J., Loubière, R., and Duvernet-Battesti, Fr. Regional variations in primary liver cancer in Ivory Coast. *J. Natl. Cancer Inst. 47:* 131–135, 1971.

8. Keen, P. Is aflatoxin carcinogenic in man? The evidence in Swaziland. *Trop. Geogr. Med. 23:* 44–53, 1971.

9. Peers, F.G., and Linsell, C.A. Dietary aflatoxins and liver cancer—a population based study in Kenya. *Br. J. Cancer 27:* 473–484, 1973.

10. Campbell, T.C., Sinnhuber, R.O., Lee, D.J., et al. Brief communication: hepatocarcinogenic material in urine specimens from humans consuming aflatoxin. *J. Natl. Cancer Inst. 52:* 1647–1649, 1974.

11. Lee, D.J. Hepatoma and renal tubule adenoma in rats fed aflatoxin and cyclopropenoid fatty acids. *J. Natl. Cancer Inst. 43:* 1037–1044, 1969.

12. Rogers, A.E., and Newberne, P.M. Aflatoxin B_1 carcinogenesis in lipotrope-deficient rats. *Cancer Res. 29:* 1965–1972, 1969.

13. Newberne, P.M., and Williams, G. Inhibition of aflatoxin carcinogenesis by diethylstilbestrol in male rats. *Arch. Environ. Hlth. 19:* 489–498, 1969.

14. Newberne, P.M., and Rogers, A.E. Rat colon carcinomas associated with aflatoxin and marginal vitamin A. *J. Natl. Cancer Inst. 50:* 439–444, 1973.

15. Anthony, P.P. Carcinoma of the liver in man. *Internatl. Path. 15:* 29–44, 1974.

16. Sebranek, J.G., and Cassens, R.G. Nitrosamines: a review. *J. Milk Food Technol. 36:* 76–91, 1973.

17. Bralow, S.P., Gruenstein, M., and Meranze, D.R. Host resistance to gastric adeno-carcinomatosis in three strains of rats ingesting N-methyl-N'-nitro-N-nitrosoguanidine. *Oncology 27:* 168–180, 1973.

18. Keefer, L.K., and Roller, P.P. N-nitrosation by nitrite ion in neutral and basic medium. *Science 181:* 1245–1247, 1973.

19. Ayanaba, A., Verstraete, W., and Alexander, M. Brief communication: possible microbial contribution to nitrosamine formation in sewage and soil. *J. Natl. Cancer Inst. 50:* 811–813, 1973.

20. Montesano, R., and Magee, P.N. Evidence of formation of N-methyl-N-nitrosourea in rats given N-methylurea and sodium nitrite. *Int. J. Cancer 7:* 249–255, 1971.

21. Mirvish, S.S. Kinetics of nitrosamide formation from alkylureas, N-alkylurethans, and alkylguanidines: possible implications for the etiology of human gastric cancer. *J. Natl. Cancer Inst. 46:* 1183–1193, 1971.

22. Hill, M.J., Hawsworth, G., and Tattersall, G. Bacteria, nitrosamines and cancer of the stomach. *Br. J. Cancer 28:* 562–567, 1973.

23. Lijinskly, W. Reaction of drugs with nitrous acid as a source of carcinogenic nitrosamines. *Cancer Res. 34:* 255–258, 1974.

24. Haenszel, W., Kurihara, M., Segi, M., et al. Stomach cancer among Japanese in Hawaii. *J. Natl. Cancer Inst. 49:* 969–988, 1972.

25. McGlashan, N.D. Oesophaegeal cancer in Northern Iran. *Bull. Int. Acad. Pathol. 11:* 5–53, 1970.

26. Zaldivar, R. Geographic pathology of oral, esophageal, gastric, and intestinal cancer in Chile. *Z. Krebsforsch. 75:* 1–13, 1970.

27. Tilgner, D.J., and Daun, H. Polycyclic aromatic hydrocarbons (polynuclears) in smoked foods. *Residue Rev. 27:* 19–41, 1969.

28. Fritz, W. Umfang und Quellen der Kontamination unserer Lebensmittel mit kreberzeugenden, Kohlenwasserstoffen. *Ernahrungsforsch 16:* 547–557, 1972.

29. Miller, J.A. Carcinogenesis by chemicals: an overview. *Cancer Res. 30:* 559–575, 1970.

30. Steinmiller, D., Lloyd, H.D., and Richmond, T.P. Lack of carcinogenic activity of 3-methylcholanthrene in the squirrel monkey. *J. Natl. Cancer Inst. 43:* 1175–1179, 1969.

31. Masuada, Y., and Kuratsune, M. Polycyclic aromatic hydrocarbons in smoked fish, "katsuobushi." *Gann 62:* 27–30, 1971.

32. Malanoski, A.J., Greenfield, E.L., Barnes, C.J., et al. Survey of polycyclic aromatic hydrocarbons in smoked foods. *J. Assoc. Off. Anal. Chem. 51:* 114–121, 1968.

33. Schmahl, D. Exogenic factors in human carcinogenesis and methods for their detection. *Neoplasma (Bratislava) 15:* 273–280, 1968.

34. Sigurjonsson, J. Occupational variations in mortality from gastric cancer in relation to dietary differences. *Br. J. Cancer 21:* 651–656, 1967.

35. Committee on Biologic Effects of Atmospheric Pollutants. *Biologic Effects of Atmospheric Pollutants: Particulate Polycyclic Organic Matter.* National Academy of Sciences, Washington, D.C., 1972.

36. Winkelstein, W., Jr., and Kantor, S. Stomach cancer: positive association with suspended particulate air pollution. *Arch. Environ. Hlth. 18:* 544–547, 1969.

37. National Clearinghouse for Smoking and Health. *The Health Consequences of Smoking.* U.S. Department of Health, Education, and Welfare, Washington, D.C., 1967.

38. Haenszel, W., Berg, J.W., Segi, M., et al. Large-bowel cancer in Hawaiian Japanese. *J. Natl. Cancer Inst. 51:* 1765–1779, 1973.

39. Laqueur, G.L., Mickelson, O., Whiting, M.G., et al. Carcinogenic properties of nuts from *Cycas circinalis* L. indigenous to Guam. *J. Natl. Cancer Inst. 31:* 919-952, 1963.

40. Miller, J.A., and Miller, E.C. Natural and synthetic chemical carcinogens in the etiology of cancer. *Cancer Res. 25:* 1292-1304, 1965.

41. Pamukcu, A.M., and Price, J.M. Induction of intestinal and urinary bladder cancer in rats by feeding bracken fern (Pteris aquilina). *J. Natl. Cancer Inst. 43:* 275-281, 1969.

42. Hirono, I., Shibuya, C., Fushimi, K., et al. Studies on carcinogenic properties of bracken, Pteridium aquilinum. *J. Natl. Cancer Inst. 45:* 179-188, 1970.

43. Evans, I.A., and Osman, M.A. Carcinogenicity of bracken and shikimic acid. *Nature (Lond.) 250:* 348-349, 1974.

44. Bohm, B.A. Shikimic acid (3, 4, 5-trihydroxy-1-cyclohexene-1-carboxylic acid). *Chem. Rev. 65:* 435-466, 1965.

45. Morton, J.F. Plant products and occupational materials ingested by esophageal cancer victims in South Carolina. *Q.J. Crude Drug Res. 13:* 2005-2022, 1973.

46. Pradhan, S.N., Chung, E.B., Ghosh, B., et al. Potential carcinogens. I. Carcinogenicity of some plant extracts and their tannin-containing fractions in rats. *J. Natl. Cancer Inst. 52:* 1579-1582, 1974.

47. Cole, P. Coffee-drinking and cancer of the lower urinary tract. *Lancet 1:* 1335-1337, 1971.

48. Schmauz, R., and Cole, P. Epidemiology of cancer of the renal pelvis and ureter. *J. Natl. Cancer Inst. 52:* 1431, 1974.

49. Donovan, P.J., and DiPaolo, J.A. Caffeine enhancement of chemical carcinogen-induced transformation of cultured Syrian hamster cells. *Cancer Res. 34:* 2720-2727, 1974.

50. Fraumeni, J.F., Jr., Scotto, J., and Dunham, L.J. Coffee-drinking and bladder cancer. *Lancet 2:* 1204, 1971.

51. Radomski, J.L. Toxicology of food colors. *Annu. Rev. Pharmac. 14:* 127-137, 1974.

52. Wolff, A.H., and Oehme, F.W. Carcinogenic chemicals in food as an environmental health issue. *J.A.V.M.A. 164:* 623-629, 1974.

53. Bryan, G.T., and Yoshida, O. Artificial sweeteners as urinary bladder carcinogens. *Arch. Environ. Hlth. 23:* 6-12, 1971.

54. Price, J.M., Biava, C.G., Oser, B.L., et al. Bladder tumors in rats fed cyclohexylamine or high doses of a mixture of cyclamate and saccharin. *Science 167:* 1131-1132, 1970.

55. Egeberg, R.O., Steinfeld, J.L., Frantz, I., et al. Report to the secretary of HEW from the medical advisory group on cyclamates. *J.A.M.A. 211:* 1358-1361, 1970.

56. Asohina, M., Yamaha, T., and Watanabe, K. Excretion of cyclohexylamine, a metabolite of cyclamate in human urine. *Chem. Pharm. Bull. 19:* 628-632, 1971.

57. Hicks, R.M., Wakefield, J.St.J., and Chowaniec, J. Co-carcinogenic action of saccharin in the chemical induction of bladder cancer. *Nature (Lond.) 243:* 347-349, 1973.

58. Kessler, I.I. Cancer and diabetes mellitus, a review of the literature. *J. Chronic Dis. 23:* 579-600, 1971.

59. Kessler, I.I. Cancer mortality among diabetics. *J. Natl. Cancer Inst. 44:* 673-686, 1970.

60. Sato, T. An approaching method for finding causative agents of human cancers of environmental origin through the analysis of the relation between the distribution of the agents and the incidence rates of the cancers, with applications to oesophagus and gastric cancers. *Bull. Inst. Public Health 12:* 160-165, 1963.

61. Hirayama, T. The epidemiology of cancer of the stomach. *Stomach Intestine 3:* 787-796, 1968.

62. MacDonald, W.C., Anderson, F.H., and Hashimoto, S. Histological effect of certain pickles on the human gastric mucosa. *Can. Med. Assoc. J. 96:* 1521–1525, 1967.

63. *Report of the Secretary's Commission on Pesticides and Their Relationship to Environmental Health. Parts I and II.* U.S. Department of Health, Education, and Welfare, Washington, D.C., December 1969.

64. Innes, J.R.M., Ulland, B.M., Valerio, M.G., et al. Bioassay of pesticides and industrial chemicals for tumorigenicity in mice: a preliminary note. *J. Natl. Cancer Inst. 42:* 1101–1114, 1969.

65. Diechmann, W.B., MacDonald, W.E., Blum, E., et al. Tumorigenicity of aldrin, dieldrin and endrin in the albino rat. *Ind. Med. Surg. 39:* 426–434, 1970.

66. Editorial. *Des Moines Register.* October 17, 1974.

67. Carter, L.J. Cancer and the environment. I. A creaky system grinds on. *Science 186:* 239–242, 1974.

68. Matsudo, H., Hodgkin, N.M., and Tanaka, A. Japanese gastric cancer. *Arch. Pathol. 97:* 366–368, 1974.

69. Mason, T.J., McKay, F.W., and Miller, R.W. Asbestos-like fibers in Duluth water supply. *J.A.M.A. 228:* 1019–1020, 1974.

70. Cunningham, H.M., and Pontefract, R.D. Asbestos fibers in beverages, drinking water, and tissues: their passage through the intestinal wall and movement through the body. *J. Assoc. Off. Anal. Chem. 56:* 976–981, 1973.

71. Jukes, T.H. Estrogens in beefsteaks. *J.A.M.A. 229:* 1920–1921, 1974.

72. Kraybill, H.F. The distribution of chemical carcinogens in aquatic environments. UICC Symposium, *Neoplasms in Aquatic Animals as Indicators of Environmental Carcinogens.* In press.

73. Brown, E.R., Hazdra, J.J., Keith, L., et al. Frequency of fish tumors found in a polluted watershed as compared to nonpolluted Canadian waters. *Cancer Res. 33:* 189–198, 1973.

74. Mertz, W. Some aspects of nutritional trace element research. *Fed. Proc. 29:* 1482–1488, 1970.

75. Schroeder, M.D., and Kraemer, A. Cardiovascular mortality, municipal water, and corrosion. *Arch. Environ. Hlth. 28:* 303–311, 1974.

76. Beattie, A.D., Moore, M.R., Devenay, W.T., et al. Environmental lead pollution in an urban soft-water area. *Br. Med. J. 2:* 491–493, 1972.

77. Schroeder, H.A., Balassa, J.J., and Vinton, W.H. Chromium, lead, cadmium, nickel and titanium in mice: effect on mortality, tumors and tissue levels. *J. Nutr. 83:* 239–250, 1964.

78. Yeh, S. Skin cancer in chronic arsenicism. *Hum. Pathol. 4:* 469–485, 1973.

79. Berg, J.W., and Burbank, F. Correlations between carcinogenic trace metals in water supplies and cancer mortality. *Ann. N.Y. Acad. Sci. 199:* 249–264, 1972.

80. Shakman, R.A. Nutritional influences on the toxicity of environmental pollutants. *Arch. Environ. Hlth. 28:* 105–113, 1974.

81. Wynder, E.L., Hultberg, S., Jacobsson, F., et al. Environmental factors in cancer of the upper alimentary tract. A Swedish study with special reference to Plummer-Vinson (Paterson-Kelly) syndrome. *Cancer 10:* 470–487, 1957.

82. Chisolm, M. The association between webs, iron and post cricoid carcinoma. *Postgrad. Med. J. 50:* 215–219, 1974.

83. Burrell, R.J., Roach, W.A., and Shadwell, A. Esophageal cancer in the Bantu of the Transkei associated with mineral deficiency in garden plants. *J. Natl. Cancer Inst. 36:* 201–214, 1966.

84. Berg, J.W., Haenszel, W., and Devesa, S.S. Epidemiology of gastrointestinal cancer. *Seventh National Cancer Conference Proceedings,* 1973, pp. 459–464.

85. Shamberger, R.J. Relationship of selenium to cancer. I. Inhibitory effect of selenium on carcinogenesis. *J. Natl. Cancer Inst. 44:* 931–936, 1970.

86. Shamberger, R.J., and Willis, C.E. Selenium distribution and human cancer mortality. *CRC Crit. Rev. Clin. Lab. Sci. 2:* 211–221, 1971.

87. Wattenberg, L.W. Inhibition of carcinogenic and toxic effects of polycyclic hydrocarbons by phenolic antioxidants and ethyoxyquin. *J. Natl. Cancer Inst. 48:* 1425–1430, 1972.

88. Black, H.S. Effects of dietary antioxidants on actinic tumor induction. *Res. Commun. Chem. Pathol. Pharmacol. 7:* 783–786, 1974.

89. Tappel, A.L. Will antioxidant nutrients slow aging processes? *Geriatrics 23:* 97–105, 1968.

90. Shamberger, R.J., Tytko, S., and Willis, C.E. Antioxidants in cereals and in food preservatives and declining gastric cancer mortality. *Cleveland Clinic Q. 39:* 119–124, 1972.

91. Poswillo, D.E., and Cohen, B. Inhibition of carcinogenesis by dietary zinc. *Nature (Lond.) 231:* 477–478, 1971.

92. Ciapparelli, L., Retief, D.H., and Fatti, L.P. The effect of zinc on 9-, 10-dimethyl-1, 2-benzanthracene (DMBA) induced salivary gland tumours in the albino rat: a preliminary study. *S. Afr. J. Med. Sci. 37:* 85–90, 1972.

93. DeWys, W., and Pories, W. Inhibition of a spectrum of animal tumors by dietary zinc deficiency. *J. Natl. Cancer Inst. 48:* 375–381, 1972.

94. Stocks, P., and Davies, R.I. Zinc and copper content of soils associated with the incidence of cancer of the stomach and other organs. *Br. J. Cancer 18:* 14–24, 1964.

95. Strain, W.H., Mansour, E.G., Flynn, A., et al. Plasma-zinc concentration in patients with bronchogenic cancer. *Lancet 1:* 1021–1022, 1972.

96. Battifora, H.A., McCreary, P.A., Hahneman, B.M., et al. Chronic magnesium deficiency in the rat. *Arch. Pathol. 86:* 610–620, 1968.

97. Bois, P., Sandborn, E.B., and Messier, P.E. A study of thymic lymphosarcoma developing in magnesium-deficient rats. *Cancer Res. 29:* 763–775, 1969.

98. Sunderman, F.W., Lau, T.J., and Cralley, L.J. Inhibitory effect of manganese upon muscle tumorigenesis by nickel subsulfide. *Cancer Res. 34:* 92–95, 1974.

99. Marjanen, H. Possible causal relationship between the easily soluble amount of manganese on arable mineral soil and susceptibility to cancer in Finland. *Ann. Agric. Fenn. 8:* 326–334, 1969.

100. Tromp, S.W. Statistical study of the possible relationship between mineral constituents in drinking-water and cancer mortality in the Netherlands (period 1900–1940). *Br. J. Cancer 8:* 585–593, 1954.

101. Articles and discussion in Section 2. *Epidemiology of Thyroid Cancers.* (Hedinger, C.E., ed.). UICC Monogr. 12, Springer-Verlag, Berlin, 1969.

102. Saffiotti, U., Montesano, R., Sellakumar, A.R., et al. Experimental cancer of the lung. *Cancer 20:* 857–864, 1967.

103. Chu, E.W., and Malmgren, R.A. An inhibitory effect of vitamin A on the induction of tumors of forestomach and cervix in the Syrian hamster by carcinogenic polycyclic hydrocarbons. *Cancer Res. 25:* 884–895, 1965.

104. Bollag, W. Prophylaxis of chemically induced papillomas and carcinomas of mouse skin by vitamin A-acid. *Experientia (Basel) 28:* 1219–1220, 1972.

105. Lasnitzki, I., and Goodman, D.S. Inhibition of the effects of methylcholanthrene on mouse prostate in organ culture by vitamin A and its analogs. *Cancer Res. 34:* 1564–1571, 1974.

106. Hill, D.L., and Shih, T. Vitamin A compounds and analogs as inhibitors of mixed-function oxidases that metabolize carcinogenic polycyclic hydrocarbons and other compounds. *Cancer Res. 34:* 564–570, 1974.

107. Bollag, W., and Ott, F. Therapy of actinic keratoses and basal cell carcinomas with local application of vitamin A acid (NSC-122758). *Cancer Chemother. Rep. 55:* 59-60, 1971.

108. Brandes, D., Rundell, J.O., and Ueda, H. Radiation response of L1210 leukemia cells pretreated with vitamin A alcohol. *J. Natl. Cancer Inst. 52:* 945-949, 1974.

109. Meltzer, M.S., and Cohen, B.E. Brief communication: tumor suppression by mycobacterium bovis (strain BCG) enhanced by vitamin A. *J. Natl. Cancer Inst. 53:* 585-587, 1974.

110. Rowe, N.H., Grammer, F.C., Watson, F.R., et al. A study of environmental influence upon salivary gland neoplasia in rats. *Cancer 26:* 436-444, 1970.

111. Rogers, A.E., Herndon, B.J., and Newberne, P.M. Induction by dimethylhydrazine of intestinal carcinoma in normal rats and rats fed high or low levels of vitamin A. *Cancer Res. 33:* 1003-1009, 1973.

112. Clifford, P. Carcinogens in the nose and throat: nasopharyngeal carcinoma in Kenya. *Proc. Roy. Soc. Med. 65:* 682-686, 1972.

113. Wynder, E.L., Kmet, J., Dungal, N., et al. An epidemiological investigation of gastric cancer. *Cancer 16:* 1461-1496, 1963.

114. Pamukcu, A.M., Yalciner, S., Price, J.M., et al. Effects of the coadministration of thiamine on the incidence of urinary bladder carcinomas in rats fed bracken fern. *Cancer Res. 30:* 2671-2674, 1970.

115. Rivlin, R.S. Riboflavin and cancer: a review. *Cancer Res. 33:* 1977-1986, 1973.

116. Wynder, E.L., and Chan, P.C. The possible role of riboflavin deficiency in epithelial neoplasia. II. Effect on skin tumor development. *Cancer 26:* 1221-1224, 1970.

117. Poirier, L.A., Wenk, M.L., Madison, R.M., et al. Vitamin B_{12} acceleration of hepatocarcinogenesis. *Proc. Amer. Assoc. Cancer Res. (Abstract) 15:* 51, 1974.

118. Blackburn, E.K., Callender, S.T., Dacie, J.V., et al. Possible association between pernicious anaemia and leukaemia: a prospective study of 1,625 patients with a note on the very high incidence of stomach cancer. *Int. J. Cancer 3:* 163-170, 1968.

119. Dungal, N., and Sigurjonsson, J. Gastric cancer and diet. A pilot study on dietary habits in two districts differing markedly in respect of mortality from gastric cancer. *Br. J. Cancer 21:* 270-276, 1967.

120. Bjelke, E. Case-control study of cancer of the stomach, colon, and rectum. *10th International Cancer Congress Proceedings.* Houston, 1970 (Clark, R.L., et al., eds.). Year Book Medical Publishers, 1971, Chicago, pp. 320-351.

121. Haenszel, W. Epidemiology of gastric cancer. *Neoplasms of the Stomach.* (McNeer, G., and Pack, G.T., eds.). J.B. Lippincott, Philadelphia, 1967, pp. 3-28.

122. Graham, S., Schotz, W., and Martino, P. Alimentary factors in the epidemiology of gastric cancer. *Cancer 30:* 927-938, 1972.

123. Ross, M.H., and Bras, G. Lasting influence of early caloric restriction on prevalence of neoplasms in the rat. *J. Natl. Cancer Inst. 47:* 1095-1113, 1971.

124. Ershoff, B.H., Bajwa, G.S., Field, J.B., et al. Comparative effects of purified diets and a natural food stock ration on the tumor incidence of mice exposed to multiple sublethal doses of total-body x-irradiation. *Cancer Res. 29:* 780-788, 1969.

125. Anderson, D.E., Pope, L.S., and Stephens, D. Nutrition and eye cancer in cattle. *J. Natl. Cancer Inst. 45:* 697-707, 1970.

126. Wynder, E.L., and Mabuchi, K. Etiological and preventive aspects of human cancer. *Prev. Med. 1:* 300-334, 1972.

127. Cheraskin, E., Ringsdorf. W.M., and Aspray, D.W. Cancer proneness profile: a study in ponderal index and blood glucose. *Geriatrics 24:* 121-125, 1969.

128. Metropolitan Life Insurance Company. *Overweight, Its Significance and Prevention.* New York, 1960.

129. Dunn, L.J., Merchant, J.A., Bradbury, J.T., et al. Glucose tolerance and endometrial carcinoma. *Arch. Intern. Med. 121:* 246-254, 1968.

130. De Waard, F., and Baanders-van Halewijn, E.A. A prospective study in general practice on breast-cancer risk in postmenopausal women. *Int. J. Cancer 14:* 153-160, 1974.

131. Brinkley, D., Carpenter, R.G., and Haybittle, J.L. An anthropometric study of women with cancer. *Br. J. Prev. Soc. Med. 25:* 65-75, 1971.

132. Wynder, E.L. Identification of women at high risk for breast cancer. *Cancer 24:* 1235-1240, 1969.

133. Hard, G.C., and Butler, W.H. Cellular analysis of renal neoplasia: induction of renal tumors in dietary-conditioned rats by dimethylnitrosamine, with a reappraisal of morphological characteristics. *Cancer Res. 30:* 2796-2805, 1970.

134. Jose, D.G., and Good, R.A. Quantitative effects of nutritional protein and calorie deficiency upon immune responses to tumors in mice. *Cancer Res. 33:* 807-812, 1973.

135. Carroll, K.K., and Khor, H.T. Effects of dietary fat and dose level of 7, 12-dimethylbenzanthracene on mammary tumor incidence in rats. *Cancer Res. 30:* 2260-2264, 1970.

136. Rogers, A.E., Sanchez, O., Feinsod, F.M., et al. Dietary enhancement of nitrosamine carcinogenesis. *Cancer Res. 34:* 96-99, 1974.

137. Lee, D.J., Wales, J.H., and Sinnhuber, R.O. Hepatoma and renal tubule adenoma in rats fed aflatoxin and cyclopropenoid fatty acids. *J. Natl. Cancer Inst. 43:* 1037-1044, 1969.

138. Chomchai, C., Bhadrachari, N., and Nigro, N.D. The effect of bile on the indication of experimental intestinal tumors in rats. *Dis. Colon Rectum 17:* 310-312, 1974.

139. Wynder, E.L., and Reddy, B.S. Metabolic epidemiology of colorectal cancer. *Cancer Res. 34:* 801-806, 1974.

140. Spiller, G.A., and Amen, R.J. Research on dietary fiber. *Lancet 2:* 1259, 1974.

141. Bowden, G.T., Slaga, T.J., Shapas, B.G., et al. The role of aryl hydrocarbon hydroxylase in skin tumor initiation by 7,12-dimethylbenzanthracene and 1,2,5,6-dibenzanthracene using DNA binding and thymidine-^{3}H incorporation into DNA as criteria. *Cancer Res. 34:* 2634-2642, 1974.

142. Czygan, P., Greim, H., Garro, A., et al. The effect of dietary protein deficiency on the ability of isolated hepatic microsomes to alter the mutagenicity of a primary and a secondary carcinogen. *Cancer Res. 34:* 119-123, 1974.

143. Venkatesan, N., Arcos, J.C., and Argus, M.F. Amino acid induction and carbohydrate repression of dimethylnitrosamine demethylase in rat liver. *Cancer Res. 30:* 2563-2567, 1970.

144. Wattenberg, L.W., and Leong, J.L. Inhibition of the carcinogenic action of benzopyrene by flavones. *Cancer Res. 30:* 1922-1925, 1970.

145. Gelboin, H.V., Kinoshita, N., and Wiebel, F.J. Microsomal hydroxylases: induction and role in polycyclic hydrocarbon carcinogenesis and toxicity. *Fed. Proc. 31:* 1298-1309, 1972.

146. Jerina, D.M., and Daly, J.W. Arene oxides: a new aspect of drug metabolism. *Science 185:* 573-582, 1974.

147. McLean, A.E.M. Diet and the chemical environment as modifiers of carcinogenesis. *Host Environment Interactions in the Etiology of Cancer in Man.* (Doll, R., Vodopija, I., eds.). IARC, Lyon, 1972, pp. 223-230.

148. Papers from Second International Symposium on Microsomes and Drug Oxidations. Stanford University, Stanford, California, July 29-31, 1972. *Drug Metabolism Distribution,* Vol. 1, January-February 1973.

149. Pamukcu, A.M., Wattenberg, L.W., Price, J.M., et al. Phenothiazine inhibition of intestinal and urinary bladder tumors induced in rats by bracken fern. *J. Natl. Cancer Inst. 47:* 155-159, 1971.

150. Yamamoto, R.S., Weisburger, J.H., and Weisburger, E.K. Controlling factors in urethan carcinogenesis in mice: effect of enzyme inducers and metabolic inhibitors. *Cancer Res. 31:* 483-486, 1971.

151. Kellermann, G., Cantrell, E., and Shaw, C.R. Variations in extent of aryl hydro-carbon hydroxylase induction in cultured human lymphocytes. *Cancer Res. 33:* 1654–1656, 1973.

152. Krieger, R.I., Feeny, P.P., and Wilkinson, C.F. Detoxication enzymes in the guts of caterpillars: an evolutionary answer to plant defenses? *Science 172:* 579–581, 1971.

153. Clemmesen, J., Fuglsang-Frederiksen, V., and Plum, C.M. Are anticonvulsants oncogenic? *Lancet 1:* 705–707, 1974.

154. Berg, J.W., Howell, M.A., and Silverman, S.J. Dietary hypotheses and diet-related research in the etiology of colon cancer. *Health Services Rep. 88:* 915–924, 1973.

155. Hill, M.J. Bacteria and the etiology of colonic cancer. *Cancer 34:* 815–818, 1974.

156. Hill, M.J., Goddard, P., and Williams, R.E.O. Gut bacteria and aetiology of cancer of the breast. *Lancet 2:* 472–473, 1971.

DISCUSSION

Dr. Nelson and other participants agreed with **Dr. Berg** on the need for cooperative efforts between epidemiologists and experimentalists. In particular, laboratory scientists should give a high priority to experiments of untested nutritional clues generated by epidemiologic studies; the reverse route of investigation was also emphasized. Several speakers agreed on the impact of diet on cancer risk, as illustrated by Dr. Wynder's estimate that about one-half of female cancer deaths and one-third of male cancer deaths may be attributed to nutritional factors. **Dr. Wynder** suggested that overnutrition may have an etiologic role in cancers of the pancreas, colon, and kidney, as well as hormone-related cancers of the breast and reproductive organs. Undernutrition, especially early in life, was suggested as a possible protective factor. An absence of high colon cancer risk in vitamin A-deficient populations was cited as an example.

Dr. Berg stressed that dietary deficiencies may produce increased susceptibility of specific tissues to nondietary carcinogens. In addition, dietary factors may promote cancer by affecting host characteristics such as age at menarche, hormone status, and composition of intestinal flora.

Despite the great difficulty and expense of accurately measuring dietary intake, the need for careful epidemiologic studies of dietary influences was stressed by **Dr. Higginson** and **Dr. Saffiotti**. The multiplicity of possible carcinogens in the diet, as well as nondietary exposure to carcinogens, complicate studies of diet-cancer relationships. Since individuals are usually exposed simultaneously to multiple carcinogens, **Dr. Kraybill** raised the possibility of synergism among dietary carcinogens.

It was suggested that epidemiologists should conduct follow-up studies on people exposed to substances that are carcinogenic in laboratory animals, even before adverse clinical effects are detected by alert practitioners. Continuous collection of survey data to quantitate the specific foods consumed by different subgroups of the population was suggested for detecting the possible risks of new food contaminants and additives.

Roland L. Phillips

14

AIR POLLUTION

Malcolm C. Pike, Ph. D., Robert J. Gordon, Ph. D., Brian E. Henderson, M.D.,
Herman R. Menck, and Jennie SooHoo

Departments of Community Medicine and Pathology
University of Southern California School of Medicine
Los Angeles, California

INTRODUCTION

The air of our cities contains varying amounts of substances known to cause cancer in experimental animals [1, Ch. 3] [1]. Tars collected from the air are carcinogenic to animals [2, 3] and transform cells in culture [4]. It appears reasonable, therefore, to assume that this air is carcinogenic to us, in particular to our lungs. The problem arises when we want to quantitate the effect. As Doll [5] stated: "Unfortunately . . . it is extremely difficult to conceive of any epidemiological study that would . . . provide a decisive answer."

Throwing up one's hands in a gesture of despair, however, does not solve the problem, and it refuses to go away. Responsible governmental and state agencies must work and, if warranted, set air pollution standards on the basis of the best estimates of effects available. It is against this background that we review the situation here.

[1]We have found this recent National Academy of Sciences report *Particulate Polycyclic Organic Matter* extremely valuable as a reference to source material and its interpretation. Rather than introduce extensive references here, we have whenever possible cited a page or chapter number from this report, where further details and specific citations can be found.

This work was conducted under Contract No. PH43-NCI-68-1030 within the Virus Cancer Program of the National Cancer Institute, National Institutes of Health, U.S. Public Health Service.

MEASUREMENT OF AIR POLLUTION

The air we breathe contains a large variety of substances that we would prefer were not there—together they constitute "air pollution." Federal standards have been set for six pollutants: carbon monoxide, sulfur dioxide, nitrogen dioxide, particulate matter, gaseous hydrocarbons, and such photochemical oxidants as ozone. In California there are also standards for lead, hydrogen sulfide, and "visibility reducing particles." These standards were determined by consideration of short-term health effects on man. There is little evidence[6, 7] that any of these pollutants is carcinogenic. It appears reasonable to ignore them here and to focus on the main class of chemically identified carcinogens in the air—the polycyclic aromatic hydrocarbons (PAH's).

At present, measurements of benzo[a]pyrene (BP) concentrations in the atmosphere provide us with the best and most widely available indicator of PAH's. Not surprisingly, BP is neither a perfect indicator of PAH's in the air nor of its carcinogenicity. Although Sawicki [8] reported that the amount of BP in the air is highly correlated with the total PAH's, this may not be true if the type of pollution in areas compared differ widely, e.g., automobile exhaust in one area and coal burning in another. In this situation, BP may not be an approximately constant proportion of the PAH's in the areas, and may be even less of a constant proportion of the carcinogenicity of the total air pollution tar [9, 10]. The latter point is particularly important since BP constitutes only a small proportion of the carcinogenicity of both air pollution and cigarette tar in experimental situations [2, 11]. Furthermore, the air pollution tar collected in Los Angeles also contained a non-PAH fraction. This fraction was as potent a cell transforming agent as the PAH fraction [10] and may be just as carcinogenic. Nevertheless, BP is the best indicator available of the potential carcinogenicity of general air pollution.

Through the late 1950's and perhaps beyond, the major sources of BP emissions in the United States were hand-stoked residential coal furnaces, refuse burning (in particular, coal refuse piles), and coke production [1, p. 23 et seq.] [2]. "That efficiency of combustion, and not the fuel used, is the controlling factor is emphasized by the low benzo[a]pyrene emission factor found in power plants burning crushed or pulverized coal" [1, p. 23]. Automobiles and trucks contributed less than 2 percent of the polycyclic organic matter in the air [1, p. 34]; however, in the outlying suburbs of many cities and in other areas, they may have been major contributors. Automobiles make a much larger contribution now. In particular, in Los Angeles County in 1971, it was officially estimated that 42 percent of the particulate emissions were caused by motor

---

[2] These quantities and others of like nature refer to the recent past but before air pollution controls began to be instituted across the country.

vehicles [12], and in downtown Los Angeles virtually all BP in the air is from this source [13]. Similar results probably hold for many other cities now.

Table 1 gives average values for BP concentrations in the air of some U.S. cities in 1959 [14]. The range is from <1 ng/m³ to around 60 ng/m³. In comparison, BP concentrations in the air at nonurban sites were almost always <1 ng/m³.

TABLE 1

BP concentrations in urban sampling sites for January through March 1959[a]

High BP		Low BP	
Urban sampling site	ng BP per m³ air	Urban sampling site	ng BP per m³ air
Montgomery, Ala.	24	Little Rock, Ark.	1.5
Indianapolis, Ind.	26	Glendale, Calif.	0.8
Des Moines, Iowa	23	San Jose, Calif.	0.6
Portland, Maine	21	Miami, Fla.	1.9
St. Louis, Mo.	54	Shreveport, La.	0.7
Charlotte, N.C.	39	Jackson, Miss.	1.2
Cleveland, Ohio	24	Las Vegas, Nev.	1.4
Youngstown, Ohio	28	Bismarck, N.Dak.	0.4
Altoona, Pa.	61	Tulsa, Okla.	1.0
Columbia, S.C.	24	Dallas, Tex.	1.4
Chattanooga, Tenn.	31	Houston, Tex.	1.6
Knoxville, Tenn.	24	Salt Lake City, Utah	0.5
Richmond, Va.	45	Burlington, Vt.	1.0
Wheeling, W.Va.	21	Cheyenne, Wyo.	1.2

[a]Data from Sawicki et al. [14].

There are a number of problems in using data of the type given in Table 1 as a measure of air carcinogenicity. First, indoor levels of PAH's tend to be about half those outside—how much less depends on many factors. One important factor is the quantity of smoking being done indoors; in a 40-m³ room, a single smoker can pollute the air with around 1 ng/m³ of BP [1, p. 29]. Second and more important, air quality varies greatly over time. For example, in Los Angeles the situation has changed dramatically over the last 25 years because of a combination of increased traffic and the imposition in the late 1950's of controls on stationary source emissions of pollutants, mainly refuse burning (Figure 1). The BP level in downtown Los Angeles changed from 31 ng/m³ in 1952-1953 to 1.6 ng/m³ in 1959 to 1.4 ng/m³ in 1971-1972 [13].

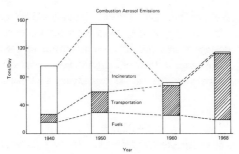

FIGURE 1. Combustion aerosol emissions in Los Angeles County:
1940-1968 [12].

Current controls on the other pollutants are having some effect on PAH's, but the relationships are complex. Figures 2 and 3, based on data from Sawicki et al. [14], show the BP concentration and total particulates (to which most of BP is adsorbed) in the air, monthly from July 1958 to June 1959, in Birmingham, Alabama, and Los Angeles, California. Birmingham had overall, compared to Los Angeles, 7.4 times the BP concentration but only 0.94 times its particulate matter.

To convert ng/m^3 BP in air to ng BP in contact with the lungs per day, we need to know how much air a person breathes per day, what proportion of BP is adsorbed onto particles that will actually reach the lungs, and what the retention characteristics are of inhaled BP.

The answer to the first question is that we breathe between 10 and 20 m^3 per day [1, p. 29;15]. The answer to the second is more complicated:

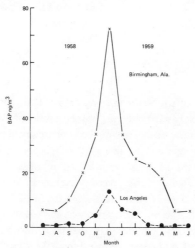

FIGURE 2. Average monthly concentrations of BP in air of
Birmingham, Alabama, and Los Angeles, California: July 1958-June 1959 [14].

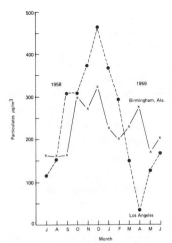

FIGURE 3. Average monthly concentrations of particulates in the air of Birmingham, Alabama, and Los Angeles, California: July 1958-June 1959 [14].

The bulk of BP now in the air is associated with particles that do reach the lungs [16, 17], but this was probably not true when large soot particles were still commonly present in the atmosphere. The third question of retention of inhaled BP is even more complex, and it does not seem useful to discuss it here [1, Ch. 4].

If one uses these estimates of air breathed and assumes no physiological filtration, the amount of BP breathed by a person in a single day in 1959 can be approximated by multiplying the values in Table 1 by 15: thus, in Montgomery, 360 ng; in St. Louis, 810 ng; and in Dallas, 21 ng. From the data in Figure 2, it can be estimated that in Los Angeles, 44 ng BP was breathed per person each day.

To translate these figures into meaningful terms, it is most useful to compare them to the amount of BP breathed in by smoking cigarettes. Clearly, we do not breathe as if we were smoking and smokers vary in their inhaling patterns, but it is estimated that a smoker of one unfiltered cigarette (85 mm) inhales approximately 30 ng of BP [1, p. 29], so that a smoker of one pack a day may be inhaling 600 ng of BP daily. If the nonsmoker in Montgomery breathed the air as if he were smoking, then in terms of BP taken in, it would be roughly equivalent to a smoker of half a pack daily in Dallas.

LUNG CANCER

Confounding Factors

The essential problem in evaluating the possible effect of air pollution on lung cancer is that it must be investigated in the presence of a powerful, known, lung carcinogen—cigarette smoke. In the United States the lung-cancer death rate in male smokers of c cigarettes per day is approximately proportional at any given age to $10 + 5c$; e.g., the lung-cancer death rate in a smoker of a pack a day is roughly 11 times that of a nonsmoker [18]. The rate is affected by inhaling practice, by the type of cigarette, by how far down the cigarette is smoked, and markedly by age at starting to smoke [18]. One can calculate this latter effect roughly by noting that the lung-cancer death rate of a smoker at any given age is approximately proportional to duration of smoking $(=^4)$; thus, at age 65 a smoker of c cigarettes per day who started smoking at age 15 will have a death rate of 2.4 $(50^4/40^4)$ times the death rate of a smoker who smoked the same amount but started at age 25 and 1.5 $(50^4/45^4)$ times that of a smoker who started at age 20 [19].

The other confounding factor is occupational exposure to lung carcinogens. The evidence for an increased risk of lung cancer in certain groups of workers is very strong [20]. Since most of these groups work in polluted cities, the lung cancer rates there would be expected to reflect this characteristic to some extent, even if the smoking habits of people in these areas were identical to those of people in less polluted towns and rural areas.

Epidemiologic Evidence

One general epidemiologic approach to minimizing the interference of confounding factors is for one to study an extreme situation, noting the results and then extrapolating them to the more relevant general situation. That is, most commonly, one assumes a simple proportional effect with dose of carcinogen and then looks for confirmatory evidence from other sources. This approach appears to be a good one to adopt in studying lung cancer and general air pollution.

An example of an extreme situation is the carbonization workers in British gasworks [21] who were exposed during their working day to average BP levels of about 2,000 ng/m^3. In a prospective study, Doll et al. [22] followed a cohort of these workers for several years. Although the results of this study were internally not completely consistent, this group had a lung cancer death rate about 80% higher than the rate for all men in England and Wales, and somewhat greater than that for unexposed workmates. The first comparison was between an age-adjusted rate of approximately $200/10^5$ for men in England and Wales and $360/10^5$ for the exposed workers. (*These estimated rates depend greatly on the age distribution of the assumed standard population*, here taken to be the surveyed gasworkers.)

A number of investigators claim the results of this study of gasworkers (and others like it) argue against any significant effect of general air pollution. Their position is summarized in a report issued by the Royal College of Physicians of London [23] as follows: "Urban air contains carcinogenic compounds, but the relatively small excess risk to men occupationally exposed to large concentrations of these compounds raises doubt about the relevance to lung cancer of the much lower levels found in the air of even the most polluted city."

In our opinion, they have misinterpreted the results. The carbonization workers were exposed to an estimated 2,000 ng/m³ BP for about 22 percent of the year (assuming a 40-hour working week, 2 weeks paid leave, 1 week sick leave); very roughly, the men were exposed to the equivalent of 440 (2000 X 0.22) ng/m³ BP general air pollution. This exposure caused an extra 160/10⁵ lung cancer cases, so that we may estimate, assuming a proportional effect, that each ng/m³ BP causes 0.4/10⁵ (160/10⁵ ÷ 440) extra lung cancer cases per year. A city with 50 ng/m³ BP air pollution might, therefore, have an extra 18/10⁵ lung cancer cases per year. These numbers are not negligible, although they are small when compared, say, to smoking a pack of cigarettes every day.

This estimate of a small, but not negligible, general air pollution effect on lung cancer agrees with most other epidemiologic evidence on the subject.

First, the effect should be fairly small as evidenced by the following: lung cancer rarely occurred until the turn of the century and did not really start to be a significant cause of death until about 1925, whereas pollution from coal smoke has been with us for generations before that [24]; and lung cancer rates in nonsmokers have been low even in heavily polluted areas [25].

Second, there should be an increased lung cancer rate in high PAH-polluted areas even allowing for cigarette smoking. Some evidence exists for a slight increase in lung cancer among nonsmokers in urban compared to rural areas [25]; the effect is magnified in most studies when we consider the joint effect of urbanization and cigarette smoking. Table 2 presents data [26] comparing rates in Liverpool to those in rural North Wales. This study by Stocks was done in an area of "stable" air pollution. A fair summary of these data is that the urban

TABLE 2

Age-standardized lung cancer mortality rates (per 100,000 per year) for men aged 35-74 by amount of cigarettes smoked in Liverpool and rural North Wales [26]

Packs/day	Mortality Rates	
(approx.)	Rural area	Liverpool
Nonsmokers	22	50
½	69	168
1	147	248
1½	232	389
2	344	327

effect produces an excess of $28/10^5$ lung cancer deaths in nonsmokers and $100/10^5$ such deaths in smokers, the latter figure being independent of the actual amount smoked. We might refer to this increase as a modified additive effect. The difference in BP levels in the air between the two areas was estimated to be 70 ng/m^3 (77 ng/m^3 compared to 7 ng/m^3); thus, we may very crudely estimate the air pollution effect in the presence of cigarette smoking at $1.4/10^5$ per ng/m^3 BP or $0.4/10^5$ per ng/m^3 BP in nonsmokers (Table 3).

Although the data of Stocks have been criticized on methodologic grounds, his estimate of BP effect for nonsmokers is remarkably consistent with that derived from the study of British gasworkers. (This comparison may be made directly, without overly insulting the data, because the $200/10^5$ estimate for England and Wales quoted in the study of gasworkers roughly corresponds to Stocks' estimate for Liverpool.) This agreement effectively answers the suggestion that the differences between rates in Liverpool and rural North Wales are the result of occupational exposure differences alone. The figure given by Stocks of $1.4/10^5$ per ng/m^3 BP for smokers appears to be 3 to 4 times too high, possibly as a result of methodological errors in his study design or execution, differences in inhaling patterns, or variations in age at starting to smoke in the two areas. However, before rejecting the figure, we should remember that the gasworkers were not shown to have been exposed to these working conditions throughout their working lives, and some of the men were retired. These effects

TABLE 3

Estimated increase in male lung cancer death rate (per 100,000 per year) per ng/m^3 BP content of air and per cigarette smoked per day

Data source		Increase per ng/m^3 BP in air	Increase per cigarette smoked per day	Estimated U.K. equivalence: ng/m^3 BP =1 cigarette/day	Estimated U.S. equivalence: ng/m^3 BP =1 cigarette/day
British carbonization workers [21, 22]		0.4	9	23	11
Liverpool and rural North Wales [26]	Non-smokers	0.4	7	17	9
	Cigarette smokers	1.4	7	5	2.5

from duration of exposure could be large and would, of course, lead to a low estimate of the effects of BP air pollution.

We conclude that, contrary to previous analyses [5,23,24], the 2 foregoing studies are quite compatible and support the notion of a simple proportional relationship between increasing BP concentration in the air and an *excess* rate of lung cancer.

Similar studies have compared areas of different BP pollution, taking into account cigarette smoking habits. However, either they do not present relevant BP levels or they are based on such small numbers that meaningful calculations cannot be made. Nevertheless, the studies of Hitosugi in Japan [27], Dean in South Africa [28], Golledge and Wicken in the Tees-side area of England [29], and Haenszel et al. in the United States [30], all fall into the same pattern as the data of Stocks, with possibly a bit of special pleading to explain a more than additive effect at the highest level of smoking. The study of Dean in Northern Ireland [31] is the only one that clearly does not fit the pattern. He found that the urban rate was a constant multiple of the rural rate independent of smoking level, but since he also reported other anomalous findings, such as no difference between small towns and Belfast, we are inclined to ignore the results.

Another approach was adopted by Carnow and Meier [1, p. 225]. They tackled the problem of estimating the effect of general air pollution in the United States by using a multiple regression approach on data from 48 states with $Y = C_0 + C_1 X_1 + C_2 X_2$, in which Y was the standardized lung cancer death rate for white males for 1959-1961, X_1 = cigarette sales (in dollars) per person over 15 years of age, and X_2 = BP concentration (in ng/m^3) averaged over each state. This approach supported an effect of general air pollution, but the inadequacy of the cigarette consumption data and the crudity of BP measurements weakened the impact of the results. Similar calculations have also been made by other investigators with corresponding results.

Some contrary evidence was recently reported by Hammond [32]. He reanalyzed the American Cancer Society's prospective study on lung cancer, separating out those men known to have been exposed to possible lung carcinogens at work. Once this had been done, there was little or no difference between lung cancer rates by city of residence size. These results certainly warn one against easy acceptance of our conclusions on the effect of air pollution; however, air pollution in towns of the same size can vary greatly, certainly as measured by BP, and the data are not given in a form allowing a more detailed evaluation.

Relative Effect of BP in Air and in Cigarette Smoke

If we assume, according to Doll et al. [22], that the average "relevant" air pollution level for England and Wales, and the unexposed British gasworkers, was 50 ng/m^3 BP, then cigarette smoking may be considered as causing roughly

$180/10^5$ lung cancer cases per year. The average cigarette consumption of both the exposed and unexposed gasworkers and of the general male population of the same age in England and Wales was 20 per day. The lung-cancer death rate per cigarette daily is, therefore, approximately $9/10^5$ per year (Table 3).

Similar calculations based on the data of Stocks [26] yield an estimated rate of $7/10^5$ per year per cigarette daily.

An average figure of $8/10^5$ per year per cigarette daily may then be compared to our figure of $0.4/10^5$ per year per ng/m^3 BP in air. That is, 1 cigarette per day is roughly equivalent to 20 ng/m^3 BP in air. Converted to terms of BP inhaled 30 ng BP in cigarette smoke is equivalent to $300(20 \times 15)$ ng BP in air. (If we take as an upper limit for the effect of BP in air the above figure of $1.4/10^5$ per year per ng/m^3 BP calculated from the results of Stocks for smokers, then these figures become: 1 cigarette per day equals 5.6 ng/m^3 BP in air, and 30 ng BP in cigarette smoke equals 84 ng BP in air.)

The effect of cigarette smoking on lung cancer mortality in the United States is probably only about half that in the United Kingdom [5]. Thus, in U.S. terms, the above equivalences are 1 cigarette per day equals 10 ng/m^3 BP in air (or 2.8 ng/m^3 using the higher figure).

Our results [33] showing an excess of lung cancer in males in south-central Los Angeles would imply an excess of BP in air of somewhere between 20 ng/m^3 (based on $1.4/10^5$) and 75 ng/m^3 (based on $0.4/10^5$) in that area some 20 or more years ago. This BP excess is perfectly reasonable considering the type of industry (mainly petroleum refining) in the area. Today, air pollution controls have reduced the level in this "worst" area to approximately 3 ng/m^3 compared to 1 ng/m^3 for all of Los Angeles County [13].

OTHER CANCERS

As stated, it is good epidemiologic practice to look first at extreme situations. The obvious extremes in air pollution are industrial exposure to high levels of similar pollution and cigarette smoking.

The authors of the British gasworkers study [22] reported an increased risk of bladder cancer, roughly $30/10^5$ compared to $17/10^5$ in England and Wales males, and about a fivefold increased risk of scrotal cancer. They went on to say: "For other causes of death the rates [in gasworkers] are . . . unremarkable, being similar to or less than the corresponding national rates." The increased scrotal cancer rate probably is specifically industrial and irrelevant to the problem of general air pollution. The increased bladder cancer rate of $13/10^5$ is roughly 8 percent of the increased annual lung cancer rate of $160/10^5$.

Cigarette smokers are reported [18] to have increased rates of cancer, not only of the lung, oral cavity, and larynx, but also of the bladder, esophagus, pancreas, and kidney. The differences, however, at sites other than lung are slight in absolute terms compared to lung cancer, and/or somewhat insecurely based as a causal connection rather than simply an association [18].

There are references [1] to studies linking air pollution to certain other cancer sites (e.g., stomach and prostate), but in the light of the industrial exposure and cigarette data, we feel that there is little to gain from discussing them here.

ARYL HYDROCARBON HYDROXYLASE

Our calculations in Table 2 showed that the excess lung cancer rate per ng/m^3 BP in air could be as much as 3.5 times greater in smokers than in non-smokers; the differential effect apparently is not related to the absolute level of smoking. A possible explanation of this finding (assuming it is not artifact)—and some other problem findings in this area—may be found in recent laboratory work on the mechanism of chemical carcinogenesis, a topic reviewed by Heidelberger [34].

For example, BP is not a carcinogen as such but must be metabolically activated to a chemically reactive electrophilic species. An enzyme system importantly involved in these changes is the aryl hydrocarbon hydroxylase (AHH) system. At least part of this system is genetically controlled in the mouse, and the level of inducibility is strongly associated with 3-methylcholanthrene (MCA)-induced sarcomas in this species [35].

In mice, inducibility is measured by the ratio of the AHH activity (measured by the hydroxylated metabolite of test PAH's, usually BP) in the liver some hours after intraperitoneal injection of MCA (the induced level) to the activity in controls of the same inbred strain that received sham injections (the constitutive level).

Man has a very similar enzyme system, but measuring it presents a problem. Kellermann et al. [36] employed an in vitro method using peripheral blood lymphocytes. They reported that inducibility in the human population appeared to be controlled by a single gene with two alleles (H-high and L-low). In a case-control study, they showed that compared to LL persons, HL persons had a 16-fold and HH persons a 36-fold increased risk of lung cancer. These relative risks are the sort epidemiologists dream about, and certainly make any comment about inadequate matching for age or smoking habits appear fatuous.

A number of groups, including ourselves, have been attempting to repeat this work. Severe technical problems have prevented obtaining repeatable measurements of AHH inducibility in a given individual. However, considerable research is in progress to develop a good assay system, since a test that correlates well with lung cancer development would be of tremendous value for screening purposes alone.

To return to the apparent differential effect of general air pollution on smokers and nonsmokers, it may be that the intense, albeit short, exposure to PAH through smoking a cigarette maximally induces the AHH system in the lung. The low-level carcinogens in the air then can be "optimally" transformed to their active form and do their most damage. On the other hand, the nonsmoker has a lower level of AHH activity in the lung, which could mean that air pollution carcinogens might be cleared via a less carcinogenic route. Thus, there is no telling reason why we should insist that the effect of air pollution on smokers and non-smokers should be the same or, alternatively, that it should be synergistic.

The attentive reader will have realized that our discussions so far have concerned only lung cancer in males. *The reason is that the relation of air pollution to lung cancer in females is very unclear.* We do not have an industrial exposure situation in which to study females, and the data of Stocks [26] and others [18] are too subject to random variation to make interpretation reliable. However, the data are compatible with a much reduced effect compared to men.

If this effect is true, it may also be related to AHH activity because the enzyme system is inducible by a variety of endogenous and exogenous compounds including steroid hormones and barbiturates, and it may be inhibited by others. AHH activity is thus quite possibly different in men and women because of hormone levels and drug usage.

The situation is further complicated because some noncarcinogenic AHH inducers enhance tumor formation, whereas others might do the exact opposite [37, 38]. There is a lot of work to be done in this area; however, it gives hope of providing not only a great deal of understanding of chemical carcinogenesis, but also useful information for the control of chemically induced cancer in man.

CONCLUSION

An analysis of the relationship between air pollution, as measured by benzo[a]pyrene concentration, and lung cancer suggests that in the United States it would be prudent to equate 10 ng/m^3 BP air pollution to 1 cigarette per day.

REFERENCES

1. National Academy of Sciences. *Particulate Polycyclic Organic Matter.* Washington, D.C., 1972.

2. Kotin, P., Falk, H.L., Mader, P., et al. Aromatic hydrocarbons. 1. Presence in the Los Angeles atmosphere and the carcinogenicity of atmospheric extracts. *AMA Arch. Ind. Health 9*:153-163, 1954.

3. Asahina, S., Andrea, J., Carmel, A., et al. Carcinogenicity of organic fractions of particulate pollutants collected in New York City and administered subcutaneously to infant mice. *Cancer Res. 32*:2263-2268, 1972.

4. Freeman, A.E., Price, P.J., Bryan, R.J., et al. Transformation of rat and hamster embryo cells by extracts of city smog. *Proc. Natl. Acad. Sci. USA 68*:445-449, 1971.

5. Doll, R. *Prevention of Cancer: Pointers from Epidemiology*. Nuffield Provincial Hospitals Trust, London, 1967.

6. Kuschner, M. The causes of lung cancer. *Am. Rev. Respir. Dis. 98*:573-590, 1968.

7. Kotin, P., and Wisely, D.V. Production of lung cancer in mice by inhalation exposure to influenza virus and aerosols of hydrocarbons. *Prog. Exp. Tumor Res. 3*:186-195, 1963.

8. Sawicki, E. Airborne carcinogens and allied compounds. *Arch. Environ. Health 14*: 46-53, 1967.

9. Hoffmann, D., and Wynder, E.L. Chemical analysis and carcinogenic bioassays of organic particulate pollutants. *In Air Pollution*, 2nd ed. *Vol. II*. Academic Press, New York, 1968.

10. Gordon, R.J., Bryan, R.J., Rhim, J.S., et al. Transformation of rat and mouse embryo cells by a new class of carcinogenic compounds isolated from particles in city air. *Int. J. Cancer 12*:223-232, 1973.

11. Wynder, E.L., and Hoffmann, D. Experimental tobacco carcinogenesis. *Science 162*: 862-871, 1968.

12. Air Pollution Control District, County of Los Angeles. *Profile of Air Pollution Control 1971*.

13. Gordon, R.J., and Bryan, R.J. Patterns in airborne polynuclear hydrocarbon concentrations at four Los Angeles sites. *Environ. Sci. Technol. 7*:1050-1053, 1973.

14. Sawicki, E., Elbert, W.C., Hauser, T.R., et al. Benzo(a)pyrene content of the air of American communities. *Am. Ind. Hyg. Assoc. J. 21*:443-451, 1960.

15. Stocks, P., and Campbell, J.M. Lung cancer death rates among non-smokers and pipe and cigarette smokers. *Br. Med. J., 2*:923-928, 1955.

16. De Maio, L., and Corn, M. Polynuclear aromatic hydrocarbons associated with particulates in Pittsburgh air. *J. Air Pollut. Control Assoc. 16*:67-71, 1966.

17. Gordon, R.J., and Bryan, R.J. Size fraction analysis of polynuclear hydrocarbons and metals in airborne particulates in Los Angeles. (Unpublished data.)

18. U.S. Department of Health, Education, and Welfare. *The Health Consequences of Smoking*. Report to the Surgeon General. U.S. Govt. Print. Off., Washington, D.C., 1971.

19. Peto, R. Personal communication, 1974.

20. Doll, R. Practical steps towards the prevention of bronchial carcinoma. *Scott. Med. J. 15*:433-447, 1970.

21. Lawther, P.J., Commins, B.T., and Waller, R.E. A study of the concentrations of polycyclic aromatic hydrocarbons in gasworkers retort houses. *Br. J. Ind. Med. 22*:13-20, 1965.

22. Doll, R., Vessey, M.P., Beasley, R.W.R., et al. Mortality of gasworkers - final report of a prospective study. *Br. J. Ind. Med. 29*:394-406, 1972.

23. Royal College of Physicians of London. *Air Pollution and Health*, Pitman, London, 1970.

24. Waller, R.E. Bronchi and lungs—air pollution. *In* Raven, R., and Roe, F.J.C., eds. *The Prevention of Cancer*. Butterworths, London, 1967.

25. Buell, P., and Dunn, J.E. Relative impact of smoking and air pollution on lung cancer. *Arch. Environ. Health 15*:291-297, 1967.

26. Stocks, P. *Cancer in North Wales and Liverpool Regions*. Supplement to British Empire Cancer Campaign Annual Report, 1957.

27. Hitosugi, M. Epidemiological study of lung cancer with special reference to the effect of air pollution and smoking habits. *Inst. Public Health Bull.* (Tokyo) *17*:237-256, 1968.

28. Dean, G. Lung cancer among white South Africans: Report on a further study. *Br. Med. J. 1*:1599-1605, 1961.

29. Golledge, A.H., and Wicken, A.J. Local variation on the incidence of lung cancer and bronchitis mortality. *Med. Officer 112*:273-277, 1964.

30. Haenszel, W., Loveland, D.B., and Sirken, M.G. Lung cancer mortality as related to residence and smoking histories: I. White males. *J. Natl. Cancer Inst. 28*:947-1001, 1962.

31. Dean, G. Lung cancer and bronchitis in Northern Ireland, 1960-2. *Br. Med. J. 1*: 1506-1514, 1966.

32. Hammond, E.C. Smoking habits and air pollution in relation to lung cancer. *In* (Lee, D.H.K., ed.) *Environmental Factors in Respiratory Disease.* Academic Press, New York, 1972.

33. Menck, H.R., Casagrande, J., and Henderson, B.E. Industrial air pollution: Possible effect on lung cancer. *Science 183*:210-212, 1974.

34. Heidelberger, C. Current trends in chemical carcinogenesis. *Fed. Proc. 32*:2154-2161, 1973.

35. Kouri, R.C., Ratrie, H., and Whitmire, C.E. Evidence of a genetic relationship between methylcholanthrene induced subcutaneous tumors and inducibility of aryl hydrocarbon hydroxylase. *J. Natl. Cancer Inst. 51*:197-200, 1973.

36. Kellermann, G., Shaw, C.R., and Luyten-Kellermann, M. Aryl hydrocarbon hydroxylase inducibility and bronchogenic carcinoma. *N. Engl. J. Med. 289:*934-936, 1973.

37. Yamamoto, R.S., Weisburger, J.H., and Weisburger, E.K. Controlling factors in urethan carcinogenesis in mice: Effect of enzyme inducers and metabolic inhibitors. *Cancer Res. 31*: 483-486, 1971.

38. Bowden, G.T., Slaga, T.J., Shapas, B.G., et al. The role of aryl hydrocarbon hydroxylase in skin tumor initiation. *Cancer Res. 34:*2634-2642, 1974.

DISCUSSION

Dr. E. C. Hammond emphasized the need for measures of absolute or attributable risks, with appropriate error estimates. On reviewing the correlation studies of Percy Stocks, he had noted marked differences in criteria used by physicians to diagnose lung cancer. For example, lung cancer seemed much more readily diagnosed in Liverpool than in rural areas. Furthermore, Stocks' data on smoking habits were based on a hospital sample and not a community sample. In Dr. Hammond's opinion, there are other more direct and precise data to evaluate the carcinogenic effects of air pollution.

Dr. Pike responded that other studies may also have deficiencies. His computations actually suggest close agreement between the data of Stocks and Doll.

Dr. Higginson asked whether air pollution could explain the urban-rural differences in cancer rates in Denmark and Sweden for sites such as the urinary bladder. **Dr. Pike** responded that the relation of air pollution to bladder cancer is unknown. He added that a lung cancer hazard is biologically plausible, inasmuch as inhalation carries pollutants into the respiratory tract. On the other hand, it is not clear why only men have shown an excess risk of lung cancer from air pollution. A possible explanation may be that women ingest drugs which affect enzymatic induction of aryl hydrocarbon hydroxylase. This type of argument is supported by animal studies.

Dr. Selikoff asked whether benzo[a]pyrene (BP) was considered as an index of pollutant exposure or as the specific causal agent. **Dr. Pike** said that it was being used as an index.

Dr. Goldsmith observed that the geographic correlation between BP levels and lung cancer mortality by state (National Academy of Science report) is merely a reflection of an urbanization effect. The data do not represent measured values of BP in rural and urban areas of each state, but rather the pooled levels of BP in all areas combined. He added that the data from Los Angeles county may not reflect general air pollution, but probably represent a large point source for industrial pollution of the surrounding community. **Dr. Pike** responded that this issue is under study and that the petroleum refineries in the area have been asked to provide employment and medical data on workers exposed over time.

John R. Goldsmith

15

VIRUSES AND OTHER MICROBES

Clark W. Heath, Jr., M.D., Glyn G. Caldwell, M.D.,
and Paul C. Feorino, Ph. D.

Cancer and Birth Defects Division and the Virology Branch
Center for Disease Control
Atlanta, Georgia

Few situations involving exposure to viruses or other infectious agents can yet be cited as unequivocally increasing human cancer risk. Many plausible hypotheses have been generated, and in several instances evidence is clearly suggestive. This review summarizes our state of knowledge and comments on possible directions that future work may take. Emphasis is given to situations in which relationships to human cancer have been seriously entertained, without undertaking any comprehensive review concerning all possible infectious agents.

VIRUSES

Viruses have received the greatest attention by far in studies concerned with infection as a cause of human cancer. Such studies cover the entire gamut of DNA and RNA viruses and can be conveniently considered in terms of viral origin, whether human, animal, or artificial.

Viruses of Human Origin

DNA Viruses—Herpesviruses and Others

At present, members of the herpesvirus family are particularly suspect in relation to human oncogenicity, partly because herpesviruses were shown

This study was supported in part by contract YO1 CP 40202 within the Virus Cancer Program of the National Cancer Institute.

conclusively [1, 2] to cause cancer in lower animals (Marek's disease in fowl, lymphoma in monkeys and rabbits, and Lucké renal carcinoma in frogs). The human viruses of particular interest are the Epstein-Barr virus (EBV), herpes simplex virus, particularly type 2 (HSV-2), and to a lesser extent varicella virus.

Epstein-Barr virus. Speculation that EBV might be oncogenic began with the initial identification of the virus in cell cultures from African Burkitt's tumor (BT) tissue [3]. Although absolute proof of oncogenicity is still lacking, considerable circumstantial evidence has been assembled, particularly in relation to BT itself and to nasopharyngeal carcinoma (NPC), and to a lesser degree to Hodgkin's disease (HD) and other lymphoproliferative tumors. With respect to BT, the virus exists in close association with lymphoid tumor cells in terms of membrane antigen, EBV-specific DNA, and the appearance of viral particles and antigens under tissue culture conditions [1]. Cases of BT in Africa, with virtually no exceptions, exhibit serum antibodies against EBV, mean titers among such patients being greatly increased over controls [4]. This phenomenon appears limited to tropical BT cases only. Whether slight elevations of anti-EBV titers may be a feature of BT elsewhere is disputed at present [5, 6], as is the concept that nontropical BT is precisely the same disease as that seen in central Africa. In this connection, tissue from nontropical BT cases appears not to contain EBV viral DNA [7].

With respect to other forms of lymphoid tumors, statistically significant elevations of geometric mean anti-EBV titers were consistently found [8-11] in lymphocyte-deficient forms of HD and in one study [12] of chronic lymphocytic leukemia (CLL). Not all individual cases show anti-EBV titers, however, and it is felt that the EBV infection in such disorders is coincidental rather than causal.

Besides tropical BT, the only other malignant disease characterized by consistent and marked elevations of anti-EBV antibody is NPC, where virtually every patient has anti-EBV antibodies with mean titers substantially higher than among controls [13]. This association is generally considered to reflect a passenger virus state rather than a causal relationship, since EBV infection in all other situations appears confined to lymphoid tissue and since NPC is basically an epithelial cell cancer, albeit heavily infiltrated with lymphocytes. However, although an early study [14] associated EBV antigens only with infiltrating lymphoid elements, more recent work [15] suggests that the epithelial cells themselves are also infected.

Whether these observations, particularly on BT and other lymphoid tumors, indicate an etiologic relationship to EBV infection is uncertain. EBV is closely associated with lymphoid cells generally; witness the virus's ability to induce lymphocyte transformation and in vitro growth [16] and its etiologic relationship to infectious mononucleosis (IM) [17]. Such observations raise the possibility that increases in anti-EBV antibody among cancer cases reflect a result rather than a cause of altered lymphoid function or morphology. Efforts to resolve this question through the suggestion that IM, known to be caused by EBV infection, may predispose to HD and other lymphomas have to date been unsuccessful. Case-control studies [18-20] have shown no association, whereas analyses of cancer risk among IM cohorts have produced conflicting results [21-23]. However, should an association exist between IM and malignancy, it may well not reflect EBV infection itself, but rather an oncogenic potential of transformed lymphocytes, perhaps activation of latent RNA viral infection in the process of transformation [24].

Clinical studies [25, 26] seeking to relate EBV infection to leukemia etiology have been negative. Some recent evidence [27], however, suggests that anti-EBV antibody levels may be elevated among healthy relatives of cancer patients in multiple-case family situations (carcinomas and sarcomas as well as lymphomas). Conceivably, such antibody patterns may reflect altered immune response in genetic settings where cancer risk is increased.

If it is assumed that EBV possesses some oncogenic potential, at least in relation to BT and NPC, the fact that EBV infection is ubiquitous, affecting most of the world's population by the time young adulthood is reached, suggests that something more than simple viral infection is required for tumor production. Present hypotheses focus on the immunologic state of the host, and perhaps the timing of EBV infection as well. The fact that tropical BT is concentrated in areas heavily infested with malaria suggests that malaria-induced alterations in reticuloendothelial structure and function enhance oncogenic response to EBV infection [28]. At present, such a sequence of events is speculative. The only information bearing directly on the question is that no differences in levels of malaria antibody were found between BT cases and controls [29]. Since such measurements may have little relationship to host immune status at time of EBV infection or BT induction, they do not necessarily refute the malaria cofactor hypothesis. In support of the hypothesis is the observation that sickle cell trait is less common among BT cases than among controls [30, 31]. Conceivably, the protective effect of sickle hemoglobin in relation to severity of falciparum malaria may lessen the intensity of host reticuloendothelial response, thus making the development of BT less likely. More definitive data on the relationship of EBV infection, host immune status, and BT development should come from an ongoing large prospective study of African children [32].

Herpes simplex virus. Considerable evidence suggests that infection with HSV-2 predisposes to cancer of the uterine cervix; as with EBV, conclusive proof of oncogenicity is lacking. After demonstration of two separate and largely site-specific herpes simplex viruses, HSV-1 (oral-pharyngeal) and HSV-2 (genital) [33], retrospective case-control serologic surveys revealed a fairly strong and consistent association between the presence of anti-HSV-2 antibodies and cervical cancer. A thorough review of these various studies has recently been compiled by Kessler [34]. The association appears to hold true not only for frank, invasive cervical cancer but also for earlier stages of carcinoma in situ and dysplasia [35-37], and it is supported by preliminary prospective observations suggesting that women who later develop invasive cancer, and possibly carcinoma in situ and dysplasia as well, have an increased prevalence of anti-HSV-2 antibodies [36, 38]. HSV-2 has also been isolated from cultures of cervical cancer cells [39] and is capable of producing malignant transformation in cell systems in vitro [40].

These findings reinforce the hypothesis, developed before knowledge of HSV-2, that cervical cancer might be a venereal disease on the strength of its close epidemiologic correlation with age at first intercourse, number of sexual partners, and socioeconomic status [34]. Despite the strength of laboratory and epidemiologic observations to date, however, it remains possible that HSV-2 infection merely accompanies malignant change and is not an essential carcinogenic ingredient. Continued laboratory research and prospective follow-up of HSV-2-infected patients should eventually clarify this crucial point.

Only cervical cancer has been studied intensively with respect to HSV, but relationships to other tumors have been considered. Specifically, nonvirion antigen-antibody studies [41, 42] suggested an association between HSV infection and cancers primarily involving the head and neck. A recent review [43] of these studies, however, failed to confirm them. With respect to HSV-1, clinical observations in Africa suggested that lesions compatible with herpes labialis precede onset of BT with unusual frequency [44]. Anti-HSV antibody studies, however, showed no unusual patterns in BT, HD, or various forms of leukemia [26, 45-47]. Elevations of anti-HSV-1 antibody have been associated with NPC, but appear to reflect reactivation of latent infection [47,48].

Other herpesviruses. Relatively little evidence suggesting oncogenicity now exists for human herpesviruses other than EBV and HSV-2. A hypothesis that varicella infection during pregnancy may heighten risk of cancer in offspring was raised by a British cohort study [49]: Among 270 children exposed in utero to varicella by maternal history, 2 developed leukemia, a statistically significant increase over expected incidence (0.15 case). Similar findings came from British case-control material [50] where 7 cases of childhood cancer (3 leukemia, 3 brain tumors—2 confirmed as medulloblastoma—and 1 Wilms' tumor) were associated with maternal history of gestational varicella compared with none among controls. Serologic studies [10, 26, 46], however, with respect to HD and leukemia showed no abnormalities related to either varicella or cytomegalovirus (CMV). Various reports have dealt with the nature and frequency of infection with these and other herpesviruses during the course of cancer, especially leukemias and lymphomas. In all such instances, however, infection probably represents a complication of the underlying malignant disease, often accompanied by varying degrees of immunologic impairment.

Finally, occasional attempts [51-53] to isolate virus material from cancer patients (specifically HD and prostatic cancer) have yielded morphologic herpes agents not yet identified as any known herpes type. These situations may, of course, reflect new or reactivated herpes infection following cancer induction. However, since EBV was discovered during just this kind of virus search, all such identifications deserve thorough investigation as possible leads toward understanding cancer etiology.

Other DNA viruses. At present, little evidence suggests that infection with human DNA viruses other than members of the herpes group increases risk of cancer. Three specific virus groups deserve mention: adenovirus, papovavirus, and hepatitis B surface antigen (HB$_S$Ag) (Australia antigen). The adenoviruses, especially adenovirus types 12, 18, and 31, produce tumors in hamsters [1]. Serologic studies [54] in human populations, however, showed no significant differences in frequency of antibody against human adenoviruses among patients with a wide range of cancers compared with controls. A search for adenovirus-specific RNA in human cancers also was negative [55].

Among papovaviruses, the wart virus has long been recognized as causing benign epidermal tumors [56]. Virus particles morphologically indistinguishable from papovavirus more recently were observed in tissue from human brain tumor (choroid papilloma) [57], whereas papovavirus was isolated from brain tumor tissue and from the urine of a patient with Wiskott-Aldrich syndrome and reticulum cell sarcoma of brain in whom serum antibodies against papovavirus were detectable for 1 year before death [58]. Human papovavirus isolated from a patient with progressive multifocal leukoencephalopathy produced malignant gliomas in hamsters [59].

Considerable attention has been paid to the possible relationship of HB$_S$Ag, first to leukemia, and more recently to liver cancer. The association with leukemia and with Down's syndrome, a leukemia-prone condition, appears to be related to altered host susceptibility to persistent HB$_S$Ag viremia [60]. Lymphocytic forms of leukemia seem involved most often, with transfusion of blood containing HB$_S$Ag being the most likely source of infection [61].

Evidence for liver cancer is conflicting. An increased frequency of HB$_S$Ag was found in African patients with hepatocellular carcinoma compared with controls [62-65], but not among cases in the United States or the Far East [66, 67]. As with other virus-cancer associations, further data will be needed before the relation of HB$_S$Ag to liver cancer etiology can be defined. It remains possible that certain cases of liver cancer reflect the end stage of a process that starts with HB$_S$Ag-caused hepatitis and cirrhosis.

RNA Viruses

Several classes of human RNA viruses have been mentioned as possible causes of human cancer. In no instance is the evidence more than suggestive. A series of recent epidemiologic studies concerns the possibility that in utero exposure to infection with the myxovirus *M. influenzae* might predispose to childhood cancer, especially childhood leukemia. The original data stem from a British cohort analysis [68] that indicated approximately a threefold increase in childhood cancer risk. Subsequent studies in England, Finland, and the United States produced conflicting results, and the question at present remains open [50, 69-72].

A possible association of reovirus infection (type 3) with BT in Africa was suggested on the basis of virus isolations and antibody studies [73-75]. At present, it is unclear whether these findings reflect an actual etiologic relationship or merely a passenger virus state.

A third RNA virus category involves the oncornaviruses. Although no such viruses have been identified specifically in man, there is morphologic and biomolecular evidence suggesting their presence, particularly in relation to leukemia, sarcoma, and breast cancer, but perhaps to other tumors as well [76]. Since 1958, when type-C particles like those seen in viral-induced murine leukemia were first described in human leukemic tissue [77], many reports have been published [1] on particle identification by electron microscopy of human tumors. However, there is little evidence in these studies for any human tumor virus; in some instances the particles seen may in fact have represented mycoplasma or normal intracellular structures [1]. None of several candidate type-C viruses isolated from human tumor material [78-81] has yet been conclusively shown to represent true human oncornavirus.

More recently, attention has focused on breast cancer with the observation in human milk and breast cancer tissue of type-B virus particles structurally similar to mouse mammary tumor virus (Bittner agent) [82]. Such particles may be more frequent in milk from women with a family history of breast cancer and from Parsi women in India, an ethnic group in which breast cancer may be unusually common. With support from enzyme and molecular hybridization experiments [83-85], evidence for a human type-B virus in the cause of breast cancer can at present be described as suggestive, although not conclusive. Epidemiologic evidence, however, makes it seem unlikely that such virus spreads from mother to child through milk [86, 87].

Viruses of Animal Origin

For most animal tumor viruses, no convincing evidence has yet been advanced that such viruses can cause tumors in man or increase the risk of human tumor development. Since several such viruses can under laboratory conditions produce tumors in various animal species, transmission to man remains a possibility that cannot be ruled out.

DNA Viruses

Of the many DNA viruses known to cause tumors in animals, only three require specific mention with respect to human oncogenesis: the simian papovavirus, SV40; the simian poxvirus, Yaba virus; and the avian herpesvirus, Marek's disease virus. Speculation that SV40 might be related to human tumors first arose when it was realized that this virus, known to be oncogenic in hamsters [88], had been in early batches of killed poliomyelitis vaccine by virtue of vaccine preparation in monkey kidney cell cultures. Follow-up studies of children receiving such vaccine have to date shown no evidence of increased cancer incidence [89, 90], although antibody response to SV40 was demonstrated in sera from at least some such children [91]. The question requires further study since one retrospective analysis suggested an increase in brain tumors among children of women receiving killed polio vaccine during gestation [92], whereas earlier observations from Australia suggested an increased risk of cancer in children immunized against poliomyelitis [93]. Also SV40 can induce transformation in human cell cultures [94].

Yaba virus, known to produce subcutaneous histiocytomas in monkeys, has been recorded as doing likewise in man and is a hazard for laboratory workers. Infection produces localized tumors after about a week's latency, with regression in 3 to 4 weeks [95, 96].

No evidence has been advanced that Marek's disease virus may infect humans, with or without clinical illness, despite widespread contact with poultry and poultry products. Serologic testing of 225 human sera, 25 from patients with BT, revealed no consistent patterns among sera reactive by immunofluorescence and no positive results by virus neutralization [97].

RNA Viruses

Knowledge that oncornaviruses cause leukemia and sarcoma in various animal species has led to considerable speculation that such viruses may, under certain conditions, cross species boundaries and infect man. To date little or no evidence, beyond anecdotal accounts of coexistent animal and human tumors [98-101], has emerged to suggest that such interspecies infection occurs under natural conditions with respect to any of the known animal tumor viruses.

Particular attention has been given to feline leukemia virus (FeLV) because of man's intimate and widespread contact with cats, because this virus can grow in human cell cultures [102], and because of evidence that the virus can pass horizontally from cat to cat [103, 104]. However, no consistent evidence of human infection has yet appeared [105]. Among sera from 626 veterinarians tested for anti-FeLV antibody, only one was positive; 8 months later, tests on a second serum specimen were negative [106]. Epidemiologically, no tendency has been found for human cancer to be more frequent in households containing tumorous animals or vice versa [107, 108]. One case-control study of human leukemia suggested an association for both adult and childhood leukemia with household presence of sick pets, particularly sick cats [109, 110]. Whether the animal illnesses involved were cancerous or not is unknown.

Similar negative data exist for murine, bovine, and avian oncornaviruses. Human serologic studies to identify murine viruses have been negative [111]. The same is true for bovine virus [112]. In addition, epidemiologic studies have shown that bovine and human cancers are not interrelated in their distribution by time and place [113, 114]. The possibility of viral spread from cow to man remains unresolved, however, particularly since virus-containing milk from a high leukemia-incidence herd may have induced a leukemia-like illness when fed to newborn chimpanzees [115].

Only faint evidence suggests human infection by avian leukemia and sarcoma viruses. Among several serologic studies done [116-122], only three instances of reactivity against such viruses were reported [119, 120]. Particular attention has been given to recipients of yellow fever vaccine, known to contain avian oncorna-virus by virtue of preparation in chick embryo. No association with vaccination was found among veterans of World War II dying of cancer when compared with surviving controls [120]. In addition, sera from yellow-fever vaccine recipients have been uniformly negative for antibody against avian leukemia-sarcoma viruses [121, 122].

Finally, with respect to avian and bovine oncornaviruses, cancer mortality studies directed at human populations with exceptionally frequent exposure to chickens and cattle have produced little if any evidence of unusual cancer experience. In a survey of veterinarians in Missouri and California, the observed numbers of cancer cases resembled those expected [123, 124]. Cancer mortality appeared decreased among farm residents in California, although a slight excess in leukemia mortality was detected [125], whereas among farmers in Oregon and Washington, mortality from leukemia and multiple myeloma, in contrast to other hematologic malignancies, was significantly increased [126]. In a study of cancer mortality in relation to poultry production among counties in the south-eastern United States, only cervical cancer showed an excess [127].

Vaccines and Viruses of Artificial Origin

There is growing concern that infectious agents, modified or produced under artificial laboratory conditions, may represent a potential oncogenic or muta-genic hazard [128]. For vaccines, no consistent evidence of increased cancer risk among vaccinated persons has yet been presented. The situations already men-tioned concerning SV40-contaminated poliomyelitis vaccine [89-93] and avian leukosis virus-contaminated yellow fever vaccine [120-122] reflect exposure both to artificially altered viral vaccine material and to naturally occurring animal viruses known to have oncogenic potential in animals.

The larger concern, however, lies with the newly developing laboratory capacity to hybridize viruses and to construct artificial viruses or virus-like nucleic acid sequences, the biologic effects of which may be quite unpredictable. Little information is yet available concerning the actual biologic performance of such materials. The potential risk, particularly for laboratory workers, is very real and may conceivably require restricted limits for viral-biomolecular experimentation in addition to stringent biohazard controls and close surveillance of potentially exposed groups [128]. No such actions have yet been taken.

OTHER MICROBES

In contrast to viruses, very little need be said concerning the relation of cancer to infection with bacteria or parasites. Despite the large number of organisms in these two microbial groups, only a handful of situations has been reported to alter cancer risk.

Bacteria

Four situations deserve mention, two of which may increase cancer risk, one may decrease risk, and one is unrelated. With regard to increased risk, indirect observations [129] have related intestinal bacterial flora to colon cancer and possibly to breast cancer [130], and urinary tract infection to gastric cancer [131]. In the first instance, the aerobic/anaerobic composition of colonic flora was found to correlate with colon cancer incidence in different parts of the world, suggesting the operation of chemical carcinogens produced by bacterial breakdown of dietary fats and bile steroids. A second study suggested that urinary tract and possibly gastrointestinal flora influence gastric cancer incidence by converting dietary nitrates to nitrosamine. In support of this idea, gastric cancer mortality rates were found to correlate with levels of nitrate in drinking water in Colombia, South America, and in Great Britain.

The second situation involving increased risk concerns cutaneous cancer in Africa. A substantial number of such tumors, particularly squamous cell carcinoma, arise in connection with tropical phagedenic ulcers [132, 133]. To the extent that such ulcers reflect chronic bacterial infection, tumors arising from them may be considered to result, indirectly at least, from bacterial causes.

Decreased risk of childhood leukemia after BCG vaccination was suggested by studies in Canada and Chicago [134, 135]. Efforts to confirm this finding, however, have been unsuccessful in Great Britain [136], Scandinavia [137], and the United States [138].

Finally, early work seeking to isolate infectious agents from malignant tissue succeeded on several occasions in demonstrating mycoplasma (PPLO) organisms. Subsequent work, however, showed that such agents are frequent contaminants of cell cultures, and it has been generally concluded that no oncogenic role is involved [1].

Parasites

Relationships between parasitic infection and cancer risk have been suggested for malaria, schistosomiasis, and infection by the oriental liver fluke, *Clonorchis sinensis*. The association of severe malarial infestation with risk of BT has already been discussed [28-31]. In this instance, the postulated mechanism is not one of direct oncogenicity but rather altered immunity within the host that may enhance viral oncogenicity.

The evidence is quite suggestive that heavy infestation by *Schistosoma haematobium* increases the risk of malignancy, although the data are not entirely consistent. Observations are primarily epidemiologic, mostly from Egypt and other parts of Africa. The first suggestion of a causal relationship was made in 1911 [139]. Several subsequent investigations revealed significant correlations, particularly in Egypt although not necessarily elsewhere in Africa, between frequency of schistosomiasis and bladder cancer incidence [140-142]. Various types of carcinoma are involved, most often squamous cell. Rather than direct parasitic oncogenicity, the mechanism of carcinogenesis seems likely to be one of chronic tissue irritation as a result of schistosomal cystitis, with possibly some related toxin production.

Primary carcinoma of the liver in oriental populations has been associated with infection by the oriental liver fluke through consumption of infested raw fish [143]. About 15 percent of all such tumors in Hong Kong has been attributed to this parasite. Conceivably, the tumor results from chronic tissue irritation or possibly toxin production by the organism. Tumors consist primarily of multifocal adenocarcinomas arising from epithelial cells lining secondary bile ducts.

UNKNOWN INFECTIOUS AGENTS

Beyond the framework of specific infectious agents, a variety of epidemiologic observations may bear on the relation of infection to cancer risk, but are not now associated with any particular agent. They include observations concerned with 1) evidence of epidemicity, such as time-space clustering, and seasonality; 2) interpersonal contact among cancer cases; and 3) the possible relationship of familial cancer to vertical viral transmission. Such work has generated intriguing epidemiologic ideas, but in no instance has it been more than suggestive.

Epidemicity

Little or no evidence exists for epidemicity in the occurrence of any form of cancer. Should such patterns exist, it is widely assumed that they would provide presumptive evidence of infectious etiology. Of course, all infectious diseases do not exhibit epidemicity [144]; therefore, the lack of such evidence need not disprove the hypothesis, especially when it is likely, as in cancer, that multiple causative factors operate simultaneously. Also, since malignant disease is generally associated with long latent periods between oncogenic event and diagnosis, it is unlikely that infection responsible for initiating cancer in the remote past will be reflected in discrete cancer epidemics. Such epidemics (using the term in the classic infectious disease sense and not as it has been applied to the modern "epidemic" of smoking-induced lung cancer or even of venereal disease) would better be interpreted, if they exist at all, as reflections of recent infection accelerating or triggering already existing malignant processes.

The question of cancer microepidemics or time-space clustering arose originally in connection with anecdotal reports of such clusters among cases of leukemia and lymphoma [145, 146]. Later reports appeared, most often concerned with leukemia [147-150] and some with BT, both in Africa [151] and the United States [152, 153], and others with multiple myeloma [154, 155] and HD [156]. Simultaneously, methodology for assessing degree of time-space clustering was developed [157-164], and numerous systematic studies employing these different methods were conducted [157-178] in relation to leukemia, BT, HD, and other lymphomas. No consistent evidence of significant time-space clustering has emerged, although several studies of acute childhood leukemia have suggested a weak tendency for cases to cluster [157-159, 163, 164, 167-169]. Initial analysis of BT data from the West Nile district of Uganda showed strong clustering across a wide range of time and space intervals [174, 175] and was widely cited as further evidence for the infectious etiology of this particular tumor. Subsequent investigations in the same region showed little if any clustering [176] and studies elsewhere in Africa were entirely negative [176, 179]. Analyses of HD and other lymphomas have been entirely negative [165, 177, 178].

Certain analyses of time-space clustering in childhood leukemia focused on time and place of birth as a test of the hypothesis that infection in utero might be responsible for initiating a considerable number of such cases and, hence, conceivably might be reflected in an epidemic pattern [180-182]. No indications of clustering were found.

Inconsistent and largely negative results have been recorded with respect to seasonality of cancer occurrence, another potential indicator of epidemicity. Again, data primarily concern hematologic malignancies: leukemias [147, 183-187], BT [188], HD [189, 190], and multiple myeloma [191], but with some data on other forms of cancer [185, 190]. Essentially negative data also resulted from studies of seasonality with respect to date of birth [192, 193].

Interpersonal Contact

Except for HD, little evidence suggests that contact with cancer patients increases the risk of cancer. Some anecdotal evidence has appeared concerning leukemia in husbands and wives [194-196] or among persons occupying the same house [197], but no supporting evidence has come from systematic analyses [198]. Firm evidence that contacts between man and domestic animals increase cancer risk has not been found [199, 200]. The occasional tendency for some forms of cancer to recur in families [201, 202] might conceivably reflect spread of infectious agents through interpersonal contact, although in most instances the influence of genetic factors seems equally, if not more, plausible.

Particular attention has been given to HD, because certain of its clinical and pathologic features are reminiscent of infectious disease and because anecdotal evidence suggests the disease may spread through interpersonal contact. In upstate New York, 34 cases of lymphoma (31 HD) linked by direct or indirect contact stemming from a single high school over a 20-year period were recorded [203, 204]. A similar episode was reported in the Los Angeles area [196]. It could not be determined from these data whether this amount of interpersonal linkage was in fact greater than might be expected in the population at large, but evidence suggesting this might be true subsequently came from a study of HD in two New York counties with respect to high-school attendance patterns [205]. Preliminary results of a comparable study in England, however, suggest no increase in linkages [206]. Possibly relevant are observations suggesting an increased frequency of HD in school teachers [207], although interpretation of these data has been questioned [208, 209].

Other epidemiologic clues to the infectious etiology of HD have come from studies of its incidence among physicians and studies of familial HD. Although the professional contact of physicians with HD patients indicates a potentially high-risk group, evidence to date is contradictory: in one study a slight but statistically significant increased risk was found [210], but in another no differences were seen [211]. In studies of familial HD, the suggestion has been raised, but not yet confirmed, that environmental causation is more likely than genetic causation, since dates of diagnosis among multiple cases within individual families correspond more closely than ages at onset [212, 213].

Familial Cancer

No evidence implicating viral infection as a cause of familial cancer has yet been developed (i.e., vertical viral transmission or spread from mother to child through milk as seen in animals). Conceivably, such viral transmission occurs and it could contribute to cancer causation in combination with genetic and immunologic factors. Present evidence is tenuous and entirely indirect. Although only two instances of leukemia developing in infants born to leukemic mothers have been recorded [214, 215], and early observations suggest no increased cancer incidence in offspring of childhood cancer survivors [216], numerous families have been studied in which several consecutive generations contain malignancy in direct line [217-225]. In several such families, immunologic and tissue culture studies have suggested immune and cellular abnormalities [222-225], which may reflect immunogenetic conditions under which viral oncogenesis is facilitated.

Other Considerations

Several other pieces of data are pertinent to the question of an infectious cause of cancer, although they do not deal with specific agents. There is no evidence for blood-borne transmission of an ubiquitous agent, since the incidence of childhood leukemia was not raised among children receiving exchange transfusions at birth [226]. A large case-control study suggested, however, that common viral infections during early childhood increase the risk of childhood leukemia in combination with other risk factors such as maternal irradiation and maternal history of reproductive wastage [227]. That childhood infections may predispose to childhood leukemia was also suggested indirectly by a study concerned with the age and birth order of leukemic children [228].

Finally, several studies examined the concept that tonsillectomy may increase the risk of HD and perhaps other cancers through removal of a functioning oropharyngeal immune barrier and, hence, facilitation of oncogenic infection. Results to date have been contradictory, some investigations suggesting that such a risk may exist [19, 229-231] and others not [20].

PROSPECTS

As the foregoing review suggests, there are many avenues that future investigations may take in exploring relationships between infection and cancer risk. Viruses, particularly EBV, HSV-2, and the various oncornaviruses, continue to hold the most promise for eventual identification of direct oncogenicity in man and thus the possibility of cancer prevention through viral manipulation or immunization. Firm evidence of causal relationships remains elusive, and it is unclear precisely how disease prevention will be achieved once proof is established.

In any case, it seems certain that future studies will increasingly require combinations of laboratory and epidemiologic observation and will, to a large extent, be shaped by progress of laboratory research and development of new laboratory techniques. With the exception, perhaps, of studies relating interpersonal contact patterns to cancer risk and continued descriptive epidemiologic work on the secular trends and geographic distributions of cancer, purely epidemiologic studies not involving laboratory observations seem less and less likely to be productive.

Laboratory/epidemiologic studies can take various forms. The most direct involve ad hoc or opportunistic studies: attempts to isolate infectious agents or to demonstrate particular immunologic or cellular responses in individual cases, especially from situations involving potentially high risk such as case clusters, human-animal aggregation, multiple-case families, or in association with chromosomal or immunologic conditions that predispose to cancer. Such studies should continue, using whatever laboratory tools seem currently most promising. Examples at present would include cell transformation studies using viral or subviral components to challenge cell cultures from particular members of multiple-case cancer families, and a search for antibody response to FeLV in persons exposed intimately to FeLV-shedding cats. In any situation where increased cancer risk is in serious question, it may be useful to obtain and store serum specimens in anticipation of possible future investigations, even if immediate use is not planned.

A more systematic and comprehensive investigation is possible by retrospective or prospective laboratory/epidemiologic surveys. They have usually been retrospective, comparing cancer patients and controls with respect to various antiviral antibody levels or other laboratory tests. In certain situations where association with particular infectious agents, such as EBV and HSV-2, seems especially strong, prospective or cohort-type studies are warranted. However, since such analyses entail much expense and time, they should be undertaken only when indications are strong.

With respect to specific infectious agents, areas most deserving of investigation at present include (in order of possible priority): 1) herpes viruses, especially EBV and HSV-2; 2) human candidate oncornaviruses, especially in relation to human breast cancer; 3) animal oncornaviruses, particularly FeLV; and 4) other agents such as HB_SAg. One common concern linking all such agent-specific studies, as well as more general investigations concerned with cancer and infection, should be for the immunologic and genetic state of the host. In particular, the potential relationship of malaria to BT deserves continued investigation, as do immunologic and genetic patterns in multiple-case cancer families.

One specific epidemiologic project, not yet undertaken, deserves comment. In view of increasing laboratory work with potential oncogenic and mutagenic agents, as well as increasing capacity to manipulate such agents and their molecular parts artificially, there is a growing possibility of hazard to laboratory workers. As a particular high-risk group, such workers and their families deserve surveillance to determine the future risk of cancer and birth defects. Through various mechanisms, this surveillance can be achieved without great effort. As a first step, a registry of exposed laboratory workers has been proposed [232], and should be established without delay.

REFERENCES

1. McAllister, R.M. Viruses in human carcinogenesis. *Prog. Med. Virol. 16:*48–85, 1973.

2. Rapp, E., and Buss, E.R. Are viruses important in carcinogenesis? *Am. J. Pathol. 77:*85–102, 1974.

3. Epstein, M.A., Achong, B.G., and Barr, Y.M. Virus particles in cultured lymphoblasts from Burkitt's lymphoma. *Lancet 1:*702–703, 1964.

4. Henle, G., Henle, W., Clifford, P., et al. Antibodies to EB virus in Burkitt's lymphoma and control groups. *J. Natl. Cancer Inst. 43:*1147–1157, 1969.

5. Levine, P.H., O'Conor, G.T., and Berard, C.W. Antibodies to Epstein-Barr virus (EBV) in American patients with Burkitt's lymphoma. *Cancer 30:*610–615, 1972.

6. Hirshaut, Y., Cohen, M.H., and Stevens, D.A. Epstein-Barr virus antibodies in American and African Burkitt's lymphoma. *Lancet 2:*114–116, 1973.

7. Pagano, J.S., Huang, C.H., and Levine, P. Absence of Epstein-Barr viral DNA in American Burkitt's lymphoma. *N. Engl. J. Med. 289:*1395–1399, 1973.

8. Johansson, B., Klein, G., Henle, W., et al. Epstein-Barr virus (EBV)–associated antibody patterns in malignant lymphoma and leukemia. I. Hodgkin's disease. *Int. J. Cancer 6:*450–462, 1970.

9. Levine, P.H., Ablashir, D.V., Berard, C.W., et al. Elevated antibody titers to Epstein-Barr virus in Hodgkin's disease. *Cancer 27:*416–421, 1971.

10. Henderson, B.E., Dworsky, R., Menck, H., et al. Case-control study of Hodgkin's disease. II. Herpesvirus group antibody titers and HL-A type. *J. Natl. Cancer Inst. 51:*1443–1447, 1973.

11. Langenhuysen, M.M.A.C., Cazemier, T., Houwen, E., et al. Antibodies to Epstein-Barr virus, cytomegalovirus, and Australia antigen in Hodgkin's disease. *Cancer 34:*262–267, 1974.

12. Levine, P.H., Merrill, D.A., Bethlenfalvay, N.C., et al. A longitudinal comparison of antibodies to Epstein-Barr virus and clinical parameters in chronic lymphocytic leukemia and chronic myelocytic leukemia. *Blood 38:*479–484, 1971.

13. Henle, W., Henle, G., Ho, H.C., et al. Antibodies to EB virus in nasopharyngeal cancer, other head and neck neoplasms and controls. *J. Natl. Cancer Inst. 44:*225–231, 1970.

14. de The, G., Ambrosini, J.C., Ho, H.C., et al. Lymphoblastoid transformation and presence of herpes type viral particles in a Chinese nasopharyngeal tumor cultured *in vitro. Nature (Lond.) 221:*770–771, 1969.

15. Wolf, H., Zur Hausen, H., and Becker, V. EB viral genomes in epithelial nasopharyngeal carcinoma cells. *Nature New Biol. 244:*245-247, 1973.

16. Henle, W., Diehl, V., Kohn, G., et al. Herpes type virus and chromosome markers in normal leukocytes after growth with irradiated Burkitt cells. *Science 157:*1064–1065, 1967.

17. Henle, G., Henle, W., and Diehl, V. Relation of Burkitt's tumor-associated herpes type virus to infectious mononucleosis. *Proc. Natl. Acad. Sci. 59:*94–101, 1968.

18. Fraumeni, J.F., Jr. Infectious mononucleosis and acute leukemia. *J.A.M.A. 215:* 1159, 1971.

19. Vianna, N.J., Greenwald, P., and Davies, J.N.P. Tonsillectomy and Hodgkin's disease. The lymphoid tissue barrier. *Lancet 1:*431–432, 1971.

20. Newell, G., Henderson, B., Rawlings, W., et al. Case control study of Hodgkin's disease. I. Results of the interview questionnaire. *J. Natl. Cancer Inst. 51:*1437–1441, 1973.

21. Miller, R.W., and Beebe, G.W. Infectious mononucleosis and the empirical risk of cancer. *J. Natl. Cancer Inst. 50:*315–321, 1973.

22. Connelly, R.R., and Christine, B.W. A cohort study of cancer following infectious mononucleosis. *Cancer Res. 34:*1172–1178, 1974.

23. Rosdahl, N., Larsen, S.O., and Clemmesen, J. Hodgkin's disease in patients with previous infectious mononucleosis: 30 years' experience. *Br. Med. J. 1:*253–256, 1974.

24. Schwartz, R.S. Immunoregulation, oncogenic viruses and malignant lymphomas. *Lancet 1:*1266–1269, 1972.

25. Miller, G., Shope, T., Heston, L., et al. Prospective study of Epstein-Barr virus infections in acute lymphoblastic leukemia of childhood. *J. Pediatr. 80:*932–937, 1972.

26. Gahrton, G., Wahren, B., Killander, D., et al. Epstein-Barr and other herpesvirus antibodies in children with acute leukemia. *Int. J. Cancer 8:*242–249, 1971.

27. Levine, P.H., Fraumeni, J.F., Jr., Reisher, J.I., et al. Antibodies to Epstein-Barr virus-associated antigens in relatives of cancer patients. *J. Natl. Cancer Inst. 52:*1037–1040, 1974.

28. O'Conor, G.T. Persistent immunologic stimulation as a factor in oncogenesis, with special reference to Burkitt's tumor. *Am. J. Med. 48:*279–285, 1970.

29. Feorino, P.M., and Mathews, H.M. Malaria antibody levels in patients with Burkitt's lymphoma. *Am. J. Trop. Med. Hyg. 23:*574–576, 1974.

30. Pike, M.C., Morrow, R.H., Kisuule, A., et al. Burkitt's lymphoma and sickle cell trait. *Br. J. Prev. Soc. Med. 24:*39–41, 1970.

31. Williams, A.O. Haemoglobin genotypes, ABO blood groups, and Burkitt's tumour. *J. Med. Genet. 3:*177, 1966.

32. Kafuko, G.W., Henderson, B.E., Kirya, B.G., et al. Epstein-Barr virus antibody levels in children from the West Nile district of Uganda. *Lancet 1:*706–709, 1972.

33. Dowdle, W., Nahmias, A., Harwell, R., et al. Association of antigenic types of *Herpesvirus hominis* to site of viral recovery. *J. Immunol. 99:*974–980, 1967.

34. Kessler I.I. Perspectives on the epidemiology of cervical cancer with special reference to the herpesvirus hypothesis. *Cancer Res. 34:*1091–1110, 1974.

35. Aurelian, L., Royston, I., and Davis, H.J. Antibody to genital herpes simplex virus: association with cervical atypia and carcinoma *in situ. J. Natl. Cancer Inst. 45:*455–464, 1970.

36. Catalano, L.W., Jr., and Johnson, L.D. Herpesvirus antibody and carcinoma *in situ* of the cervix. *J.A.M.A. 217:*447–450, 1971.

37. Nahmias, A.J., Josey, W.E., Naib, Z.M., et al. Antibodies to *Herpesvirus hominis* types 1 and 2 in humans. II. Women with cervical cancer. *Am. J. Epidemiol. 91:*547–552, 1970.

38. Nahmias, A.J., Naib, Z.M., Josey, W.E., et al. Prospective studies of the association of genital herpes simplex infection and cervical anaplasia. *Cancer Res. 33:*1491–1497, 1973.

39. Aurelian, L., Standberg, J.D., Melendez, L.V., et al. Herpesvirus type 2 isolated from cervical tumor cells grown in tissue culture. *Science 174:*704–707, 1971.

40. Duff, R., and Rapp, F. Oncogenic transformation of hamster cells after exposure to herpes simplex virus type 2. *Nature New Biol. 223:*48-50, 1971.

41. Hollinshead, A.C., and Tarro, G. Soluble membrane antigens of lip and cervical carcinomas: reactivity with antibody for herpesvirus nonvirion antigens. *Science 179:*698–700, 1973.

42. Hollinshead, A.C., Lee, O., Chretien, P.B., et al. Antibodies to herpesvirus nonvirion antigens in squamous carcinomas. *Science 182:*713–715, 1973.

43. Sabin, A.B. Herpes simplex-genitalis virus nonvirion antigens and their implication in certain human cancers: unconfirmed. *Proc. Natl. Acad. Sci. 71:*3248–3252, 1974.

44. Dean, A.G., Williams, E.H., Attobua, G., et al. Clinical events suggesting herpes-simplex infection before onset of Burkitt's lymphoma. *Lancet 2:*1225–1228, 1973.

45. Henle, G., and Henle, W. Studies on cell lines derived from Burkitt's lymphoma. *Trans. N.Y. Acad. Sci. 29:*71–79, 1966.

46. Catalano, L.W., Jr., and Goldman, J.M. Antibody to *Herpesvirus hominis* types 1 and 2 in patients with Hodgkin's disease and carcinoma of the nasopharynx. *Cancer 29:*597-602, 1972.

47. Feorino, P., Palmer, E.L., and Martin, M.L. Incidence of herpesvirus antibody among leukemic and nasopharyngeal carcinoma patients. *Proc. Soc. Exp. Biol. Med. 139:*913-915, 1972.

48. Palmer, E.L., Feorino, P.M., and Martin, M.L. Increased antibody to herpes simplex virus in patients with nasopharyngeal cancer. *J. Infect. Dis. 126:*186-188, 1972.

49. Adelstein, A.M., and Donovan, J.W. Malignant disease in children whose mothers had chickenpox, mumps, or rubella in pregnancy. *Br. Med. J. 2:*629-631, 1972.

50. Bithell, J.F., Draper, G.J., and Gorbach, P.D. Association between malignant disease in children and maternal virus infections. *Br. Med. J. 1:*706-708, 1973.

51. Stewart, S.E., Mitchell, E.Z., Whang, J.J., et al. Viruses in human tumors. I. Hodgkin's disease. *J. Natl. Cancer Inst. 43:*1-14, 1969.

52. Eisinger, M., Fox, S.M., de Harven, E., et al. Virus-like agents from patients with Hodgkin's disease. *Nature (Lond.) 233:*104-108, 1971.

53. Centifanto, Y.M., Kaufman, H.E., Zam, S., et al. Herpesvirus particles in carcinoma of the prostate. *J. Virol. 12:*1608-1611, 1974.

54. Gilden, R.V., Kern, J., Lee, Y.K., et al. Serologic surveys of human cancer patients for antibody to adenovirus T antigens. *Am. J. Epidemiol. 91:*500-509, 1970.

55. McAllister, R.M., Gilden, R.V., and Green, M. Adenoviruses in human cancer. *Lancet 1:*831-833, 1972.

56. Rowson, K.E.K., and Mahy, B.W.J. Human papova (wart) virus. *Bacteriol. Rev. 31:* 110-131, 1967.

57. Bastian, F.O. Papova-like virus particles in a human brain tumor. *Lab. Invest. 25:*169-175, 1971.

58. Takemoto, K.K., Rabson, A.S., Mullarkey, M.F., et al. Isolation of papovavirus from brain tumor and urine of a patient with Wiskott-Aldrich syndrome. *J. Natl. Cancer Inst. 53:*1205-1207, 1974.

59. Walker, D.L., Padgett, B.L., and ZuRhein, G.M. Human papovavirus (JC): Induction of brain tumors in hamsters. *Science 181:*674-676, 1973.

60. Blumberg, B.S., Gerstley, B.J.S., Hungerford, D.A., et al. A serum antigen (Australia antigen) in Down's syndrome, leukemia and hepatitis. *Ann. Intern. Med. 66:*924-930, 1967.

61. Sutnick, A.I., Levine, P.H., London, W.T., et al. Frequency of Australia antigen in patients with leukaemia in different countries. *Lancet 1:*1200-1202, 1971.

62. Vogel, C.L., Anthony, P.P., Mody, N., et al. Hepatitis-associated antigen in Ugandan patients with hepatocellular carcinoma. *Lancet 2:*621-624, 1970.

63. Vogel, C.L., Anthony, P.P., Sadikali, F., et al. Hepatitis-associated antigen and antibody in hepatocellular carcinoma: results of a continuing study. *J. Natl. Cancer Inst. 48:*1583-1588, 1972.

64. Prince, A.M. The high voltage immunoelectroosmophoretic (IEOP) technique for detection of SH antigen: application to blood donor screening and to study of liver disease. *Vox Sang. 19:*205-210, 1970.

65. Sherlock, S., Fox, R.A., Niazi, S.P., et al. Chronic liver disease and primary liver cell cancer with hepatitis-associated (Australia) antigen in serum. *Lancet 1:*1243-1247, 1970.

66. Smith, I.B., and Blumberg, B.S. Letter to editor. *Lancet 2:*953, 1969.

67. Simons, M.J., Yap, E.H., Yu, M., et al. Australia antigen in Singapore Chinese patients with hepatocellular carcinoma. *Lancet 1:*1149-1151, 1971.

68. Fedrick, J., and Alberman, E.D. Reported influenza in pregnancy and subsequent cancer in the child. *Br. Med. J. 1:*485–488, 1972.

69. Leck, I.,and Steward, J.K. Incidence of neoplasms in children born after influenza epidemics. *Br. Med. J. 2:*631–634, 1972.

70. Hakulinen, T., Hovi, L., Karkinen-Jaaskelainen, M., et al. Association between influenza during pregnancy and childhood leukaemia. *Br. Med. J. 2:*265–267, 1973.

71. Randolph, V.L., and Heath, C.W., Jr. Influenza during pregnancy in relation to subsequent childhood leukemia and lymphoma. *Am. J. Epidemiol. 100:*399–409, 1974.

72. Curnen, M.G.M., Varma, A.A.O., Christine, B.W., et al. Childhood leukemia and maternal infectious diseases during pregnancy. *J. Natl. Cancer Inst. 53:*943–947, 1974.

73. Bell, T.M., Massie, A., Ross, M.G.R., et al. Isolation of a reovirus from a case of Burkitt's lymphoma. *Br. Med. J. 1:*1212–1213, 1964.

74. Bell, T.M., Massie, A., Ross, M.G.R., et al. Further isolations of reovirus type 3 from cases of Burkitt's lymphoma. *Br. Med. J. 1:*1514–1517, 1966.

75. Levy, J.A., Tanabe, E., and Curnen, E.C. Occurrence of reovirus antibodies in healthy African children and in children with Burkitt's lymphoma. *Cancer 21:*53–57, 1968.

76. Cuatico, W., Cho, J.R., and Spiegelman, S. Evidence of particle-associated RNA–directed DNA polymerase and high molecular weight RNA in human gastrointestinal and lung malignancies. *Proc. Natl. Acad. Sci. 71:*3304–3308, 1974.

77. Dmochowski, L., Grey, C.E., Sykes, J.A., et al. Studies in human leukemia. *Proc. Soc. Exp. Biol. Med. 101:*686–690, 1959.

78. Morton, D.L., Hall, W.T., and Malgrem, R.A. Human liposarcomas: tissue cultures containing foci of transformed cells with virus particles. *Science 165:*813–815, 1969.

79. Priori, E.S., Dmochowski, L., Myers, B., et al. Constant production of type C virus particles in a continuous tissue culture derived from pleural effusion cells of a lymphoma patient. *Nature New Biol. 232:*61-62, 1971.

80. Stewart, S.E., Kasnic, G., Jr., Draycott, C., et al. Activation *in vitro* by 5-iododeoxyuridine, of a latent virus resembling C-type virus in a human sarcoma line. *J. Natl. Cancer Inst. 48:*273–277, 1972.

81. McAllister, R.M., Nicolson, M., Gardner, M.B., et al. C-type virus released from cultured human rhabdomyosarcoma cells. *Nature New Biol. 235:*3-6, 1972.

82. Moore, D.H., Charney, J., Kramarsky, B., et al. Search for a human breast cancer virus. *Nature (Lond.) 229:*611–614, 1971.

83. Schlom, J., Spiegelman, S., and Moore, D. RNA-dependent DNA polymerase activity in virus-like particles isolated from human milk. *Nature (Lond.) 231:*97–100, 1971.

84. Moore, D.H. Evidence in favor of the existence of human breast cancer virus. *Cancer Res. 34:*2322–2329, 1974.

85. Axel, R., Schlom, J., and Spiegelman, S. Presence in human breast cancer of RNA homologous to mouse mammary tumour virus RNA. *Nature (Lond.) 235:*32–36, 1972.

86. Fraumeni, J.F., Jr., and Miller, R.W. Letter to editor. *Lancet 2:*1196–1197, 1971.

87. Henderson, B.E., Powell, D., Rosario, I., et al. An epidemiologic study of breast cancer. *J. Natl. Cancer Inst. 53:*609–614, 1974.

88. Eddy, B.E., Borman, G.S., Berkeley, W.H., et al. Tumors induced in hamsters by injection of rhesus monkey kidney cell extracts. *Proc. Soc. Exp. Biol. Med. 107:*191–197, 1961.

89. Fraumeni, J.F., Jr., Ederer, F., and Miller, R.W. An evaluation of the carcinogenicity of simian virus 40 in man. *J.A.M.A. 185:*713–718, 1963.

90. Fraumeni, J.F., Jr., Stark, C.R., Gold, E., et al. Simian virus 40 in polio vaccine: follow-up of newborn recipients. *Science 167:*59–60, 1970.

91. Gerber, P. Patterns of antibodies to SV40 in children following the last booster with inactivated poliomyelitis vaccines. *Proc. Soc. Exp. Biol. Med. 125:*1284–1287, 1967.

92. Heinonen, O.P., Shapiro, S., Monson, R.R., et al. Immunization during pregnancy against poliomyelitis and influenza in relation to childhood malignancy. *Int. J. Epidemiol. 2:*229–235, 1973.

93. Innis, M.D. Oncogenesis and poliomyelitis vaccine. *Nature (Lond.) 219:*972–973, 1968.

94. Todaro, G.J., Green, H., and Swift, M.R. Susceptibility of human diploid fibroblast strains to transformation by SV40 virus. *Science 153:*1252–1254, 1966.

95. Grace, J.T., Jr., Mirand, E.A., Millian, S.J., et al. Experimental studies of human tumors. *Fed. Proc. 21:*32–36, 1962.

96. Griesemer, R.A., and Manning, J.S. Simian tumor viruses. *In* Hellman, A., Oxman, M.N., and Pollack, R., eds. *Biohazards in Biological Research.* Cold Spring Harbor Laboratory, New York, 1973, pp. 179–190.

97. Sharma, J.M., Witter, R.L., Burmester, B.R., et al. Public health implications of Marek's disease virus and herpesvirus of turkeys. Studies on human and subhuman primates. *J. Natl. Cancer Inst. 51:*1123–1128, 1973.

98. Drusin, L.M., Finkbeiner, J.A., McCoy, J.R., et al. Malignant lymphoma occurring in patient and pet. *J.A.M.A. 196:*99–101, 1966.

99. Viola, M.V. Hematological malignancies in patients and their pets. *J.A.M.A. 205:*567–568, 1968.

100. Van Hoosier, G.L., Jr., Stenback, W.A., Mumford, D.M., et al. Epidemiological findings and electron microscopic observations in human leukemia and canine contacts. *Int. J. Cancer 3:*7–16, 1968.

101. Heath, C.W., Jr. Human leukaemia: genetic and environmental clusters. *Bibl. Haematol. 36:*649–653, 1970.

102. Jarrett, O., Laird, H.M., and Hay, D. Growth of feline leukaemia virus in human cells. *Nature (Lond.) 224:* 1208–1209, 1969.

103. Hardy, W.D., Jr., Old, L.J., Hess, P.W., et al. Horizontal transmission of feline leukaemia virus. *Nature (Lond.) 244:*266–269, 1973.

104. Jarrett, W., Jarrett, O., Mackey, L., et al. Horizontal transmission of leukemia virus and leukemia in the cat. *J. Natl. Cancer Inst. 51:*833–841, 1973.

105. Gardner, M.R. Current information on feline and canine cancers and relationship or lack of relationship to human cancer. *J. Natl. Cancer Inst. 46:*281–290, 1971.

106. Schneider, R., and Riggs, J.L. A serologic survey of veterinarians for antibody to feline leukemia virus. *J.A.V.M.A. 162:*217–219, 1973.

107. Schneider, R. Human cancer in households containing cats with malignant lymphoma. *Int. J. Cancer 10:*338–344, 1972.

108. Hanes, G., Gardner, M.B., Loosli, C.G., et al. Pet association with selected human cancers: a household questionnaire survey. *J. Natl. Cancer Inst. 45:*1155–1162, 1970.

109. Bross, I.D.J., and Gibson, R. Cats and childhood leukemia. *J. Med. 1:*180–187, 1970.

110. Bross, I.D.J., Bertell, R., and Gibson, R. Pets and adult leukemia. *Am. J. Public Health 62:*1520–1531, 1972.

111. Charman, H.P., Kim, N., White, M., et al. Failure to detect, in human sera, antibodies cross-reactive with group-specific antigens of murine leukemia virus. *J. Natl. Cancer Inst. 52:*1409–1413, 1974.

112. Olson, C. Bovine lymphosarcoma (leukemia)—a synopsis. *J.A.V.M.A. 165:*630–632, 1974.

113. Khokhlova, M.P., and Rakhmanin, P.P. Comparative study on geographical distribution of human and cattle leukosis. *Bibl. Haematol. 36:*654–658, 1970.

114. Priester, W.A., Oleinick, A., and Conner, G.H. Letter to editor. *Lancet 1:*367–368, 1970.

115. McClure, H.M., Keeling, M.E., Custer, R.P., et al. Erythroleukemia in two infant chimpanzees fed milk from cows naturally infected with the bovine C-type virus. *Cancer Res. 34:*2745–2757, 1974.

116. Solomon, J.J., Purchase, H.G., and Burmester, B.R. A search for avian leukosis virus and antiviral activity in the blood of leukemic and nonleukemic adults and children. *J. Natl. Cancer Inst. 42:*29–33, 1969.

117. Roth, F.K., and Dougherty, R.M. Search for group-specific antibodies of avian leukosis virus in human leukemic sera. *J. Natl. Cancer Inst. 46:*1357–1360, 1971.

118. Morgan, H.R. Antibodies for Rous sarcoma virus (Bryan) in fowl, animal, and human populations of East Africa. II. Antibodies in domestic chickens, wildfowl, primates, and man in Kenya, and antibodies for Burkitt lymphoma cells in man. *J. Natl. Cancer Inst. 39:*1229–1234, 1967.

119. Cohen, S., Weiner, L.M., Baechler, C.A., et al. Immunologic cross-reaction between human leukemic plasma and avian leukosis group-specific antiserum. *Proc. Soc. Exp. Biol. Med. 135:*800–803, 1970.

120. Waters, T.D., Anderson, P.S., Jr., Beebe, G.W., et al. Yellow fever vaccination, avian leukosis virus, and cancer risk in man. *Science 177:*76–77, 1972.

121. Harris, R.J.C., Dougherty, R.M., Biggs, P.M., et al. Contaminant viruses in two live virus vaccines produced in chick cells. *J. Hyg. 64:*1–7, 1966.

122. Piraino, F., Krumbiegel, E.R., and Wisniewski, H.J. Serologic survey of man for avian leukosis virus infection. *J. Immunol. 98:*702–706, 1967.

123. Botts, R.P., Edlavitch, S., and Payne, G. Mortality of Missouri veterinarians. *J.A.V.M.A. 149:*499–504, 1966.

124. Fasel, E., Jackson, E.W., and Klauber, M.R. Mortality in California veterinarians. *J. Chronic Dis. 19:*293–306, 1966.

125. Fasel, E., Jackson, E.W., and Klauber, M.R. Leukemia and lymphoma mortality and farm residence. *Am. J. Epidemiol. 87:*267–274, 1967.

126. Milham,S.,Jr. Leukemia and multiple myeloma in farmers. *Am. J. Epidemiol. 94:* 307–310, 1971.

127. Priester, W.A., and Mason, T.J. Human cancer mortality in relation to poultry population, by county in 10 southeastern states. *J. Natl. Cancer Inst. 53:*45–49, 1974.

128. Berg, P., Baltimore, D., Boyer, H.W., et al. Letter to editor. *Science 185:*303, 1974.

129. Hill, M.J., Crowther, J.S., Drasar, B.S., et al. Bacteria and aetiology of cancer of large bowel. *Lancet 1:*95–100, 1971.

130. Hill, M.J., Goddard, P., and Williams, R.E.Q. Gut bacteria and aetiology of cancer of the breast. *Lancet 2:*472–473, 1971.

131. Hill, M.J., Hawksworth, G., and Tattersall, G. Bacteria, nitrosamines and cancer of the stomach. *Br. J. Cancer 28:*562–567, 1973.

132. Davies, J.N.P., Tauk, R., Meyer, R., et al. Cancer of the integumentary tissues in Uganda Africans: the basis for prevention. *J. Natl. Cancer Inst. 41:*31–51, 1968.

133. Camain, R., Tuyns, A.J., Sarrat, H., et al. Cutaneous cancer in Dakar. *J. Natl. Cancer Inst. 48:*33–49, 1972.

134. Davignon, L., Lemonde, P., Robillard, P., et al. BCG vaccination and leukaemia mortality. *Lancet 2:*638, 1970.

135. Rosenthal, S.R., Crispen, R.G., Thorne, M.G., et al. BCG vaccination and leukemia mortality. *J.A.M.A. 222:*1543–1544, 1972.

136. Kinlen, L.J., and Pike, M.C. BCG vaccination and leukaemia. *Lancet 2:*398–402, 1971.

137. Waaler, H.T. Letter to editor. *Lancet 2:*1314, 1970.

138. Comstock, G.W., Livesay, V.T., and Webster, R.G. Leukaemia and BCG. *Lancet 2:*1062-1063, 1971.

139. Ferguson, A.R. Associated bilharziasis and primary malignant disease of the urinary bladder, with observations on a series of forty cases. *J. Pathol. Bacteriol. 16:* 76-94, 1911.

140. Dimmette, R.M., Sproat, H.F., and Klimt, C.R. Examination of smears of urinary sediment for detection of neoplasms of bladder. *Am. J. Clin. Pathol. 25:*1032-1042, 1955.

141. Mustacchi, P., and Shimkin, M.B. Cancer of the bladder and infestation with *Schistosoma hematobium. J. Natl. Cancer Inst. 20:*825-842, 1958.

142. Gelfand, M., Weinberg, R.W., and Castle, W.M. Relation between carcinoma of the bladder and infestation with *Schistosoma haematobium. Lancet 1:*1249-1251, 1967.

143. Hou, P.C. The relationship between primary carcinoma of the liver and infestation with *Clonorchis sinensis. J. Pathol. Bacteriol. 72:*239-246, 1956.

144. Nye. F.J., and Spicer, C.C. Space-time clustering in infectious mononucleosis. *Br. J. Prev. Soc. Med. 26:257-258, 1972.*

145. Wood, E.E. A survey of leukaemia in Cornwall 1948-1959. *Br. Med. J. 1:* 1760-1764, 1960.

146. Heath, C.W., Jr., and Hasterlik, R.J. Leukemia among children in a suburban community. *Am. J. Med. 34:*796-812, 1963.

147. Kessler, I., and Lilienfeld, A.M. Perspectives in the epidemiology of leukemia. *Adv. Cancer Res. 12:*225-302, 1969.

148. Heath, C.W., Jr., Manning, M.D., and Zelkowitz, L. Case clusters in the occurrence of leukaemia and congenital malformations. *Lancet 2:*136-137, 1964.

149. Flynt, J.W., Doto, I.L., McCullough, R.J., et al. Epidemiologic studies of childhood leukemia in Green Bay, Wisconsin. *J. Natl. Cancer Inst. 44:*489-495, 1970.

150. Powell, D.E.B. Incidence and distribution of acute leukaemia in one district general hospital area. *Lancet 2:*350-352, 1971.

151. Morrow, R.H., Pike, M.C., Smith, P.C., et al. Burkitt's lymphoma: a time-space cluster of cases in Bwamba county of Uganda. *Br. Med. J. 1:*491-492, 1971.

152. Levine, P.H., Sandler, S.G., Kemp, D.M., et al. Simultaneous occurrence of "American Burkitt's lymphoma" in neighbors. *N. Engl. J. Med. 288:*562-563, 1973.

153. Brown, T.M., Jr., and Heath, C.W., Jr. Time-space clustering among cases of Burkitt's tumor. *Cancer Res. 34:*1216-1218, 1974.

154. Kyle, R.A., Herber, L., Evatt, B.L., et al. Multiple myeloma, a community cluster. *J.A.M.A. 213:*1339-1341, 1970.

155. Kyle, R.A., Finkelstein, S., Elveback, L.R., et al. Incidence of monoclonal proteins in a Minnesota community with a cluster of multiple myeloma. *Blood 40:*719-724, 1972.

156. Klinger, R.J., and Minton, J.P. Case clustering of Hodgkin's disease in a small rural community with associations among cases. *Lancet 1:*168-170, 1973.

157. Pinkel, D., and Nefzger, D. Some epidemiologic features of childhood leukemia in the Buffalo, New York, area. *Cancer 12:*351-358, 1959.

158. Pinkel, D., Dowd, J.E., and Bross, I.D.J. Some epidemiologic features of malignant solid tumors of children in the Buffalo, New York, area. *Cancer 16:*28-33, 1963.

159. Knox, G. Epidemiology of childhood leukaemia in Northumberland and Durham. *Br. J. Prev. Soc. Med. 18:*17-24, 1964.

160. Ederer, F., Myers, M.H., and Mantel, N. A statistical problem in space and time: do leukemia cases come in clusters? *Biometrics 20:*626-638, 1964.

161. David, F.N., and Barton, D.E. Two space-time interaction tests for epidemicity. *Br. J. Prev. Soc. Med. 20:*44-48, 1966.

162. Mantel, N. The detection of disease clustering and a generalized regression approach. *Cancer Res. 27:*209-220, 1967.

163. Evatt, B.L., Chase, G.A., and Heath, C.W., Jr. Time-space clustering among cases of acute leukemia in two Georgia counties. *Blood 41:*265-272, 1973.

164. Larsen, R.J., Holmes, C.L., and Heath, C.W., Jr. A statistical test for measuring unimodal clustering: a description of the test and of its application to cases of acute leukemia in metropolitan Atlanta, Georgia. *Biometrics 29:*301-309, 1973.

165. Ederer, F., Myers, M.H., Eisenberg, H., and Heath, C.W., Jr. Temporal-spatial distribution of leukemia and lymphoma in Connecticut. *J. Natl. Cancer Inst. 35:*625-629, 1965.

166. Lock, S.P., and Merrington, M. Leukaemia in Lewisham (1957-1963). *Br. Med. J. 3:*759-760, 1967.

167. Till, M.M., Hardesty, R.M., Pike, M.C., et al. Childhood leukaemia in greater London: a search for evidence of clustering. *Br. Med. J. 3:*755-758, 1967.

168. Gunz, F.W., and Spears, G.F.S. Distribution of acute leukaemia in time and space. Studies in New Zealand. *Br. Med. J. 4:*604-608, 1968.

169. Glass, A.G., Mantel, N., Gunz, F.W., et al. Time-space clustering of childhood leukemia in New Zealand. *J. Natl. Cancer Inst. 47:*329-336, 1971.

170. Glass, A.G., and Mantel, N. Lack of time-space clustering of childhood leukemia in Los Angeles county 1960-1964. *Cancer Res. 29:*1995-2001, 1969.

171. Merrington, M., and Spicer, C.C. Acute leukaemia in New England, an investigation into the clustering of cases in time and place. *Br. J. Prev. Soc. Med. 23:*124-127, 1969.

172. Browning, D., and Gross, J. Epidemiological studies of acute childhood leukemia. *Am. J. Dis. Child. 116:*576-585, 1968.

173. Klauber, M.R., and Mustacchi, P. Space-time clustering of childhood leukemia in San Francisco. *Cancer Res. 30:*1969-1973, 1970.

174. Pike, M.C., Williams, E.H., and Wright, B. Burkitt's tumour in the West Nile District of Uganda. 1961-5. *Br. Med. J. 2:*395-399, 1967.

175. Williams, E.H., Spit, P., and Pike, M.C. Further evidence of space-time clustering of Burkitt's lymphoma patients in the West Nile District of Uganda. *Br. J. Cancer 23:*235-246, 1969.

176. Morrow, R.H. Burkitt's lymphoma in Africa. *Cancer Res. 34:*1211-1215, 1974.

177. Alderson, M.R., and Nayak, R. A study of space-time clustering in Hodgkin's disease in the Manchester region. *Br. J. Prev. Soc. Med. 25:*168-173, 1971.

178. Kryscio, R.J., Myers, M.H., Prusiner, S.T., et al. A study of the time-space distribution of Hodgkin's disease in Connecticut 1940-69. *J. Natl. Cancer Inst. 50:*1107-1110, 1973.

179. Brubaker, G., Geser, A., and Pike, M.C. Burkitt's lymphoma in the north Mara district of Tanzania, 1964-70: failure to find evidence of time-space clustering in a high-risk isolated rural area. *Br. J. Cancer 28:*469-472, 1973.

180. Fraumeni, J.F., Jr., Ederer, F., and Handy, V.H. Temporal-spatial distribution of childhood leukemia in New York State. *Cancer 19:*995-1000, 1966.

181. Stark, C.R., and Mantel, N. Temporal-spatial distribution of birth dates for Michigan children with leukemia. *Cancer Res. 27:*1749-1775, 1967.

182. Klauber, M.R. A study of clustering of childhood leukemia by hospital of birth. *Cancer Res. 28:*1790-1792, 1968.

183. Hayes, D.M. The seasonal incidence of acute leukemia. *Cancer 14:*1301-1305, 1961.

184. Lee, J.A.H. Seasonal variation in the clinical onset of leukaemia in young people. *Br. Med. J. 1:*1737-1738, 1962.

185. Lee, J.A.H., and Gardner, M.J. Season and malignant disease. *In* Hayhoe, E.G.J., ed. *Current Research in Leukaemia*. London, Cambridge, 1965, pp. 266-273.

186. Fraumeni, J.F., Jr. Letter to editor. *Br. Med. J. 2:*1408-1409, 1963.

187. Fekety, F.R., Jr., and Carey, J.J.H. Season and the onset of acute childhood leukemia. *Md. State Med. J. 18:*73-77, 1969.

188. Williams, E.H., Day, N.E., and Geser, A.G.: Seasonal variation in onset of Burkitt's lymphoma in the West Nile district of Uganda. *Lancet 2:*19-22, 1974.

189. Cridland, M.D. Seasonal incidence of clinical onset of Hodgkin's disease. *Br. Med. J. 2:*621-623, 1961.

190. Newell, G.R. Letter to editor. *Lancet 1:*1024-1025, 1974.

191. McPhedran, P., Heath, C.W., Jr., and Garcia, J. Multiple myeloma incidence in metropolitan Atlanta, Georgia: Racial and seasonal variations. *Blood 39:*866-873, 1972.

192. Bailar, J.C., III, and Gurian, J.M. Month of birth and cancer mortality. *J. Natl. Cancer Inst. 33:*237-242, 1964.

193. Ederer, F., Miller, R.W., Scotto, J., et al. Letter to editor. *Lancet 2:*185-186, 1965.

194. Street, W.W., and Allen, E.G. Leukemia occurring in man and wife. *N.Y. State J. Med. 50:*1621-1622, 1950.

195. Amos, D.A., Wellman, W.E. Bowie, E.J.W., et al. Acute leukemia in a husband and wife. *Mayo Clin. Proc. 42:*468-472, 1967.

196. Dworsky, R.L., and Henderson, B.E. Hodgkin's disease clustering in families and communities. *Cancer Res. 34:*1161-1163, 1974.

197. McPhedran, P., and Heath, C.W., Jr. Multiple cases of leukemia associated with one house. *J.A.M.A. 209:*2021-2025, 1969.

198. Milham, S., Jr. Leukemia in husbands and wives. *Science 148:*98-100, 1964.

199. Schneider, P., Dorn, C.R., and Klauber, M.R. Cancer in households: a human-canine retrospective study. *J. Natl. Cancer Inst. 41:*1285-1292, 1968.

200. Norris, F.D., Jackson, E.W., and Aaron, E. Prospective study of dog bite and childhood cancer. *Cancer Res. 31:*383-386, 1971.

201. Lilienfeld, A.M. Formal discussion—Genetic factors in the etiology of cancer: an epidemiologic view. *Cancer Res. 25:*1330-1335, 1965.

202. Fraumeni, J.F., Jr. Genetic factors. *In* Holland, J.F., Frei, E. eds., *Cancer Medicine*. Lea and Febiger, Philadelphia, 1973, pp. 7-15.

203. Vianna, N.J., Greenwald, P., and Davies, J.N.P. Extended epidemic of Hodgkin's disease in high-school students. *Lancet 1:*1209-1211, 1971.

204. Vianna, N.J., Greenwald, P., Grady, J., et al. Hodgkin's disease: cases with features of community outbreak. *Ann. Intern. Med. 77:*169-180, 1972.

205. Vianna, N.J., and Polan, A.K. Epidemiologic evidence for transmission of Hodgkin's disease. *N. Engl. J. Med. 289:*499-502, 1973.

206. Smith, P.G., and Pike, M.C. Case clustering in Hodgkin's disease: a brief review of the present position and report of current work in Oxford. *Cancer Res. 34:*1156-1160, 1974.

207. Milham, S., Jr. Letter to editor. *N. Engl. J. Med. 290:*1329, 1974.

208. Bahn, A.K. Letter to editor. *N. Engl. J. Med. 291:*207, 1974.

209. Hoover, R. Letter to editor. *N. Engl. J. Med. 291:*473, 1974.

210. Vianna, N.J., Polan, A.K., Keogh, M.D., et al. Hodgkin's disease mortality among physicians. *Lancet 2:*131-133, 1974.

211. Smith, P.J., Kinlen, L.J., and Doll, R. Letter to editor. *Lancet 2:*525, 1974.

212. MacMahon, B. Epidemiology of Hodgkin's disease. *Cancer Res. 26:*1189-1200, 1966.

213. Vianna, N.J., Davies, J.N.P., Polan, A.K., et al. Familial Hodgkin's disease: an environmental and genetic disorder. *Lancet 2:*854-857, 1974.

214.   Cramblett, H.G., Friedman, J.L., and Najjar, S. Leukemia in an infant born of a mother with leukemia. N. Engl. J. Med. 259:727-729, 1958.

215.   Bernard, J., Jacquillat, C., Chavelet, F., et al. Leucémie aiguë d'une enfant de 5 mois née d'une mère atteinte de leucémie aiguë au moment de l'accouchement. Nouv. Rev. Fr. Hematol. 4:140-146, 1964.

216.   Li, F.P., and Jaffe, N. Progeny of childhood-cancer survivors. Lancet 2:707-709, 1974.

217.   Zuelzer, W.W., and Cox, D.E. Genetic aspects of leukemia. Semin. Hematol. 6:4-25, 1969.

218.   Heath, C.W., Jr., and Moloney, W.C. Familial leukemia. Five cases of acute leukemia in three generations. N. Engl. J. Med. 272:882-887, 1965.

219.   Li, F.P., and Fraumeni, J.F., Jr. Soft tissue sarcomas, breast cancer and other neoplasms. Ann. Intern. Med. 71:747-752, 1969.

220.   McPhedran, P., Heath, C.W., Jr., and Lee, J. Patterns of familial leukemia. Ten cases of leukemia in two interrelated families. Cancer 24:403-407, 1969.

221.   Ferguson, S.W., and Lynn, T.N. Familial leukemia: A report of 4 cases of acute leukemia in 4 consecutive generations. South. Med. J. 63:1337-1340, 1970.

222.   Snyder, A.L., Li, F.P., Henderson, E.S., et al. Possible inherited leukaemogenic factors in familial acute myelogenous leukaemia. Lancet 1:586-589, 1970.

223.   Fraumeni, J.F., Jr., Vogel, C.L., and DeVita, V.T. Familial chronic lymphocytic leukemia. Ann. Intern. Med. 71:279-284, 1969.

224.   Potolsky, A.I., Heath, C.W., Jr., Buckley, C.E., et al. Lymphoreticular malignancies and immunologic abnormalities in a sibship. Am. J. Med. 50:42-48, 1971.

225.   Levine, P.H., Fraumeni, J.F., Jr., Reisher, J.I., et al. Antibodies to Epstein-Barr virus-associated antigens in relatives of cancer patients. J. Natl. Cancer Inst. 52:1037-1040, 1974.

226.   Dawson, P.J., and Meighan, S.S. Neonatal exchange transfusion and childhood leukemia. Pediatrics 41:1128-1130, 1968.

227.   Gibson, R.W., Bross, I.D.J., Graham, S., et al: Leukemia in children exposed to multiple risk factors. N. Engl. J. Med. 279:906-909, 1968.

228.   Spiers, P.S., and Quade, D. On the question of an infectious process in the origin of childhood leukemia. Biometrics 26:723-738, 1970.

229.   Gross, L. Incidence of appendectomies and tonsillectomies in cancer patients. Cancer 19:849-852, 1966.

230.   Johnson, S.K., and Johnson, R.E. Tonsillectomy history in Hodgkin's disease. N. Engl. J. Med. 287:1122-1125, 1972.

231.   Gutensohn, N., Li, F.P., Johnson, R.E., et al. Hodgkin's disease, tonsillectomy and family size. N. Engl. J. Med. 292:22-25, 1975.

232.   Cole, P. Epidemiologic studies and surveillance of human cancers among personnel of virus laboratories. In Hellman, A., Oxman, M.N., Pollack, R., eds. Biohazards in Biological Research, Cold Spring Harbor Laboratory, New York, 1973, pp. 309-315.

DISCUSSION

Several discussants commented on the strengths of evidence for the oncogenic role of Schistosoma haematobium in bladder cancer and of Clonorchis sinensis in primary liver cancer. Dr. Shimkin said that, although the mechanism was poorly understood, S. haematobium was a well-established cause of bladder cancer in man. **Dr. Cole** was not convinced, particularly in light of **Dr. Shubik's** reference to possible confounding by ingestion of potentially carcinogenic drugs. **Dr. Shimkin** pointed out that the association between schistosomiasis and bladder carcinoma was observed as early as the 19th century, long before antischistosomal drugs were available. **Dr. Higginson** noted that the diagnosis of schistosomal infection is often arbitrary, and in some studies cases are more thoroughly examined for infection than are controls. However, he felt that the relationship of *C. sinensis* to cholangiocarcinoma of the liver is well established.

Dr. Cole made several points: 1) efforts have begun to establish a registry of laboratory workers exposed to potentially oncogenic viruses, 2) the frequency of breast cancer in Parsi women is high compared with other Indian women but is only about two-thirds that of American women, 3) although many sib pairs of Hodgkin's disease have been reported, conjugal pairs seem to be very rare. This finding suggests that environmental determinants in familial Hodgkin's disease act very early in life. **Dr. Greenwald** commented that the Albany studies of Hodgkin's disease utilized the acquaintance-network method to evaluate "clustering" because standard epidemiologic techniques were inadequate for a disease with a long latent period and possible carrier state. The method is still being perfected, and future studies will be better designed. **Dr. Heath** stated that his group had attempted to use the acquaintance-network method but found it very difficult, time-consuming, and costly.

Dr. Pike commented that the specificity of antibody tests for herpes simplex was low and that Dr. Sabin had recently retracted his earlier papers on the usefulness of nonvirion antigens. In addition, the Canadian studies indicating a protective effect of BCG vaccine against childhood leukemias may be incorrect because recent data from the Province of Quebec are not confirmatory. **Dr. Kessler** considered that some tests for herpes simplex viruses are acceptable. Although most antibody surveys done since 1968 utilized neutralization tests which distinguished poorly between type 1 and type 2 forms of herpes simplex, Aurelian's test for Ag4 antigen offers some hope of distinguishing between the two types. **Dr. Heath** replied that all the serologic tests present problems that have to be resolved. **Dr. Rabson** concluded by noting that newly identified human papovaviruses should be appropriately studied in seroepidemiologic surveys. He also noted that radioimmune assays for oncornaviruses may soon be available for studies of high-risk groups.

Thomas Mack

16

SEXUAL FACTORS AND PREGNANCY

Brian E. Henderson, M.D., Veeba R. Gerkins,
and Malcolm C. Pike, Ph. D.

Departments of Pathology and Community Medicine
University of Southern California School of Medicine
Los Angeles, California

INTRODUCTION

Sex differences in risk are commonly observed for most cancers. Some of these differences are probably related to peculiarities of habit such as cigarette smoking and cancer of the respiratory tract. Another group of malignancies in which one sex has a higher rate than the other, for relatively unknown reasons, involves cancers of the thyroid and kidney, and Hodgkin's disease. Finally, there is a group of cancers in which sexual factors and/or pregnancy are thought to contribute substantially to pathogenesis; they are classified in Table 1. It is these cancer sites of concern to us here.

The etiology of cancers of the female breast, corpus uteri, and ovary probably focuses around the hormone excretion of the pituitary-gonad axis (Figure 1). These three cancers have certain epidemiological features in common. As shown in Table 2, the risk of all three cancers is lowest in Asian women and highest in white women in the United States and Western Europe [1]. The rates for cancers of the breast and corpus uteri are low also in Africans. As racial and ethnic groups migrate to the United States (or, as with blacks, adopt a living pattern associated with a higher economic status), their incidence rates move toward those of the white population. Our incidence data for Los Angeles

This study was conducted under Public Health Service contract PH43-NCI-68-1030 within the Virus Cancer Program of the National Cancer Institute.

TABLE 1

Cancers related to sexual factors and pregnancy
according to presumed major etiological mechanism

Presumed etiologic mechanism	Cancer site
Pituitary-gonadal hormones	Breast
	Uterus
	Ovary
Sexual activity	Cervix
	Penis
Unknown	Gallbladder
	Prostate
	Testis

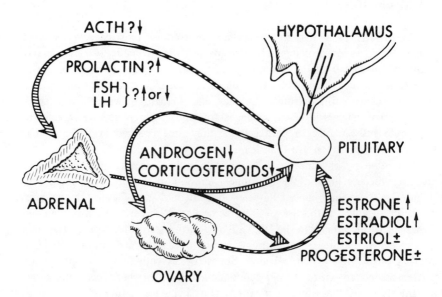

FIGURE 1.   Hypothalamic-pituitary and end organ axis in etiology of breast
cancer.

TABLE 2

Selected international age-standardized
incidence rates[a] in females for cancers of the
breast, corpus uteri, and ovary

Site	U.S. whites Alameda County	England (Oxford)	Japan	Ibadan
Breast	62.4	44.0	11.0	13.7
Corpus uteri	16.8	9.1	1.3	1.9
Ovary	12.6	10.1	1.9	7.5

[a]Standardized to Segi's world population distribution (1); rates given per 100,000 per year.

County for 1972 (Table 3) show this trend particularly for cancers of the breast and corpus uteri in two migrating populations: Mexican-Americans and Japanese [2]. Finally, relative infertility (e.g., nuns, single women) is a common characteristic of women with these cancers [3]. The protective effect of early pregnancy has been demonstrated for cancers of the breast and ovary [4,5].

We have no clear understanding of the hormonal basis of the altered risk in migrating populations resulting from changes in diet or reproductive behavior, nor do we understand the changes related to early pregnancy. However, recent studies in breast cancer have opened the door to possible underlying mechanisms, and we expect a rapid expansion of our knowledge of the pathogenesis of these cancers.

TABLE 3

Age-standardized female cancer incidence rates[a]
by racial and ethnic group, Los Angeles County, 1972 (2)

Site	Blacks	Mexican-Americans U.S.-born	Mexican-Americans Mexican-born	Other whites	Japanese
Breast	52.3	69.1	31.6	68.4	32.5
Corpus uteri	12.2	20.1	9.9	25.9	13.9
Ovary	6.6	9.1	5.5	11.1	3.3

[a]Standardized to Segi's world population distribution (1); rates given per 100,000 per year.

Breast

The important known risk factors associated with female breast cancer are summarized in Table 4. Although the relatives of premenopausal women with bilateral breast cancers have a sixfold to ninefold increased risk [4,6], the risks associated with most factors are between 2 and 3. These factors are interrelated and interdependent. For example, while most previous studies suggested an increased risk of breast cancer related to increased age at marriage and first pregnancy [7,8], MacMahon and co-workers [4,9] demonstrated that these variables reflected a more important relationship with age at first full-term delivery. More recently, we found [10] the influence of early age at menarche was so strong that for women with menarche prior to age 13, the effect of age at first delivery was not apparent.

The nature of several risk factors, such as the decreased age at menarche [10,11], increased age at first delivery [4,9,10,12], late natural menopause [4,10,13], and decreased risk after artificial menopause [4,14], has centered attention on ovarian activity. As a result, much research has been carried out in efforts to identify an abnormality of ovarian function.

Several studies [4,15-17] have focused on the relative amounts of the three estrogen fractions. Two fractions, estradiol and estrone, regularly produce mam-

TABLE 4

Known risk factors in female breast cancer

Category	Risk factors
Demographic	Old age Higher socioeconomic status Caucasian
Menstrual	Earlier age at menarche Later age at menopause Decreased frequency of artificial menopause
Reproductive	Never married Increased age at first full-term delivery Fewer pregnancies
Hormonal	Decreased use of exogenous estrogens (oral contraceptives, hormones at menopause)?
Other	History of benign breast disease Family history of breast cancer Increased total body size

mary tumors in rats; apparently the third, estriol, does not [4,18,19]. The suggestion is that estriol may be an antagonist of the other two fractions by competing for binding sites in breast tissue; therefore, the estriol ratio—the ratio of estriol to estrone plus estradiol—might be a measure of risk to breast cancer [15]. Case-control studies [20-22] of pre- and postmenopausal women have not supported this hypothesis. However, the estrogen profile of a woman with breast cancer may not reflect the hormonal status that increased her risk earlier in life; thus, these studies may be regarded as noninformative rather than negative [4,17]. Indirect support for the role of estrogen fractions has come from comparative international studies [23]. American women have a lower urinary estriol ratio than their Asian counterparts, generally accounted for by an increased amount of estradiol and estrone. More recently, these investigators found [24] that Asian women in Hawaii, whose breast cancer rates are intermediate between their homeland rates and those of Caucasian Americans, have a similarly elevated estriol ratio.

Several other hypotheses have been suggested. The pituitary hormones are important regulators of susceptibility to breast cancer in rodents [4,25], and prolactin enhances dimethylbenz[a]anthracene (DMBA)-induced breast cancer in the rat [26]. In most human studies [27,28], however, no difference has been found in the basal levels of serum prolactin between breast cancer cases and controls, although one recent study [29] found increased serum prolactin in patients with advanced breast cancer. Kwa and co-workers [30] reported increased prolactin levels in members of nine families with a high frequency of breast cancer. Further study of the role of prolactin in the etiology of breast cancer is indicated.

Recently, it was suggested [31-33] that women taking reserpine have an increased risk of breast cancer. Earlier, reserpine had been found to block the release of a prolactin-inhibiting factor in rats, leading to raised serum prolactin levels [34]. However, other antihypertensive drugs similarly affect prolactin secretion (methyldopa, phenothiazines), and no increased risk is associated with their use [31,33].

Several workers [35-37] reported that patients with benign and malignant breast cancer have decreased levels of plasma androgens and urinary androgen metabolites and that these changes can be detected several years before onset of disease. The decreased androgen excretion may not be of etiologic significance per se, but may reflect a fundamental alteration in endocrine status [4]. It has been proposed [38] that the primary defect in breast cancer patients is in corpus luteum formation, with decreased cyclic excretion of progesterone in the presence of estrogenic stimulation. Recent data bearing on this hypothesis are presented later in this section. Finally, relative thyroid deficiency has been suggested as a characteristic of breast cancer patients [39]. Whether the thyroid disorder exists before the onset of clinical disease and how it relates to the pathogenesis of breast cancer are unclear.

In attempting to define the hormonal patterns associated with the risk to breast cancer, we observed [10] that the patients and their mothers tend to be older at first pregnancy and menopause. Recently, we found that the sisters of patients tend to be younger at onset of menarche and first delivery and have fewer pregnancies when compared to sisters of controls (Henderson, B.E., Gerkins, V., Pike, M.C., and Casagrande, J., unpublished data). These findings suggest that any hormonal pattern predisposing to breast cancer may be familial as well, and possibly detected in the daughters of patients. Therefore, we are studying estrogen and progesterone levels in teenage offspring of patients and matched controls. By examining teenage girls, we hope to avoid alterations in the basic hormonal pattern that might be obscured in older women by pregnancy and exogenous hormones.

Preliminary results show that the mean levels of estrone and estradiol are slightly elevated in the follicular phase (sixth day) plasma of case daughters compared to control daughters (Table 5); the difference for estrone plus estradiol approaches statistical significance ($P = 0.08$). The levels of estrogen and progesterone in the luteal phase specimens are not different. These findings suggest that the case daughters have a relative hyperestrogenemia and are consistent with those of MacMahon and co-workers [23, 24]. We were unable to obtain reproducible plasma estriol levels (values too low); therefore, estriol ratios could not be calculated for direct comparison with the findings of MacMahon et al.

TABLE 5

Geometric means of the estrone, estradiol, and progesterone levels[a]
(ngm/100cc) in teenage daughters of breast cancer patients and controls

| | Daughters | |
Phase	Cases (*n*=35)	Controls (*n*=33)
Follicular (sixth day)		
Estrone	4.54	4.00
Estradiol	4.46	3.67
Estrone plus estradiol	9.19	7.82
Luteal (22nd day)		
Estrone	8.11	7.77
Estradiol	11.11	11.28
Progesterone[b]	345.72	337.90

[a]Measured by specific radioimmunoassay by D. M. Mayes at Endocrine Science Laboratory, Tarzana, California.
[b]For cases *n*=32; for controls *n*=35.

If this finding of hyperestrogenemia in certain daughters of breast cancer patients can be confirmed, we may have a method of early case detection for at least one subgroup of women at increased risk of breast cancer. The data in Table 5 do not support the hypothesis of Sherman and Korenman [38], because there was no difference in mean levels of progesterone in the luteal phase.

In summary, a woman's risk of breast cancer may result from an underlying abnormality of hormone excretion, one manifestation of which is an increase in circulating estradiol and estrone. The increased excretion of certain pituitary hormones might also be related to this abnormality. The apparent increased secretion of the hypothalamic–pituitary–gonadal axis may not be the only mechanism of breast cancer pathogenesis. Other variations in hormone excretion need to be sought before it is assumed that all breast cancer has the same etiology.

Further clues to the etiology of breast cancer may be found by studies of this cancer as it occurs in males. Male breast cancer has been associated with gonadal dysgenesis (Klinefelter's syndrome, XXY), an antecedent history of orchitis or orchiectomy, and the use of various exogenous hormones [8,40-42]. These features suggest that the risk of this disease is increased by a decrease in functioning male gonadal tissue. The mechanism would be an increase in hypothalamic-pituitary excretion from decreased gonadal feedback and a relative increase in the amount of circulating estrogens compared to androgens. It is still unclear whether the administration of exogenous estrogens to patients with prostatic cancer increases the risk of breast cancer [43].

Ovary

There are many epidemiologic similarities between cancers of the ovary and breast [5,44]. A twofold excess risk of ovarian cancer occurs among breast cancer patients and vice versa [45-47]. In a recent case-control study [5], the risk of ovarian cancer was associated with delayed age at first pregnancy and with a smaller number of pregnancies. As with breast cancer, these risk factors suggest an abnormality of endocrine secretion as an important component of ovarian carcinogenesis. This abnormality is associated with difficulty in achieving fertility and may reside in the pituitary or ovary. Unfortunately, endocrine studies like those reported above for breast cancer are not available. Elevated urinary estrogen levels and pregnanediol levels were found in almost half of the ovarian cancer cases studied. These increases are probably the result of proliferation of ovarian tumor cells and stimulation of the adjacent ovarian stroma, since the levels return to normal after oophorectomy [48].

Experimental work in animals demonstrated that unchecked production of pituitary gonadotropins is associated with ovarian cancer. Increased gonadotropin levels can result from decreased estrogen feedback control because of ovarian atrophy after ionizing radiation or chemical carcinogens, or from estrogen inactivation by the liver [5,49-50].

We will not know whether the hormonal defect lies in the pituitary or the ovary until suitable endocrinological studies have been made. The relative infertility of ovarian cancer patients may reflect a basic imbalance in excretion patterns of ovarian and pituitary hormones, perhaps evidenced by frequent anovulatory cycles and decreased pituitary feedback control by estrogens and progesterone. Determination of pituitary gonadotropin levels in persons with ovarian cancer would clarify this point.

Corpus Uteri

Only a few studies [3,51-52] concern the epidemiology of cancer of the corpus uteri, but the data available suggest many features in common with breast and ovarian cancers. Relative infertility, irregular menses, delayed menopause, and obesity have all been associated with this cancer [51,52]. Excessive menstrual bleeding and premenstrual breast swelling are also characteristic [52].

Patients with endometrial cancer have an increased frequency of diabetes and hypertension [51]; both factors probably reflect the tendency to obesity. Certain histologic types of ovarian tumors predispose to endometrial cancer, presumably because of the excessive estrogens excreted [53,54]. In addition, a twofold increased risk of ovarian cancer in patients with cancers of the corpus uteri or breast and vice versa was reported [45-47]. Presumably, relative hyperestrogenism, whether of gonadal or pituitary origin, predisposes to endometrial cancer. Hausknecht and Gusberg [55] reported that postmenopausal women with endometrial carcinoma excrete less estriol in relation to estrone. These workers also found increased conversion rates of androstenedione to estrone. The net result of this pattern of excretion would be an increase in circulating total estrogens. Further study of the endocrinopathy associated with endometrial carcinoma should be most revealing.

Cervix

The results of many epidemiological studies [56-60] have defined several risk factors for cervical cancer, the most important of which are:

Early age of coitus	Multiple marriages and pregnancies
Multiple sexual partners	(?) Hormone factors
Low socioeconomic status	(?) Herpes simplex virus type 2

The most significant factor appears to be age at first coitus; celibate women are at very low risk [3]. In Los Angeles County, cervical cancer is most common among Mexican-Americans and least common among other whites (Table 6).

The etiologic mechanism of cervical cancer has been the subject of considerable speculation. The importance of age at first coitus is thought to be related to increased susceptibility of the cervical epithelium in young women

TABLE 6
Cervix cancer incidence rates[a]
for Los Angeles County, 1972-73

Racial and ethnic group	Rate
Mexican-Americans	
U.S.-born	17.4
Mexico-born	31.4
Blacks	16.1
Other whites	8.8

[a] Age-standardized to Segi's world population distribution (1); rates given per 100,000 per year.

[60]. Cervical cancer has certain characteristics of a venereal disease [60]; in particular, the risk has been associated with sexual promiscuity. The search for a venereally transmitted agent has focused on herpes simplex virus type 2 (HSV-2) [60-65]. Several case-control studies showed higher antibody titers to HSV-2 in patients with cervical dysplasia, carcinoma in situ, and invasive carcinoma. However, with current serological methods, it is not possible to determine whether all women with cervical carcinoma have antibodies to HSV-2. Whether infection with HSV-2 is causally responsible for all or some cervical carcinoma or is merely a coincidental event remains unresolved.

Penile Cancer

Penile cancer occurs most frequently in areas of the world where circumcision is not practiced and where penile hygiene is poor [66,67]. Experimental and clinical evidence points to smegma as the leading etiological factor, although the specific substances and mechanism involved are unknown [68].

Gallbladder

Cancer of the gallbladder is more common in women and is strongly associated with cholelithiasis [69-71]. Incidence rates vary considerably by geographical area, being higher in European-born than Asian-born Jews in Israel [71] and in those of Mexican-American and American Indian descent in the United States (Table 7). Although little more is known about the etiology of gallbladder cancer, there have been several studies of the epidemiology of cholelithiasis [72-75]. This disease is associated with obesity and probably high

TABLE 7

Gallbladder cancer incidence rates[a]

for Los Angeles County, 1972-73

Racial and ethnic group	Male	Female
Mexican-Americans		
U.S.-born	2.6	4.1
Mexico-born	0.7	9.5
Blacks	0.7	1.6
Other whites	1.4	1.7

[a]Standardized to Segi's world population distribution (1); rates given per 100,000 per year.

parity in women, with the relationship to parity being more marked in young women [73]. It is unclear whether the parity effect is caused primarily by some hormonal factor or by the bile stasis that occurs during pregnancy [74,76]. It is known, however, that prolonged administration of estrogen and progesterone produces cholelithiasis in rabbits [77]. Recently, a relationship between oral contraceptive use–menopausal estrogen therapy and an increased risk of gallbladder disease was reported [78]. The role of dietary factors in the pathogenesis of cholelithiasis is equally unclear.

Prostate

The incidence of prostatic cancer has increased over the past 30 years [79]. The rate of increase is higher among blacks than whites, with the incidence among blacks now almost double that in whites (Table 8). The risk of prostatic cancer is considerably lower among Mexican-Americans (particularly those born in Mexico) than among blacks and similar to that of the other white population.

In Africa and Asia prostatic cancer is relatively uncommon. It is also less frequent in Israel among Jews born in Asia compared to those born in Europe [80]. Japanese migrants to the United States have an increased incidence of prostatic cancer [81,82]. Since this cancer may be a coincidental finding at autopsy, some of these international variations in rates may reflect differences in medical practice.

There are few epidemiological studies of prostatic cancer; however, there seems to be an excess risk among ever-married men as compared to single men [83]. A recent study [84] reported an excess of venereal disease and multiple sexual partners among prostatic cancer cases compared to age-matched hospital controls. The investigators concluded that patients with prostatic cancer exhibit

TABLE 8
Prostatic cancer incidence rates[a]
for selected countries and for Los Angeles County, 1972-73

International rates (1)		Los Angeles County rates	
U.S. (Alameda County)		Mexican-Americans	
Whites	38.0	U.S.-born	48.5
Blacks	65.3	Mexico-born	32.4
England (Oxford)	19.2	Blacks	72.0
Japan	3.2	Other whites	40.5
Ibadan	9.7	Japanese	14.0

[a]Standardized to Segi's world population distribution (1); rates given per 100,000 per year.

a greater sexual drive, suggesting that a venereally transmitted agent might be an important etiological factor. Recently, an increased risk of cervical cancer was reported among spouses of prostatic cancer patients, thus suggesting a common etiology [85]. However, the lower rate of prostatic cancer among Mexican-Americans compared to blacks, occurring when the rate of cervical cancer among Mexican-Americans exceeds that among blacks, argues against a common viral-venereal origin for these two cancers.

Decreased excretion of estrone and estradiol compared to estriol was reported for persons with prostatic cancer [86]. Similar findings were reported for other types of cancer; these hormonal abnormalities probably reflect the nutritional and metabolic response to carcinomatous disease rather than a pre-existing endocrinopathy.

Testis

Grumet and MacMahon [87] described three basic features of the epidemiology of testicular cancer in the United States: 1) an age curve showing a peak incidence in young adults, 2) low rates for blacks compared to whites (most conspicuous is the absence of a young adult peak among blacks), and 3) an increasing secular trend. An increasing incidence in young adults has been seen also in Danish and Japanese men [88,89]. In addition, testicular cancer seems more common in higher socioeconomic groups, although there is some variability in this finding [87,90].

Cryptorchidism and other genitourinary tract anomalies are highly associated with testicular cancer in children and adults [91]. Interestingly, orchiopexy does not necessarily protect against the increased risk of cancer of the involved testis [92,93]. The contralateral scrotal testis also is at increased risk

[94]. There is some evidence that the frequency of testicular maldescent has increased during the past 150 years [95]. The percentage of American army recruits with maldescent increased from 0.31 to 0.44 percent between 1927 and 1947. At least some of the recent secular increase in testicular cancer could be related to this increase.

These observations also suggest there is a factor that predisposes to both testicular maldescent and cancer. It has been proposed that fetal pituitary gonadotropin excretion is involved in testicular descent [96], since maldescent is found in some hypogonadotropic patients [97]. However, hormonal assays in a limited number of cases of testicular cancer showed an increase in gonadotropin levels [98]. It is unclear whether this increase was of pituitary origin or a by-product of the tumor, although the gonadotropin levels tended to return to normal after surgery and remain low unless recurrent disease developed. Urinary 17-oxysteroids were reported [98] as normal in patients with benign and malignant tumors of the testis. A follow-up study [99] of persons with repaired maldescent revealed elevated follicle-stimulating hormone (FSH) and luteinizing hormone (LH) levels when compared to normal controls. Clearly, further study of the endocrinological status of patients with testicular cancer is necessary.

SUGGESTIONS FOR FURTHER RESEARCH TO DEFINE HIGH RISK GROUPS

Current research shows that levels of certain estrogenic fractions are elevated in populations at high risk of breast cancer. Definition of the nature of this difference should provide valuable leads to the control of breast cancer. Further research on hormone levels (estrogens, androgens, prolactin, etc.) is particularly needed in high-risk populations (e.g., relatives of young women with bilateral breast cancer).

Using the altered estrogen fractions as a measure of population susceptibility, we need information on the effect of diet and other environmental variables (drugs, exercise, etc.) on the level of the circulating estrogen fractions and other hormones.

After obtaining the results of the preceding suggestion, an approach may be made to lower the circulating estrogen level in susceptible teenagers and young adults using dietary manipulation and/or exogenous hormones and noting the incidence of benign breast disease.

An expanded effort is needed to understand the basic mechanism responsible for the onset of menarche and the influence of a variety of environmental variables (e.g., diet, drugs, activity).

It seems clear that the etiology of ovarian and endometrial cancers is related to a mechanism similar to but probably not identical with that of breast cancer. More studies are needed on the endocrine profile of women with these cancers or with predisposing conditions.

We need to know the relationship of exogenous hormones to the risk of cancers of the breast, ovary, and corpus uteri in pre- and postmenopausal women. Our own experience in attempting to gain information on the risk associated with hormones at menopause suggests that a randomized prospective clinical trial may be the only way of obtaining a clear answer to the harmful or beneficial effect of postmenopausal estrogen therapy.

We need further information on factors that influence the susceptibility of the cervical and vaginal epithelium to metaplasia.

The relationship of HSV-2 to cervical carcinoma needs further clarification. Further seroepidemiologic studies are not likely to'resolve the central issue. If an approach to therapy is available, then a randomized prospective clinical study of persons infected with HSV-2 might provide a definitive answer.

We need basic epidemiologic and endocrinologic information on prostatic and testicular cancers.

REFERENCES

1. International Union Against Cancer. (Doll, R., Muir, C., and Waterhouse, J., eds.) *Cancer Incidence in Five Continents.* Vol. 2, Springer-Verlag, Berlin, 1970.

2. Menck, H.R., Henderson, B.E., Pike, M.C., et al. Cancer incidence in the Mexican-American. *J. Natl. Cancer Inst.* (submitted).

3. Fraumeni, J.F., Jr., Lloyd, J.W., Smith, E.J., et al. Cancer mortality among nuns: Role of marital status in etiology of neoplastic disease in women. *J. Natl. Cancer Inst. 42:* 455–468, 1969.

4. MacMahon, B., Cole, P., and Brown, J. Etiology of human breast cancer: A review. *J. Natl. Cancer Inst. 50:* 21–42, 1973.

5. Joly, D., Lilienfeld, A.J., Diamond, E.L., et al. An epidemiologic study of the relationship of reproductive experience to cancer of the ovary. *Am. J. Epidemiol. 99:* 190–209, 1974.

6. Anderson, D.E. Some characteristics of familial breast cancer. *Cancer 28:* 1500–1504, 1971.

7. Wynder, E.L., Bross, I.J., and Hirayama, T. A study of the epidemiology of cancer of the breast. *Cancer 13:* 559–601, 1960.

8. Lilienfeld, A.M. The epidemiology of breast cancer. *Cancer Res. 23:* 1503–1513, 1963.

9. MacMahon, B., Cole, P., Lin, T.M., et al. Age at first birth and breast cancer risk. *Bull. W.H.O. 43:* 209–221, 1970.

10. Henderson, B., Powell, D., Rosario, I., et al. An epidemiological study of breast cancer. *J. Natl. Cancer Inst. 53:* 609–614, 1974.

11. Staszewski, J. Age at menarche and breast cancer. *J. Natl. Cancer Inst. 47:* 935–940, 1971.

12. Valaoras, V.G., MacMahon, B., Trichopoulos, D., et al. Lactation and reproductive histories of breast cancer patients in Greater Athens, 1965-1967. *Int. J. Cancer 4:* 350-363, 1969.

13. Trichopoulos, D., MacMahon, B., and Cole, P. The menopause and breast cancer risk. *J. Natl. Cancer Inst. 48*:605–613, 1972.

14. Lilienfeld, A.M. Relationship of cancer of the female breast to artificial menopause and marital status. *Cancer 9:*927–934, 1956.

15. Lemon, H.M., Wotiz, H.H., Parsons, L., et al. Reduced estriol excretion in patients with breast cancer prior to endocrine therapy. *J.A.M.A. 196:*1128–1136, 1966.

16. Lemon, H.M. Endocrine influences on human mammary cancer formation. A critique. *Cancer 23:*781–790, 1969.

17. Cole, P., and MacMahon, B. Estrogen fractions during early reproductive life in the etiology of breast cancer. *Lancet 1:*604–606, 1969.

18. Dunning, W.F., Curtis, M.R., and Segaloff, A. Strain differences in response to estrone and the induction of mammary gland, adrenal and bladder cancer in rats. *Cancer Res. 13:*147–152, 1953.

19. Cutts, J.H., and Nobel, R.L. Estrone-induced mammary tumors in the rat. *Cancer Res. 24:*1116–1123, 1964.

20. Gronos, M., and Aho, A.J. Estrogen metabolism in postmenopausal women with primary and recurrent breast cancer. *Eur. J. Cancer 4:*523–527, 1968.

21. Marmorston, J., Crowley, L.G., Myers, S.M., et al. II. Urinary excretion of estrone, estradiol and estriol by patients with breast cancer and benign breast disease. *Am. J. Obstet. Gynecol. 92:*460-467, 1965.

22. Arguelles, A.E., Poggi, U.L., Saborida, C., et al. Endocrine profiles and breast cancer. *Lancet 1:*165–167, 1973.

23. MacMahon, B., Cole, P., Brown, J.B., et al. Urine estrogen profiles of Asian and North American women. *Int. J. Cancer 14:*161–167, 1974.

24. Dickinson, L.E., MacMahon, B., Cole, P., et al. Estrogen profiles of Oriental and Caucasian women in Hawaii. *N. Engl. J. Med. 291:*1211–1213, 1974.

25. Smith, O.W., and Smith, G.V. Urinary estrogen profiles and etiology of breast cancer. *Lancet 1:*1152–1155, 1970.

26. Talwalker, P.K., Meites, J., and Mizieno, H. Mammary tumor induction by estrogen or anterior pituitary hormones in ovariectomized rats given 7,12-dimethy-1,2-benzanthracene. *Proc. Soc. Exp. Biol. Med. 116:*531–534, 1962.

27. Mittra, I., Hayward, J.L., and McNeilly, A.S. Hypothalamic-pituitary-prolactin axis in breast cancer. *Lancet 1:*889–891, 1974.

28. Wilson, R.G., Buchans, R., Roberts, M.M., et al. Plasma prolactin and breast cancer. *Cancer 33:*1325–1327, 1974.

29. Rolandi, E., Barreca, T., Masturzo, P., et al. Plasma-prolactin in breast cancer. *Lancet 2:*845–846, 1974.

30. Kwa, H.G., Engelsman, E., DeJong-Bakker, M., et al. Plasma-prolactin in human breast cancer. *Lancet 1:*433–435, 1974.

31. Boston Collaborative Drug Surveillance Program. Reserpine and breast cancer. *Lancet 2:*669–671, 1974.

32. Armstrong, B., Stevens, N., and Doll, R. Retrospective study of the association between use of Rauwolfia derivatives and breast cancer in English women. *Lancet 2:*672–674, 1974.

33. Heinonen, O.P., Shapiro, S., Tuominen, L., et al. Reserpine use in relation to breast cancer. *Lancet 2:*675–677, 1974.

34. Welsch, C.W., and Meites, J. Effects of reserpine on development of carcinogen-induced mammary tumors in rats. In *24th International Congress on Physiological Science,* Washington, D.C., 1968.

35. Bulbrook, R.D., and Hayward, J.L. Abnormal urinary steroid excretion and subsequent breast cancer. A prospective study in the Island of Guernsey. *Lancet 1:*519–522, 1967.

36. Brennan, M.J., Bulbrook, R.D., Deshpande, N., et al. Urinary and plasma androgens in benign breast disease. *Lancet 1:*1076-1079, 1973.

37. Bulbrook, R.D., Hayward, J.L., and Spicer, C.C. Relation between urinary androgen and corticoid excretion and subsequent breast cancer. *Lancet 2:*395-398, 1971.

38. Sherman, B., and Korenman, S.G. Inadequate corpus luteum function: A pathophysiological interpretation of human breast cancer epidemiology. *Cancer 33:*1306-1312, 1974.

39. Mittra, I., and Hayward, J.L. Hypothalamic-pituitary-thyroid axis in breast cancer. *Lancet 1:*885-888, 1974.

40. Schottenfeld, D., Lilienfeld, A.M., and Diamond, H. Some observations on the epidemiology of breast cancer among males. *Am. J. Public Health 53:*890-897, 1963.

41. Cuenca, C.R., and Becher, K.L. Klinefelter's syndrome and cancer of the breast. *Arch. Intern. Med. 121:*159-162, 1968.

42. Jackson, A.W., Muldal, S., Ockey, C.H., et al. Carcinoma of the male breast in association with the Klinefelter's syndrome. *Br. Med. J. 5429:*223-225, 1965.

43. Salyer, W.R., and Salyer, D.C. Metastases of prostatic carcinoma to the breast. *J. Urol. 109:*671-675, 1973.

44. Wynder, E., Dodo, H., and Barber, H. Epidemiology of cancer of the ovary. *Cancer 23:*352-369, 1969.

45. Schottenfeld, D., and Berg, J. Incidence of multiple primary cancers. IV. Cancers of the female breast and genital organs. *J. Natl. Cancer Inst. 46:*161-170, 1971.

46. Lynch, H., and Krush, A.J. Carcinoma of the breast and ovary in three families. *Surg. Gynecol. Obst. 133:*644-648, 1971.

47. Schoenberg, B., Greenberg, R.A., and Eisenberg, H. Occurrence of certain multiple primary cancers in females. *J. Natl. Cancer Inst. 43:*15-32, 1969.

48. Edwards, R., Nicholson, H., Zoidis, T., et al. Endocrine studies in post menopausal women with ovarian tumors. *J. Obstet. Gynaecol. Br. Commonw. 78:*467-477, 1971.

49. Biskind, G.R., and Biskind, M.S. Experimental ovarian tumors in rats. *Am. J. Clin. Pathol. 19:*501-521, 1949.

50. Gardner, W.U. Tumorigenesis in transplanted irradiated and nonirradiated ovaries. *J. Natl. Cancer Inst. 26:*829-852, 1961.

51. Stewart, H., Dunham, L., Casper, J., et al. Epidemiology of cancers of the uterine cervix and corpus, breast and ovary in Israel and New York City. *J. Natl. Cancer Inst. 37:*1-95, 1966.

52. Wynder, E.L., Escher, G.C., and Mantel, N. An epidemiological investigation of cancer of the endometrium. *Cancer 19:*489-520, 1966.

53. Marcus, C.C. Ovarian cortical stromal hyperplasia and carcinoma of the endometrium. *Obstet. Gynecol. 21:*175-186, 1963.

54. Kistner, R.W., Duncan, C.J., and Mansell, H. Suppression of ovulation by tri-p-anisylchlorethylene (TACE). *Obstet. Gynecol. 8:*399-407, 1956.

55. Hausknecht, R.U., and Gusberg, S.B. Estrogen metabolism in patients at high risk for endometrial carcinoma. *Am. J. Obstet. Gynecol. 116:*981-984, 1973.

56. Wynder, E.L., Cornfield, J., Shroff, P.D., et al. A study of environmental factors in carcinoma of the cervix. *Am. J. Obstet. Gynecol. 68:*1015-1052, 1954.

57. Terris, M. and Oalmann, M.C. Carcinoma of the cervix: An epidemiological study. *J.A.M.A. 174:*1847-1851, 1960.

58. Lundin, F.E., Erickson, C.C., and Sprunt, D.H. Socioeconomic distribution of cervical cancer. *Public Health Monograph No. 73,* Washington, D.C., Govt. Print. Off., 1964.

59. Stern, E. Epidemiology of dysplasia. *Obstet. Gynecol. Survey 24:*711-723, 1969.

60. Rotkin, I.D. A comparison review of key epidemiological studies in cervical cancer related to current searches for transmissible agents. *Cancer Res. 33:*1353-1367, 1973.

61. Naik, M., Hahmias, A.J., Josey, W.E., et al. Genital herpetic infection: Association with cervical dysplasia and carcinoma. *Cancer 23:*940–945, 1969.

62. Aurelian, L., Davis,H.J.,and Julian,C.G. Herpesvirus type 2 induced, tumor-specific antigen in cervical carcinoma. *Am. J. Epidemiol. 98:*1–9, 1973.

63. Adam, E., Kaufman, R.H., Melnick, J.L., et al. Sero-epidemiologic studies of herpesvirus type 2 and carcinoma of the cervix. IV. Dysplasia and carcinoma in-situ. *Am. J. Epidemiol. 98:*77–87, 1973.

64. Nahmias, A.J., Josey, W.E., Naik, Z.M., et al. Antibodies to *Herpesvirus hominis* types 1 and 2 in humans. II. Women with cervical cancer. *Am. J. Epidemiol. 91:*547–552, 1970.

65. Alexander, E.R. Possible etiologies of cancer of the cervix other than herpesvirus. *Cancer Res. 33:*1458–1496, 1973.

66. Schmauz, R., and Jain, D.K. Geographical variation of carcinoma of the penis in Uganda. *Br. J. Cancer 25:*25–32, 1971.

67. Reviros, M., and Lebron, R.F. Geographical pathology of cancer of the penis. *Cancer 16:*798, 1963.

68. Shabad, A.L. The experimental production of the penis tumours. *Neoplasma (Bratisl.) 12:*635, 1965.

69. Gerst, P.H. Primary carcinoma of the gallbladder. A thirty year summary. *Ann. Surg. 153:*369–372, 1961.

70. Lieber, M.M. The incidence of gallstones and their correlation with other diseases. *Ann. Surg. 135:*394–405, 1952.

71. Hart, J., Shani, M., and Modan, B. Epidemiological aspects of gallbladder and biliary tract neoplasm. *Am. J. Public Health 62:*36–39, 1972.

72. Large, A.M., Lofstrom, J.E., and Stevenson, C.S. Gallstones and pregnancy. *Arch. Surg. 78:*966–968, 1959.

73. Bernstein, R.A., Werner,L.H.,and Rimm, A.A. Relationship of gallbladder disease to parity, obesity and age. *Health Serv. Rep. 88:*925–936, 1973.

74. Friedman, G.D., Kannel, W.B., and Dawber, T.R. The epidemiology of gallbladder disease: Observations in the Framingham study. *J. Chronic Dis. 19:*273–292, 1966.

75. Horn, G. Observations on the aetiology of cholelithiasis. *Br. Med. J. 2:*732–737, 1956.

76. Gerdes, M.M., and Bryden, E.A. The rate of emptying of the human gallbladder in pregnancy. *Surg. Gynecol. Obst. 66:*145–156, 1938.

77. Imamoglu, K., Wangensteen, S.L., Root, H.D., et al. Production of gallstones by prolonged administration of progesterone and estradiol in rabbits. *Surg. Forum:*246–249, 1959.

78. Boston Collaborative Drug Surveillance Program. Surgically confirmed gallbladder disease, venous thromboembolism, and breast tumors in relation to postmenopausal estrogen therapy. *N. Engl. J. Med. 290:*15–19, 1974.

79. Cutler, S.J., and DeVesa, S.S. Trends in cancer incidence and mortality in the USA. In Doll, R., and Vodopija, I., eds, *Host Environment Interaction in th Etiology of Cancer in Man.* pp. 15-34, 1973.

80. Kook, H., and Kook, H. Carcinoma of the prostate in Israel. *Br. J. Urol. 34:*322–325, 1962.

81. Haenszel, W. Cancer mortality among the foreign born in the United States. *J. Natl. Cancer Inst. 26:*37–132, 1961.

82. Dorn, H.F.,and Cutler, S.J. Morbidity from cancer in the United States. *Public Health Monograph No. 56,* 1959.

83. Moriyama, I.M. Deaths from selected causes by marital status, by age and sex, United States, 1940. *Vital Statist. Spec. Rep. 23*, No. 7, 1945.

84. Steele, R., Lees, R.E., Krause, A.S., et al. Sexual factors in the epidemiology of cancer of the prostate. *J. Chron. Dis. 24:*29-37, 1971.

85. Feminella, J.G., Jr., and Lattimer, J.K. An apparent increase in genital carcinomas among wives of men with prostatic carcinomas: An epidemiologic survey. *Pirquet Bull. Clin. Med. 20:*3-10, 1974.

86. Marmorston, J., Lombardo, L.J., Jr., Myers, S.M., et al. Urinary excretion of estrone, estradiol and estriol by patients with prostatic cancer and benign prostatic hypertrophy. *J. Urol. 93:*287-295, 1965.

87. Grumet, R.F., and MacMahon, B. Trends in mortality from neoplasms of the testes. *Cancer 2:*790-797, 1958.

88. Clemmesen, J. A doubling of morbidity from testes carcinoma in Copenhagen, 1943-1962. *Acta Pathol. Microbiol. Scand. 72:*348-349, 1968.

89. Lee, J.A., Hitosugi, M., and Petersen, G.R. Rise in mortality from tumors of the testis in Japan, 1947-1970. *J. Natl. Cancer Inst. 51:*1485-1490, 1973.

90. Graham, S., and Gibson, R.W. Social epidemiology of cancer of the testes. *Cancer 29:*1242-1249, 1972.

91. Li, F.P., and Fraumeni, J.F., Jr. Testicular cancers in children: Epidemiologic characteristics. *J. Natl. Cancer Inst.* 48:1575-1582, 1972.

92. Campbell, H.F. Incidence of malignant growth of the undescended testicle. *Arch. Surg. 44:*353-369, 1942.

93. Altman, B.L., and Malanent, M. Carcinoma of the testis following orchiopexy. *J. Urol. 97:*498-504, 1967.

94. Dow, J.A., and Mostofi, F.K. Testicular tumors following orchiopexy. *South. Med. J. 60:*193-195, 1967.

95. Campbell, H.E. The incidence of malignant growth of the undescended testicle: A reply and re-evaluation. *J. Urol. 81:*663-668, 1959.

96. Turner, R.C. Maldescended testes. *Lancet 2:*174-175, 1974.

97. Turner, R.C., Bobrow, M., Bobrow, L.G., et al. Cryptorchidism in a family with Kallman's syndrome. *Proc. R. Soc. Med. 67:*33-35, 1974.

98. Symington, T., and Wallace, N. Hormone investigations in cases of testicular tumour. *In* Collins, D.H., and Pugh, R.C.B., eds. *Pathology of Testicular Tumors.* E. and S. Livingston, Edinburgh and London, 1965, pp. 103-106.

99. Bramble, F.J., Haughton, A.L., Eccles, S., et al. Reproductive and endocrine function and surgical treatment of bilateral cryptorchidism. *Lancet 2:*311-314, 1974.

DISCUSSION

Dr. Wynder commented on the 3:1 ratio of breast cancer rates before menopause in American as compared with Japanese women, and the 8:1 ratio in later life, and asked for possible explanations. He also wondered whether dietary factors might be important in familial aggregations of breast cancer. **Dr. Henderson** responded that many epidemiologic patterns of breast cancer may be linked with dietary factors, but this hypothesis has not been adequately tested. In explaining the racial and familial tendencies of breast cancer, it is still difficult to separate environmental and genetic factors.

Dr. Blattner suggested future studies of breast cancer incorporate questions on the use of marijuana, which has been linked recently with gynecomastia.

Dr. Lynch proposed that genetic analyses of breast cancer assess the familial risk of other cancer sites, since recent pedigree studies indicate that breast cancer aggregates with leukemia and brain tumors and with ovarian cancer. Such studies could also have important implications for cancer control.

Dr. Rawson raised three questions: 1) Are estrogens carcinogenic or permissive? 2) What is the role of estrogen and prolactin binders? and 3) Could the protective effect of estriol be related to immune function? **Dr. Henderson** responded that very little is known about these issues. Studies are needed to assess the influence of exogenous hormones on endogenous estrogen activity and on the effect of diet in females with hyperestrogenemia. **Dr. Wynder** asked whether our present knowledge permits recommendations on the possible dietary control of breast cancer in the United States. **Dr. Henderson** replied that little is known about the effect of diet on estrogen levels in females and that such studies should be given high priority. **Dr. A. B. Miller** suggested these studies separate premenopausal from postmenopausal patients with breast cancer, since obesity may be an important risk factor for breast cancer in postmenopausal women. Finally, **Dr. Koss** urged that the present studies of hormonal and other factors in breast cancer be extended to other endocrine-dependent neoplasms, particularly those of the endometrium and prostate.

Nicholas J. Vianna

17

OVERVIEW: ENVIRONMENTAL FACTORS

Brian MacMahon, M.D.

Department of Epidemiology
Harvard School of Public Health
Boston, Massachusetts

In this review of environmental factors related to cancer risk we have been presented with examples of true carcinogens, cocarcinogens, tumor initiators, tumor promoters, and a great many substances whose modes of action are unknown. From a practical viewpoint, the distinction between these classes of compounds—all of which I will loosely refer to as carcinogens—is often unimportant. Their common characteristic is that, empirically, they produce an increase in tumor risk; by inference, prevention of exposure to them would result in a decrease in cancer risk.

VARIETY OF ENVIRONMENTAL FACTORS

A striking feature emerging from these papers is the large number and variety of known carcinogens—even if the list is limited to those known for humans. This variety has many dimensions. There is, first, variety in the *nature* of the substances. Physical, chemical, and biologic agents are all represented. Physical agents are most clearly represented by ionizing radiation, as described by Jablon [1], but other forms of solar radiation were also implicated. The variety of known chemical agents is in itself startling, ranging through tobacco in its several forms [2], alcoholic beverages [3], food contaminants and perhaps deficiencies [4], therapeutic drugs [5], and the myriad of industrial chemicals [6]. Biological agents include the microbiologic agents reviewed by

Heath [7] and the many biological characteristics of the potential host, such as patterns of endocrine metabolism [8].

There is variety, too, in the modes of action of these agents. Some act by the induction of germinal genetic mutation, as in the relatively rare single-gene cancers of man. Some act by the production of aberrations during normal anatomic development, as in the tumors occurring in undescended testes or the diethylstilbestrol (DES)-induced vaginal adenocarcinomas. Others act through their effect on physiologic development, most notable perhaps being the many environmental influences that determine the rate and pattern of endocrine development. A number of agents act as true carcinogens, which is probably the case with ionizing radiation and the aflatoxins. Some appear to act through several mechanisms. Thus, it seems likely that the tumors induced by chewing tobacco, snuff, and cigarettes have different etiologic mechanisms. It is unlikely that the mechanism of action of cigarette smoke in inducing lung cancer is the same as that whereby the same agent produces cancer of the bladder.

One sees also great variety in the age at which these substances exert their effects: It may involve ancestral times, as with the genetic determinants; in utero, as with the DES-induced vaginal carcinomas and, inferentially, many of the tumors of early childhood; or any point in childhood or adult life. Again, some agents seem capable of action at several different age periods. The estrogens, including DES for example, appear to alter cancer risk at many periods from early in utero life to late middle age [9].

The picture is further complicated by the interactions between environmental agents, discussed in more detail in a later chapter of this volume [10], but whose significance is so clearly illustrated in Rothman's description of the roles of tobacco and alcohol in the etiology of cancer of the mouth [3]. Such interactions are undoubtedly much more extensive than we now understand. As we have often seen, however, it is not necessary to understand the etiology of a disease in its entirety to take effective preventive action. For example, the pattern of interaction of tobacco and alcohol in mouth cancer appears to be such that substantial prevention could be accomplished by knowledge of and effective action against either one, and not necessarily both, of the two factors.

IMPLICATIONS FOR PREVENTION

No single known measure would lengthen the life or improve the health of the American population more than eliminating cigarette smoking. While the benefits of such action would be most striking with regard to cancer—notably in reduction of lung cancer rates to about one-tenth of those now prevailing—they would not be restricted to this disease. As Hammond [2] pointed out, the persons attending this conference are not the ones who need to be convinced. Nevertheless, it provides a forum for stressing to the public and the government the significance of this problem. It seems almost beyond comprehension that the problem remains, 40 years after suspicion was first directed to cigarettes as carcinogens and more than 20 years after the definitive evidence began to appear.

Beyond that, the reviews presented contain numerous examples, less important quantitatively but nevertheless significant for substantial parts of the population, of ways in which knowledge of environmental factors has led to preventive possibilities. Two of most practical significance are the recognition of the need for reduction of radiation exposure and the reduction of exposure to known carcinogens in industry.

IMPLICATIONS FOR CONTROL

These reviews clearly demonstrated that there are a few population subgroups at relatively high risk of cancers of certain sites. If there were equally clear evidence that early diagnosis and treatment of these cancers led to improved survival, the knowledge that such high-risk groups exist would have important implications for these individuals. However, while cancers as a class are common, most individual cancers are uncommon and, even in a group that is at high risk relative to the rest of the population, the absolute tumor rate may be quite small. Therefore, the yield from screening such groups may be small and the cost substantial. The financial, personal, and psychologic costs must be weighed against the possible benefits derived by the cases found. For the one tumor for which a survival advantage associated with early diagnosis and treatment has been demonstrated, cancer of the breast, no environmental determinants are known that would lead to restriction of screening to exposed individuals. For the most common tumor with a clear environmental determinant, cancer of the lung, there is no evidence that early detection and treatment lead to improved survival, much less warrant the human and financial costs involved.

In short, current knowledge of environmental factors in cancer might alert physicians and others, including the exposed individuals themselves, to the significance of particular symptoms in certain population subgroups. Overall, however, present knowledge contributes little to the possibility of control through identification of high-risk groups for screening and early treatment.

IMPLICATIONS FOR RESEARCH

Indirect evidence—sharp time trends, abrupt frequency changes over short geographic distances, changes in cancer rates following migration, and so on—

makes it apparent that environmental causes of cancer must be far more numerous than those identified. The nature and variety of recognized factors suggest some of the difficulties facing research efforts to uncover causes. Almost nothing can be above suspicion. Separation of "likely" and "unlikely" candidates on the basis of a priori reasoning is of limited value. The biochemists are becoming better at predicting carcinogenic potential from chemical structure, and the development of in vitro tests for mutagenicity will be enormously helpful in focusing research on likely candidates. Ultimately, the potential for carcinogenicity of an agent for humans will have to be evaluated from empiric data collected in humans. When it comes to the cocarcinogens, promoters, and causal environmental factors other than the true carcinogens, the basis for a priori selection is even less secure.

Further difficulties arise from the ubiquity of some of the possible determinants and the problems of identifying and measuring factors that are often seemingly trivial and present in minute amounts. Lastly, there is the problem of the time scale involved in this disease, or group of diseases, and the rapidity of environmental change. For some cancers, the latent or induction period may be quite short; for others, it must be measured in decades. Empiric evidence collected in man will always reflect the situation of previous years or decades; because of the rapidity with which man's ecosystem is changing, the evidence may not be relevant to the present scene.

The complexity of this situation presents yet another argument for continuing to support the individual investigator with the imagination and initiative to explore new fields. The last decade has seen an increasing trend toward large-scale collaborative research, directed toward questions posed by a committee or group of administrators. Valuable information has come from such research, and many questions can only be answered in this manner. Such research must continue, but not at the expense of the free-wheeling investigator who asks questions that committees do not. No committee asked whether Hodgkin's disease might be infectious or whether exposure to DES in utero caused vaginal carcinoma.

In this symposium, Miller referred to the need for trained investigators [11]. This need deserves to be reemphasized. It relates to investigators with sound capability for testing hypotheses quantitatively in humans, as well as those with the knowledge and insights of the clinician and experimentalist. In addition, the unexpectedness of some of the relationships that have emerged between environmental factors and cancer should prompt us to examine our information resources to determine whether investigators, and the funds they expend, are being used to maximum efficiency. Even a superficial examination reveals that the information resources at hand are, in fact, far from adequate.

To determine cancer risks among persons exposed to particular environmental factors, we need to be able to link information relating to the same individual at different times in his life and to determine whether an individual exposed in the past is now dead or alive and in what state of health. Proposals to improve procedures to accomplish these ends have been made by several study groups [12]. They include wider use of the Social Security number on medical and vital records (to facilitate linkage), inclusion of parental Social Security numbers on birth certificates, the assignment of Social Security numbers at birth, and the establishment of a National Death Index.

Opposition to such relatively simple proposals seems to stem, not from doubts as to desirability, feasibility, or cost, but from a concern for privacy and confidentiality of medical and social information. Such concerns are real and legitimate. However, a tradeoff is involved. Maximum confidentiality means minimum epidemiologic information and minimal effectiveness in identifying new cancer hazards. In my opinion, we are well beyond the point at which concern for confidentiality seriously impairs the extraction of valuable knowledge, even from routinely collected information. Working as an epidemiologist, one comes to recognize the readiness with which most people, patients or nonpatients, will supply even sensitive information if they believe the cause is reasonable. Somehow, the issue of confidentiality becomes more difficult when it is institutionalized or politicized. We must attempt to convince the public's representatives that a reasonable balance can be achieved.

REFERENCES

1. Jablon, S. Radiation. This volume, 1975.
2. Hammond, E.C. Tobacco. This volume, 1975.
3. Rothman, K.J. Alcohol. This volume, 1975.
4. Berg, J.W. Diet. This volume, 1975.
5. Hoover, R., and Fraumeni, J.F., Jr. Drugs. This volume, 1975.
6. Cole, P., and Goldman, M.B. Occupation. This volume, 1975.
7. Heath, C.W., Caldwell, G.G., and Feorino, P.C. Viruses and other microbes. This volume, 1975.
8. Henderson, B.E., Gerkins, V.R., and Pike, M.C. Sexual factors and pregnancy. This volume, 1975.
9. MacMahon, B., Cole, P., and Brown, J. Etiology of human breast cancer: A review. *J. Natl. Cancer Inst. 50:*21-42, 1973.
10. Selikoff, I.J., and Hammond, E.C. Multiple risk factors in environmental cancer. This volume, 1975.
11. Miller, R.W. Overview: Host factors. This volume, 1975.
12. National Center for Health Statistics. *Use of Vital and Health Records in Epidemiologic Research.* NCHS Series 4, No. 7. Public Health Service Publication No. 1000, U.S. Govt. Print. Off., Washington, D.C., 1968.

DISCUSSION

Dr. MacMahon concluded his paper by urging establishment of a National Death Index. At present, mortality records are maintained by over 50 jurisdictions in the United States, mostly State vital records departments; therefore, search for a death certificate is tedious and costly. The Death Index would make it possible to determine quickly on a national level if a person has died and where the death record can be found. It would greatly facilitate the conduct of many epidemiologic studies without threatening privacy, because the States would retain the certificates. **Dr. R. W. Miller** cited an example of a costly and lengthy mortality study of an occupational cohort (American steelworkers) which could have been easily completed through use of a Death Index. **Dr. Peters** indicated that a working group has been formed at the National Institutes of Health to facilitate the development of this Index.

A lively discussion followed on the uses and potential misuses of data files compiled for epidemiologic studies. Several discussants commented favorably on the record-linkage approach; others encouraged creation of new files on occupational cohorts and other high-risk groups and improvement in quality of existing records such as hospital charts. **Dr. Schneiderman** related his concern that currently proposed legislation on protection of confidentiality may limit opportunities for epidemiologic research. He indicated that alternate proposals are being submitted to legislators and sought help in formulating the intent and language of the new legislation. **Dr. Shapiro** stated that cost-benefit analysis should be applied to weigh socially useful epidemiologic research against possible invasion of privacy. **Dr. Bahn** favored establishing a unique numbering system to identify individuals for record-linkage studies; she felt appropriate safeguards against abuses can be maintained. **Dr. Shimkin** offered another viewpoint. He supported establishment of a Death Index but thought that extensive linkage of records may pose excessive risks to society.

Several discussants indicated the need to preserve and strengthen data resources. **Dr. Hirohata** cited the follow-up studies of persons exposed to ionizing radiation and the importance of continued monitoring. Because the risk of various cancers remains excessive among Japanese survivors of the atomic blast over 25 years ago, estimates of radiation hazard would have been falsely low if studies had terminated 20 years after the bombing.

Frederick P. Li

DEMOGRAPHIC LEADS TO
HIGH-RISK GROUPS

18

INTERNATIONAL VARIATION IN HIGH-RISK POPULATIONS

Calum S. Muir, M.B.

International Agency for Research on Cancer
Lyon, France

INTRODUCTION

The very considerable differences in cancer levels that exist among countries and groups within a nation (high-risk groups) should be considered largely the result of environmental factors until proved otherwise. As etiological hypotheses are all too few, this axiom implies that such differences should be systematically sought, recorded, and ensuing hypotheses tested.

This chapter outlines some of the major international variations in risk that exist and how they may be used to advantage in the elucidation of etiology, indicates how comparison of national high-risk groups with those in other countries may improve understanding of pathogenesis, and suggests occasionally where control measures may be applied. This approach to environmental carcinogenesis has great potential. There is an urgent need to fill in the large gaps in our knowledge on high-risk populations at the international level, particularly for certain cancer sites.

DATA ON INTERNATIONAL CANCER RISK VARIATION

Incidence

Despite the large gaps in the cancer incidence map of the world [1], the most cursory glance at the age-adjusted cancer incidence figures contained in both volumes of the UICC monograph, *Cancer Incidence in Five Continents*

293

[2, 3], reveals that the reported incidence of cancer taken as a whole varies by a factor of around 3. When individual anatomical sites are considered, however, the differences may be more than a hundredfold (Table 1). While such extremes, which can be further accentuated by consideration of restricted age groups, are unusual, for many common sites such as breast, stomach, and cervix uteri, risk ratios of 10 to 30 obtain. Differences within regions (e.g., Western Europe or North America) are usually much less pronounced.

The incidence data published in *Cancer Incidence in Five Continents* represent a sample of the best available [4]. There are other registries, not included in the cited monograph, that have data of significance. They comprise:

1) High-quality registries that have recently started operation (e.g., New South Wales, Australia)
2) High-quality registries (e.g., Geneva, Switzerland) whose findings currently exist only in the form of reports that are not readily available [5]
3) Registries that, despite the existence of considerable underreporting for at least some sites, have convincing evidence of high risk for others (e.g., the extraordinary variation in esophageal cancer risk noted within the area covered by the Caspian Cancer Registry [6]). Knowledge of much of this additional material on incidence is not widespread; thus, publication of an annotated catalog would be of considerable value.

Mortality

An estimate can be made from mortality data for many, but by no means all, of the lacunae in cancer incidence. Segi's invaluable series contain mortality data for 24 selected countries [7]. The World Health Organization (WHO), Geneva, maintains a data bank for mortality and periodically publishes the numbers of cancer deaths by site and 10-year age group together with the populations-at-risk; however, it provides neither age-specific, crude, nor age-adjusted rates [8]. The quality of mortality figures varies; further, in areas for which neither morbidity nor mortality data are available, many of which have distinctive cultural patterns, numerous high-risk populations probably exist.

A recent detailed comparative analysis of the material in *Cancer Incidence in Five Continents* and Segi's and WHO publications is available [9].

Relative Frequency

In many parts of the world, it is unlikely that either mortality or morbidity data can be made available without considerable expense. Under such circumstances, it may be worthwhile to systematically examine the relative frequency information available in pathologists' files; Dunham and Bailar [10] collated such data in 1968. It is usually unwise to proclaim the rarity of the occurrence

TABLE 1
Range of incidence and ratio of highest to lowest[a] recorded age-adjusted
incidence rate for cancers of selected sites[b]

			Males	
ICD No.			Range of incidence	
(7th rev.)	Site[c]	Ratio	High	Low
150	Esophagus	176	Bulawayo 75.6	Vas 0.6
155.0	Liver	95	Bulawayo 47.5	Bombay 0.5
162 - 163	Bronchus, lung	72	Liverpool 86.6	Ibadan 1.2
145, 147, 148	Pharynx	53	Bombay 16.0	Norway, rural 0.3
141	Tongue	47	Bombay 14.0	Israel (Jews born in Europe) 0.3
154	Rectum	44	Saskatchewan 22.2	Ibadan 0.5
153	Colon	30	Hawaii (Chinese) 35.9	Ibadan 1.2
140	Lip	24	Newfoundland 28.6	Israel (Jews born in Africa) 1.2
177	Prostate	21	Alameda (Negro) 65.3	Israel (non-Jews) 3.1
193	Brain[d]	14	Israel (Jews born in Europe) 13.8	Ibadan 1.0
161	Larynx	13	Bombay 13.8	El Paso (non-Latin) 1.1
151	Stomach	12	Miyagi 95.3	Ibadan 8.0
181	Bladder	9	Connecticut 19.9	Bombay 2.3
157	Pancreas	8	Hawaii (Chinese) 11.8	Ibadan 1.4

TABLE 1 (Continued)

Females

ICD No. (7th rev.)[a]	Site[c]	Ratio	Range of incidence High	Low
181	Bladder	190	Rhodesia 56.9	Szabolcs Szatmar 0.3
155.0	Liver	171	Bulawayo 34.2	Norway, rural 0.2
191	Other skin	76	El Paso (Latins) 106.1	Miyagi 1.4
153	Colon	60	Saskatchewan 30.0	Bulawayo 0.5
162-163	Bronchus, lung	37	New Zealand (Maori) 37.7	Ibadan 1.0
155.1	Gallbladder	34	Bulawayo 26.9	Bombay 0.8
171	Cervix uteri	30	Bulawayo 80.1	Israel (Jews born in Israel) 2.7
194	Thyroid	30	Hawaii (Chinese) 20.7	Szabolcs Szatmar 0.7
150	Esophagus	29	South Africa (Bantu) 14.3	Katowice 0.5
193	Brain[d]	16	Israel (Jews born in Europe) 14.3	Ibadan 0.9
157	Pancreas	15	Hawaii (Hawaiian) 13.8	Ibadan 0.9
151	Stomach	11	Natal (Indians) 30.0	Nevada 2.7
172	Corpus uteri	11	New Zealand (Maori) 21.0	Ibadan 1.9
154	Rectum	9	Saskatchewan 13.6	Israel (non-Jews) 1.6
170	Breast	8	Hawaii (Caucasians) 62.9	Israel (non-Jews) 8.1
175	Ovary	6	Israel (Jews born in Europe) 15.3	Israel (non-Jews) 2.7

[a]Rates based on less than five cases are excluded. For leukemia in females the highest rate (Bulawayo) has been excluded as rate depends on a few cases aged 65-plus.
[b]Data from *Cancer Incidence in Five Continents, Volume II* [3], which contains further information about the location and characteristics of the registries. The incidence rates are adjusted to the "world" population and are per 100,000 per annum.
[c]By rank order of ratio.
[d]Some registries include benign and unspecified neoplasms.

of a particular type of cancer from relative frequency information unless a thorough study of possible bias has been made, but it is remarkable how often a high frequency has been confirmed after a cancer registry was established; to cite one example, cancer of the nasopharynx in Singapore [11].

Risk by Anatomical Subsite

Few cancer registries or national vital statistics offices publish data by fine anatomical detail, a notable exception being *Statistics Canada* [12, 13]. Such tabulations could reveal shifts in the distribution of neoplasms within a site and hence suggest differences in etiology.

Camain et al. [14] drew attention to the existence of different site and histology patterns for skin cancer in Africans, Europeans, and Asians and suggested etiological reasons.

De Jong et al. [15] looked at the distribution of subsites of large-bowel cancer in 13 cancer registries where overall risk for this disease in males varied from 5.5 to 33.2 per 100,000 per annum; they noted that irrespective of overall incidence the proportion of cancer at any subsite was much the same, a finding with which any theory of etiology must be in consonance. The pattern was one of a gradual decrease from cecum and ascending colon to transverse and descending colon with a sharp increase at the sigmoid colon, the rates for the sigmoid colon being, in turn, less than those for the rectum. Denmark had disproportionately high rates for rectal cancer in relation to the rates for sigmoid colon, which indicated that an additional causal factor probably exists. Subsequent work [16] shows that the differences observed between Denmark and Finland are unlikely to result from differences in diagnostic criteria.

The ninth revision of the *International Classification of Diseases, Injuries, and Causes of Death (ICD)* will provide finer anatomical detail than the eighth but as in previous revisions, use of the fourth digits will not be mandatory for member governments of WHO. The cancer epidemiologist cannot realistically expect publication of tabulations with large numbers of zero frequencies in the cells, and how these data can be made available to the research worker will have to be considered. Perhaps an international organization could be persuaded to maintain an appropriate catalog and data bank.

Risk by Histologic Type

For most sites, the ICD does not distinguish between the various histological types of neoplasms that may occur (choriocarcinoma and malignant melanoma of skin excepted). Conversely for the malignant lymphomas, morphology is given in considerable detail but the primary site is not.

It is now well recognized that the emergence of a hitherto unusual histologic type of cancer indicates the introduction of a new environmental carcinogen.

Recently, considerable attention has been paid to the collection, on an international basis, of rare neoplasms to determine whether the underlying cause was the same. Interest has focused on pleural and peritoneal mesothelioma (asbestos), adenocarcinoma of the vagina (diethylstilbestrol, DES), benign hepatoma of the liver (hormonal contraceptive pills), and angiosarcoma of the liver (vinyl chloride monomer).

With modern technology, the number of persons exposed in one country, let alone in one plant, to a carcinogen may be small; hence, mechanisms for the international collection of the occurrence of unusual cancer types need to be developed. The International Association of Cancer Registries has made a start in this direction on an *ad hoc* basis, but these efforts need to be systematized.

Much less attention has been paid to differences in the distribution of the more common histological types of cancer. Munoz and associates [17-19] studied the ratio of the "intestinal" and "diffuse" types of gastric cancer in populations in Norway, Connecticut, Colombia, and Israel, noting that the major differences in risk apply to the intestinal type of cancer, a fall in risk being largely the result of disappearance of this variant. The dissociation of the two types of cancer may make etiological studies easier since they may have different causes.

Volume II of *Cancer Incidence in Five Continents* [3] contains detailed information on the histological type of cancer of the testis, ovary, bladder, and thyroid, and the leukemias for several countries. Tulinius [20] noted considerable differences in the incidence of squamous and other bladder cancers (sarcoma excluded) in South Africa, America, and Europe. The predominance of squamous carcinoma in Bulawayo and Natal was expected, but the considerable differences between Birmingham and Sweden were not anticipated and may indicate, if confirmed, different etiological factors. The Cancer Registry of Sweden in its pioneer publication, *Cancer Incidence in Sweden, 1959-1965* [21] also provides such information for all cancer sites. However, neither of these publications is strictly comparable because they did not use a common coding scheme. Fortunately, WHO has agreed that the ninth revision of the ICD shall contain a comprehensive morphology code, which should do much to facilitate valid international comparison. It must be stressed that any difference that emerges must be checked by examining a sample of the material, itself a formidable undertaking.

Use of this proposed international morphology coding scheme is not mandatory, but it is hoped that at least the cancer registries will use it. Implications for the future are the availability of large bodies of data that are unlikely to merit routine publication. Thus, it is important that this material be cataloged, stored centrally, and analyzed periodically.

DISCUSSION

In general terms, international differences in cancer risk, when sizable, result from a widespread exposure in one population compared to another (e.g., the chewing of the betel quid throughout India) rather than to high-risk groups (such as radium ore miners) within one of the countries under comparison.

Intercountry Differences

Even crude comparison can, if soundly based, be of great etiological significance. Thus, Kennaway [22], comparing primary liver cancer in the Bantu population of Africa and in blacks in the United States, concluded that: " .... the very high incidence of primary cancer of the liver found among Negroes in Africa does not appear in Negroes in the United States of America, and is therefore not of a purely racial character. Hence, the prevalence of this form of cancer in Africans may be due to some extrinsic factor, which could be identified." The report on high-risk migrant groups given at this workshop underscores the truth of this conclusion.

While primary liver cancer is not currently a problem in Occidental societies, there is evidence that it may become so. Thus, in Geneva, Switzerland, an age-adjusted incidence rate of 9 per 100,000 per annum was recorded for males [23]. It is of some importance for cancer control to determine whether this increase results from an increased survival of persons with alcohol-related cirrhosis or to other causes such as postnecrotic scarring following infectious hepatitis or the import of aflatoxin-contaminated foodstuffs. Some of these questions can probably best be answered, at a time when the disease is still infrequent in the Occident, by study in areas where suspected causal agents and the cancer are common. In Kenya, Peers and Linsell [24] showed that aflatoxin consumption parallels the incidence of primary liver cancer. The study is open to criticism on the grounds that aflatoxin ingestion and primary liver cancer were estimated contemporaneously, but conditions as far as *Aspergillus flavus* contamination is concerned probably have not changed much over the past 20 years.

In West Africa, where high levels of primary liver cancer have been recorded, the prevalence of hepatitis B antigen (HBAg) in the blood is around 9 percent in the general population [25], in contrast to 40 to 50 percent in patients with primary liver cancer and around 1 percent in Occidental populations. A prospective study of a population of known high aflatoxin consumption and high HBAg levels would resolve the question.

The Kenya study showed that in an area where the daily aflatoxin intake was 4.9 and 3.5 nanograms per kilogram of body weight, the recorded incidence of primary liver cancer was 3.1 per 100,000 in males and nil in females, respectively. Such information is of great value when one attempts to set rational permissible limits for aflatoxin, not only for foods imported from Africa but in the protein supplements given to malnourished African children. These supplements have been withheld because, being contaminated with aflatoxin, they might cause cancer in later life.

The recent rise in esophageal cancer in the U.S. black population [26] may be the result of increased use of alcohol and tobacco; on the other hand, the rise may be caused by a hitherto unsuspected risk factor. This factor may be uncovered in the current studies in Iran where, despite a very high incidence of this cancer in both sexes, alcohol and tobacco use are of little significance [27]. Appropriate control measures then can be instituted.

The flow of information is not all one way. The developing countries have much to learn about industrial hazards uncovered elsewhere.

The existence of differences in risk between countries is a valuable check on hypotheses emerging from one population. The finding by MacMahon and his colleagues [28, 29] that breast cancer risk is influenced by the age at first full-time pregnancy is all the more impressive when it was reproduced in seven countries. The demonstration that the degree of protection varied from population to population shows that this factor is not the only one in the genesis of the disease. The repeated demonstration that lung cancer is linked with cigarette smoking strengthens the hypothesis, so much so that the discovery that half of the lung cancers in Singapore Cantonese women occur in nonsmokers [30] can today only be interpreted as indicating the existence of another causal agent. The sequential introduction of a new environmental hazard should be mirrored in the incidence time trends for the exposed population; if not, the agent cannot be the sole factor involved.

International Comparison of High-Risk Groups

The comparison of the experience of international high-risk groups has yielded significant information on risk factors. Thus, the risks associated with exposure in chrysotile mines and mills in Canada, crocidolite and amosite mines in South Africa, and anthophyllite mines in Finland were reviewed in a series of papers in the IARC publication, *Biological Effects of Asbestos* [31]. This evidence and other data suggest that crocidolite is the most dangerous fiber. Without international study of national high-risk groups, it would have been exceedingly difficult to reach this conclusion; without further international study, it is unlikely that accurate assessment of the cancer risk following exposure to only one type of fiber will be feasible.

The large international differences in lung cancer incidence are well known. It is now accepted that they result in large part from the differences in the amount of tobacco, notably cigarettes, smoked. Nevertheless, there appear to be differences in the carcinogenicity of the various smokes. International comparative studies of high-risk groups (cigarette smokers) of the type undertaken in

Finland and Norway [32] may identify the responsible factors. Black tobacco used in France, Spain, and Italy may be less carcinogenic for the lung than the blonde types—a point that could be resolved by international comparison. However, it would be a disservice to examine lung cancer in isolation, since black tobaccos may be responsible for the increased levels of laryngeal cancer found in the countries mentioned.

The value of such studies can be enhanced immensely if a common protocol is followed (taking into account local variation) by a group of investigators who meet regularly to standardize procedures. Regrettably, judgment often has to be made from data collected in a noncomparable fashion.

SUGGESTIONS FOR FUTURE WORK

Table 2 lists the problems of cancer epidemiology considered to need the most urgent attention. Comments on each problem area stress that for nearly all the sites considered there *still* exist major differences in risk throughout the world, differences that for the most part await exploitation and explanation in terms of environmental carcinogens.

As stated earlier, there are large areas of the world for which no information on cancer risk is available; further, data for nearly all countries on anatomical subsite and histologic type are lacking. Even if this information should become available, it would be useless unless examined. Thus, there is a need for a body to collate and publish existing data, to fill the gaps systematically, and to analyze the material drawing attention to interesting high-risk groups.

Yet if all this information became available, it would swamp us; there are not enough epidemiologists available to exploit present opportunities. Perhaps the training of chronic disease epidemiologists should be accorded top priority.

IMPLICATIONS FOR CANCER CONTROL

The implications for cancer control of the existence of international variations in high-risk populations lie in their utilization to elucidate etiology: without knowledge of cause there can be no rational prevention.

TABLE 2

Priority areas for etiological research utilizing
international risk differentials

Site	Comments
Esophagus	Vast esophageal cancer belt stretches across Central Asia, from east Turkey to north China; problem in East Africa and Transkei of South Africa, U.S. blacks, France, and Switzerland
Stomach	Disappearing in U.S. and Western Europe. Still a major problem in Eastern Europe, U.S.S.R., Japan, and Latin America
Large bowel	Increasing in industrialized societies but still rare in much of the world
Liver	Major problem in Africa and Southeast Asia; possible increase in Europe
Pancreas	Probably increasing in industrial societies
Larynx, hypopharynx	Larynx increasing in Western Europe and cancer of both sites a major problem in Assam, Burma, north Thailand, and Egypt
Breast	Increasing in Occidental populations and probably in populations that now have comparatively low incidence
Cervix uteri	Very common in Asia, Latin America, and Africa
Prostate	Now the most frequent cancer in Sweden but still rare in China and Japan; will become increasingly common as populations age

REFERENCES

1. Muir, C.S. Geographical differences in cancer patterns. *In* Doll, R., Vodopija, I., eds. *Host Environment Interactions in the Etiology of Cancer in Man.* I.A.R.C. Scientific Publications No. 7. I.A.R.C., Lyon, 1973.

2. Doll, R., Payne, P., and Waterhouse, J., eds. U.I.C.C. *Cancer Incidence in Five Continents. A Technical Report.* Springer-Verlag, Berlin, 1966.

3. Doll, R., Muir, C.S., and Waterhouse, J., eds. U.I.C.C. *Cancer Incidence in Five Continents.* Vol. II. Springer-Verlag, Berlin, 1970.

4. Tuyns, A.J. Techniques of registration. *In* Doll, R., Muir, C.S., and Waterhouse, J., eds. U.I.C.C. *Cancer Incidence in Five Continents.* Vol. II. Springer-Verlag, Berlin, 1970, pp. 5-8.

5. Riotton, G., and Raymond, L. *Incidence du cancer à Genève 1970/1971.* Registre Genevois des Tumeurs, Geneva, 1974.

6. Mahboubi, E., Kmet, J., Cook, P.J., et al. Oesophageal cancer studies in the Caspian littoral of Iran: The Caspian Cancer Registry. *Br. J. Cancer 28:*197-214, 1973.

7. Segi, M., and Kurihara, M. *Cancer Mortality for Selected Sites in 24 Countries. No. 6 (1966-1967).* Japan Cancer Society, Tokyo, 1972.

8. World Health Organization. *Mortality from Malignant Neoplasms, 1955-1965. Number of Deaths by Site, Sex and Age.* Vols. I and II. W.H.O., Geneva, 1970.

9. Muir, C.S., Nectoux, J., and Hansluwka, H. *Cancer Morbidity and Mortality Statistics. [Comparison of material published by W.H.O., Segi, and Kurihara and Cancer Incidence in Five Continents.]* I.A.R.C., Lyon, 1975.

10. Dunham, L.J., and Bailar, J.C. World maps of cancer mortality rates and frequency ratios. *J. Natl. Cancer Inst. 41:*155-203, 1968.

11. Muir, C.S. Nasopharyngeal carcinoma in non-Chinese populations with special reference to Southeast Asia and Africa. *Int. J. Cancer 8:*351-363, 1971.

12. Statistics Canada. *New Primary Sites of Malignant Neoplasms in Canada, 1971.* Catalogue 82-207. Information Canada, Ottawa, 1973.

13. Statistics Canada. *Causes of Death. Provinces by Sex and Canada by Age and Sex. Detailed Categories of the International Classification of Diseases, Adapted – I.C.D.A. 1973.* Catalogue 84-203. Information Canada, Ottawa, 1974.

14. Camain, P., Tuyns, A.J., Sarrat, H., et al. Cutaneous cancer in Dakar. *J. Natl. Cancer Inst. 48:*33-49, 1972.

15. de Jong, U.W., Day, N.E., Muir, C.S., et al. The distribution of cancer within the large bowel. *Int. J. Cancer 10:*463-477, 1972.

16. Jensen, O.M., Mosbech, J., Salaspuro, M., et al. A comparative study of the diagnostic basis for cancer of the colon and rectum in Denmark and Finland. *Int. J. Epidemiol. 3:*183-186, 1974.

17. Munoz, N., Correa, P., Cuello, C., et al. Histologic types of gastric carcinoma in high- and low-risk areas. *Int. J. Cancer 3:*809-818, 1968.

18. Munoz, N., and Connelly, R. Time trends of intestinal and diffuse types of gastric cancer in the United States. *Int. J. Cancer 8:*158-164, 1971.

19. Munoz, N., and Steinitz, R. Comparative histology of gastric cancer in migrant groups in Israel. *Israel J. Med. Sci.* 7:1479-1487, 1971.

20. Tulinius, H. Frequency of some morphological types of neoplasms of five sites. *In* Doll, R., Muir, C.S., and Waterhouse, J., eds. U.I.C.C. *Cancer Incidence in Five Continents.* Vol. II. Springer-Verlag, Berlin, 1970, pp. 23-83.

21. National Board of Health and Welfare. *Cancer Incidence in Sweden, 1959-1965.* Stockholm, 1971, pp. 76-81.

22. Kennaway, E.L. Cancer of the liver of the Negro in Africa and America. *Cancer Res.* 4:571-577, 1944.

23. Tuyns, A.J., and Obradovic, M. Unexpected high incidence of primary liver cancer in Geneva. *J. Natl. Cancer Inst.* 54:61-64, 1975.

24. Peers, F.G., and Linsell, C.A. Dietary aflatoxins and liver cancer – a population-based study in Kenya. *Br. J. Cancer* 27:473-484, 1973.

25. Tuyns, A.J., Rive, J., Zuckermann, A., et al. Prevalence de l'antigène de l'hépatite B dans une population rurale en Côte d'Ivoire. *Med. Afr. Noire* 21:507-512, 1974.

26. Cutler, S.J., and Devesa, S.S. Trends in cancer incidence and mortality in the USA. *In* Doll, R., Vodopija, I., eds. *Host Environment Interactions in the Etiology of Cancer in Man.* I.A.R.C. Scientific Publications No. 7. I.A.R.C., Lyon, 1973, pp. 15-34.

27. Kmet, J., and Mahboubi, E. Esophageal cancer studies in the Caspian Littoral of Iran. Initial observations. *Science* 175:846-853, 1972.

28. MacMahon, B., Cole, P., Lin, T.M., et al. Age at first birth and breast cancer risk. *Bull. W.H.O.* 43:209-221, 1970.

29. MacMahon, B., Cole, P., Lin, T.M., et al. Lactation and cancer of the breast. *Bull. W.H.O.* 43:185-194, 1970.

30. MacLennan, R.M., da Costa, J., Day, N.E., et al. Etiological factors in lung cancer in Singapore Chinese. *In Proceedings of the 11th International Cancer Congress.* Excerpta Medica, Int. Congr. Ser. In press, 1975.

31. Bogowski, P., Gilson, J.C., Timbrill, V., et al. *Biological Effects of Asbestos.* I.A.R.C. Scientific Publication No. 8. I.A.R.C., Lyon, 1973.

32. Pedersen, E., Magnus, K., Mork, T., et al. Lung cancer in Finland and Norway. An epidemiological study. *Acta Pathol. Microbiol. Scand. Suppl. 199*:1-74, 1969.

DISCUSSION

Dr. **Hirayama** recommended further studies of international variation in cancer. He suggested that attention be paid to high-risk groups in areas of generally low risk, such as groups prone to stomach cancer in the United States. Around the world there are "belts'" of countries with similar cancer patterns, and these countries should be considered jointly, rather than individually, for epidemiologic studies. On the other hand, Dr. **Hirayama** noted the etiologic importance of within-country variations, such as differences in the risk of nasopharyngeal cancer between north and south China and in the risk of stomach cancer between Okinawa and Japan's main islands. International comparisons should not involve cancer alone but also diseases related to cancer. Finally, he felt we should not ignore the dynamic aspects of cancer, namely, the temporal changes in incidence and mortality that carry important implications for cancer etiology and control.

During his presentation, Dr. **Muir** commented that his agency, the IARC, could do more with increased support. Dr. **S. Cutler** questioned whether additional staffing or funding was required; if the former, how could the supply of people be increased? Dr. **Muir** answered that the agency needed both, but offered no solution to the problem of recruitment.

Dr. **Saffiotti** emphasized the need to define population exposures more accurately, and cited the collaborative efforts between the IARC and the National Cancer Institute to assess the carcinogenicity of a large number of chemicals. He stressed the need to document new occupational exposures to potential carcinogens, since the excess risk of cancer may follow by many years the development of the industry. By way of example, **Dr. Saffiotti** traced the history of aromatic amine production in western Europe. He noted that several governments have stopped production of aromatic amines, suggesting that this experience be used in taking corrective actions elsewhere.

William J. Blot

19

DEMOGRAPHIC PATTERNS OF CANCER INCIDENCE IN THE UNITED STATES

Sidney J. Cutler, Sc.D., and John L. Young, Jr., Dr. P.H.

Biometry Branch, National Cancer Institute
Bethesda, Maryland

The Third National Cancer Survey, organized by the National Cancer Institute, provides updated information on the incidence of cancer in the United States and variation in incidence by race, sex, and geographic area. The first survey provided data for the period 1937-1939,[1] the second for 1947-1948. No survey was conducted during the 1950's.

In planning the third survey, it was decided to collect data in each geographic area for the 3-year calendar period 1969-1971. Collection of data for a full 3-year period in each area was undertaken to obtain enough cases to allow meaningful comparisons of cancer incidence among various segments of the population, particularly for the less common forms of cancer. This 3-year period made possible direct use of detailed population data from the 1970 census.

This chapter provides data on the annual incidence rate of cancer among male and female members of the white and black populations of the United States, and on the variation in incidence among the seven metropolitan areas and two entire states included in the survey (Table 1). The data are not grouped into broad geographic regions such as North or South; rather, for the nine survey areas, the data are presented in a sequence that suggests a regional concept.

---

[1] Data were collected for 1 calendar year in each of the 10 survey areas, but different years were covered in different areas.

TABLE 1

Populations of survey areas by race and sex, 1970

All areas	Total[a]	White males	White females	Black males	Black females
Detroit	4,199,931	1,673,124	1,746,596	362,846	394,237
Pittsburgh	2,401,245	1,066,036	1,158,985	79,815	90,069
Atlanta	1,390,164	523,949	552,194	144,338	166,294
Birmingham	739,274	248,586	272,050	100,396	117,051
Dallas-Ft. Worth	2,318,036	959,262	1,012,509	156,332	173,363
Iowa	2,824,376	1,352,567	1,430,195	15,958	16,638
Minneapolis-St. Paul	1,813,647	849,551	914,218	15,984	16,134
Colorado	2,207,259	1,041,364	1,070,988	34,047	32,364
San Francisco-Oakland	3,109,519	1,256,291	1,318,511	160,984	169,123

[a]Includes other races.

The observed variation in the incidence of cancer in individual organ sites by sex, race, and geographic area provides one approach to the identification of groups at both high and low risk. Such information is useful in planning the targeting of cancer control programs and as a source of clues for epidemiologic research.

METHODS

In each area, a local, medically oriented, nonprofit organization such as a Department of Health or School of Public Health carried out the survey. The staff of each field office identified cases and abstracted information from hospital charts, pathology reports, autopsy reports, radiotherapy records, outpatient clinic records, cancer registries, and medical record indices. Copies of all death certificates that mentioned cancer were obtained from state offices of vital statistics. Almost all death certificates were traced to hospital or other medical records to confirm the date and the accuracy of the diagnosis. Medical records provided the information in 97.9 percent of the cases. The remaining 2.1 percent were identified from death certificates only. Periodic reviews of case finding, including rechecking all sources within each hospital, were carried out in each field office to insure completeness of reporting.

The tumor type and site are coded according to the *Manual of Tumor Nomenclature and Coding* (American Cancer Society, 1968). Selected histologies, such as carcinoids and tumors not specified as benign or malignant and carcinoma in situ, were reportable but were not included in routine tabulations. Over 90 percent of all cancers were microscopically confirmed.

The abstracts were reviewed for compatibility of such items as site/sex, site/histologic type, and birth date/age. All the documents for each individual were compared for consistency of birth date, age, race, sex, primary site, histologic type, and date of diagnosis. Wherever possible, the comparison was done by computer. Duplicate cases were identified by both manual operations in the field offices as well as by computer. All records for an individual were then consolidated.

FINDINGS

There were 281,056 active cases reported for the 3-year period 1969-71. Of this number, 41,709 were not residents of the areas under study, and 58,230 of the resident patients had been diagnosed in an earlier year. Subtracting these cases leaves a total of 181,027 newly diagnosed resident cases. The annual crude incidence rate of invasive cancer (excluding nonmelanoma skin cancers) among the residents of the survey areas was 287.3 per 100,000 population.

To facilitate comparison of cancer risk by sex, race, and geographic area, the calculated incidence rates were all adjusted to the U.S. age distribution in 1950. The year 1950 was selected as a standard to permit comparison with a sizable body of previously published data.

Figures 1 through 14 show the average annual cancer incidence rates for the period 1969-1971 by race, sex, and geographic area. The 95 percent confidence interval is shown for each rate. As shown in Figure 1 and Tables 2 through 6, the highest rate for all cancers combined was observed among black males (354 invasive cancers per 100,000 population per year), followed by white males (301), white females (252), and black females (243). This wide range, in which the highest rate is 50% higher than the lowest, reflects a different mix of sites in which cancer occurs in males and females and differences in the incidence of specific forms of cancer in the white and black populations.

In Figures 1 through 14, rates are presented for all nine survey areas for white persons. For the black population, rates are shown only for six of the nine areas. The excluded areas, Iowa, Minneapolis-St. Paul, and Colorado, all have small black populations; thus, the calculated rates are based on small numbers of cases and are subject to wide variation.

Within a race-sex group, the variation in reported incidence of all cancers combined is moderate. Nevertheless, the relative position of an area with respect to the total incidence of cancer provides a useful frame of reference for assessing its relative position with respect to the incidence of cancer in an individual site.

The figures present age-adjusted rates for all cancers and for a selected number of primary sites and histologic types, which account for 80 percent of all the cancers identified in the survey. The selected sites, by organ system are:

Digestive	Stomach, colon, rectum
Respiratory	Lung
Reproductive	Breast, uterine cervix,[1] uterine corpus, ovary, prostate
Urinary	Bladder, kidney
Skin	Melanoma only
Hematopoietic	Lymphoma, leukemia

These figures are supplemented by Tables 2 through 6 which show age-adjusted rates for 52 specific sites and types of cancer and for 12 organ systems.

Stomach (Figure 2)

The incidence of stomach cancer is markedly higher in males than in females and in blacks than in whites. As previously reported [1,2] the incidence of stomach cancer has been decreasing among both blacks and whites, but the rate of decrease has been slower among blacks.

[1] Data are presented for in situ as well as for invasive cancers of the uterine cervix.

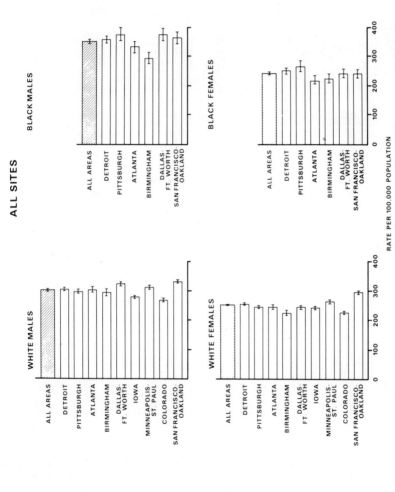

FIGURE 1. All sites: Average annual cancer incidence rates, by race, sex and geographic area.

311

TABLE 2

Age adjusted (1950 standard) cancer incidence rates[a] by site and by area: all races, both sexes Third National Cancer Survey 1969-1971

	All areas	Detroit SMSA[b]	Pittsburgh SMSA	Atlanta SMSA	Birmingham SMSA	Dallas/ Ft. Worth SMSA	State of Iowa	Minneapolis/ St. Paul SMSA	State of Colorado	San Francisco/ Oakland SMSA
All sites	272.4	277.1	269.9	263.3	251.6	275.8	255.5	281.1	247.1	300.3
Buccal cavity & pharynx	10.0	9.1	8.8	10.0	8.6	15.2	8.9	8.6	7.6	12.6
Lip	1.7	0.6	0.1	1.2	1.5	5.2	2.8	1.5	1.9	1.4
Tongue	1.9	2.0	2.1	2.3	2.0	2.2	1.2	1.7	1.3	2.3
Salivary gland	1.0	0.9	0.9	1.2	0.8	1.3	1.0	0.9	0.9	1.3
Gum & mouth	2.6	2.5	2.9	2.6	2.3	3.3	2.0	2.3	1.6	3.3
Nasopharynx	0.5	0.6	0.5	0.6	0.3	0.5	0.4	0.2	0.4	1.0
Tonsil	1.0	1.1	1.0	1.0	0.7	1.0	0.6	0.9	0.6	1.6
Other pharynx	1.3	1.4	1.2	1.2	1.0	1.6	1.0	1.0	0.8	1.7
Digestive system	65.9	70.4	71.1	57.2	53.4	58.6	62.5	70.8	54.7	73.6
Esophagus	3.0	3.8	3.4	3.8	2.9	2.8	2.0	2.7	1.7	3.8
Stomach	8.9	10.2	10.6	6.9	7.4	7.1	7.3	9.1	7.1	10.5
Small intestine	0.9	0.9	0.7	0.6	0.7	0.9	1.1	1.2	0.8	0.9
Colon excluding rectum	26.6	27.0	27.8	24.8	21.2	22.7	28.1	30.1	22.7	28.3
Transverse colon	4.3	4.6	3.8	4.2	3.4	3.6	4.3	4.6	3.7	5.1
Descending colon	2.4	2.4	2.6	2.4	2.6	2.1	2.3	2.5	1.8	2.5
Sigmoid colon	9.2	9.5	9.7	9.1	6.0	7.3	9.9	9.5	8.0	10.5
Cecum	4.7	4.7	4.1	4.0	3.3	4.2	4.8	6.9	4.2	5.0
Appendix	0.3	0.2	0.2	0.4	0.2	0.4	0.2	0.2	0.2	0.3
Ascending colon	3.5	3.7	3.1	3.4	2.9	3.5	3.5	3.7	2.7	3.9
Large intestine NOS[c]	2.3	1.9	4.4	1.2	2.8	1.6	3.1	2.7	2.1	0.9
Rectum & rectosigmoid	12.0	13.1	13.9	8.5	7.6	10.7	11.8	13.1	8.8	13.5
Rectosigmoid junction	3.4	3.6	3.6	2.1	2.3	3.3	3.3	3.3	2.7	4.4
Rectum	8.6	9.5	10.3	6.4	5.3	7.4	8.5	9.7	6.1	9.2
Liver	2.0	2.1	2.1	1.8	2.3	2.0	1.4	1.5	1.6	2.8
Gallbladder	1.4	1.7	1.9	0.8	0.7	0.6	1.5	1.9	1.6	1.1
Other biliary	1.1	1.2	0.9	0.7	0.7	1.3	0.9	1.2	1.2	1.4
Pancreas	8.4	8.8	8.1	7.9	8.8	9.1	7.0	8.3	8.1	9.2
Retroperitoneum	0.7	0.8	0.7	0.7	0.3	0.7	0.7	0.8	0.6	1.1
Other digestive organs	0.9	0.8	0.9	0.8	0.8	0.8	0.7	0.8	0.6	1.1
Respiratory system	41.9	44.9	43.6	43.5	46.1	47.8	34.8	36.0	32.3	47.1
Larynx	3.9	4.4	4.3	4.1	3.9	3.9	3.2	3.6	3.2	4.3
Lung, bronchus, trachea	36.9	39.5	38.4	38.1	40.9	42.8	30.8	31.4	28.4	41.6
Other respiratory organs	1.0	1.0	0.9	1.3	1.3	1.1	0.7	1.0	0.7	1.3
Bones & joints	0.7	0.7	1.0	0.7	0.8	0.6	0.7	0.7	0.6	0.9
Soft tissue	1.9	1.8	1.8	2.0	1.7	2.3	1.6	2.1	2.1	2.1
Melanoma skin	4.2	2.8	2.9	5.5	4.4	7.1	3.3	3.5	5.2	5.2
Breast	38.4	37.7	36.9	37.3	31.8	35.7	37.0	42.5	37.1	43.6
Female genital system	29.4	30.3	27.8	30.0	30.3	28.3	29.2	31.3	25.8	31.5
Cervix	9.1	9.9	8.1	10.2	15.1	10.6	9.3	9.0	7.0	7.5
Corpus	10.3	10.9	9.9	8.8	7.1	8.3	9.5	10.9	9.3	13.9
Uterus NOS	1.2	1.2	1.6	1.9	0.7	0.8	1.7	1.1	1.1	0.9
Ovary	7.2	6.8	6.7	7.2	5.3	7.1	7.5	8.5	7.2	7.4
Vagina	0.3	0.3	0.2	0.4	0.5	0.3	0.3	0.3	0.2	0.4
Vulva	0.9	0.8	0.9	1.2	1.3	0.9	0.8	1.2	0.7	0.8
Other female genital	0.3	0.3	0.3	0.4	0.4	0.3	0.3	0.3	0.3	0.5

TABLE 2 (Continued)

	All areas	Detroit SMSA[b]	Pittsburgh SMSA	Atlanta SMSA	Birmingham SMSA	Dallas/ Ft. Worth SMSA	State of Iowa	Minneapolis/ St. Paul SMSA	State of Colorado	San Francisco/ Oakland SMSA
Male genital	22.5	22.5	18.9	23.4	22.9	22.3	21.4	24.0	26.4	23.5
Prostate	20.4	20.6	17.0	21.5	21.6	20.3	19.1	21.7	24.2	20.8
Testis	1.6	1.4	1.4	1.4	0.9	1.3	1.9	1.8	1.9	2.2
Penis	0.4	0.4	0.4	0.5	0.3	0.5	0.4	0.4	0.3	0.4
Other male genital	0.1	0.1	0.1	0.0	...	0.1	0.1	0.0	0.1	0.1
Urinary system	17.5	18.9	17.9	14.1	12.7	15.6	16.7	19.5	18.3	18.4
Bladder	11.4	12.4	12.7	8.4	8.0	9.0	10.8	11.6	12.3	12.3
Kidney, renal pelvis	5.5	5.9	4.7	5.0	4.1	5.8	5.4	7.4	5.3	5.5
Other urinary	0.6	0.6	0.4	0.6	0.6	0.7	0.5	0.6	0.6	0.6
Eye & orbit	0.8	0.7	0.7	0.6	0.6	1.2	0.7	0.8	0.8	0.9
Brain & other nervous system	4.9	4.6	4.2	5.4	4.7	4.7	4.6	5.8	4.4	5.8
Brain	4.5	4.1	3.8	4.9	4.3	4.4	4.3	5.4	3.9	5.4
Other nervous system	0.4	0.5	0.4	0.6	0.4	0.4	0.3	0.5	0.5	0.4
Endocrine system	4.2	4.1	3.3	3.6	3.3	4.4	3.2	4.0	4.9	5.5
Thyroid	3.7	3.6	3.1	3.1	3.1	4.0	2.8	3.5	4.6	5.0
Other endocrine	0.4	0.5	0.2	0.6	0.2	0.4	0.4	0.5	-0.4	0.5
Lymphomas	9.2	8.7	8.5	7.6	8.6	9.2	10.1	10.4	7.9	10.3
Lymphosarcoma & RCS	4.4	4.1	3.5	3.4	4.6	4.6	4.9	4.4	4.4	5.2
Hodgkin's disease	3.2	3.0	3.6	2.7	2.0	3.0	3.4	3.6	2.5	3.6
Other lymphoma	1.6	1.6	1.4	1.5	1.9	1.6	1.8	2.4	1.1	1.5
Multiple myeloma	3.1	3.1	2.9	3.5	3.3	3.4	2.8	3.6	2.9	3.2
Leukemia	8.7	8.4	8.6	8.3	6.9	9.7	9.6	9.3	8.6	7.8
Acute lymphocytic	1.1	0.6	1.3	1.2	1.0	1.3	1.6	0.9	1.1	1.2
Chronic lymphocytic	2.2	2.0	2.0	2.0	1.5	2.4	2.9	2.6	1.9	1.7
Other lymphocytic	0.3	0.2	0.2	0.3	0.3	0.3	0.4	0.5	0.4	0.3
Acute granulocytic	2.1	1.9	2.3	2.5	1.0	2.7	1.7	2.2	2.2	2.3
Chronic granulocytic	1.3	1.4	1.2	1.1	1.1	1.5	1.4	1.6	1.4	1.0
Other granulocytic	0.5	0.4	0.4	0.1	0.5	0.7	0.4	0.8	0.6	0.4
Monocytic leukemia	0.3	0.5	0.2	0.4	0.4	0.1	0.5	0.2	0.2	0.2
Other acute leukemia	0.4	0.9	0.7	0.3	0.2	0.3	0.2	0.1	0.3	0.4
Other chronic leukemia	0.0	...	0.0	...	0.0	0.0	0.0	...	0.0	0.0
Other leukemia	0.4	0.4	0.4	0.4	0.3	0.7	0.4	0.5	0.4	0.3
Unknown	9.1	8.4	11.2	10.7	11.5	9.8	8.6	8.2	7.4	8.4

[a]Excluding carcinoma in situ and nonmelanoma skin cancer. Organ specific lymphomas are distributed among the sites.
[b]SMSA = Standard Metropolitan Statistical Area.
[c]NOS = Not Otherwise Specific.

TABLE 3

Age-adjusted (1950 standard) cancer incidence rates[a] by site and by area: white male
Third National Cancer Survey 1969-1971

	All areas	Detroit SMSA[b]	Pittsburgh SMSA	Atlanta SMSA	Birmingham SMSA	Dallas/ Ft. Worth SMSA	State of Iowa	Minneapolis/ St. Paul SMSA	State of Colorado	San Francisco/ Oakland SMSA
All sites	300.9	302.9	298.9	303.9	293.7	321.4	278.8	310.9	268.1	330.1
Buccal cavity & pharynx	15.8	14.1	14.3	17.3	16.8	26.1	14.6	13.2	11.4	18.1
Lip	3.8	1.5	0.3	2.8	3.8	11.5	5.9	3.0	3.9	2.8
Tongue	2.9	3.0	3.6	3.2	4.3	3.5	1.6	2.8	1.9	3.6
Salivary gland	1.2	0.9	1.0	1.7	0.9	1.6	1.0	1.3	1.2	1.3
Gum & mouth	3.6	3.7	4.8	4.0	3.7	4.0	2.8	3.0	1.9	4.4
Nasopharynx	0.7	0.8	0.8	1.1	0.4	1.0	0.6	0.3	0.7	0.8
Tonsil	1.5	1.8	1.6	1.7	1.4	1.6	0.9	1.2	0.9	2.4
Other pharynx	2.2	2.4	2.3	2.8	2.2	2.9	1.8	1.6	1.1	2.9
Digestive system	78.2	84.5	86.3	64.8	57.7	67.9	72.5	88.4	63.5	88.6
Esophagus	4.1	4.6	5.0	4.3	3.2	3.5	3.3	4.6	2.9	4.7
Stomach	12.0	13.5	14.5	7.4	7.6	9.2	10.4	13.3	10.1	14.2
Small intestine	1.1	1.1	0.7	0.9	0.6	1.0	1.4	1.9	0.9	1.1
Colon excluding rectum	28.5	30.0	31.3	26.7	21.1	23.2	28.1	33.2	22.6	31.7
Transverse colon	4.4	4.7	3.9	5.2	3.3	4.1	4.0	5.2	3.3	5.8
Descending colon	2.5	2.4	2.8	2.2	2.0	2.0	2.5	2.9	1.5	3.0
Sigmoid colon	10.5	11.2	11.5	9.6	6.7	7.5	11.4	10.5	8.8	11.6
Cecum	4.9	5.0	4.4	4.9	4.0	4.3	4.1	8.0	4.1	5.6
Appendix	0.2	0.3	0.2	0.2	0.2	0.3	0.2	0.2	0.2	0.3
Ascending colon	3.5	4.2	3.4	3.5	2.6	3.4	3.0	3.7	2.7	4.1
Large intestine NOS[c]	2.5	2.1	5.2	1.1	2.5	1.7	2.9	2.7	1.9	1.3
Rectum & rectosigmoid	15.5	18.0	17.6	11.3	9.5	13.3	14.7	17.7	11.1	16.9
Rectosigmoid junction	4.3	5.0	4.2	2.9	2.8	4.5	3.9	4.4	3.4	5.5
Rectum	11.2	13.0	13.3	8.3	6.6	8.8	10.8	13.3	7.7	11.5
Liver	2.6	2.9	3.2	2.4	2.6	2.6	1.8	2.2	2.0	3.3
Gallbladder	0.9	1.1	1.3	0.4	0.1	0.3	0.9	1.6	0.9	0.8
Other biliary	1.4	1.5	1.1	0.9	0.9	1.8	1.2	1.7	1.5	1.8
Pancreas	10.5	10.2	10.2	9.4	11.3	11.3	9.5	10.9	10.0	11.9
Retroperitoneum	0.8	0.9	0.7	0.8	0.4	0.8	0.6	1.0	0.7	1.2
Other digestive organs	0.7	0.8	0.7	0.5	0.4	0.8	0.6	0.4	0.7	1.1
Respiratory system	73.2	77.1	76.0	82.4	93.5	87.8	63.6	65.2	56.4	78.4
Larynx	7.5	8.4	8.0	8.0	8.9	8.0	6.4	6.9	5.8	8.2
Lung, bronchus, trachea	64.3	67.3	66.8	72.3	82.9	78.2	56.2	56.9	49.6	68.4
Other respiratory organs	1.4	1.3	1.3	2.0	1.7	1.7	1.1	1.4	1.0	1.8
Bones & joints	0.9	0.8	1.2	0.7	0.9	0.7	0.8	0.9	0.7	1.1
Soft tissue	2.2	1.9	2.1	2.2	1.6	2.9	1.6	2.3	2.2	2.6
Melanoma skin	4.7	3.1	3.0	6.5	6.1	8.3	3.6	3.6	5.5	5.7
Breast	0.7	0.9	0.8	0.6	0.6	0.5	0.5	0.4	0.3	0.8
Male genital	50.6	46.2	41.9	54.8	47.8	49.3	49.3	59.0	58.7	55.4
Prostate	45.9	41.9	37.5	50.2	44.8	45.3	44.4	54.1	54.1	49.3
Testis	3.7	3.4	3.2	3.5	2.3	3.0	4.0	3.7	3.8	5.1
Penis	0.8	0.9	1.0	1.0	0.7	0.8	0.8	1.1	0.6	0.8
Other male genital	0.2	0.1	0.2	0.1	...	0.2	0.1	0.1	0.2	0.2

TABLE 3 (Continued)

	All areas	Detroit SMSA[b]	Pittsburgh SMSA	Atlanta SMSA	Birmingham SMSA	Dallas/ Ft. Worth SMSA	State of Iowa	Minneapolis/ St. Paul SMSA	State of Colorado	San Francisco/ Oakland SMSA
Urinary system	28.9	31.6	28.6	25.4	23.1	26.4	27.3	30.1	29.5	30.4
Bladder	20.3	22.6	21.8	16.5	16.5	16.8	18.7	19.5	21.1	21.6
Kidney, renal pelvis	7.8	8.1	6.3	7.9	5.4	8.6	7.8	9.8	7.6	8.0
Other urinary	0.8	0.9	0.5	1.0	1.3	1.0	0.8	0.7	0.8	0.8
Eye & orbit	0.9	1.0	0.6	0.8	1.0	1.3	0.7	0.6	0.9	0.9
Brain & other nervous system	5.8	5.4	5.3	7.9	6.9	6.1	5.1	6.6	5.1	6.8
Brain	5.4	5.0	4.9	7.3	6.3	5.8	4.8	6.2	4.6	6.5
Other nervous system	0.4	0.4	0.4	0.6	0.6	0.3	0.3	0.4	0.5	0.3
Endocrine system	2.7	2.4	1.8	2.7	1.1	3.8	2.0	2.1	2.8	4.2
Thyroid	2.2	2.0	1.6	1.9	0.6	3.0	1.6	1.6	2.6	3.5
Other endocrine system	0.5	0.4	0.2	0.8	0.5	0.7	0.5	0.5	0.3	0.7
Lymphomas	11.4	10.7	9.9	9.9	13.2	12.0	12.1	12.8	9.4	13.6
Lymphosarcoma	5.4	4.9	4.1	4.3	7.0	6.2	5.6	5.3	5.2	6.7
Hodgkin's disease	4.0	3.7	4.3	3.4	3.4	4.0	4.2	4.5	3.0	4.9
Other lymphomas	2.0	2.1	1.5	2.3	2.8	1.8	2.3	3.0	1.2	2.0
Multiple myeloma	3.4	3.0	3.6	3.0	2.9	4.0	3.1	3.8	3.5	3.6
Leukemia	11.4	11.4	10.9	12.4	9.3	11.9	12.6	12.7	9.9	10.6
Acute lymphocytic	1.4	0.9	1.7	1.4	1.7	1.4	2.2	1.2	1.2	1.4
Chronic lymphocytic	3.0	2.8	2.6	3.3	2.2	3.1	4.0	4.1	2.1	2.6
Other lymphocytic	0.4	0.2	0.1	0.5	0.5	0.4	0.6	0.8	0.6	0.4
Acute granulocytic	2.7	2.6	2.9	3.7	1.2	3.4	1.9	2.8	2.5	3.1
Chronic granulocytic	1.7	2.1	1.6	1.5	1.3	1.7	1.8	1.7	1.7	1.4
Other granulocytic	0.6	0.4	0.7	0.4	0.5	0.8	0.6	1.2	0.8	0.4
Monocytic leukemia	0.4	0.6	0.2	0.6	0.7	0.1	0.5	0.3	0.2	0.3
Other acute leukemia	0.5	1.1	0.7	0.5	0.3	0.5	0.3	0.2	0.3	0.6
Other chronic leukemia	0.0	...	...	...	...	...	0.1	...	0.1	0.0
Other leukemia	0.5	0.6	0.4	0.4	0.8	0.4	0.7	0.5	0.5	0.4
Unknown	10.1	9.0	12.6	12.3	11.3	12.2	9.4	9.2	8.1	9.4

[a]Excluding carcinoma in situ and nonmelanoma skin cancer. Organ specific lymphomas are distributed among the sites.
[b]SMSA = Standard Metropolitan Statistical Area.
[c]NOS = Not Otherwise Specific.

TABLE 4

Age adjusted (1950 standard) cancer incidence rates[a] by site and by area: black male
Third National Cancer Survey 1969-1971

	All areas	Detroit SMSA[b]	Pittsburgh SMSA	Atlanta SMSA	Birmingham SMSA	Dallas/ Ft. Worth SMSA	San Francisco/ Oakland SMSA
All sites	354.3	360.0	378.8	333.4	295.9	376.5	365.1
Buccal cavity & pharynx	12.8	13.5	13.0	12.0	7.9	14.1	13.7
Lip	0.2	0.1	...	...	0.3	...	1.0
Tongue	3.3	3.6	4.4	6.0	1.8	3.2	1.2
Salivary gland	1.2	1.5	...	1.6	1.0	1.4	0.9
Gum & mouth	3.7	3.7	4.7	1.0	3.2	5.3	4.0
Nasopharynx	0.5	0.2	0.2	0.9	0.4	0.6	1.3
Tonsil	1.6	1.9	2.1	1.0	0.3	1.4	2.5
Other pharynx	2.2	2.6	1.6	1.4	0.9	2.2	2.8
Digestive system	97.8	103.0	108.9	90.1	73.9	100.4	106.7
Esophagus	15.5	15.8	20.8	20.1	7.4	15.0	15.4
Stomach	19.7	18.1	20.6	19.2	21.4	19.1	22.0
Small intestine	1.5	1.5	2.1	1.5	0.7	1.9	1.1
Colon excluding rectum	24.6	27.9	22.6	21.3	18.0	24.1	27.7
Transverse colon	5.5	7.4	3.0	4.5	3.0	4.6	5.3
Descending colon	3.2	2.6	3.8	3.0	3.2	2.9	3.8
Sigmoid colon	7.0	7.7	6.7	7.5	3.4	8.6	7.4
Cecum	4.0	4.1	4.5	1.5	3.9	3.1	6.3
Appendix	0.2	0.1	...	0.7	...	...	0.2
Ascending colon	2.5	2.8	1.0	2.9	1.4	2.6	4.2
Large intestine NOS[c]	2.3	3.1	3.6	1.2	3.0	2.3	0.5
Rectum & rectosigmoid	13.1	14.9	17.7	10.2	6.8	13.3	14.4
Rectosigmoid junction	3.0	3.4	3.6	0.7	2.9	3.2	4.3
Rectum	10.1	11.5	14.1	9.6	3.9	10.1	10.1
Liver	5.2	5.0	4.1	4.9	6.2	6.1	5.7
Gallbladder	0.5	0.3	0.7	0.7	0.7	0.6	1.0
Other biliary	1.0	1.0	1.6	...	0.6	1.8	1.0
Pancreas	15.1	16.9	16.7	11.1	10.7	17.7	16.3
Retroperitoneum	0.8	0.6	1.3	0.8	0.3	0.5	1.3
Other digestive organs	0.8	1.0	0.7	0.3	1.2	0.3	0.8
Respiratory system	93.0	96.9	106.8	82.3	76.8	95.7	92.5
Larynx	7.9	8.6	5.9	6.0	5.1	7.4	11.8
Lung, bronchus, trachea	83.8	87.1	99.8	74.9	70.1	87.1	79.0
Other respiratory organs	1.3	1.2	1.2	1.4	1.6	1.2	1.7
Bones & joints	0.9	0.8	0.3	0.6	1.0	1.1	1.6
Soft tissue	2.6	2.8	3.2	1.7	2.2	3.3	2.4
Melanoma skin	0.9	0.6	1.2	1.3	1.4	0.6	0.8
Breast	0.8	1.1	1.1	0.5	0.3	0.3	1.2
Male genital	81.2	80.3	70.7	81.9	72.7	93.2	85.8
Prostate	78.1	77.1	69.4	79.9	70.5	87.1	81.9
Testis	0.9	1.0	...	0.3	1.1	1.0	1.5
Penis	1.9	1.9	1.2	1.7	1.1	4.5	1.9
Other male genital	0.3	0.3	...	...	...	0.7	0.5

TABLE 4 (Continued)

	All areas	Detroit SMSA[b]	Pittsburgh SMSA	Atlanta SMSA	Birmingham SMSA	Dallas/ Ft. Worth SMSA	San Francisco/ Oakland SMSA
Urinary system	18.3	18.1	21.5	13.0	15.9	18.9	20.1
Bladder	10.7	10.0	12.9	8.4	9.4	9.6	11.2
Kidney, renal pelvis	7.1	7.4	8.1	4.6	6.1	7.2	8.8
Other urinary	0.6	0.7	0.5	...	0.4	2.1	...
Eye & orbit	0.4	0.2	...	0.5	0.4	0.6	0.2
Brain & other nervous system	3.9	4.5	4.1	3.7	1.7	3.0	5.2
Brain	3.4	3.7	3.2	3.3	1.7	2.4	5.0
Other nervous system	0.6	0.7	1.0	0.5	...	0.6	0.2
Endocrine system	1.7	1.8	0.8	1.8	0.7	0.9	2.4
Thyroid	1.1	1.1	0.8	0.9	0.7	0.3	2.0
Other endrocrine	0.6	0.7	...	0.9	...	0.6	0.4
Lymphomas	8.6	8.8	9.2	7.5	11.0	7.5	7.3
Lymphosarcoma & RCS	3.9	3.9	4.2	3.3	4.8	3.4	3.4
Hodgkin's disease	3.2	3.4	3.1	3.6	3.8	2.4	2.5
Other lymphomas	1.6	1.5	1.9	0.6	2.4	1.7	1.4
Multiple myeloma	7.2	6.2	5.7	8.7	7.2	7.9	7.3
Leukemia	9.5	8.9	10.9	9.4	7.6	12.0	8.8
Acute lymphocytic	0.9	1.0	0.8	1.4	0.7	1.0	0.8
Chronic lymphocytic	2.9	2.7	3.8	2.2	2.3	3.6	2.8
Other lymphocytic	0.2	0.1	...	0.3	0.3	0.3	0.7
Acute granulocytic	2.0	1.5	1.7	2.5	0.7	3.7	1.5
Chronic granulocytic	1.7	1.4	2.0	2.0	2.3	1.8	1.7
Other granulocytic	0.4	0.4	...	...	0.3	0.8	1.0
Monocytic leukemia	0.3	0.5	0.7	0.7	...	...	...
Other acute leukemia	0.6	0.9	1.1	...	0.4	0.3	0.2
Other chronic leukemia	...	...	...	...	...	...	...
Other leukemia	0.5	0.4	0.7	0.3	0.6	0.3	...
Unknown	14.8	12.5	21.5	18.4	15.3	16.9	9.1

[a]Excluding carcinoma in situ and nonmelanoma skin cancer. Organ specific lymphomas are distributed among the sites.
[b]SMSA = Standard Metropolitan Statistical Area.
[c]NOS = Not Otherwise Specific.

TABLE 5

Age adjusted (1950 standard) cancer incidence rates[a] by site and by area: white fema[...] Third National Cancer Survey 1969-1971

	All areas	Detroit SMSA[b]	Pittsburgh SMSA	Atlanta SMSA	Birmingham SMSA	Dallas/ Ft. Worth SMSA	State of Iowa	Minneapolis/ St. Paul SMSA	State of Colorado	San Francisco/ Oakland SMSA
All sites	252.0	254.6	244.1	243.5	224.0	242.9	240.3	262.6	227.2	291.0
Buccal cavity & pharynx	5.2	4.8	4.0	5.3	4.8	7.4	4.0	4.7	4.1	8.0
Lip	0.2	0.1	0.0	0.3	0.3	0.9	0.1	0.3	0.2	0.2
Tongue	1.0	0.9	0.9	1.2	1.0	1.4	0.7	0.9	0.7	1.5
Salivary gland	0.9	1.0	0.7	0.8	0.6	1.1	0.9	0.7	0.7	1.4
Gum & mouth	1.7	1.5	1.4	2.0	1.6	2.6	1.3	1.5	1.4	2.4
Nasopharynx	0.3	0.4	0.3	0.1	0.1	0.2	0.2	0.1	0.1	0.5
Tonsil	0.6	0.4	0.3	0.6	0.6	0.4	0.4	0.5	0.5	1.2
Other pharynx	0.5	0.5	0.3	0.2	0.5	0.8	0.3	0.6	0.5	0.8
Digestive system	54.0	55.5	57.0	47.1	47.6	48.0	54.3	56.9	45.7	60.1
Esophagus	1.2	1.3	1.0	1.0	1.3	1.1	0.8	1.2	0.6	2.1
Stomach	5.7	6.6	7.1	4.2	3.4	4.3	4.8	6.1	4.3	6.7
Small intestine	0.7	0.7	0.7	0.4	0.9	0.7	0.9	0.7	0.7	0.7
Colon excluding rectum	25.3	24.9	25.2	24.1	22.7	22.1	28.2	27.5	21.9	26.6
Transverse colon	4.0	4.0	3.7	3.7	3.5	3.2	4.5	4.1	3.9	4.8
Descending colon	2.2	2.4	2.3	2.4	2.5	2.0	2.1	2.2	1.9	2.1
Sigmoid colon	8.5	8.8	8.6	9.1	6.4	7.1	8.9	8.5	7.2	10.0
Cecum	4.6	4.6	3.8	3.8	3.7	4.3	5.3	6.1	4.2	4.7
Appendix	0.3	0.2	0.3	0.6	...	0.5	0.2	0.3	0.2	0.2
Ascending colon	3.5	3.4	3.0	3.4	3.8	3.6	3.9	3.7	2.5	4.0
Large intestine NOS[c]	2.2	1.5	3.6	1.1	2.8	1.5	3.4	2.6	2.1	0.8
Rectum & retrosigmoid	9.4	9.4	10.9	6.8	7.9	9.1	9.4	9.7	6.5	11.2
Rectosigmoid junction	2.8	2.7	3.1	2.0	2.4	2.8	2.8	2.4	2.1	3.7
Rectum	6.6	6.6	7.8	4.9	5.4	6.3	6.6	7.3	4.4	7.5
Liver	1.2	1.2	1.2	0.8	1.3	1.1	1.1	1.0	1.2	1.5
Gallbladder	1.8	2.2	2.4	1.3	1.1	0.7	1.9	2.1	2.1	1.2
Other biliary	0.9	1.0	0.8	0.8	0.6	0.9	0.6	0.9	0.9	1.2
Pancreas	6.2	6.5	5.9	6.1	7.1	6.7	5.1	6.1	6.5	6.8
Retroperitoneum	0.7	0.9	0.7	0.6	0.3	0.6	0.7	0.6	0.5	0.8
Other digestive organs	0.9	0.9	1.1	1.0	0.9	0.8	0.8	1.0	0.6	1.2
Respiratory system	15.1	14.7	15.3	16.5	13.8	17.1	10.2	13.0	11.4	22.5
Larynx	0.9	0.9	1.1	1.5	0.9	0.8	0.4	0.8	0.8	1.1
Lung, bronchus, trachea	13.5	13.0	13.6	14.2	11.9	15.7	9.3	11.4	10.2	20.6
Other respiratory organs	0.7	0.7	0.6	0.8	1.0	0.7	0.4	0.8	0.5	0.8
Bones & joints	0.6	0.7	0.8	0.8	0.8	0.6	0.6	0.5	0.4	0.7
Soft tissue	1.7	1.7	1.4	2.0	1.1	1.6	1.5	1.9	1.9	1.7
Melanoma skin	4.5	3.4	3.1	6.6	5.2	7.3	3.0	3.5	5.1	5.9
Breast	72.0	73.0	67.8	71.4	59.4	66.4	68.9	76.7	68.3	83.2

TABLE 5 (Continued)

	All areas	Detroit SMSA[b]	Pittsburgh SMSA	Atlanta SMSA	Birmingham SMSA	Dallas/ Ft. Worth SMSA	State of Iowa	Minneapolis/ St. Paul SMSA	State of Colorado	San Francisco/ Oakland SMSA
Female genital system	54.0	56.1	50.9	53.0	52.2	49.8	54.8	56.2	47.6	60.0
Cervix	15.5	15.8	14.1	15.8	24.0	17.1	17.5	16.4	12.7	13.1
Corpus	20.0	22.4	18.8	17.5	13.8	16.0	17.8	19.3	17.0	27.7
Uterus NOS	2.2	2.1	2.9	3.1	0.7	1.2	3.2	2.0	2.1	1.6
Ovary	13.6	13.3	12.5	13.3	10.2	12.9	14.1	15.5	13.6	14.7
Vagina	0.5	0.6	0.4	0.6	0.5	0.5	0.4	0.4	0.4	0.6
Vulva	1.6	1.6	1.6	2.0	2.1	1.6	1.3	2.1	1.2	1.4
Other female genital	0.6	0.5	0.6	0.7	0.9	0.5	0.5	0.6	0.5	0.9
Urinary system	9.4	10.3	9.8	8.1	6.5	8.2	8.2	11.6	8.9	10.5
Bladder	5.3	5.9	6.1	4.2	3.1	4.1	4.3	5.8	5.2	6.4
Kidney, renal pelvis	3.7	4.1	3.3	3.3	3.0	3.6	3.5	5.4	3.3	3.6
Other urinary	0.4	0.3	0.3	0.6	0.4	0.4	0.3	0.5	0.4	0.5
Eye & orbit	0.8	0.6	0.7	0.7	0.4	1.2	0.8	0.9	0.7	1.0
Brain & other nervous system	4.3	4.2	3.3	4.3	4.6	3.8	4.1	5.3	3.8	5.4
Brain	3.9	3.7	2.9	4.1	3.9	3.5	3.8	4.8	3.4	4.9
Other nervous system	0.4	0.5	0.4	0.3	0.7	0.4	0.3	0.5	0.4	0.5
Endocrine system	5.8	6.2	4.6	5.1	5.8	5.7	4.3	5.6	6.6	7.3
Thyroid	5.4	5.7	4.4	4.7	5.7	5.6	4.0	5.1	6.2	7.0
Other endocrine	0.3	0.5	0.2	0.4	0.1	0.1	0.3	0.5	0.4	0.3
Lymphomas	7.7	7.8	7.2	7.1	6.0	7.9	8.4	8.2	6.7	8.3
Lymphosarcoma & RCS	3.8	3.7	2.9	3.6	3.8	3.7	4.2	3.8	3.6	4.2
Hodgkin's disease	2.6	2.7	3.0	2.4	0.9	2.6	2.7	2.7	2.1	3.1
Other lymphomas	1.3	1.3	1.3	1.1	1.2	1.6	1.5	1.7	0.9	1.1
Multiple myeloma	2.4	2.3	2.1	2.3	1.6	2.4	2.4	3.3	2.1	2.5
Leukemia	6.8	6.3	6.9	6.0	5.5	8.6	7.1	6.5	7.4	6.1
Acute lymphocytic	0.9	0.4	1.0	1.1	0.5	1.4	1.0	0.7	1.1	1.2
Chronic lymphocytic	1.5	1.5	1.4	1.2	0.8	1.9	2.0	1.4	1.8	1.2
Other lymphocytic	0.3	0.2	0.3	0.3	0.2	0.3	0.3	0.3	0.2	0.2
Acute granulocytic	1.8	1.5	1.9	1.8	1.1	2.5	1.5	1.8	1.9	1.8
Chronic granulocytic	1.0	0.9	0.8	0.8	1.0	1.3	1.1	1.3	1.0	0.6
Other granulocytic	0.4	0.4	0.2	. . .	0.6	0.6	0.3	0.5	0.5	0.4
Monocytic leukemia	0.3	0.3	0.1	0.4	0.5	0.1	0.5	0.1	0.3	0.2
Other acute leukemia	0.4	0.8	0.7	0.2	0.1	0.2	0.1	0.1	0.2	0.3
Other chronic leukemia	0.0	. . .	0.0	. . .	0.1	0.1	. . .	. . .	. . .	. . .
Other leukemia	0.3	0.3	0.5	0.1	0.7	0.3	0.4	0.2	0.4	0.2
Unknown	7.7	7.1	9.4	7.2	8.5	7.0	7.8	7.6	6.5	7.8

[a]Excluding carcinoma in situ and nonmelanoma skin cancer. Organ specific lymphomas are distributed among the sites.
[b]SMSA = Standard Metropolitan Statistical Area.
[c]NOS = Not Otherwise Specific.

TABLE 6
Age adjusted (1950 standard) cancer incidence rates[a] by site and by area: black fema
Third National Cancer Survey 1969-1971

	All areas	Detroit SMSA[b]	Pittsburgh SMSA	Atlanta SMSA	Birmingham SMSA	Dallas/ Ft. Worth SMSA	San Francisco/ Oakland SMSA
All sites	243.0	250.4	266.9	219.7	226.2	241.7	241.7
Buccal cavity & pharynx	5.1	5.6	5.7	5.0	3.4	4.6	5.0
Lip	0.1	...	...	...	0.2	0.5	...
Tongue	1.3	1.7	1.5	1.3	0.7	0.5	1.1
Salivary gland	1.0	0.6	1.8	1.1	1.0	0.8	0.9
Gum & mouth	1 5	1.6	1.4	1.4	0.8	1.9	2.0
Nasopharynx	0.3	0.4	...	0.5	0.2	0.3	0.4
Tonsil	0.5	0.4	0.4	0.8	0.3	0.7	0.6
Other pharynx	0.4	0.8	0.7	...	0.2	...	...
Digestive system	58.8	61.8	72.9	52.4	47.2	59.6	60.9
Esophagus	3.6	4.0	5.6	3.0	2.9	2.7	3.8
Stomach	8.2	9.0	8.0	7.5	6.8	8.7	9.0
Small intestine	0.7	0.7	1.1	...	0.5	1.2	0.7
Colon excluding rectum	24.9	25.7	32.2	24.0	20.8	25.3	22.3
Transverse colon	4.2	4.6	6.1	3.5	3.9	4.2	2.8
Descending colon	3.2	3.3	3.2	2.2	3.6	3.6	3.9
Sigmoid colon	7.2	6.8	9.9	8.3	5.9	7.2	6.5
Cecum	3.8	4.2	4.2	3.9	1.0	4.4	5.0
Appendix	0.5	0.7	0.3	0.7	0.7	0.2	...
Ascending colon	3.0	3.6	1.0	3.0	2.3	3.5	3.5
Large intestine NOS[c]	2.8	2.5	7.5	2.5	3.4	2.0	0.6
Rectum & rectosigmoid	7.7	8.6	12.5	6.9	4.7	6.9	7.2
Rectosigmoid junction	1.8	2.2	3.1	1.7	0.7	0.5	2.1
Rectum	6.0	6.5	9.4	5.2	4.0	6.4	5.1
Liver	1.4	1.0	0.7	1.3	1.3	1.7	2.2
Gallbladder	1.4	2.4	1.7	0.5	0.7	0.8	1.1
Other biliary	0.8	1.0	0.7	...	0.7	1.0	0.9
Pancreas	8.6	8.3	8.8	8.1	7.4	9.2	10.3
Retroperitoneum	0.5	0.3	...	0.2	0.3	0.5	2.1
Other digestive organs	1.1	0.7	1.5	1.3	1.2	1.6	1.3
Respiratory system	15.1	16.7	15.7	9.9	12.2	10.5	22.5
Larynx	1.0	1.1	1.9	1.0	0.2	0.8	1.0
Lung, bronchus, trachea	13.6	15.3	13.8	8.5	11.1	9.4	20.7
Other respiratory organs	0.5	0.3	...	0.4	0.9	0.3	0.7
Bones & joints	0.6	0.6	1.8	0.3	0.5	0.3	0.8
Soft tissue	2.0	1.7	2.6	1.5	2.9	2.4	2.1
Melanoma skin	0.7	0.7	1.3	0.8	0.6	0.9	0.5
Breast	56.4	57.7	61.5	50.2	51.5	55.8	59.6

TABLE 6 (Continued)

	All areas	Detroit SMSA[b]	Pittsburgh SMSA	Atlanta SMSA	Birmingham SMSA	Dallas/ Ft. Worth SMSA	San Francisco/ Oakland SMSA
Female genital system	61.8	64.3	58.4	59.0	62.8	67.6	53.0
Cervix	34.1	36.2	30.2	30.7	36.9	40.0	26.5
Corpus	11.2	11.8	10.4	9.6	10.3	9.7	12.9
Uterus NOS	2.7	2.6	2.6	4.0	2.4	2.7	2.1
Ovary	10.3	10.9	11.8	10.8	8.3	12.0	7.5
Vagina	1.0	0.9	0.4	1.3	1.7	0.5	0.9
Vulva	1.7	1.1	2.6	1.8	2.6	1.3	2.0
Other female genital	0.9	0.8	0.5	0.9	0.5	1.3	1.1
Urinary system	7.6	7.7	9.4	6.8	6.6	8.2	8.0
Bladder	3.6	3.2	4.6	3.5	3.8	3.3	4.3
Kidney, renal pelvis	3.6	4.0	3.8	3.0	2.8	4.1	3.5
Other urinary	0.4	0.4	1.1	0.3	...	0.8	0.2
Eye & orbit	0.4	0.6	0.5	...	0.4	0.5	0.2
Brain & other nervous system	3.4	3.1	3.1	3.8	3.0	3.9	3.5
Brain	2.9	2.6	2.8	2.3	3.0	3.5	3.1
Other nervous system	0.6	0.4	0.2	1.5	...	0.4	0.4
Endocrine system	3.7	4.5	4.7	3.4	4.1	2.5	2.6
Thyroid	3.3	3.8	4.3	3.1	4.1	1.8	2.6
Other endocrine	0.4	0.8	0.4	0.2	...	0.7	...
Lymphomas	4.7	5.0	6.5	2.9	4.1	4.0	4.1
Lymphosarcoma & RCS	2.3	2.8	2.4	1.0	1.8	2.3	1.9
Hodgkin's disease	1.2	1.3	2.9	0.7	0.9	1.0	0.9
Other lymphoma	1.1	0.9	1.1	1.3	1.4	0.7	1.3
Multiple myeloma	5.8	5.4	5.4	5.6	5.2	4.9	6.2
Leukemia	5.5	5.2	5.3	4.5	5.6	3.8	6.2
Acute lymphocytic	0.5	0.3	...	0.2	0.9	0.6	0.8
Chronic lymphocytic	1.2	1.0	1.2	1.7	1.6	0.8	1.2
Other lymphocytic	0.1	...	...	...	0.2	0.2	...
Acute granulocytic	1.3	1.5	1.6	1.5	0.8	0.1	1.6
Chronic granulocytic	1.2	1.2	2.0	0.4	0.2	0.8	1.3
Other granulocytic	0.2	0.1	...	...	0.7	0.2	0.2
Monocytic	0.1	0.2	...	...	...	0.2	0.3
Other acute leukemia	0.3	0.6	0.5	0.1	0.4	0.3	...
Other chronic leukemia	...	...	...	...	...	...	...
Other leukemia	0.5	0.3	...	0.5	0.7	0.5	0.8
Unknown	11.4	10.0	12.1	13.3	16.1	12.0	6.8

[a]Excluding carcinoma in situ and nonmelanoma skin cancer. Organ specific lymphomas are distributed among the sites.
[b]SMSA = Standard Metropolitan Statistical Area.
[c]NOS = Not Otherwise Specific.

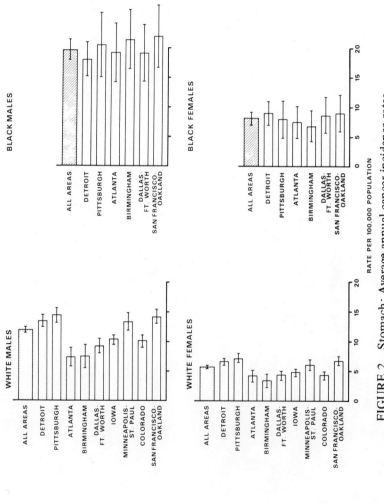

FIGURE 2. Stomach: Average annual cancer incidence rates, by race, sex and geographic area.

The area rates for the white population, for both males and females, may be grouped into two clusters: high in Detroit, Pittsburg, Minneapolis-St. Paul, and San Francisco-Oakland; and low in Atlanta, Birmingham, Dallas-Fort Worth, Iowa, and Colorado. No consistent pattern emerges from examination of the rates for the black population.

Colon, Excluding Rectum (Figure 3)

Variation in the incidence of colon cancer among the four race-sex groups is moderate, from a high of 28.5 in white males to a low of 24.6 in black males.

For the white population, the areas with low rates—Birmingham, Dallas-Ft. Worth, and Colorado—are more distinct than the ones with higher rates. For the black population, the rates in Birmingham are the lowest.

Rectum and Rectosigmoid (Figure 4)

Within each racial group, the rates for males are clearly higher than for females, with somewhat higher rates for white persons of each sex.

The incidence rates tend to be high in Detroit, Pittsburgh, Minneapolis-St. Paul and San Francisco-Oakland, and low in Atlanta, Birmingham, and Colorado.

Lung, Bronchus, and Trachea (Figure 5)

Lung cancer occurs much more frequently in males than in females. The incidence ratio is 5 to 1. Among males, incidence is clearly higher in blacks (83.8 vs 65.3). As previously reported [1,2], the incidence has been increasing more rapidly among black than among white persons of both sexes.

Among males, the relative positions of the areas are not consistent for whites and blacks. For example, Birmingham has the highest rate among white men and the lowest among black men. In contrast, Pittsburgh with an average incidence level for white men has the highest lung cancer rate for black men. However, it is worth noting that Dallas-Fort Worth ranks second in incidence of lung cancer among both white and black men.

Among females, the San Francisco-Oakland rates are highest. Among white persons of both sexes, lung cancer occurs less frequently in Iowa, Minneapolis-St. Paul, and Colorado.

COLON (EXCLUDING RECTUM)

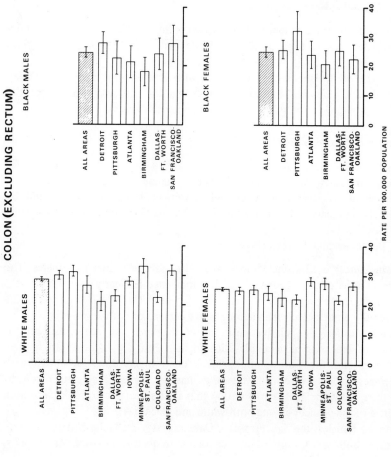

FIGURE 3. Colon (excluding rectum): Average annual cancer incidence rates, by race, sex and geographic area.

324

RECTUM AND RECTOSIGMOID

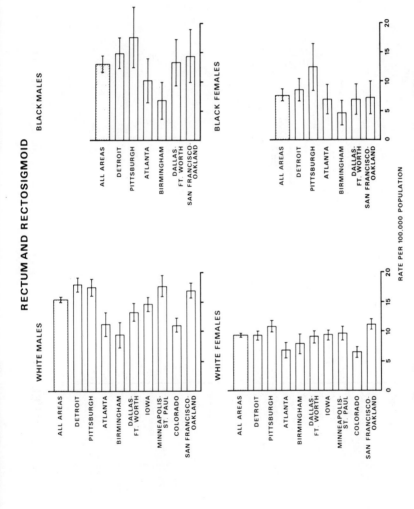

FIGURE 4. Rectum and rectosigmoid: Average annual cancer incidence rates, by race, sex and geographic area.

325

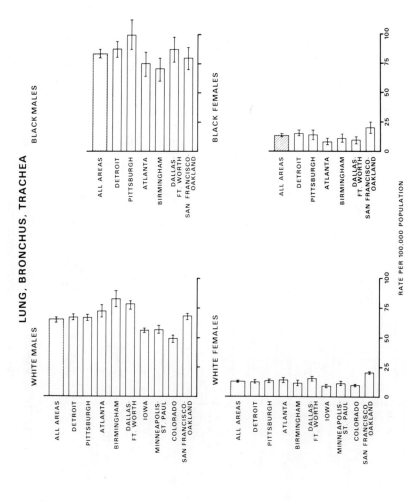

FIGURE 5. Lung, bronchus and trachea: Average annual cancer incidence rates, by race, sex and geographic area.

326

Breast (Figure 6)

Cancer of the breast is occurring more frequently in white than in black women, but the rate has been increasing more rapidly among black women [1,2].

In comparing the areas, it is clear that the reported incidence of breast cancer is low in Birmingham for women of both races. Among white women, the two highest rates were reported from San Francisco-Oakland and Minneapolis-St. Paul. Among black women, the two highest rates were in Pittsburgh and San Francisco. Thus, San Francisco had a high incidence of breast cancer for both black and white women.

Uterine Cervix (Figure 7)

The incidence of invasive cancer of the uterine cervix is twice as high in black as in white women. Among white women, the rate in Birmingham is clearly higher than in any of the other areas. Among black women, the rate in Birmingham is a close second to the high rate in Dallas-Ft. Worth. The high rates for cervical cancer in Birmingham are particularly noteworthy in view of the generally low level of reported cancer incidence for this area. Conversely, the low rates in San Francisco-Oakland contrast with the relatively high rates in this area for all cancers combined.

The incidence of carcinoma in situ of the uterine cervix varies widely among both white and black females. The observed differences may be more apparent than real as a result of increased case finding from organized community screening programs and variation caused by the lack of uniformity in classification of cervical lesions by pathologists.

Uterine Corpus (Figure 8)

In contrast to the pattern for cervical neoplasms, cancers of the uterine corpus occur more frequently in white than in black women, and among white women Birmingham has the lowest rather than the highest rate. The highest rates were reported in San Francisco-Oakland, which also has high rates for cancers of the breast.

BREAST

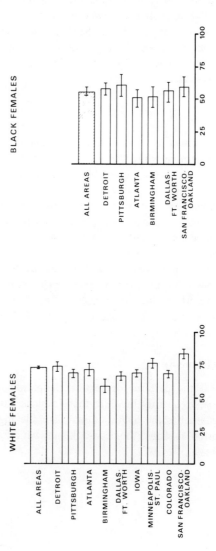

RATE PER 100,000 POPULATION

FIGURE 6. Breast: Average annual cancer incidence rates, by race and geographic area.

328

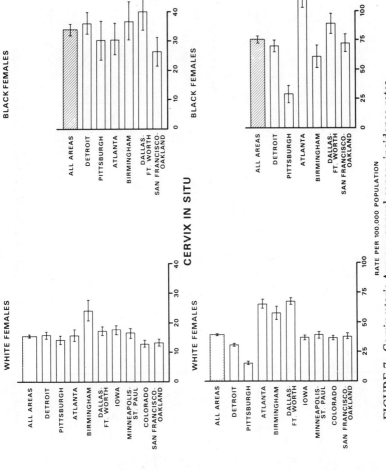

FIGURE 7. Cervix uteri: Average annual cancer incidence rates, by race and geographic area.

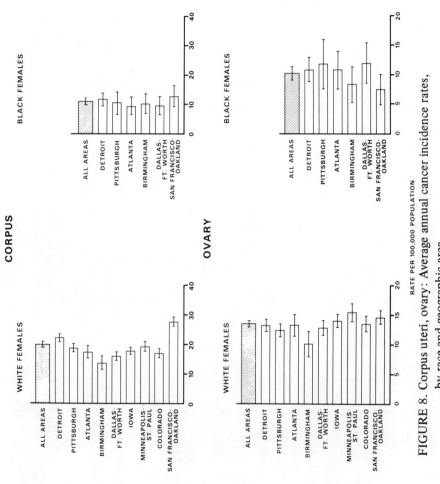

CORPUS

BLACK FEMALES

WHITE FEMALES

OVARY

BLACK FEMALES

WHITE FEMALES

RATE PER 100,000 POPULATION

FIGURE 8. Corpus uteri, ovary: Average annual cancer incidence rates, by race and geographic area.

Ovary (Figure 8)

Among white women the highest incidence rates were reported in Minneapolis-St. Paul and San Francisco-Oakland, the lowest in Birmingham. Incidence of ovarian cancer in Birmingham was also low among black women, but the rate for black women in San Francisco-Oakland was low rather than high.

The incidence of cancers of the reproductive system among white women in Birmingham exhibits a unique pattern. The incidence of cancers of the breast, corpus, and ovary are uniformly low, whereas the incidence of cervical cancer is high. This pattern may reflect socioeconomic characteristics of the white population in Birmingham; that is, high incidence of cervical cancer has been found to be associated with low socioeconomic status.

Prostate (Figure 9)

The incidence of prostate cancer is much higher in black than in white men and has been increasing more rapidly over time [1,2]. Among the survey areas, there is no clear pattern of variation except that rates in Pittsburgh were relatively low for both races.

Bladder (Figure 10)

The incidence of bladder cancer is highest among white males and lowest among black females. In both races, cancer of the bladder occurs much more frequently among males. The trend of bladder cancer incidence in males and females differs markedly [1,2]. Among both white and black men the incidence has been increasing, in contrast to a decrease in incidence among women.

Among the nine survey areas, Pittsburgh reported the highest or second highest incidence rate for the four race-sex groups. The rates in Detroit and San Francisco-Oakland were also generally high. In contrast, the rates in Atlanta, Birmingham, and Dallas-Fort Worth were generally low.

Kidney and Renal Pelvis (Figure 11)

Cancers of the kidney occur more frequently in males than females, and are at the same levels in the white and black populations.

For the white population, the rates in Minneapolis-St. Paul are clearly high and the rates in Birmingham are low. For the black population, the relationship among the areas is more distinct at the low end of the range. Reported incidence was low in Atlanta and Birmingham for both sexes.

PROSTATE

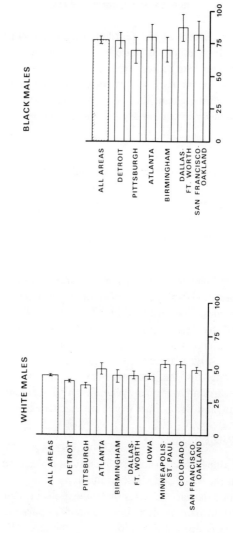

WHITE MALES

BLACK MALES

RATE PER 100,000 POPULATION

FIGURE 9. Prostate: Average annual cancer incidence rates, by race and geographic area.

332

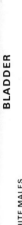
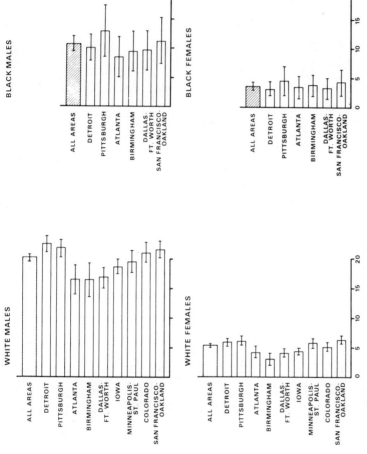

FIGURE 10. Bladder: Average annual cancer incidence rates, by race, sex and geographic area.

333

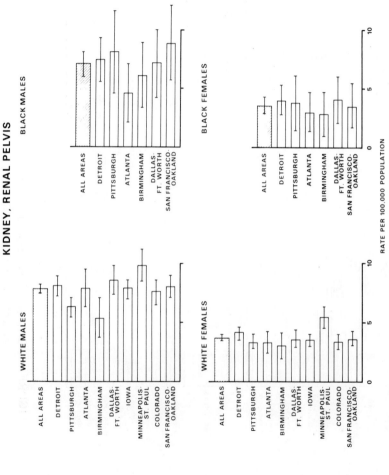

FIGURE 11. Kidney and renal pelvis: Average annual cancer incidence rates, by race, sex and geographic area.

334

Melanoma of the Skin (Figure 12)

Melanoma of the skin is relatively rare among black people. In the white population, the incidence rates are similar in the two sexes.

Among whites, the highest rates for both sexes were reported in Dallas-Ft. Worth. Relatively high rates were also reported in Atlanta and Birmingham; also in Colorado and San Francisco-Oakland. Low rates were reported in Detroit, Pittsburgh, Iowa, and Minneapolis-St. Paul. In general, low rates were reported from northern areas and high rates from southern and western areas.

Lymphomas (Figure 13)[1]

Within each race, lymphomas occur more frequently in males than in females, and within each sex the rates are higher among whites. In comparing the rates for the nine survey areas, the high rate among both white and black males in Birmingham stands out. This fact is noteworthy because the overall level of cancer incidence reported in Birmingham is low. There was no distinct geographic pattern of lymphoma incidence in females.

Leukemias (Figure 14)

The incidence of leukemia is greater in males than females of both races. Within each sex, incidence is somewhat higher among whites. Among males, the rates in Birmingham were low in contrast to the high rates in this area for lymphoma. Among females, no clear geographic pattern is evident.

DISCUSSION

The findings herein are derived from the extensive collection of data contained in the first monograph reporting the results of the Third National Cancer Survey [3]. The monograph provides detailed data on the incidence of cancer in the nine survey areas, which in 1970 had a combined population of 21 million people. Subsequent monographs and reports will deal with a variety of subjects, including duration and cost of hospitalization of cancer patients.

---

[1] The data presented in Figure 13 exclude lymphomas arising in specific organ sites.

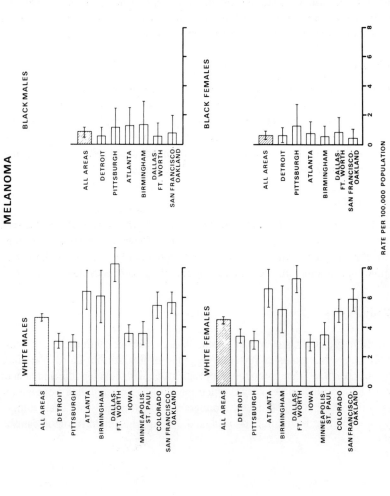

FIGURE 12. Melanoma of the skin: Average annual cancer incidence rates, by race, sex and geographic area.

336

LYMPHOMAS

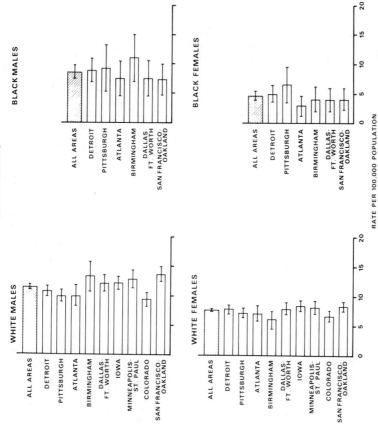

FIGURE 13. Lymphomas: Average annual incidence rates, by race, sex and geographic area. Data exclude lymphomas arising in specific organ sites.

LEUKEMIAS

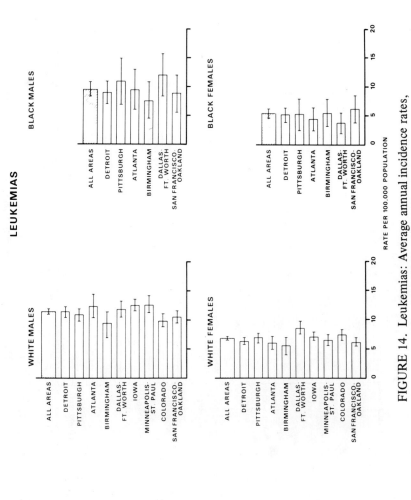

FIGURE 14. Leukemias: Average annual incidence rates, by race, sex and geographic area.

The data in this chapter can serve as a convenient reference regarding demographic and geographic variation in the reported incidence of the various forms of cancer in the United States. The data pertaining to the more frequently occurring cancers were presented in a series of charts and briefly discussed in the previous section. To recapitulate those findings, some of the highlights are:

1) Cancer occurs more frequently in males than in females and more frequently in black than in white males.

2) Among males, incidence rates in blacks are significantly higher for cancers of the esophagus, stomach, pancreas, lung, and prostate, and for multiple myeloma. Although total cancer incidence is higher in black males, rates for a number of malignancies are significantly higher in whites; namely, cancers of the colon, rectum and bladder, melanoma of the skin, lymphoma, and leukemia.

3) Among females, cancer occurs somewhat more frequently in whites, but incidence is clearly higher in blacks for cancers of the esophagus, stomach, and pancreas, and is markedly higher for cancer of the uterine cervix. In contrast to the race relationship with respect to cervical cancer, the incidence of cancer in the breast, uterine corpus, and ovary is more frequent among whites.

4) Comparison of cancer incidence for the white population in the nine survey areas discloses a regional pattern for a number of sites; that is, the three southern areas (Atlanta, Birmingham, and Dallas-Ft. Worth) had high rates for cervical cancer in females (invasive plus in situ), lung cancer in males, and melanoma of the skin in both sexes. The same three areas had low rates for cancers of the stomach, colon, rectum, and bladder.

The 95 percent confidence interval for each rate shown in the figures provides one means for assessing the statistical reliability of observed differences. However, it must be remembered that formal tests of statistical significance do not provide an assessment of the impact of a "seek and show" procedure. We are here examining data for 15 individual forms of cancer. The data for each are subdivided by race and sex, and then by geographic area. Thus, by chance alone, in this very large set of data, some incidence rates are likely to appear to be high or low. In this type of exploration of data, consistency of a pattern is more convincing than a formal test of statistical significance. For example, the reported incidence of cancer of the rectum is substantially lower in Atlanta and Birmingham than in the other survey areas for each of the four race-sex groups. In contrast, the highest lung cancer rate for black males was reported from Pittsburgh, but the rates in Pittsburgh for white males and for white and black females were not unusual. Thus, on the basis of general considerations of probability, the above observations regarding rectal cancer can be accepted with more confidence than the observation regarding lung cancer. On the other hand, it is unwise to be a statistical purist in looking for epidemiologic clues. One should not ignore the observation that lung cancer appears to occur with unusual frequency in Pittsburgh in only one race-sex group, namely, black males. The high rate may well be a reflection of specific occupational exposure.

Another consideration in assessing the reliability of reported geographic differences is completeness of case finding. Identification of every diagnosed case of cancer in a community is a tedious task. Considerable effort was expended in each of the survey areas to insure complete case finding, but some variation in success of case identification probably occurred.

A further and difficult issue pertains to possible variation in diagnostic criteria; that is, the criteria for differentiating between benign and malignant lesions. For example, is the difference in the reported incidence rates for bladder cancer among white males in Detroit and Pittsburgh (high) compared to Atlanta and Birmingham (low) a reflection of variation in the criteria used to differentiate between benign and invasive lesions? This type of issue could be assessed through a review of biopsy specimens.

Each reported case of cancer is being assigned to a census tract of residence. By use of information from the 1970 census, certain characteristics of the population residing within each tract can be ascertained. This tract-by-tract information will be used to explore the variation in cancer incidence with respect to income, educational level, and so forth. Of particular interest will be the consistency of relations among the survey areas. For example, will the analysis disclose a consistent association between high incidence of cancer of the uterine cervix and low socioeconomic status?

Descriptive information to provide "community profiles" for each of the survey areas will be developed. These profiles should help in the interpretation of the reported variation in incidence among the areas and may suggest the relevance for investigation of factors such as specific industrial exposures and ethnic characteristics.

Further leads regarding etiologic factors associated with variation of cancer incidence among population groups may be obtained through examination of the available data on the histologic characteristics of tumors of various sites. For example, the survey data indicated that cancer occurs more frequently in the uterine corpus in white than in black women. However, examination of information on histology revealed that in black women 25 percent of corpus cancers are sarcomas of the myometrium compared to only 7 percent in white women [4]. In fact, the incidence rate of sarcoma of the myometrium is twice as high in black as in white women (2.9 vs 1.5 per 100,000 per year). The inverse relationship between white and black women in the occurrence of carcinoma and sarcoma of the uterine corpus suggests racially related etiologic factors.

Many findings of the Third National Cancer Survey are probably applicable to many communities. For example, it is likely that the high incidence of bladder cancer in white males, as compared to black males and both white and black females, is a widespread phenomenon in the United States and is not limited to the nine areas included in the survey. This type of observation provides a guide to the targeting of screening and other cancer control programs. On the other hand, the high incidence of cancers of the uterine cervix among white women in Birmingham appears to be associated with specific community characteristics. Whether these characteristics can be defined with sufficient specificity to permit selection of additional areas in which incidence is likely to be high remains to be seen. Perhaps to a large extent communities will have to assess the magnitude and nature of their cancer problem on an individual basis. Since information on cancer mortality is available for all 50 states, the survey data on cancer incidence, plus data on cancer mortality in the survey areas, provide a means for making rough estimates of cancer incidence levels in broad geographic regions of the United States.

The survey method is a way to collect a wide variety of data, as exemplified by the Third National Cancer Survey [5]. Periodic surveys can provide information on changes over time. However, since a survey is discontinuous, it does not facilitate following up on leads for further investigation. The personnel experience and community contacts built up during the survey cannot be exploited for further work, because the field organization is dissolved upon completion of a survey.

In contrast, a continuing reporting system can provide all the descriptive information obtainable through a survey, plus much more. Thus, a population-based, continuous, cancer reporting system can provide all the types of data collected in the Third National Cancer Survey, and in addition can provide an operational framework for a variety of ad hoc epidemiologic studies and for planning and assessing community-oriented cancer control programs.

Three of the areas included in the survey (Detroit, Iowa, and San Francisco-Oakland) are now participating in a collaborative, continuous, cancer reporting system sponsored by the National Cancer Institute. Six other areas with population-based cancer reporting systems (Connecticut, Hawaii, New Mexico, New Orleans, Seattle, and Utah) are participating in the collaborative program sponsored by the National Cancer Institute. This reporting network, with representation of a variety of geographic areas and demographic groups, is known as the Surveillance, Epidemiology, and End Results Reporting (SEER) Program. All participants report data on cancer incidence, case management, and patient survival according to a uniform set of definitions and codes. The program is designed to stimulate both local and collaborative research within the framework of a uniform reporting system. Thus, it will be possible to design and carry out ad hoc studies to pursue the kinds of epidemiologic leads uncovered by the recently completed survey.

REFERENCES

1. Cutler, S.J., Report on the Third National Cancer Survey. *In Proceedings of the Seventh National Cancer Conference.* J.B. Lippincott, Philadelphia, 1972, pp. 639-652.
2. Cutler, S.J., and Devesa, S.S., Trends in cancer incidence and mortality in the USA. *In* Doll, R., and Vodopija, I., eds., *Host Environment Interactions in the Etiology of Cancer in Man.* I.A.R.C. Scientific Publications No. 7, I.A.R.C., Lyon, 1973, pp. 15-34.
3. Biometry Branch, National Cancer Institute. Third National Cancer Survey: Incidence data. *Natl. Cancer Inst. Monogr.* 41: In press, 1975.
4. Cramer, D.W., Cutler, S.J., and Christine, B., Trends in the incidence of endometrial cancer in the United States. *Gynecol. Oncol.* 2:130-143, 1974.
5. Cutler, S.J., Scotto, J., Devesa, S.S., et al., Third National Cancer Survey: An overview of available information. *J. Natl. Cancer Inst.* 53:1565-1575, 1974.

DISCUSSION

Dr. Keller reported some recent findings on cancer among blacks treated at Veterans Administration hospitals in the United States. Deficits were found for cancers of the lip, nasopharynx, and bladder; excesses were found for cancers of the esophagus and stomach. Among patients with bladder cancer there was significantly less cigarette smoking than reported in the literature. **Dr. S. Cutler** encouraged Dr. Keller to use the Veterans hospitals for case-control studies of such cancers among blacks. **Dr. Selikoff** wondered if the deficiency of bladder cancer might be related to the fact that few blacks were employed as skilled chemical workers in the past. Blacks have had limited occupational exposure also to other carcinogens, such as vinyl chloride and asbestos. However, blacks contributed largely to the reported excess of lung cancer among coke-oven workers.

Dr. J. Cutler remarked that some variability in cancer risk between the areas included in the Third National Cancer Survey could be due to screening procedures used in the respective areas and should be investigated. **Dr. Wynder** remarked that studies of breast cancer among black women should be conducted. Nutritional factors and obesity have been linked to breast cancer, but the risk is low in black women, among whom obesity is prevalent. He also stressed that the very high rate of prostatic cancer among black males is an important etiologic lead, which is now being pursued at his institution.

Thomas J. Mason

20

GEOGRAPHIC PATTERNS OF CANCER MORTALITY IN THE UNITED STATES

Robert Hoover, M.D., Thomas J. Mason, Ph.D., Frank W. McKay, and
Joseph F. Fraumeni, Jr., M.D.

Epidemiology Branch, National Cancer Institute
Bethesda, Maryland

INTRODUCTION

The geographic variation in cancer mortality in the United States usually has been evaluated on a state-by-state basis. The paucity of clues arising from such surveys can be traced to the heterogeneity of statewide populations. Recently, we acquired 20 years of cancer mortality data (1950-1969) for the 3,056 individual counties of the contiguous United States [1]. Counties may represent an ideal compromise between the need for units small enough to be homogeneous for demographic and environmental characteristics that might influence cancer risk, and yet large enough to provide stable estimates of site-specific cancer mortality. An initial evaluation confirms this opinion, and we have begun to use the county data for studies to formulate and test hypotheses pertaining to high-risk groups. This chapter summarizes some preliminary findings that will be refined and expanded as we gain experience with this resource.

DEMOGRAPHIC CHARACTERISTICS

Urban-Rural and Socioeconomic Differences

The wealth of demographic data characterizing county populations permits detailed analyses of characteristics that may influence the geographic variation of cancer. Preliminary results are available on the effects of urbanization and social class, based on a comparison of counties with extreme values for these factors. Using census-derived data, we compared the mortality rates for the 957 counties listed as 100 percent rural in the 1960 census with the rates for the 13 counties listed as 100 percent urban. Since urbanization is related to social class, we removed these areas from the total 3,056 counties in the United States, and ranked the remaining counties by social class, based on the median number of school years completed by the adult population. We then compared the rates in the top 10 percent of counties ranked on this variable with those in the bottom 10 percent. The 35 cancer sites were then ordered according to the magnitude of the urban-rural ratios (Table 1) and social-class ratios (Table 2). Most of the urban-rural differences are in the direction expected from previous studies [2,3], but in both sexes a surprisingly large urban effect is observed for cancers of the nasopharynx, larynx, colon, and rectum. The social-class ratios also are as anticipated for many tumors [4,5], but with certain peculiarities. In some instances, urbanization may confound the social-class associations, or the extremes may not be representative of the total social-class gradient. To evaluate these possibilities, the age-adjusted death rates were calculated for cross-classified categories of social-class and urbanization for the entire country. Table 3 shows examples of these analyses. Several interesting associations emerge from these more detailed classifications. Positive social-class and urbanization effects are seen for breast cancer and Hodgkin's disease (HD) in females, whereas the urbanization effect for colon cancer disappears when we control for social-class differences. Noteworthy also is the lack of either effect for stomach cancer, which confirms the unexpected lack of association noted when the extremes on these variables are compared.

The patterns for skin cancer mortality in Tables 1 and 2 illustrate potentialities for cancer control. Skin cancer other than melanoma is strongly and inversely related to both social class and urbanization, but no gradients are observed for melanoma. If both tumors have the same cause (sunlight), perhaps the discrepancy is related to variations in treatment and survival. Further studies should evaluate the possibility that segments of the population are experiencing delays in the diagnosis and adequate treatment of an essentially curable cancer; if so, control measures should be instituted.

Thus far, we have moved from demographic variables to cancer mortality. The reverse approach is illustrated in Figure 1 by the geographic distribution of mortality from cancer of the uterine cervix among white women. There is an obvious clustering of high rates in counties in the southeastern portion of the United States. Socioeconomic and urbanization data for the groups of counties having very high rates and for the total United States are given in Table 4. These data suggest that the excess mortality in the southeastern United States can be attributed to the predominance of this cancer in the rural lower socioeconomic classes.

TABLE 1

Urban-rural ratios of age-adjusted cancer mortality rates[a] among whites in the contiguous United States, according to cancer site and sex, 1950-1969

Male		Female	
Site	Urban/rural	Site	Urban/rural
Esophagus	3.08	Esophagus	2.12
Larynx	2.96	Rectum	2.11
Mouth and throat	2.88	Larynx	1.92
Rectum	2.71	Nasopharynx	1.66
Nasopharynx	2.17	Lung	1.64
Bladder	2.10	Breast	1.61
Colon	1.97	Bladder	1.58
Lung	1.89	Other endocrine glands	1.52
Breast	1.77	Ovary	1.52
All malignant neoplasms	1.56	Colon	1.51
Thyroid gland	1.56	Non-Hodgkin's lymphoma	1.42
Other endocrine glands	1.53	Hodgkin's disease	1.39
Stomach	1.45	Thyroid	1.38
Kidney	1.44	All malignant neoplasms	1.36
Non-Hodgkin's lymphoma	1.39	Stomach	1.35
Other and unspecified	1.38	Pancreas	1.34
Connective tissue	1.35	Mouth and throat	1.29
Pancreas	1.34	Connective tissue	1.28
Biliary passages and liver (primary)	1.34	Brain	1.26
Salivary glands	1.31	Multiple myeloma	1.25
Hodgkin's disease	1.25	Other and unspecified	1.17
Brain	1.21	Leukemia	1.15
Multiple myeloma	1.12	Kidney	1.12
Nasal sinuses	1.10	Salivary glands	1.12
Leukemia	1.07	Nasal sinuses	1.08
Bone	1.05	Biliary passages and liver	1.04
Melanoma of skin	1.01	Corpus uteri	1.00
Prostate	.96	Cervix uteri	1.00
Testis	.96	Eye	.92
Eye	.77	Bone	.89
Other skin	.67	Melanoma of skin	.87
Lip	.57	Other skin	.65
		Lip	.29

[a]Rates were calculated for 100 percent urban and 100 percent rural counties.

TABLE 2

Social-class ratios of age-adjusted cancer mortality rates[a] among whites in the
contiguous United States, according to cancer site and sex, 1950-1969

Male Site	Social-class ratio (high/low)	Female Site	Social-class ratio (high/low)
Rectum	2.13	Rectum	1.67
Thyroid gland	1.72	Breast	1.54
Colon	1.67	Ovary	1.52
Bladder	1.67	Other endocrine glands	1.52
Other endocrine glands	1.59	Non-Hodgkin's lymphoma	1.49
Connective tissue	1.54	Colon	1.45
Kidney	1.49	Connective tissue	1.43
Esophagus	1.49	Multiple myeloma	1.39
Non-Hodgkin's lymphoma	1.37	Hodgkin's disease	1.37
Multiple myeloma	1.35	Brain	1.35
Mouth and throat	1.19	Nasopharynx	1.28
Testis	1.18	Lung	1.27
Breast	1.18	Bladder	1.19
Brain	1.18	All malignant neoplasms	1.18
All malignant neoplasms	1.16	Kidney	1.14
Hodgkin's disease	1.14	Eye	1.12
Leukemia	1.11	Pancreas	1.10
Lung	1.10	Thyroid gland	1.09
Nasopharynx	1.10	Leukemia	1.06
Prostate	1.09	Stomach	1.03
Stomach	1.09	Nasal sinuses	1.01
Larynx	1.02	Esophagus	.97
Pancreas	1.01	Corpus uteri	.94
Melanoma of skin	.98	Biliary passages and liver	.94
Nasal sinuses	.96	Salivary glands	.86
Biliary passages and liver	.88	Other and unspecified	.85
Eye	.87	Melanoma of skin	.85
Other and unspecified	.85	Mouth and throat	.78
Salivary glands	.83	Cervix uteri	.74
Lip	.81	Bone	.69
Bone	.81	Larynx	.67
Other skin	.53	Other skin	.47
		Lip	.32

[a]*See* text for method of choosing high and low social-class counties.

TABLE 3

Age-adjusted mortality rates (1950-1969) for selected cancers among whites in counties, grouped according to the percent of the population living in an urban area and the median number of years of school completed by the adult population (1960)

Site and sex	Years of schooling	Percent urban		
		0–39.9	40–69.9	70–100
Colon (females)	≤ 8.5	11.52	11.07	9.23
	8.6–10.0	14.88	14.88	18.71
	> 10.0	16.04	15.36	16.72
Esophagus (males)	≤ 8.5	2.13	2.56	3.09
	8.6–10.0	2.46	3.12	5.65
	> 10.0	2.69	3.24	5.07
Breast (females)	≤ 8.5	17.17	18.05	16.84
	8.6–10.0	21.55	22.17	27.32
	> 10.0	23.42	24.03	28.28
Hodgkin's disease (females)	≤ 8.5	0.97	1.02	0.79
	8.6–10.0	1.18	1.22	1.45
	> 10.0	1.28	1.28	1.44
Nasopharynx (males)	≤ 8.5	0.32	0.39	0.19
	8.6–10.0	0.27	0.30	0.53
	> 10.0	0.24	0.30	0.41
Stomach (males)	≤ 8.5	12.31	12.59	14.47
	8.6–10.0	14.09	13.64	16.88
	> 10.0	13.58	13.77	16.30

North-South Variation

Variation in cancer mortality by latitude has always intrigued etiologists, particularly those seeking evidence of infectious agents. A constant dilemma in such analyses has been the inability to separate North-South differences from urban-rural or social-class effects. Our efforts to clarify the associations are illustrated by two cancer sites.

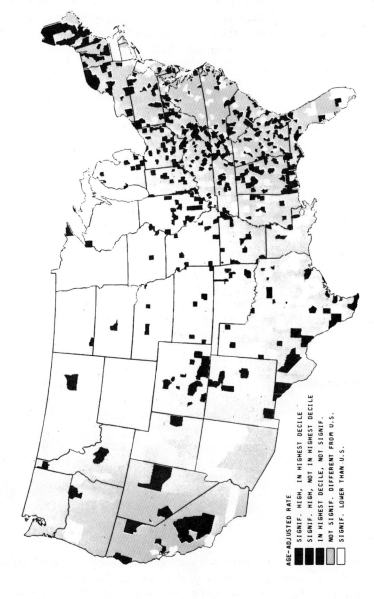

FIGURE 1. Mortality from cancer of cervix among white females by U.S. county, 1950-69.

AGE-ADJUSTED RATE

SIGNIF. HIGH, IN HIGHEST DECILE

SIGNIF. HIGH, NOT IN HIGHEST DECILE

IN HIGHEST DECILE, NOT SIGNIF.

NOT SIGNIF. DIFFERENT FROM U.S.

SIGNIF. LOWER THAN U.S.

TABLE 4

Measures of urbanization and socioeconomic class (1960) for the total United States, and for counties with an upper-decile mortality rate for cervical cancer among white females, 1950–1969

Area	Percent urban[a]	Median school yrs.[b]	Median family income($)
Total United States	69.9	10.2	5,741
Counties in highest decile for cervical cancer, statistically significant[c]	52.9	9.4	4,402
Counties in highest decile for cervical cancer, not statistically significant	25.4	8.7	3,316

[a]Percent of the population living in urban areas (1960 census definition).
[b]Median number of years of schooling completed by the adult population, 25 years old and older.
[c]Significantly different from the rate for the total United States ($p<0.05$).

Melanoma previously has been related to latitude (sunlight exposure) [6], and Figure 2 confirms an excess in the South in mortality from this tumor. This figure illustrates the distribution of rates by state economic areas. There are 506 of these areas, which are groups of counties with similar geographic, demographic, and economic characteristics. We found these units provide more stable rates for relatively uncommon cancers than do counties. Figure 3 illustrates mortality rates from melanoma for eight zones of latitude, standardized for age, urbanization, and social-class differences. There is a striking trend of increasing mortality as one moves from North to South. Also presented are the relationships for HD, a neoplasm of unknown etiology, previously shown to predominate in the North [7]. As shown for white females, there is a gradient of declining mortality from North to South independent of urbanization and social class. Since the bimodal age distribution of HD suggests epidemiologic heterogeneity, the data are being reanalyzed by age group.

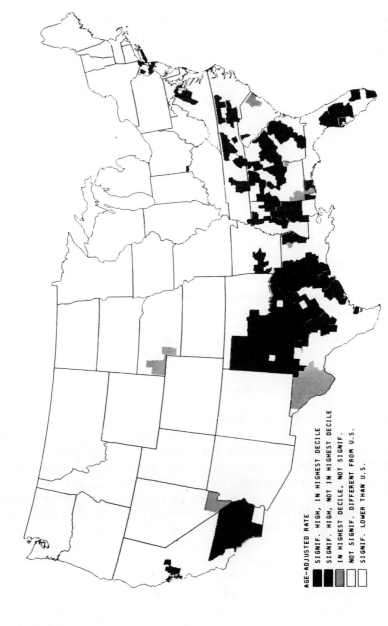

AGE-ADJUSTED RATE

SIGNIF. HIGH, IN HIGHEST DECILE

SIGNIF. HIGH, NOT IN HIGHEST DECILE

IN HIGHEST DECILE, NOT SIGNIF.

NOT SIGNIF. DIFFERENT FROM U.S.

SIGNIF. LOWER THAN U.S.

FIGURE 2.   Mortality from skin melanoma among white males by U.S. state economic area, 1950-69.

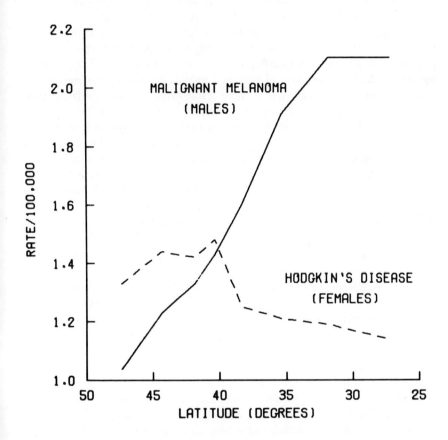

FIGURE 3. Mortality rates for malignant melanoma (males) and Hodgkin's disease (females) according to latitude in United States, 1950-69.

Concomitant Variation

Detection of a strong geographic correlation between different cancers may suggest a related etiology and potentiality for control programs targeted toward certain constellations of cancer. Pearson product-moment correlation coefficients were calculated between cancer sites for white males and females in all 3,056 counties. We computed two sets of coefficients: 1) the first allows each county to contribute equally to the comparison and 2) the other is a weighted correlation, with the weight being the proportion of the total U.S. population (race- and sex-specific) in the individual counties. The weighted correlation has the advantage of increased stability because of the greater contribution from large counties with more stable rates, and the disadvantage of accentuating urban correlations and masking those that are unrelated to urbanization. When the results from the two methods are synthesized, we find among males that cancers of the lung, larynx, and mouth and throat are highly correlated and might be thought of as a "smoking complex." Another group of correlated sites consists of cancers of the colon, rectum, esophagus, and bladder, and might be considered an "urbanization complex." Although bladder and esophageal cancers correlate also with the smoking complex, the association is not as strong as with the urbanization group. This finding is consistent with evidence for independent smoking and urbanization components for these two cancers [8,9]. Stomach and kidney cancers correlate with the urban complex, but at lower levels. Pancreatic cancer correlates with the smoking complex, but also at a considerably lower level. Further correlations include melanoma with other skin cancers, and non-Hodgkin's lymphoma with several sites in the urban complex (particularly bladder cancer). On the other hand, no impressive between-site correlations were found for leukemia, testicular cancer, or prostatic cancer.

Among white females, cancers of the colon, rectum, breast, and ovary are all highly correlated, and probably reflect both urbanization and social-class determinants of these tumors. Stomach cancer, bladder cancer, and lymphomas join this complex at successively lower magnitudes of association. However, contrary to the experience in males, esophageal cancer is not part of this urban complex, but correlates mainly with lung and pancreatic cancers to form a possible "smoking complex" for women. Notably absent from this complex are cancers of the oropharynx and larynx, possibly underscoring the interaction of heavy alcohol consumption with smoking in the induction of these tumors, particularly in males [10]. In women, mouth and throat cancer correlates with melanoma, other skin cancer, and cervical cancer—a complex of tumors with a lower socioeconomic class, southern predominance.

One provocative finding involved two cancers of obscure etiology—multiple myeloma and brain tumor. In the unweighted analysis, these cancers had the strongest correlation achieved by white males ($r = 0.5$). This association was not present among white females, but was one of the few detected among nonwhite males (the analysis in nonwhites was hindered by small county populations). In the weighted analysis, the myeloma-brain tumor correlation remained, but at a greatly reduced level (0.19). This reduction in the magnitude of the correlation can be traced to two factors. First, the magnitude of the unweighted coefficient is artifactually inflated because a few very small counties have very high rates for both tumors. When these counties are eliminated (or given small weights), the association remains, but at a much lower level. Second, the association is generally much stronger in the smaller, rural counties that do not carry much weight in the weighted correlations. These analyses do not necessarily signify that the two cancers are rural diseases. Indeed, the rates are higher in cities than in rural areas. These observations indicate, however, that in rural settings brain tumors and multiple myeloma among males may vary concomitantly. This correlation may be related in some way to the reported excess of both tumors in farmers [11,12], but the finding remains to be clarified by further study.

For further clues to etiologic factors and control measures, county correlations were made between the male and female cancer rates for whites. Both the unweighted and the weighted correlations show an impressive range in the magnitude of the coefficients (Table 5). The low correlations for some rare tumor sites may be due to artifact, but this explanation is unlikely to apply to the low values obtained with both methods for cancers of the larynx and kidney, HD, multiple myeloma, and leukemia. Also noteworthy are the high correlations for cancers of the stomach, colon, rectum, and lung.

ENVIRONMENTAL EXPOSURES

Hypothesis Testing

Although population-based mortality data are a crude means of testing hypotheses concerning public health hazards, geographic correlations with environmental measurements can be done quickly and inexpensively, and may be a valuable first step in evaluation of possible dangers. For example, cancer mortality patterns were not unusual among people residing in counties where drinking water is contaminated by asbestos [13], or where homes are built upon radioactive tailings from uranium mines [14]. Caution is necessary, however, since the latent period between exposure and disease may not have been sufficiently long for manifestation of risk. On the other hand, in a recent survey of counties where the chemical industry is highly concentrated [15], we found among males, excessive mortality from cancers of the bladder, lung, liver, and certain other sites. The correlation could not be explained by confounding variables such as urbanization, socioeconomic class, or employment in nonchemical industries. If the excess cancer mortality in

TABLE 5

Unweighted and weighted correlation coefficients $(r)^a$ between white men and
women, using age-adjusted sex-specific mortality rates for
individual counties of the contiguous United States,
according to cancer site, 1950-1969

Site	Unweighted r	Weighted r
Lip	-.01	.01
Salivary gland	.03	.05
Nasopharynx	.01	.08
Mouth and throat	.14	.25
Esophagus	.12	.39
Stomach	.34	.77
Colon	.39	.80
Rectum	.41	.81
Liver and biliary passages	.13	.39
Pancreas	.09	.37
Nasal sinus	-.02	.03
Larynx	.07	.19
Lung	.24	.62
Breast	.03	.20
Kidney	.06	.19
Bladder	.12	.45
Melanoma	.07	.24
Other skin	.14	.31
Eye	.00	.02
Brain	.04	.28
Thyroid	.01	.12
Other endocrine	.04	.06
Bone	.02	.11
Connective tissue	.01	.05
Hodgkin's disease	.06	.18
Non-Hodgkin's lymphoma	.08	.34
Multiple myeloma	.01	.11
Leukemia	.10	.21
Other and unspecified	.24	.57
All sites combined	.45	.82

[a]Pearson product-moment correlation coefficients. In the unweighted comparison each of
the 3,056 counties contributed equally. In the weighted comparison, the weights used were
the proportion of the total population that resided in each county during the 20-year
period.

these areas were due to industrial exposures, the actual risk of cancer among certain chemical workers must be very high. Indeed, the correlation was limited to counties associated with specific categories of the chemical industry; many involve known occupational hazards, whereas others suggest new leads to chemically induced cancer in man.

Hypothesis Formulation

The major contribution of the county resource probably will be to identify geographic clusters suggesting etiologic clues, which can then be pursued by analytic studies. The distribution of stomach cancer was one of the first examined, since the expected social-class gradient was absent (*see* above), suggesting important confounding variables. Figure 4 shows the geographic distribution of stomach cancer among white males. Elevated mortality is prominent in the major cities and in areas characterized by low social class (e.g., certain counties in Pennsylvania and Kentucky). Overshadowing those areas, however, is an impressive cluster of excessive mortality in primarily rural counties in the north-central region (Minnesota, the Dakotas, Michigan, and Wisconsin). Concentrated in these areas are people of Russian, Austrian, Scandinavian, and German descent. In fact, the 306 counties with the highest rates (highest decile) had three times as many first- and second-generation Finns, Austrians, and Russians as expected, and 40 to 60 percent more Norwegians, Swedes, and Germans than expected, based on the national percentages for these ethnic groups. Susceptibility of these migrant groups to stomach cancer would be compatible with the high incidence of this tumor in their countries of origin [16,17]. The smaller cluster in New Mexico and Colorado seems consistent with reports of elevated stomach cancer rates among Spanish-Americans in this area [18]. Thus, although urbanization and socioeconomic factors affect mortality from stomach cancer, ethnicity seems to be the major determinant of geographic variation within the United States.

A different array of geographic clustering is seen with bladder cancer mortality among white males (Figure 5). The clusters of elevated mortality correlate well with industrial exposures previously linked to this tumor. Since it seems likely that new occupational factors remain to be identified, the clusters can provide clues to industries that should be evaluated. To help isolate these areas, we selected a group of counties with the following criteria: 1) a significantly high mortality from bladder cancer among males compared to the national rate, 2) a greater male-to-female ratio of bladder cancer than found nationally, and 3) a lung cancer rate among males not significantly different than the national average (to reduce the confounding influence of cigarette smoking). The industrial makeup of this group of counties was determined from the 1950 census of workers by county employed in various industries. The percentage of workers employed in 41 separate industries was calculated for the

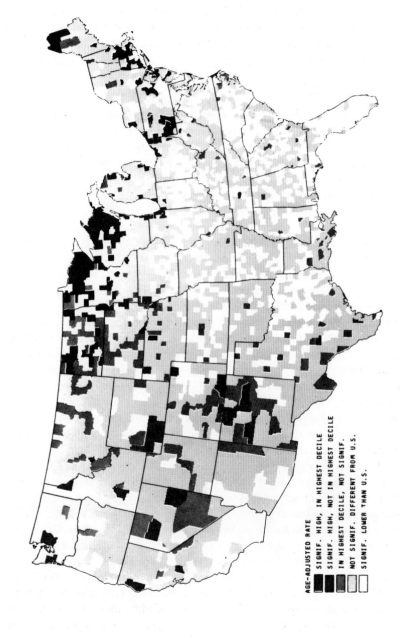

FIGURE 4. Mortality from stomach cancer among white males by U.S. county, 1950-69.

AGE-ADJUSTED RATE

SIGNIF. HIGH, IN HIGHEST DECILE

SIGNIF. HIGH, NOT IN HIGHEST DECILE

IN HIGHEST DECILE, NOT SIGNIF.

NOT SIGNIF. DIFFERENT FROM U.S.

SIGNIF. LOWER THAN U.S.

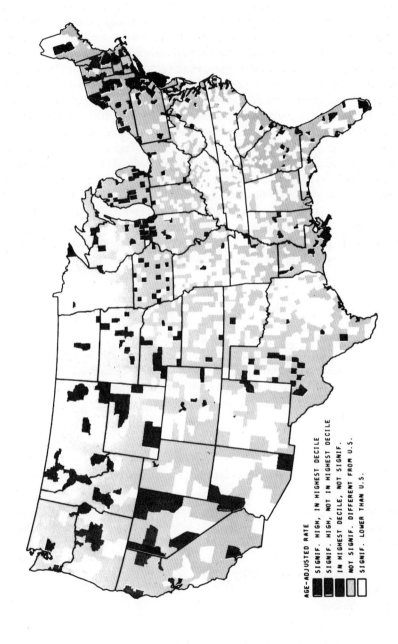

FIGURE 5. Mortality from bladder cancer among white males by U.S. county, 1950-69.

AGE-ADJUSTED RATE

SIGNIF. HIGH, IN HIGHEST DECILE

SIGNIF. HIGH, NOT IN HIGHEST DECILE

IN HIGHEST DECILE, NOT SIGNIF.

NOT SIGNIF. DIFFERENT FROM U.S.

SIGNIF. LOWER THAN U.S.

study counties and compared with corresponding percentages for the entire United States. Statistically significant differences occurred for only six industrial categories (Table 6). For three categories, the percentage employed in the study counties was significantly lower than the national experience, but the industries were mainly in rural areas, where the risk of bladder cancer is low. However, the percentage of workers in the study counties was significantly high for three categories: machinery manufacturing (except electrical), electrical machinery manufacturing, and motor vehicle manufacturing. These industries have not been previously implicated in bladder carcinogenesis, and would be a logical place to search for occupational determinants. Suspicions regarding the automobile industry were deepened by recent results from the Third National Cancer Survey, 1969–1971 [19]. Detroit had the highest incidence rate for bladder cancer (but only the fifth highest rate for lung cancer) among white men in the seven cities and two states participating in the Survey. Wayne County (Detroit) was excluded from our correlation study because of a significantly elevated rate for lung cancer. However, its mortality rate for bladder cancer is significantly high among men, but not among women.

TABLE 6

Industrial categories in which the percent of persons employed in counties with a high bladder cancer risk[a] differed significantly ($p < 0.05$) from the percent of such persons employed nationwide

Type of industry	Total U.S. (expected)	High-risk counties (observed)	Observed/ expected
Agriculture	15.5	4.2	0.3
Mining	2.2	0.3	0.1
Manufacturing	27.0	42.2	1.6
Furniture, lumber, wood	2.7	1.4	0.5
Machinery (except electrical)	2.8	6.3	2.3
Electrical machinery	1.3	2.8	2.2
Motor vehicles	1.9	4.8	2.5

[a]*See* text for method of selecting "high-risk" counties.

Unusual Counties

Because of the many comparisons involved with data for 3,056 counties over 20 years, it may be dangerous to single out a particular county or even a small group of counties for special attention. In certain situations, however, the unusual mortality experience of a county would seem to warrant further investigation. For example, Salem County, New Jersey, leads the nation in bladder cancer mortality among white men. The excess risk is surely due to occupational exposures, since about 25 percent of the employed persons in this county work in the chemical industry, primarily the manufacturing of organic chemicals with a potential for causing bladder tumors. This finding indicates the need for surveys of cancer risk and programs in cancer control among workers in this area.

Another rationale for studying individual counties is the identification of a highly unusual occurrence not easily explained. For example, in Nebraska there are two adjacent counties (Butler and Colfax) that have very high death rates for colon cancer. Although this tumor predominates in the upper social class and urban northeast, these two counties are predominantly low social class, rural, and midwestern. Over 25 percent of the population in these counties are foreign born or have foreign-born parents, mainly of Czechoslovakian descent [20]. The rates for colon cancer are reportedly not high in Czechoslovakia [17], but further studies of colon cancer in these Nebraskan counties seem warranted. ·

REFERENCES

1. Mason, T.J., and McKay, F.W. *U.S. Cancer Mortality by County: 1950-1969.* DHEW Publication (NIH) 74-615. U.S. Govt. Print. Off., Washington, D.C., 1973.

2. Haenszel, W., Marcus, S.C., and Zimmerer, E.G. *Cancer Morbidity in Urban and Rural Iowa.* Public Health Monograph 37. U.S. Govt. Print. Off., Washington, D.C., 1956.

3. Clemmesen J., and Nielsen, A. Age distribution figures for cancer in Danish towns and country, 1943 to 1947. *Acta Un. Int. Contra Cancer. 8:*140-159, 1952.

4. *The Registrar-General's Decennial Supplement, England and Wales, 1951.* Part I. Her Majesty's Stat. Off., London, 1968.

5. Dorn, H.F., and Cutler, S.J. *Morbidity from Cancer in the United States,* Part II. Public Health Monograph 56. U.S. Govt. Print. Off., Washington, D.C., 1959.

6. Movshovitz, M. and Modan, B. Role of sun exposure in the etiology of malignant melanoma: Epidemiologic inference. *J. Natl. Cancer Inst. 51:*777-779, 1973.

7. Cole, P., MacMahon, B., and Aisenberg, A. Mortality from Hodgkin's disease in the United States, *Lancet 2:*1371-1376, 1968.

8. Cole, P. Lower urinary tract. *In* Schottenfeld, D., ed. *Cancer Epidemiology and Prevention: Current Concepts.* Charles C. Thomas, Springfield, Ill., 1974, pp. 233-262.

9. Schoenberg, B.S., Bailar, J.C., III, and Fraumeni, J.F., Jr. Certain mortality patterns of esophageal cancer in the United States, 1930-67. *J. Natl. Cancer Inst. 46:*63-73, 1971.

10. Rothman, K. Alcohol. This volume, 1975.

11. Choi, N.W., Schuman, L.M., and Gullen, W.H. Epidemiology of primary central nervous system neoplasms. *Am. J. Epidemiol. 91:*238–259, 1970.

12. Milham, S. Leukemia and multiple myeloma in farmers. *Am. J. Epidemiol., 94:* 307–310, 1971.

13. Mason, T.J., McKay, F.W., and Miller, R.W. Asbestos-like fibers in the Duluth water supply. *J.A.M.A. 228:*1019–1020, 1974.

14. Mason, T.J., Fraumeni, J.F., Jr., and McKay, F.W., Jr. Uranium mill tailings and cancer mortality in Colorado. *J. Natl. Cancer Inst. 49:*661–664, 1972.

15. Hoover, R., and Fraumeni, J.F., Jr. Cancer mortality in U.S. counties with chemical industries. *Environ. Res.* In press.

16. Doll, R., Muir, C., and Waterhouse, J. *Cancer Incidence in Five Continents.* Vol. II. Springer-Verlag, New York, 1970.

17. Dunham, L.J., and Bailar, J.C. III. World maps of cancer mortality rates and frequency ratios. *J. Natl. Cancer Inst. 41:*155–203, 1968.

18. Weitzner, S., and Smith, D.E. Carcinoma of the stomach in New Mexico: A preliminary report. *Am. Surg. 40:*161–163, 1974.

19. Cutler, S.J., and Young, J.L. Demographic patterns of cancer incidence in the United States. This volume, 1975.

20. U.S. Bureau of the Census: *U.S. Census of the Population: 1960.* Vol. 1, Part 29. U.S. Govt. Print. Off., Washington, D.C., 1963.

DISCUSSION

Dr. Peters noted that "bedroom communities"—counties on the fringes of urban areas—might be expected to have cancer patterns similar to those of urban areas. **Dr. Hoover** responded that this was generally so, and that such communities are not necessarily contiguous to the urban areas. For example, Dade County, Florida (Miami), with high cancer rates for a number of sites, could be pictured as the bedroom community for New York, Chicago, or a number of Northeastern and Midwestern cities.

Dr. Mack commented that Dr. Hoover's county correlation studies between cancer mortality and environmental-demographic exposures represent a prime example of what record-linkage can accomplish.

William J. Blot

21

MIGRANT STUDIES

William Haenszel

Biometry Branch, National Cancer Institute
Bethesda, Maryland

INTRODUCTION

Several studies have delineated differences in site-specific cancer risks between the native- and foreign-born populations of the United States [1-8]. Similar observations have been assembled in New Zealand [9], South Africa [10], and most recently in Australia [11]. The motivation for these efforts is the desire to take advantage of the natural experiment represented by population migration to investigate host and environmental factors as determinants of cancer risk [11].

Migration does not have to cross national boundaries to be of value. Information that has been vital in deciphering some steps in the etiology of stomach cancer has come from studies of migrants from the countryside to a large urban center in Colombia [12].

Cancer mortality for foreign-born residents of the United States as of 1959-61 was reported by Lilienfeld et al. [8]. The following list of ethnic groups with site-specific mortality exceeding that for U.S. native-born whites is abstracted from that source:

Buccal cavity and pharynx   *Large bowel*
  Ireland (males)   Ireland (males)
  Finland (females)

Esophagus
  Ireland
  Poland
  U.S.S.R. (females)

Stomach
  Austria
  Czechoslovakia
  Finland
  Hungary
  Ireland
  Japan
  Norway
  Poland
  Sweden
  U.S.S.R.
  Yugoslavia

Larynx
  Ireland
  Sweden (females)

Thyroid
  Poland
  Norway (females)
  U.S.S.R.

Contrasts of native- and foreign-born populations in the country of destination provide only a partial picture of migration effects. For complete, rounded assessment, the migrant experience must be related to that prevailing in both home and host countries. Lombard and Doering [1] attempted this assessment in the United States, using the limited range of mortality data from foreign countries at their disposal. More extensive compilations of mortality data and the improved quality of death certifications in the countries of origin have permitted later investigators to make more precise descriptions of the direction and probable magnitude of changes in risks. The available evidence is based on migration to the United States and British Commonwealth countries, which share a characteristic site profile of risks. Thus, the migrant observations reflect unidirectional shifts from high-risk countries to a low-risk host population (for cancer of the stomach) or from low-risk countries to a high-risk host population (for cancer of the large bowel). The data indicate the migrant effects to be specific for both site and country of origin; for many sites, no obvious pattern of relationships can be discerned.

For cancer of the stomach, lung, large bowel, breast, ovary, corpus uteri and prostate, sizable consistent effects for several key migrant groups lend themselves to the following generalizations:

Stomach   The migrants from high-risk areas show some reduction
                 in rates, but still display the characteristic experience of
                 the country of origin.

Lung

The rates for migrants from countries with high and low risks are displaced to a level intermediate to home and host populations.

Large bowel, breast, ovary, corpus uteri, prostate

Migrants from low-risk areas attain in their lifetime the rates prevailing in the host population; the breast cancer experience of Japanese migrants is an exception to this general rule.

CANCER CONTROL

Direct application of migrant studies to the planning and conduct of cancer control activities in the United States has limited scope. The major streams of migration to this country from Europe and Japan took place in the late nineteenth and early twentieth centuries. Many of the original migrants are dead, so that efforts to identify high-risk groups would be focused on persons disappearing from our midst. This approach may prove more valuable in Canada and Australia, where migrants have arrived more recently.

Even when migrants from individual countries can be identified to be at high risk for a specific site, the utility of such an observation will depend on the concentration and accessibility of the population. For example, the knowledge that migrants from the United Kingdom have above-average lung cancer risks is not very helpful in view of their wide dispersion throughout the United States. The well-known excess liability of Chinese to nasopharyngeal cancer might suggest that screening and detection programs be undertaken in the Chinese communities of New York, San Francisco, and Honolulu, but efforts to reach the large numbers of Chinese dispersed throughout the United States would have a low benefit-cost yield, even if the available control measures for nasopharyngeal cancer were effective and productive. The Japanese migrants and their U.S.-born offspring, who still exhibit elevated risks for stomach cancer, are a more accessible target population for control measures represented by Japanese communities concentrated in Honolulu, Los Angeles, and other Pacific Coast metropolitan areas.

The nature of the migrant effects can provide some clues to appropriate control activities. Since the migrant studies indicate that the level of stomach cancer risk is determined primarily by events in early life, primary prevention of the disease through modification of environmental exposures, including changes in diet, offers limited prospects for success. A preferable strategy would seem to be a screening program to detect lesions in a very early stage in the gastric mucosa before penetration of the submucosa, since favorable survival is limited to small lesions confined to the gastric mucosa. A screening program developed in Japan and based on radiography, in which paraprofessional personnel were used, has reported success in detection of very early lesions, associated with 5-year survival rates of 90 percent. Extension to Japanese communities in the United States is at least conceptually feasible.

We have enumerated some sites (large bowel, breast, ovary, corpus uteri, prostate) for which the risks in the migrants' lifetime have risen to the prevailing level of the U.S. host population. In a real sense the total U.S. population is at high risk to these diseases, and one value of migrant studies and interpopulation comparisons is that they provide perspective and highlight the arbitrary nature of any definition of "high risk." However, the knowledge that the total U.S. population is at high risk to large-bowel cancer does not help to delineate a target population; it merely indicates size. Screening methods on a mass scale to detect precursor lesions or early large-bowel cancers will be enormously expensive. One must look to epidemiologic studies to identify risk factors that can circumscribe a target population of manageable dimensions. Age is a valuable criterion for this purpose, but it must be combined with other parameters.

For implementation of cancer control activities, it is more important to identify high-risk populations; however, the knowledge that the earlier low risk for certain migrant groups has been altered unfavorably subsequent to their arrival in the United States suggests a long-range approach to control of large-bowel cancer through primary prevention, i.e., identification and removal of the factors responsible. The great contribution of migrant studies to cancer control is still to be realized and should come through epidemiologic studies to develop new knowledge. Migrant populations seem particularly suited for investigation of diet-related etiologies suspected as factors in cancers of the stomach and large bowel. Dietary practices tend to be relatively homogeneous in individual localities or countries, which makes it difficult to detect differences in case-control or prospective studies conducted within the confines of a single population as pointed out by Wynder et al. [12]. In other situations when environmental exposures and/or habits are unevenly distributed throughout a population (e.g., cigarette smoking), work in a single locality can detect effects. For studies of interaction effects (air pollution and cigarette smoking), migrant populations possess attractive advantages. English and Norwegian migrants to the United States have been used in this context for studies of cardiorespiratory diseases [13,14].

EPIDEMIOLOGY OF STOMACH CANCER

This section is devoted to the epidemiologic facet of migrant studies, particularly their use in generating a sequence of epidemiologic investigations. We chose stomach cancer to illustrate some advantages in the exploitation of observational situations represented by migrant populations. A resumé of the sequence of events in stomach cancer epidemiology since 1960 follows:

1)   The persistence in the United States of high stomach cancer risks among migrants from high-risk countries pointed to factors in the

environment of the home country. Migrants from Japan and Norway to the United States and their U.S.-born offspring were designated as study populations. Plans called for case-control studies using the same questionnaire and procedure in the home and host countries, accompanied by surveys of a representative sample of households in the countries of origin and destination. The household survey data provided comparative estimates on the prevalence of suspect factors in the migrant and sedent populations and an alternate set of general population controls for contrasts with the series of cases.

Effective coordination in collecting epidemiologic and pathologic observations on the Japanese populations was made possible through close collaboration with pathologists in Japan and Hawaii.

2) Muñoz et al. [15], Correa et al. [16], and others typed stomach cancers in Latin-America populations at high and low risk to the disease using the criteria of Jarvi and Lauren. They reported that the intestinal type predominated among cases in high-risk areas. From this observation, they inferred the intestinal type to be an "epidemic" component of stomach cancer responsible for most of the difference between high- and low-risk areas.

3) The cancer registry in Cali, Colombia, described marked variation in stomach cancer risk among residents of that city by birthplace, the marked excess of cases occurring among migrants from the Department of Nariño. Intestinal-type tumors accounted for most of the excess incidence in this subpopulation [16]. The next critical step in Cali was to elaborate the registry findings by autopsy studies, which showed intestinal metaplasia to be more prevalent among the migrants from Nariño [16]. For the several migrant populations in Cali, the prevalence of intestinal metaplasia was more closely correlated with intestinal-type stomach cancer than with the diffuse type, thus incriminating intestinal metaplasia as a precursor lesion for at least some types of stomach cancer.

Other broadly based studies of autopsy materials [17,18] confirmed the greater prevalence of intestinal metaplasia in populations at high risk to stomach cancer. A variety of other observations—coincidence of sites of maximal intestinalization and gastric cancer, observation of transitional states between metaplasia and cancer—strengthened the case for intestinal metaplasia as a precursor lesion [19].

4) The case-control study of Hawaiian Japanese [20] revealed that migrants from the Japanese prefectures with highest stomach cancer risks continued to experience an excess risk in Hawaii, but this effect did not persist among their Nisei offspring. Lower risks were suggested for the Nisei, but not Issei, who had adopted Western-style diets. These

nativity distinctions reinforced earlier inferences from migrant study data on the critical nature of exposures in childhood.

The Hawaiian Japanese study deviated from a long line of earlier studies conducted among sedentes in many countries that had failed to uncover case-control differences in food histories. The favorable observational situation presented by the Hawaiian Japanese—two distinct patterns of Japanese and Western foods, heterogeneity in food habits arising from variation in timing and degree of transition from Japanese-to Western-style customs—facilitated the detection of differences. Elevated risks of stomach cancer were noted for users of pickled vegetables and dried/salted fish, with the suggestion of risks rising with increased use. In the absence of similar associations for raw fish and unprocessed vegetables, suspicion was directed to methods of preparation. Low risks were described for several Western-type vegetables (lettuce, celery, corn, etc.) and the latter appeared to be independent of the high risks for pickled Japanese foods, raising the possibility of some protective food effects.

5)   The companion case-control studies [21] conducted in Japan (Hiroshima and Miyagi prefectures) did not reproduce the associations with the pickled vegetables and salted/dried fish reported for the Hawaiian Japanese; a homogeneous background of food habits in early life during the pre-World War II period operated against their detection. Controls in Japan reported a greater frequency of use of lettuce and celery which suggests that the concept of protective food effects in stomach cancer etiology warrants continued attention.

Characterization of the farm population as the group at highest risk of stomach cancer may be the important finding from work in Japan. Traditional Japanese customs have persisted in the farm population, and the household surveys showed higher use of dried/salted fish and some pickled vegetables, particularly radishes, among farmers. The gradients might be construed as secondary evidence reinforcing the associations with these foods noted for the Hawaiian Japanese.

6)   The pathology studies [22] on stomach cancer cases in Miyagi prefecture and Hawaii elaborated earlier distinctions for intestinal and diffuse types. Since tumor registries provide incidence data for both populations, type- and age-specific incidence rates could be estimated. The incidence for diffuse carcinomas was substantially the same in both localities, but the incidence for intestinal, mixed and other types was markedly lower in Hawaii, providing further documentation for the conjecture of Muñoz et al. discussed earlier.

The slopes of the age curves of log incidence for the diffuse and intestinal types were distinctly different, the slope for the diffuse type rising more slowly with age. The same slope of log incidence by age for intestinal type was observed in both areas; the difference between Miyagi and Hawaii being the lateral displacement of the curve to the right (to older ages) in Hawaii, a feature reproduced in the separate data for males and females. The constant slope values suggest that the forces contributing to the rise in incidence with age are similar once some critical age has been reached. The lateral displacement of the Hawaii curve to an older age could arise from a later onset of carcinogenic insults or variable incubation periods. Given the evidence for the close association between intestinal metaplasia with intestinal-type tumors, the latter appears more plausible.

7) Case-control studies of diet and stomach cancer have been complicated by problems of informant recall and accuracy of histories. The interval between exposure and onset of disease might be reduced by substitution of observations on a precursor condition and the findings on intestinal metaplasia suggested the transformation of the epidemiology of stomach cancer into the epidemiology of intestinal metaplasia to be a reasonable line of attack. A cohort of Japanese males in Hawaii assembled and under surveillance by the National Heart and Lung Institute was chosen for this purpose. A variety of physiological, anthropometric, blood chemistry, and dietary observations had already been assembled. Another round of examinations collected data relevant to gastro-intestinal cancers. Tests for gastrin bioassay, parietal-cell antibodies, and pepsinogens I and II were included to provide information on the presence and degree of intestinalization of the gastric mucosa. Unfortunately, the sensitivity and specificity of the tests do not yield an adequate classification for intestinal metaplasia. For this purpose, direct visual and histologic observations of the gastric mucosa via gastroscopy seem required. A limited amount of such information for cohort members is available.

8) More promising opportunities for gastroscopic studies of intestinal metaplasia have been presented in Colombia. The high stomach cancer risks for Cali residents born in Nariño also prevail within Nariño. Because of the exceptionally high risks (equal to or exceeding those described for Japan and the altiplano of Costa Rica), a proposal to study the distribution of intestinal metaplasia was supported by local health authorities and medical groups. A preliminary assessment of hospital admissions and discharges confirmed the clinical impressions of local physicians that stomach cancer risks were not uniformly distributed throughout Nariño, but instead were concentrated in certain localities [23]. This information was taken into account in the conduct of field work. The primary objective of the examination of a popu-

lation of apparently well individuals by gastroscopy was to determine the prevalence of intestinal metaplasia and/or chronic atrophic gastritis, but individuals examined were also questioned with respect to residence history, food history, and sources of water supply. The distribution of intestinal metaplasia and chronic atrophic gastritis by place of birth agreed well with the previously noted clustering of stomach cancer cases. Persistence of the high prevalence of intestinal metaplasia among individuals born in the high-risk communities, but later moving to low-risk areas (by Nariño standards), reinforced the pervasive theme on importance of exposures in early life for this disease.

The presence of wells with nitrate-rich water in several of the high-risk (for both stomach cancer and intestinal metaplasia) communities in Nariño is provocative in view of other evidence tentatively linking nitrates with stomach cancer [24,25]. Weisburger [26] has reported the conversion of nitrates in foods stored overnight at room temperatures by bacterial action to nitrites, thus raising the possibility of in vivo conversion of nitrites to nitrosamine-type compounds. The subsequent discovery that users and nonusers of these wells in high-risk communities have the same prevalence of precursor lesions may detract from the attractiveness of this line of speculation. A modified hypothesis that well water may be an index of local soil composition, so that locally grown foods may be the source of nitrate, can be entertained. Elevated urinary nitrate levels (an index of nitrate intake) have been observed among residents of high-risk areas who do not use well water [23].

An advantage of the observational microcosm of circumscribed geographical differences in prevalence of precursor lesions delineated in Nariño is that it may facilitate search and refinement of detailed differences in diet and related exposures, such as soil effects mediated through locally grown foods.

9)   The divergent experience of the Hawaiian Japanese with respect to gastric cancer and gastric ulcer offers opportunities to clarify the function of intestinal metaplasia in these diseases. Whereas the stomach cancer experience of the original Japanese migrants remained close to the level prevailing in Japan, available evidence [6] indicates that the gastric ulcer risks among these same migrants have diminished markedly in their lifetime to approximate the risks of U.S. whites. Close co-incidence in anatomical sites of maximal intestinalization and gastric cancer has been observed [27] ; metaplasia also shares sites in common with gastric ulcer, except for ulcers just proximal to the duodenum. The latter are rarely associated with metaplasia, and their etiology may have more in common with duodenal ulcers.

If intestinal metaplasia is a precursor lesion for both gastric ulcer and cancer, a supposition supported by the data on site localization, an explanation for the contrary trends of gastric ulcer and gastric cancer among the Japanese migrants may require postulation of two distinct pathways. Contrary to an inverse association of stomach cancer and a Western diet limited to the second-generation Nisei, a recent case-control study [28] of gastric ulcer among the Hawaiian Japanese suggests this association to hold for both Issei and Nisei. The Issei finding points to protective effects that can suppress acute changes culminating in gastric ulcer. The Miyagi and Hawaii pathology studies [22] of stomach cancer indicate that the effect of migration on intestinal-type carcinomas has been to lengthen long latent periods preceding onset and diagnosis.

DISCUSSION AND SUMMARY

If the precedent set by the recent history of stomach cancer epidemiology is a reliable guide, one might predict that the contributions of migrant studies to cancer control will be expressed primarily through development of new knowledge by epidemiologic research. Reviews of the state of stomach cancer epidemiology in the 1950's leave the distinct impression that much earlier work undertaken within populations sharing homogeneous backgrounds of environmental exposures had come to a dead end [29, 30]. Within the past 15 years, ideas derived from migrant populations have infused new life into this subject. The great virtue of the migrant population approach has been its ability to correlate observations over a wider spectrum of environmental exposures in home and host populations, which have clarified the following features of stomach cancer:

1) The critical role of exposures in early life in determining the level of risk.

2) The important distinction between intestinal and diffuse types of the disease for descriptive and analytical epidemiology. This statement does not imply that the final word has been said on the meaning and significance of the morphologic distinctions.

3) Documentation of intestinal metaplasia as a candidate precursor lesion.

4) Detection of associations with certain classes of foods that had escaped attention in studies confined to sedentes.

These results were achieved by quite straightforward epidemiologic methods demanding no novel analytical techniques. The new elements were the selection of suitable observational settings that might be expected to yield fruitful leads and the coordinated collection of epidemiologic and pathologic data.

In turn, a foundation has been laid for the transformation of stomach cancer epidemiology into the epidemiology of intestinal metaplasia and allied precursor conditions. The latter will require endoscopic observations of the gastric mucosa to delineate differences in prevalence within small geographic areas and to relate them to specific local factors. Animal work to test associations revealed by epidemiological studies is needed, particularly the development of suitable animal models for intestinalization of the gastric mucosa. Continued pursuit of these lines of attack may yield information on how the chain of events leading to stomach cancer can be interrupted.

REFERENCES

1. Lombard, H.L., and Doering, C.R. Cancer studies in Massachusetts. Cancer mortality in nativity groups. *J. Prev. Med. 3:*343–361, 1929.

2. Mancuso, T.F., and Coulter, E.J. Cancer mortality among native white, foreign-born white, and nonwhite male residents of Ohio: Cancer of the lung, larynx, bladder, and central nervous system, *J. Natl. Cancer Inst. 20:*79–105, 1958.

3. MacMahon, B. The ethnic distribution of cancer mortality in New York City, 1955. *Acta Unio Int. Contra Cancrum 16:*1716–1724, 1960.

4. Haenszel, W. Cancer mortality among the foreign-born in the United States. *J. Natl. Cancer Inst. 26:*37–132, 1961.

5. Staszewski, J., and Haenszel, W. Cancer mortality among the Polish-born in the United States. *J. Natl. Cancer Inst. 35:*291–297, 1965.

6. Haenszel, W., and Kurihara, M. Studies of Japanese migrants. I. Mortality from cancer and other diseases among Japanese in the United States. *J. Natl. Cancer Inst. 40:*43–68, 1968.

7. King, H., and Haenszel, W. Cancer mortality among foreign- and native-born Chinese in the United States. *J. Chron. Dis. 26:*623–646, 1973.

8. Lilienfeld, A.M., Levin, M.L., and Kessler, I.I. *Cancer in the United States.* Cambridge, Mass. Harvard Univ. Press, 1972.

9. Eastcott, D.F. *Report of the B.E.C.C. (N.Z.) Branch, Cancer Registration Scheme.* Department of Health, Wellington, New Zealand, 1954.

10. Dean, G. The causes of death among the South African-born and immigrants to South Africa. *So. Afr. Med. J. 39:* (Supplement) 1–20, 1965.

11. Staszewski, J., McCall, M.G., and Stenhouse, N.S. Cancer mortality in 1962-66 among Polish migrants to Australia. *Br. J. Cancer 25:*599–610, 1971.

12. Wynder, E.L., Kmet, J., Dungal, N., et al.: An epidemiological investigation of gastric cancer, *Cancer 16:*1461–1496, 1963.

13. Reid, D.D. Studies of disease among migrants and native populations in Great Britain, Norway, and the United States. I. Background and design. *In* Haenszel, W., ed. *Epidemiological Approaches to the Study of Cancer and Other Chronic Diseases. Natl. Cancer Inst. Monogr. 19:*287–299, 1966.

14. Reid, D.D., Cornfield, J., Markush, R.E., et al. Studies of disease among migrants and native populations in Great Britain, Norway, and the United States. III. Prevalence of cardiorespiratory symptoms among migrants and native-born in the United States. *In* Haenszel, W., *Epidemiological Approaches to the Study of Cancer and Other Chronic Diseases. Natl. Cancer Inst. Monogr. 19:*321–346, 1966.

15. Muñoz, N., and Connelly, R. Time trends of intestinal and diffuse types of gastric cancer in the United States. *Int. J. Cancer 8:*158–164, 1971.

16. Correa, P., Cuello, C., and Duque, E. Carcinoma and intestinal metaplasia of the stomach in Colombian migrants. *J. Natl. Cancer Inst. 44:*297–306, 1970.

17. Imai, T., Kubo, T., and Watanabe, H. Chronic gastritis in Japanese with reference to high incidence of gastric carcinoma. *J. Natl. Cancer Inst. 47:*179–195, 1971.

18. Kubo, T., and Imai, T. Intestinal metaplasia of gastric mucosa in autopsy materials in Hiroshima and Yamaguchi districts. *Gann 62:*49–53, 1971.

19. Morson, B., and Dawson, I.M.P. *Gastrointestinal Pathology.* Blackwell Scientific Publications, London, 1973, p. 136.

20. Haenszel, W., Kurihara, M., Segi, M., et al. Stomach cancer among Japanese in Hawaii. *J. Natl. Cancer Inst. 49:*969–988, 1972.

21. Haenszel, W., and Segi, M. Unpublished data.

22. Correa, P., Sasano, N., Stemmermann, G.N., et al. Pathology of gastric carcinoma in Japanese populations: Comparisons between Miyagi prefecture, Japan, and Hawaii. *J. Natl. Cancer Inst. 51:*1449–1459, 1973.

23. Cuello, C. Personal communication.

24. Hill, M.J., Hawksworth, G., and Tattersall, G. Bacteria, nitrosamines and cancer of the stomach. *Br. J. Cancer 28:*562–567, 1973.

25. Hawksworth, G. Hill, M.J., Gordillo, G., et al. Possible relationship between nitrates, nitrosamines and gastric cancer. *In Proceedings of the Third International Meeting on the Analysis and Formation of N-Nitroso Compounds.* I.A.R.C. Scientific Publications, Lyon. (In press, 1975.)

26. Weisburger, J., and Raineri, R. Assessment of human exposure and response to N-nitroso compounds. A new view on the etiology of digestive tract cancers. *Toxicol. Appl. Pharmacol.* In press.

27. Stemmermann, G.N. The epidemiologic pathology of gastric carcinoma. *Excerpta Med.* In press.

28. Stemmermann, G.N., and Haenszel, W. Unpublished data.

29. Doll, R. Environmental factors in the aetiology of cancer of the stomach. *Gastroenterologia 86:*320–328, 1956.

30. Haenszel, W. Variation in incidence of and mortality from stomach cancer, with particular reference to the United States. *J. Natl. Cancer Inst. 21:*213–262, 1958.

DISCUSSION

The discussion centered around the relative usefulness of homogeneous versus heterogeneous populations. **Dr. A. B. Miller** suggested that populations with heterogeneous characteristics may often appear quite homogeneous due to inappropriate or unrefined methods of study. He also asked whether future research should concentrate on heterogeneous migrant and international populations, or on the more readily available homogeneous populations to which we wish to apply control measures. **Mr. Haenszel** replied that populations with widely varying characteristics are very useful in initially detecting etiologic relationships. Subsequently, more refined studies in a relatively homogeneous population can corroborate and possibly amplify the relationships.

Roland L. Phillips

22

OVERVIEW: GEOGRAPHIC OPPORTUNITIES
AND DEMOGRAPHIC LEADS

J.N.P. Davies, D. Sc., M.D.

Department of Pathology
Albany Medical College
Albany, New York

INTRODUCTION

The intent of this overview is not to emphasize the details of the situations described in the preceding four chapters—all by eminent authorities in the fields they have reviewed—but to stress certain aspects and lessons to be learned by considering some of the geographic differences in cancer incidence. A most important point was made by Haenszel [1] who noted that in the 1950's the epidemiologic studies of gastric cancer in homogeneous communities, subjected to the same environmental factors, had just about reached a dead end. The escape route was by study of gastric cancer and the circumstances under which it developed in communities having very different experiences with this disease, the changes consequent upon migration within such areas, and the different histologic types of gastric cancer. There are certainly lessons to be learned here that have relevance for other cancers [2]. Surely, the vital need for specificity in the diagnosis of cancers to be studied, in the different sites in which they arise in the body, and in the epidemiological distribution of the various histologic subtypes has become evident from many of the contributions made here, and cannot be overemphasized.

Research support is acknowledged from the National Institutes of Health grant NIH 71 2426; from the Brown-Hazen Fund; and from the Damon Runyan Memorial Fund for Cancer Research (DRG 830).

In the two volumes of *Cancer in Five Continents,* we have preliminary observations in this respect and a mass of data on the varied experience of cancers in numerous countries. To the earlier comparisons of Doll [3], we have the figures that Muir [4] put before us in his Table 1 of Chapter 18. In it we see remarkable variations in the major cancers of mankind which emphasize the tremendous importance of environmental factors that epidemiologists should endeavor to uncover. Just as a half-full glass is viewed differently by pessimists and optimists, Dr. Muir's figures can be similarly regarded. Those interested in establishing the causative factors and students of carcinogenesis will dwell on the highest rates; those concerned with public health and cancer prevention will consider the lowest rates. The differences are measures of the task before us in respect to prevention, but the lowest rates are as worthy of consideration as the highest, for they represent populations that by some means protect themselves or are not exposed to those factors that produce high rates. How they achieve this protection is worthy of study. Of course, there is no guarantee that the high rates in any two communities are the result of the same factors. Since we have to monitor the cost-effectiveness of preventive measures, it is important that they be concentrated where they can be most beneficial.

INTEGUMENTARY CANCER IN AFRICA

To illustrate these points, it is worth examining certain aspects of integumentary cancer in Africa based on two independent studies in Uganda [5,6] and a further study in West Africa [7]. The results of these studies are remarkably similar. At one level of measurement, integumentary cancer in Uganda is a major cancer problem causing virtually a quarter of all cancers diagnosed. Those to be considered are cancers of the skin, penis, and the external ocular tissues, major problems in the Uganda male [15 percent] and only a slightly lesser problem in the female because of high prevalence of carcinoma of the uterine cervix (Table 1). Clearly, squamous cell carcinomas, melanomas, and Kaposi's sarcoma are the major problems, and basal cell carcinomas and other individual skin cancers are relatively unimportant. We cannot here consider Kaposi's sarcoma, although there can be no question that it is environmentally determined and thus must be preventable.

If we consider the squamous carcinomas, there is a vast problem with penile carcinoma that is totally preventable by circumcision, even in Uganda [8]. This statement is true despite the fact that we do not know the pathogenic mechanisms of penile carcinoma in relation to lack of circumcision. Elimination of penile cancer, which seems to be occurring in Uganda through social progress, would considerably alter the cancer picture there.

With squamous carcinoma of the skin, we see that the site distribution is not uniform over the body surface (Table 2). In a personal series of 410

TABLE 1
Integumentary cancers–Uganda, 1964-1968

		No. of cases
Total cancers:		10,945
Integumentary:	Penis	474
	Cervix	751
	Skin	
	Squamous	663
	Melanoma	195
	Kaposi's	334
	Other	86
	Eye	
	Squamous	93
	Melanoma	6
	Other	26
	Total	2,628

squamous skin cancers [5] and in a larger series studied by the Iversens [6], the findings are virtually identical. At least four of every five squamous cancers of the skin developed on the leg, and around 80 percent of them developed from the knee down. Data in all these series show that about 80 percent of these cancers develop on a basis of tropical phagedenic ulceration and that almost every squamous cancer of the legs and arms and many of the trunk and head and neck have clearly defined antecedent lesions (Table 3). Thus, in a personal series of 400 squamous leg cancers there were only four without a defined antecedent lesion [5]. Apart from the tropical ulcer lesions on the limbs, scars on the head and neck, albinism, and xeroderma pigmentosum complete the list of antecedents. Evidently a major factor is tropical phagedenic ulceration [9,10]. Direct causative factors are trauma and infection with Vincent's organisms, so classically associated, as in tropical ulcers, with malnutrition and debility. We can be certain of trauma as a factor because in Ugandan children tropical ulcers of the shin develop equally in both sexes; in adults, it is a disease predominantly of males because females wear long dresses that protect the front of the legs [5]. The wearing of shoes also reduces the frequency of such ulcers. The resulting acute infection is a rapidly developing necrotizing hemorrhagic ulceration with rapid destruction of skin and subcutaneous tissues, exposure or destruction of bone joints and tendons, and development of secondary infections (e.g., osteomyelitis). Healing is very slow and chronicity common. The microbiological causes

TABLE 2

Site and type distribution—Uganda, 1947-1960 in males

Cancer	Penis	Skin	No. of cases Eyelid	Eyebulb	Lacrimal	Total
Squamous	503	323	9	58	0	893
Basal	–	15	2	2	0	19
Melanoma	–	102	0	13	0	115
Kaposi's	–	239	5	0	0	244
Other	–	2	0	0	7	9
					Total	1,280

TABLE 3

Squamous skin cancer—Uganda, 1964-1968

	Head and Neck	Trunk	Upper Limb	No Record	Lower Limb	Total
No. of cases	29	31	18	32	553	663
% total	4.4	4.7	2.7	4.8	83.4	100
Tropical ulcer (%)	20.7	32.3	61.0	71.8	77.0	
Burn (%)	3.4	0	16.7	0	0.9	
Albino (%)	13.8	0	0	0	0	
Some AL[a] (%)	27.9	25.5	83.3	93.7	87.5	

[a] AL = antecedent lesion.

of these ulcers should be considered for their possible carcinogenic powers. As Dr. Templeton [11] mentioned, in osteomyelitis, in the sinuses and fistulas in which carcinomas develop, staphylococci do not cause the bone infection.

If we examine the distribution of squamous carcinomas of the head and neck skin not associated with scars, sinuses, albinism, or xeroderma pigmentosum, the distribution is not uniform. There is a concentration on the upper aspect of the infraorbital ridge [5]. Clearly, we have reason to think that sunlight is the causative factor in the cancers of this site, as it is with genetic skin conditions. It is probably the causative factor with most cases of ocular squamous carcinoma, so similar to the cancer eye of cattle in Texas, and other sunny cattle-raising climes, for casual observation suggests that many affected in Uganda were rather popeyed compared to their fellows. Thus, we have direct or indirect evidence of the causative factors in well over 90 percent of all the skin squamous cancers in Ugandan natives.

A contrasting pattern is seen for melanomas in Uganda; there is little overlap with the distribution of squamous carcinomas [12], and the antecedent factors are distinct. Melanomas are virtually confined to the soles of the feet and are preceded by black spots in areas of lighter pigmentation [12]; melanomas of the uveal tract are rare and if any causative factor is under suspicion it is local heat rather than light. Further, the causative association with tropical ulceration is a factor in Uganda and other areas of the tropics, but is of no importance whatsoever in this country where leg ulcers (e.g., varicose ulcers) rarely become malignant. Thus, there may be some causative factors common to various countries with a high incidence of cancer, but the specific local factors may be totally different. As noted, alcoholism, highly suspect as a factor in esophageal carcinoma in some countries, appears to be quite unimportant in Iran [4].

Equally important is the observation that tropical phagedenic ulceration is almost totally preventable by the wearing of shoes and clothing that protects the legs and is so prevented in Africa. These measures are totally acceptable to the population. But should such ulceration develop, adequate and complete treatment by well established medical-surgical means [10] can eliminate the ulceration and subsequent cancer formation. Medical care of burn and other scars and the wearing of hats and sun-protective clothing would almost totally eliminate squamous skin and eye carcinomas, just as circumcision eliminates penile carcinoma. Clearly, it is not the duty or within the ability of the medical services of the country to shoe, hat, and clothe the population. Circumcision would make demands on the medical services; more specific measures to cope with ulcers and scars would also pose considerable demands. We can make some measure of the risks involved, however, and here again there are valuable lessons to be learned.

The black Ugandan is not at any great risk of skin cancer; overall average annual incidence rates are 1.7 per 100,000 [6], and the highest rates at certain ages are about 6.7 per 100,000. These rates are trivial compared with established rates for Caucasians in Africa, let alone in this country. But when the Ugandan does develop a tropical ulcer, the situation alters abruptly. Cancerous ulcers (2–8 percent) were found in a series of cases with established tropical ulcers [5,10]. With ulcers present for more than 2 years, far higher percentages are recorded. Thus, the development of a tropical ulcer means at least a ten-thousandfold increased risk of cancer. The sufferer has jumped from a low- to a high-risk group, toward which specific cancer preventive measures should be directed.

These observations reinforce two further points. The precise carcinogenic mechanisms by which tropical ulcers became carcinomatous are unknown, and much time could be spent discussing them. The mechanisms are no doubt of immense scientific interest but quite irrelevant to the prevention of the ulcer cancers. It is of course a truism in preventive medicine that prevention can be effective when causative factors are known, or even suspected, regardless of the precise mechanisms of pathogenesis. We can recognize situations where causative factors are known or suspected, or where we have no satisfactory evidence and the causative factors are totally unknown. Even where they are unknown, we can often see them at work by recognizing antecedent or precancerous lesions that may be local or generalized. As Koss [13] suggested, there are probably many more than have been recognized so far. As with noncancerous tropical ulcers, we can hope to intervene and eliminate the antecedent lesions before a cancer develops. The importance of searching for such lesions should be considered. However, it will only be successful if we study the separate cell types individually, rather than cancer at specific sites or in organs. We have high hopes, in the light of experience, that such studies will be informative.

CHILDHOOD CARCINOMAS

There is another field in which more precise knowledge is urgently needed, and it involves the induction time of many cancers. Virtually every writer on the subject of childhood carcinomas has stressed the importance of such studies because they may provide valuable clues concerning corresponding carcinomas in adults. That so little has been done is a measure of the paucity of these occurrences in childhood, even in the largest centers. In some areas of the world, however, the risk of certain carcinomas is increased during late childhood and adolescence. Thus, in Mozambique [14], the incidence of primary hepatocellular carcinoma (Table 4) starts to rise in childhood to fantastically high levels in adult life. Comparable situations occur in Hong Kong for nasopharyngeal carcinoma, hepatocellular carcinoma, and perhaps thyroid cancer, but not for biliary cancer. Gallbladder carcinoma may begin its incidence rise in childhood in certain Amerindian groups, as does oropharyngeal cancer in Asian populations. For many carcinomas occurring with very high incidence in some countries, there seems to be no reflection of the high adult rates in childhood; however, this situation needs to be clearly established. Where the carcinomas are common in children and young adults, induction times might be established; and, in the more limited environmental experience of children, potential causative factors might be identified more easily.

Colonic carcinoma is one of the more common carcinomas of childhood. Although some carcinomas arise in connection with ulcerative colitis, multiple

TABLE 4

Age-specific annual incidence rates per 100,000 for certain
childhood carcinomas (information from various sources)

Age, yr.	Hepatocellular carcinoma (Mozambique) Male	Female	Nasopharyngeal carcinoma (Hong Kong) Male	Hepatocellular carcinoma (Hong Kong) Male	Cholangiocellular carcinoma (Hong Kong) Male
0	0.0	0.0	0.0	0.1	0.0
5	3.7	0.0	0.0	0.0	0.0
10	51.1	17.6	0.4	0.6	0.0
15	77.2	10.8	1.1	0.7	0.0
20	181.5	47.6	2.5	1.2	0.0
25	151.9	35.0	5.4	2.7	0.0
30	162.5	36.9	16.6	3.7	0.0
35	192.9	25.9	21.9	9.0	0.5
40	264.7	81.5	29.6	15.8	0.0
45	117.6	51.9	35.5	18.9	0.8
50	80.0	16.5	35.7	25.7	2.3
55	90.9	75.5	—	—	—
60	87.9	54.1	—	—	—

polyposis, and other genetically determined disorders, many tumors develop
in the absence of precursor lesions, thus paralleling the situation in adults. In
other circumstances, antecedent states appear to explain most of the childhood
risk of cancer. Recently established [15] is a belt from Morocco to Iraq, and
perhaps to the borders of India and beyond, where about 10 percent or more of
childhood cancers are skin cancers developing on xeroderma pigmentosum;
Arabic genes may be responsible. The same defect occasionally seems responsible
for some carcinomas of the tongue and penis in children. In this field, our
ignorance is so great that detailed discussion is worthless.

SUMMARY

At present we have overwhelming evidence of remarkable variations in the
overall cancer incidence and of specific types between countries and within
countries even, as Hoover et al. [16] showed, down to the county level. It is
these differences we must explore. Whatever the prospects for purely epidemiologic studies, the outlook for combined epidemiologic-laboratory studies has

never been better. Others have touched on the need for the support and assistance of the public, which in my personal experience is almost always most fully and generously accorded. We need, too, the fullest cooperation of members of the profession in all branches. From my own experience, there is a difference in the professional's outlook in this country and in other countries. Cancer and cancer studies are regarded much more pessimistically in the United States than elsewhere. As a student in the 1930's I attended the cancer clinic in the radiotherapy department of my medical school; a considerable proportion of the patients passing through the clinic were healthy men and women reporting their healthy state 5, 10, or more years after surgery and radiotherapy. I had the impression then that a high proportion of cancer was curable by surgery and radiotherapy, because I saw the successes. But when I visit cancer clinics attended by students today, I see the failures of therapy, failures that are mitigated or relieved by chemotherapy, but failures of treatment nevertheless. Where are the successes? They stay with their private physicians and radiotherapists. If our students are surrounded chiefly by the failures of treatment, can we expect them to be optimistic until they have gained the experience of success over time?

REFERENCES

1. Haenszel, W. Migrant studies. This volume, 1975.

2. Munoz, N. and Connelly, R. Time trends of intestinal and diffuse types of gastric cancer in the U.S. *Int. J. Cancer 8:*158–164, 1971.

3. Doll, R. The geographical distribution of cancer. *Br. J. Cancer 23:*1–8, 1969.

4. Muir, C. International variation in high risk populations. This volume, 1975.

5. Davies, J.N.P., Tank, R., Meyer, R., et al. Cancer of the integumentary tissues in Uganda Africans: the basis for prevention. *J. Natl. Cancer Inst.* 41:31–51, 1968.

6. Iversen, U., and Iversen, O.H. Tumours of the skin. *In* Templeton, A.C., ed. *Tumours in a Tropical Country. A Survey of Uganda 1964-1968.* Springer-Verlag, Berlin, 1973, pp. 180–199.

7. Camain, R., Tuyns, A., Sarratt, H., et al. Cutaneous cancer in Dakar, *J. Natl. Cancer Inst. 48:*33–50, 1972.

8. Dodge, O.G., Linsell, A.C., and Davies, J.N.P. Circumcision and the incidence of carcinoma of the penis and cervix. A study in Kenya and Uganda Africans. *E. Afr. Med. J.40:*444, 1963.

9. Shepherd, J.J. Tribal variation in cutaneous tumours of the leg. *E. Afr. Med. J. 44:* 600-602, 1966.

10. Nelson, G.S., and Semambo, Y.B. The treatment of tropical ulcers in Uganda with special reference to an easily organised itinerant skin grafting team. *E. Afr. Med. J. 33:*189–202, 1956.

11. Templeton, A.C. Acquired diseases. This volume, 1975.

12. Lewis, M.D. Melanoma. *In* Templeton, A.C., ed. *Tumours in a Tropical Country. A Survey of Uganda 1964-1968.* Springer-Verlag, Berlin, 1973, pp. 171–179.

13. Koss, L.G. Precancerous lesions. This volume, 1975.

14. Prates, M.D., and Torres, F.O. A cancer survey in Lourenso Marques, Portuguese East Africa. *J. Natl. Cancer Inst. 35:*729–757, 1965.
15. Miller, R.W. Personal communication, 1974.
16. Hoover, R., Mason, T.J., McKay, F.W., et al. Geographic patterns of cancer mortality in the United States. This volume, 1975.

DISCUSSION

Dr. Greenwald seconded the suggestion for further etiologic study of adult cancers occurring in childhood, then commented on the need for better, more complete patient histories, particularly with respect to occupation. Even with refined statistical methods, one may not recognize a cluster of industrial cancer unless appropriate histories are taken.

Dr. Kessler agreed with Dr. Davies that more epidemiologic studies should emanate from clinical, pathology, and radiology departments but felt we should not reduce the number of such studies conducted by schools of public health.

Dr. Shubik indicated that the search for antecedent factors is only a first step in unraveling the carcinogenic mechanism. He suggested that before treating antecedent conditions, we need to clarify how cancer develops, using experimental approaches when applicable. In response, **Dr. Davies** noted that what is important for prevention is to identify the causative factor; we do not need to know precisely how or why this factor works before taking preventive measures.

William J. Blot

IMPLICATIONS OF HIGH-RISK GROUPS

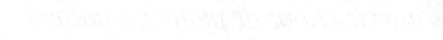

23

CANCER ETIOLOGY AND PREVENTION

John Higginson, M.D.

International Agency for Research on Cancer
Lyon, France

INTRODUCTION

The evidence that 80 percent of human neoplasms directly or indirectly depend on environmental factors carries important implications for prevention of cancer. It is widely assumed that if the etiology of a cancer can be identified, primary control is possible through either elimination or reduced exposure to such factors. Epidemiology is an essential tool in investigation of the role of environmental hazards in man. Such studies help identify carcinogenic agents already in the environment, permit suspected new carcinogenic stimuli entering the environment to be monitored, and provide necessary data for determining the degree of risk required for so-called cost-benefit calculations. Finally, the epidemiological technique is the only way hypotheses derived from animal experiments can be evaluated in man. This chapter reviews the role of high-risk groups, and their limitations, in studies of cancer etiology.

THE CONCEPT OF THE HIGH-RISK GROUP

A suspected carcinogenic agent usually is tested in an animal at the highest dose level compatible with reasonable health and life expectancy, because these conditions have proved the most favorable for demonstrating a carcinogenic effect. In contrast to animal experiments during which the observer can modify external conditions, epidemiology in man usually implies observational studies of naturally occurring situations (the so-called "natural experiment"). In man, further factors give rise to logistic and technical problems for the observer in demonstrating an etiological association between a suspected carcinogen and a specific cancer. These factors include the long latent period between first identifiable exposure and cancer development—this period tends to be much longer for carcinogens than for other chronic toxic agents. As modern societies become increasingly homogeneous, exposure to potential carcinogens in the general population tends to be multiple and to occur at low levels over prolonged periods. Thus, measurement of the total carcinogenic load at either the individual or the group level often presents the investigator with almost insurmountable practical problems and consequent difficulties in establishing etiological relationships. The examination of so-called "high-risk groups," either in terms of cancer risk or level of exposure, has many attractions. Not only can the conditions found in animal experimentation be theoretically reproduced, but also some of the logistic difficulties can be eliminated. Furthermore, after an agent is identified, the effects of exposure at varying dose levels often can be determined more easily than in the general population. Under some circumstances, the effects of man-made modifications of the microenvironment may be noted, e.g., a lowered risk of bladder cancer following reduction of industrial exposure.

The success of examining high-risk groups has been demonstrated by a number of classical studies on cultural and occupational groups, as more fully described by other authors in this monograph. However, certain inherent logistic and scientific limitations merit further discussion; these have prevented this approach from being successful for several types of cancer.

Classically, the term "high-risk group" describes a population (set) that differs from the general population (universe set) because it is composed either of: 1) individuals who show an unusual frequency of a specific cancer; or 2) individuals who are exposed to an unusually high concentration of a suspected carcinogenic stimulus. In practice, a group may initially be identified by both characteristics. The term "risk" implies axiomatically that these differences between the set and the universe set can be expressed in terms of mathematical significance. However, the terms "unusual groups" or "different groups" might describe the situation in real life more accurately. In some circumstances, the risk may be so high that the etiological relationship can be established beyond reasonable doubt by case reports alone, even if the level of risk cannot be expressed mathematically [1]. Moreover, the distinction from the general population may only involve a subgroup within a larger group or set, in whom the observation was first made, e.g., nickel workers [2]. These various combinations can be readily illustrated by Venn diagrams and the use of set theory [3].

Identification of a population showing an unusual frequency of cancer at a specific site or sites generally implies that the group is exposed to an unusual carcinogenic hazard that theoretically can be identified and measured and the level of risk calculated. However, there are different levels or kinds of risk, which may be expressed in terms of a whole population or strength of the carcinogenic stimulus. Thus, a strong carcinogen may be so limited in distribution that the level of risk in the general population is very low, but the risk for the exposed individual is very high. Conversely, a exposure or a large population to a weak carcinogen may produce a large number of cancers; the risk is low for the individual but high for the general population. Therefore, it is justifiable to consider high-risk populations separately according to the number of individuals at risk.

Small Population Groups

The term "high-risk group" most frequently refers to a population exposed to such a strong carcinogenic stimulus that a significant increase in cancer can be demonstrated even though the number of individuals at risk is small. In the ideal situation, such groups can be clearly distinguished from the general population by a single variable, e.g., drug exposure, occupation, or cultural habit. Further, when this variable itself is responsible for or is closely associated with the carcinogenic stimulus, the possibility of identification and measurement of the hazard is increased considerably. Such studies most closely approximate those in experimental animals and are the least complex to investigate. Some of the better-known situations are summarized briefly in Table 1. It should be emphasized that it is in these high-risk groups that satisfactory preventive efforts most often can be developed. Thus, appropriate action in cases such as those involving an occupational hazard may lead to effective control. The small size of such groups, however, presents considerable problems when one attempts to extrapolate the effects of low levels of exposure to the general population. The numbers of individuals at risk may be quite inadequate to estimate any degree of safety.

Large Population Groups

Whereas large populations may not be considered to be high-risk groups in the generally accepted sense, the wide extent of the hazard, the large number of cancers observed, and the fact that other populations do not carry equally high risks for the cancer would, in my opinion, justify such terminology. Thus, cigarette smokers could be described as being at high risk to lung cancer, African populations to primary carcinoma of the liver, and most Western industrial populations to neoplasms of the large intestine or breast. Identification and evaluation of the carcinogenic stimulus, however, pose problems quite different from those in small populations. Large populations at high risk may

TABLE 1

Summary of high-risk groups indicating nature of exposure, potential risk, and organs involved[a]

Chemical	Epidemiology[b] C	R	P	CR	Exposure patterns[c]	Daily intake[d]	Latency period, yr. (mean)	Relative risk	Site of neoplasm
Aflatoxin				+	General population (high in Africa): 0.12-0.35 μg/kg in food + 0.05-0.17 μg/liter in beer in Kenya	0.15 ng/kg bw/day	Unknown since childhood	$\frac{23 \text{ Obs}}{19 \text{ Exp}} = 1.3$	Liver
4-Aminobiphenyl	+	+			Ind—Past use as rubber antioxidant 1935-1955 (studies on 503 workers up to 1968)	Unknown	Unknown	Unknown	Bladder
Arsenic	+	+		+	Ind-Vineyards, miners, copper smelters (8,047) Med.-Fowlers solution Env-Water (Total number of persons exposed unknown)	Ind-4 mg/ m³ air Med-Unknown Env-3 ppm in drinking water	34-41 heavy & light exposure	$\frac{147 \text{ Obs}}{44 \text{ Exp}} = 3.3$	Respiratory tract
Asbestos	+	+		+	Ind-Miners, insulation and brake-lining workers (total number of persons exposed unknown)	Mills:100 mpppcf in 1952	10-50 (33)	$\frac{213 \text{ Obs}}{44 \text{ Exp}} = 4.8$	Lung

[a]Table I is a selected summary from Volumes 1-7 of the IARC Monographs on the Evaluation of the Carcinogenic Risk of Chemicals to Man, IARC, Lyon. It is not intended to be a complete coverage of the literature.

[b]C = case reports; R = retrospective studies; P = prospective studies; CR = correlation studies; + = positive.

[c]Ind = occupational; Env = environmental; Med = drug.

388

TABLE 1 (Continued)

Chemical	Epidemiology[b] C R P CR	Exposure patterns[c]	Daily intake[d]	Latency period, yr. (mean)	Relative risk	Site of neoplasm
Asbestos (cont.)		Env-Air, water, beverages, pharmaceuticals	0.1-100mg/ m^3 of air	10-50+ (33)	Very high	Pleura
Auramine	+	Ind-Exposure during manufacture (total number of workers exposed unknown)	Unknown	9-28 (19)	$\frac{6 \text{ Obs}}{0.45 \text{ Exp}} = 13$	Bladder
Benzene	+ +	Ind-Shoemaking, solvents (total number of workers exposed unknown, but in the thousands)	Unknown, but probably > 80 mg/m^3 (25 ppm) in air	Un- known expos- ures <20	One study $\frac{30 \text{ Obs}}{12 \text{ Exp}} = 2.5$	Leukemia
Benzidine	+ +	Ind-Manufacture of dyes and rubber (total number of workers exposed unknown)	Unknown	16	$\frac{10 \text{ Obs}}{0.72 \text{ Exp}} = 14$	Bladder
Bis (chloro-methyl) ether	+	Ind-Intermediate (total number of workers exposed unknown)	Unknown	8-16	Unknown	Lung

389

TABLE 1 (Continued)

Chemical	Epidemiology[b] C R P CR	Exposure patterns[c]	Daily intake[d]	Latency period, yr. (mean)	Relative risk	Site of neoplasm
Cadmium oxide	+	Ind-One study of 240 workers Env-Food, cigarettes	Unknown 1.5-2 µg/day	Unknown	$\frac{4 \text{ Obs}}{0.5 \text{ Exp}}=8$	Prostate
N,N-bis(2-chloro-ethyl)-2-naph-thylamine	+ +	Med-61 polycythemia patients studied	400 mg/day (total dose= 4-350 g)	See Table 2	Unknown, 7 of 61 cases developed cancer	Bladder
Chromate production	+ +	Ind-Production of chromate pigments	Unknown	11-31	$\frac{12 \text{ Obs}}{3.3 \text{ Exp}}=4$	Lung
Diethylstilbestrol (DES)	+	Med-In one study 49 of 66 cases developing vaginal cancers had been exposed to DES in utero	1.5-150 mg/day to mothers	Approx. 8-25 (17)	Unknown	Vagina
Hematite	+ +	Ind-Mining of hematite, underground workers (more than 5000 studied)	Unknown	Unknown	2-10 times increase in miners com-pared with nonminers or surface workers	Lung

TABLE 1 (Continued)

Chemical	Epidemiology[b] C R P CR	Exposure patterns[c]	Daily intake[d]	Latency period, yr. (mean)	Relative risk	Site of neoplasm
2-Naphthyla-mine	+ +	Ind-Manufacture and use as antioxidant in rubber (total number of exposed workers unknown)	Unknown	5-45 (18)	$\dfrac{26\ \text{Obs}}{0.3\ \text{Exp}} = 80$	Bladder
Nickel	+ +	Ind-Refining, mainly in workers exposed prior to 1925 Env-Air, food (very small)	Unknown	See Table 3	5-10 100-900 times expected figures	Lung Nasal cavity
Soot and tars	+ +	Ind-Mainly to tars (thousands of workers exposed)	Tars 3 $\mu g/m^3$ BP in retort houses	Unknown	One study $\dfrac{15\ \text{Obs}}{1.5\ \text{Exp}} = 10$	Skin (scrotum)
Vinyl chloride monomer	+	Ind-Cleaning of poly-merization reactors (exposures of 500-2,000 ppm 13 cases; >20,000 workers exposed)	Unknown	12-29 (20)	$\dfrac{13\ \text{Obs}}{0.03\ \text{Exp}} = 400$	Liver (blood vessels)

differ from populations with lower risks by so many variables that etiological comparisons become difficult or impossible. In this event, the epidemiological approach may be quite different from that of the small high-risk population groups.

Occasionally, a subgroup showing an unusual risk may be so diluted within the general population that it is not readily identifiable. Thus, an increase in a common cancer, e.g., lung cancer, may not readily be appreciated if it occurs in a subgroup showing few other differences from the general population. Identification of an unusually rare tumor, however, may provide clues to the existence of a group in the general population exposed to an unusual environmental hazard. For example, in the United Kingdom, the appearance of isolated mesotheliomas drew attention to the dangers of asbestos in the shipbuilding industry [4]. In this context, the existence of a well-organized morbidity cancer registry is of great value, especially if combined with a record linkage system [5].

ROLE OF ANIMAL EXPERIMENTATION IN EVALUATION OF EPIDEMIOLOGICAL INVESTIGATIONS OF HIGH-RISK GROUPS

Despite the limitations of direct extrapolation from animals to man, the principles of carcinogenesis developed from animal experimentation have considerable significance for human studies. The organization of such studies in chemical carcinogenesis was reviewed extensively by Weisburger and Weisburger [6]. Among the factors of importance to the human situation are: 1) the number of animals—sufficient animals must be used to ensure the appearance of enough tumors for evaluation; 2) the dose levels of the carcinogen under study; 3) the latent period between exposure and appearance of the neoplasm—if the period exceeds the lifespan of the animal, no tumors will be observed; and 4) the susceptibility of the species of animal involved, e.g., age, nutritional status.

In relating these factors to the epidemiological study of high-risk groups, the following points require consideration:

Tumor incidence. Age-specific rates in epidemiological studies have led to the mistaken belief that cancer is a rare disease in man. The lifetime figures indicate that cancer is fairly common, e.g., lung cancer causes 8 percent of all deaths in the United Kingdom. Thus, an increase of only a few cases of cancer per year within the general population would be difficult to identify unless the increase could be shown to be confined to an identifiable subgroup. Continuing evaluation of large population groups according to different variables may lead to the identification of a high-risk subgroup. For example, reserpine therapy was implicated recently in the causation of breast carcinoma by such an approach [7].

Dose and latent period. The latent period for most experimentally induced cancers appears to be related to the lifespan of the species. Druckrey [8] demonstrated a close relationship between dose and the length of the latent period for certain carcinogens. Tomatis et al. [9] showed that in mice, however, increasing exposure to DDT from 2 ppm to 50 ppm did not significantly increase the rate of liver tumors or change the length of the latent period. However, increasing exposure to 250 ppm shortened the latent period and increased the tumor incidence. The significance of such observations in man, in whom the level of exposure may be low, is unclear. Thus, the increased risk for individuals smoking cigarettes is relatively slight for the first 20 years of exposure, but then becomes obvious (Table 2).

Some of the data available from other studies on the relationship of carcinogenic stimulus to dose level and latent period are summarized in Tables 1, 3, and 4. Although inadequate, the data support the view that no definitive association exists between the strength of a carcinogen and the latent period. Clearly, in man, the absence of exposure to a strong carcinogenic stimulus cannot be assumed if examination of a small group fails to show tumors within one or two decades. Such a dichotomy between latent period and dose level is illustrated by atomic-bomb survivors in whom a high incidence of leukemia appeared within the first 10 years after the explosion, whereas an increased incidence of other cancers appeared much later [10]. The biological mechanisms (such as the role of DNA repair) behind such observations are beyond the scope of this paper, but they carry significant epidemiological implications. The existence, however, of a long latent period does permit application of the concept of "personnel engineering" in industry.

TABLE 2

Mean age at onset of lung cancer relative to number of cigarettes[a]

No. of cigarettes per day	Age at onset (yr.)
1 - 10	58.6
11 - 20	57.0
21 - 30	57.1
31 - 40	55.9
41 - 80	56.6

[a]Passey, R.D. Some problems of lung cancer. *Lancet 2:* 107–112, 1962.

TABLE 3

Interval between first treatment and diagnosis of bladder tumor
after chlornaphazine (N,N-bis(2-chloroethyl)-2-naphthylamine)[a]

Total dose (g)	No. of cases	Range of doses (g)	Latent period Mean	Range
49	1	4	5 yr 10 mo	–
50-149	3	50-100	5 yr 8 mo	4 yr 3 mo-7 yr 2 mo
150-249	5	160-200	5 yr 11 mo	2 yr 7 mo-10 yr
250	1	350	2 yr 9 mo	–
All cases	10	4-350	5 yr 6 mo	2 yr 7 mo-10 yr

[a]Thiede, T. and Christensen, B.C. Bladder tumors induced by chlornaphazine, *Acta. Med. Scand.* 185:133–137, 1969.

TABLE 4

Latent period for cancer of the respiratory
organs among workers at a nickel refinery [2]

Year of first employment	No. of cases	Duration of employment (yr.) Mean	Range	Latent period (yr.) Mean	Range
Lung cancer					
1910 - 29	10	26.8	13-33	35.6	26-47
1930 - 40	11	13.6	4-32	31.6	20-39
Cancer of nasal cavities					
1910 - 29	6	30.0	23-42	36.8	26-49
1930 - 39	8	18.3	7-33	27.8	18-36

Individual susceptibility. In a group exposed to a carcinogen at approximately the same level, those individuals who develop cancer are generally believed to be unduly susceptible to the agent. This situation clearly offers attractive theoretical possibilities for prevention [11]. So far, objective techniques to measure individual susceptibility in epidemiological studies are still in the development phase. Factors affecting susceptibility may be either exogenous or endogenous. The former includes other carcinogens; thus, asbestos workers who smoke cigarettes are at a much higher risk than those who do not smoke [12]. Both epidemiological and experimental studies [13] also suggest that transplacental transmission of carcinogens or viruses gives rise to individuals with increased susceptibility to cancer. Iatrogenically induced immunodeficiency increases tumors of reticular tissues in patients receiving renal transplants. Studies on cancer of the breast, cervix, and uterus indicate that high-risk subgroups exist, with the overall population differing according to such variables as age at first child, etc., which cannot as yet be expressed objectively. On the other hand, the use of long-term oral steroid contraceptives has created definable, large high-risk populations that can be used for etiological studies [14].

The relatively minor importance of genetic, compared to environmental, factors in cancer has been discussed [11], with certain exceptions such as the role of skin pigmentation in skin cancer. Special attention is now being paid to the inducibility of aryl hydrocarbon hydroxylase in lung cancer, and to certain HL-A antigens in nasopharyngeal cancer, which may permit the identification of genetically susceptible individuals. However, in at least one experiment in rats [15], in which mammary tumors were induced by irradiation, the development of cancer was governed by Poisson probability, indicating that the animals developing cancer were not more susceptible than the cancer-free animals; this possibility cannot be excluded for man.

MISCELLANEOUS HIGH-RISK GROUPS

These groups include people with benign tumors or premalignant lesions, e.g., polyposis coli. Many such lesions, however, may merely reflect the first stages of a response to a carcinogen, e.g., papilloma in shale oil workers. Hence, they may provide indices of more serious carcinogenic hazards. Such groups contribute to secondary prevention by permitting earlier diagnosis. In practice, the progression of benign to malignant tumors seems less frequent than in experimental animals. This may be because most cancers occur at inaccessible sites.

The Geographic Isolate

This group probably represents most closely the situation in inbred animals and, theoretically, should permit assessment of hereditary factors. In many instances, the groups are exposed to relatively primitive conditions with poor hygiene and a high frequency of communicable disease. Best studied is the population of Tristan da Cunha, which came to the United Kingdom after a volcanic eruption in the early sixties [16]. Although hereditary diseases were identified, there was no evidence of an exceptional risk of cancer. Other groups studied include isolates in Sweden [17], Eskimos in North America, and natives in New Guinea.

MONITORING OF PREVENTIVE MEASURES

Active measures to eliminate a presumed carcinogen from a population produce a situation most closely corresponding to the experimental model, since the observer modifies the conditions of the experiment. When only a few individuals are exposed and the strength of the carcinogen is high, the observer has no special difficulties in evaluating the effect of action [18].

With larger populations, however, it is important to ensure that the effects of action are not diluted out, and to direct monitoring toward specific subgroups, as shown by the relation of cigarette smoking to lung cancer. The feasibility of prevention was clearly illustrated by examination of a subgroup, e.g., British doctors who stopped smoking [19]. Such studies are useful in assessing the effects of educational techniques.

ROLE OF HIGH-RISK GROUPS IN DEDUCING "NONEFFECT" LEVELS

When a high-risk group is exposed to a strong carcinogen at varying dose levels, it may be possible to determine whether a "noneffect" level exists. This is especially true if reducing exposure to the carcinogen lowers the incidence to a level comparable to that in the general population. However, in view of the inherent limitations due to small numbers and long latent period, as described above, complete safety may never be guaranteed.

CONCLUSIONS

It is clear that the examination of small high-risk populations offers unusual opportunities for the identification of environmental carcinogens, especially when such groups are readily identified within the general population, e.g., occupational groups. When there is evidence that such populations are exposed to putative carcinogens, these observations carry very significant implications in terms of prevention. In most situations in which a carcinogen was so identified, it was possible to take appropriate action to reduce or eliminate the suspected agent. Furthermore, the possibilities are enhanced for monitoring the situation following such action. This not only helps confirm the etiological role of the potential carcinogen but also emphasizes the feasibility of practical prevention. Although the risk of a carcinogen to a total population may appear to be low, the risk for the exposed individual may be so high as to be completely unacceptable. Thus, it is desirable to distinguish between the level of risk for the total population and that for an individual.

REFERENCES

1. Bradford Hill, A. The statistician in medicine. Alfred Watson Memorial Lecture. *J. Inst. Actuaries 88:*178-191, 1962.

2. Pederson, E., Hogetveit, A.N., and Andersen, A. Cancer of respiratory organs among workers at a nickel refinery in Norway. *Int. J. Cancer 12:*32-41, 1973.

3. Higginson, J. The role of geographical pathology in environmental carcinogenesis. *In Proceedings of the 1971 Symposium on Fundamental Cancer Research, Environment and Cancer.* Williams and Wilkins, Baltimore, 1972, pp. 69-92.

4. Gilson, J.C. Wyers Memorial Lecture 1965: Health hazards of asbestos—recent studies on its biological effects. *Trans. Soc. Occup. Med. 16:*62-74, 1966.

5. Acheson, E.D. *Medical Record Linkage.* Oxford University Press, London, 1967.

6. Weisburger, J.H., and Weisburger, E.K. Tests for chemical carcinogens. *Methods Cancer Res. 1:*307-397, 1967.

7. Boston Collaborative Drug Surveillance Program. Reserpine and breast cancer. *Lancet 2:*669-671, 1974.

8. Druckrey, H. Quantitative aspects in chemical carcinogenesis. U.I.C.C. Monograph Series Vol. 7. *In* Truhaut, R., ed. *Potential Carcinogenic Hazards from Drugs.* Springer-Verlag, Berlin, 1967, pp. 60-78.

9. Tomatis, L., Turosov, V., Day, N., et al. The effect of long-term exposure to DDT on CF-1 mice. *Int. J. Cancer 10:*489-506, 1972.

10. Jablon, S., and Kato, H. Studies of the mortality of A-bomb survivors. 5. Radiation dose and mortality: 1950-1970. *Radiat. Res. 50:*649-698, 1972.

11. Doll, R., and Vodopija, I., eds. *Host Environment Interactions in the Etiology of Cancer in Man.* I.A.R.C. Scientific Publications No. 7, Lyon, 1973, p. 464.

12. Selikoff, I.J., Hammond, E.C., and Churg, J. Asbestos exposure, smoking and neoplasia. *J.A.M.A. 204:*106-112, 1968.

13. Tomatis, L., and Mohr, U., eds. *Transplacental Carcinogenesis.* I.A.R.C. Scientific Publications No. 4, Lyon, 1973, p. 181.

14. Royal College of General Practitioners. *Oral Contraceptives and Health. An interim report.* Pitman Medical, London, 1974, p. 100.

15. Krebs, J.S. Ionizing radiation. *Life Sci. Res. Rep. 6:*August 1974.

16. Black, J.A., Thacker, C.K.M., Lewis, H.E., et al. Tristan da Cunha: General medical investigations. *Br. Med. J. 2:*1018-1024, 1963.

17. Henschen, F. Hereditary disease in the four Nordic countries. *Schweiz. Z. Allg. Pathol. Bacteriol. 18:*385-408, 1955.

18. Fox, A.J., Lindars, D.C., and Owen, R. A survey of occupational cancer in the rubber and cablemaking industries: Results of five-year analysis, 1967-71. *Br. J. Ind. Med. 31:*140-151, 1974.

19. Doll, R., and Hill, A.B. Mortality in relation to smoking: Ten years' observations of British doctors. *Br. Med. J. 1:*1399-1410, 1460-1467, 1964.

DISCUSSION

Dr. R. W. Miller pointed out that both Dr. Higginson and Dr. Davies seemed to agree that a high-risk group may provide opportunities for cancer prevention even when the responsible carcinogenic agent or mechanism is obscure.

Some environmental determinants of cancer (e.g., smoking, alcohol, certain industries, tropical ulcers) are amenable to preventive measures, although the precise carcinogens remain to be identified.

Dr. Schneiderman commented on the pitfalls of statistical analysis in evaluating high-risk groups. He discussed the recent report by Clemmesen, who claimed no evidence of a cancer hazard when a group of epileptics in Denmark were treated with anticonvulsant drugs, mainly phenobarbital. Animal experimentation indicates that phenobarbital induces liver tumors, but the excess of liver cancer in the survey of epileptics was reported as not statistically significant. In analyzing the data, however, **Dr. Schneiderman** found that the excess was significant, suggesting that phenobarbital or possibly another anticonvulsant may indeed be a liver carcinogen in man.

Joseph F. Fraumeni, Jr.

24

CANCER DETECTION PROGRAMS

David Schottenfeld, M.D.

Memorial Hospital for Cancer and Allied Diseases
New York, N. Y.

INTRODUCTION

It seems desirable to identify presymptomatic and early unrecognized symptomatic cancer in entire population groups (mass screening) or selected high-risk groups (selective screening). The assumption is that early case-finding and therapeutic intervention will restore health, diminish disability, or postpone death. A program of early cancer detection would focus on predisposing pathologic conditions, precursor lesions, and early cancerous lesions. A preventive program of health maintenance would be concerned with the likelihood of developing cancer and would seek initially to identify specific risk factors in various target populations. The expected rates of morbidity and mortality could then be reduced by providing health counseling and future surveillance.

The concept of "at risk" implies that the individual, family, cohort, or community is either unusually susceptible or has been exposed to a potentially hazardous substance. As a consequence, there is an increased probability of developing a pathologic condition. A risk factor is some antecedent attribute or characteristic, either a causal factor or precursor manifestation, that is associated with incurring a disease. A subset of risk factors or attributes that influence the incidence of a disease may be distinctive from those that affect mortality or the degree of disability. Excessive mortality may arise from

---

The author is grateful to Professor Mary E.W. Goss for her thoughtful review and comments.

behavioral and attitudinal factors that interfere with the utilization of available preventive services or from societal factors that deter effective and efficient delivery of medical care. Age, sex, race, social class, residence, and marital status may determine selectively the distribution of established risk factors and probable magnitude of unrecognized disease, and thereby facilitate the design and allocation of limited resources of a screening program.

The presentation of an "early" cancer has been described in terms of its size, noninvasiveness or confinement to the organ of origin, and its occurrence in the absence of symptoms or with minimal patient delay. However, without knowing the time of biologic onset or the prior rate of growth of a tumor, the duration of disease before detection is not known. The rate of growth of a cancer is irregular and, with increasing size, frequently departs from a simple exponential growth function [1-3]. Human solid tumors have varying doubling times, and, for those biologically more indolent, longer observation will be needed after treatment before the benefits of early detection can be established.

Wilson and Jungner [4] have reviewed the fundamental principles which should guide the planning and development of a program of screening and early detection within any given population. These principles are summarized as follows:

1) Select a disease that is an important public health problem.
2) Have facilities available for diagnosis and treatment, an accepted treatment, and a clearly defined policy about the indications for treatment.
3) Be sure the natural history of the disease is understood. A suitable screening test would identify preclinical or early symptomatic disease.
4) Keep the cost of case-finding and treatment reasonable in relation to total health expenditures.
5) Make the screening program a continuing and health-maintaining process, acceptable to the target population.

I will describe these principles in the context of evaluating a program of early cancer detection and of identifying the determinants of preventive behavior in high-risk groups.

EVALUATING THE SCREENING PROCESS

The effectiveness of any screening procedure may be determined by assessment of validity, predictiveness, reproducibility, yield in relation to cost, ease of administration, and patient compliance. The United States Commission on Chronic Illness defined validity as the percentage frequency with which the result of the screening test was later confirmed by an acceptable diagnostic procedure, or in terms of the ability of the test to separate those who have the disease from those who do not. Validity may be determined by measurement of sensitivity and specificity. Sensitivity is whether the test can give a positive finding when the person tested truly has the disease under study. Specificity is whether the test can give a negative finding when the person tested is free of the disease under study. The predictive value of a positive test — the likelihood that a positive individual has disease — increases with increasing specificity and with increasing frequency of disease in the screened population (Table 1).

TABLE 1

Predictive value of a positive test in relation to
disease frequency, sensitivity, and specificity

Percent sensitivity	Percent specificity	Prevalance per 1,000	Percent predictive value of positive test
95	95	0.5	0.9
		2.0	5.3
		5.0	8.7
95	80	0.5	0.2
		2.0	0.9
		5.0	2.3
80	95	0.5	0.8
		2.0	3.1
		5.0	7.4
80	80	0.5	0.2
		2.0	0.8
		5.0	2.0
70	95	0.5	0.7
		2.0	2.7
		5.0	7.0
70	80	0.5	0.2
		2.0	0.7
		5.0	1.7

The sensitivity of a screening program or instrument can be increased in one or more of the following ways:

1) Move the screening level to a lower point or closer to the nondiseased segment on the scale; allow the screening criteria to be less restrictive.

2) Use two or more screening tests in parallel and label as positive any subject with a positive response to any of the tests.

3) Refine and standardize the screening instrument and the method of administration by trained screeners. These factors also influence specificity and the precision or reproducibility of a screening procedure.

Alternatively, the level of specificity can be raised, but usually at the cost of diminishing sensitivity and increasing the ratio of false negatives. Specificity can be enhanced in one or more of the following ways:

1) Move the screening level to a higher point or closer to the diseased segment on the scale; allow the screening criteria to be more restrictive.

2) Rescreen, with the same screening method, all subjects found positive on initial screening, and refer only those who were positive on two occasions.

3) Use two or more screening tests in series, and label as positive any subject with a positive response to all tests.

A method of summarizing sensitivity and specificity is by deriving a validity score or the Youden index. The Youden index, expressed as a percent, equals the sum of the sensitivity and specificity minus 100. Thus a sensitivity of 85 percent and a specificity of 80 percent minus 100 percent equals a Youden index of 65 percent. If the Youden index is 50 percent or less, the screening test results are no better than random chance.

With what frequency should the target population be rescreened? Mainly, this should be a function of the rate of progression through the latent period to early clinical disease and the validity of the screening procedure. A practical limitation is imposed by economic, social, and administrative considerations. Annual examination schedules have evolved empirically, and proposed alternative models for optimizing the frequency of screening will require experimental trial. An optimal schedule should have high yield and achieve early detection, or minimal detection delay, but not have an excessive number of examinations per person. Obviously, the limits of "early," "minimal," and "excessive" must be specified in relation to the expected outcome of the screening process. For example, Kirch and Klein [5] developed a mathematical model for the periodicity or nonperiodicity of screening for breast cancer. They assumed that tumor volumetric doubling time is constant for a given tumor and that tumor size and axillary node involvement are correlated with duration of disease. With the application of appropriate estimates of volumetric doubling time and of age-specific incidence of breast cancer in the general population and in selected high-risk groups, they will attempt to predict the efficiency of regular screening at six-month intervals, as compared with annual or biannual examinations.

DETERMINANTS OF HEALTH-MAINTAINING
BEHAVIOR IN GROUPS AT HIGH RISK

Whereas mass screening is cumbersome and costly, selected screening of groups at high risk appears to be more efficient if such target groups were readily identified and reached. Periodic screening is difficult to accomplish within an unstable or highly mobile population, and high-risk characteristics do not generally aggregate within accessible units of the population, except in the familial and industrial settings. Perhaps a central or population-based registry, such as those conceived under the SEER (Surveillance, Epidemiology, and End Results Reporting) program, will serve to identify and motivate high-risk individuals and population subgroups to receive periodic and prescriptive screening.

By identifying groups or individuals at increased risk of incurring cancer at a specific site, the epidemiologist facilitates the selective application of optimal screening methods. For cost-benefit considerations, the principle would be to concentrate the greatest proportion of potentially new cases into the smallest proportion of the total population at risk. For example, in approaching women at risk of breast cancer, we may at first consider three variables – age, marital status, and parity. Among women 45 years of age and older (approximately 35 million women in the United States), we would expect to find, based upon the preliminary report of the Third National Cancer Survey, 85 percent of the incident cases within 32 percent of the United States population at risk. Between the ages 45 to 74 years, the annual incidence approximates 2 per 1,000 (Table 2). Among single women 35 years of age and older, we would expect to find 11-15 percent of the incident cases within 7 percent of the population at risk. Among married nonparous women 35 years of age and older, we would expect to find 10-20 percent of the incident cases within 16 percent of the population at risk [6]. In principle, the risk factors of age and parity, when combined with family history of breast cancer or prior personal history of benign breast dysplasia, should increase the predictive value of a positive screening test. However, in the breast cancer screening program of the Health Insurance Plan [7], joint consideration in the experimental group of family history, parity and age at first pregnancy, age at menarche, and benign breast disease was not sufficiently discriminating with respect to the total yield, 33 percent, of diagnosed cases in 21 percent of the population at risk. The validity and epidemiologic application of various screening procedures for carcinoma of the uterus, breast, lung, and large intestine are summarized in Table 2 and have been reviewed previously [8].

Even with effective and efficient screening procedures and our ability to define risk factors and target populations, there are formidable behavioral barriers in asymptomatic patients. In 1966, a study of those factors that deter-

TABLE 2

The validity and application of screening procedures for selected cancer sites

Site	Method	Validity			High-risk features							Comments	References
					age-specific incidence at .05% or greater, U.S. 1969			% total population at risk, U.S. 1970					
		percent sensitivity	percent specificity	percent false negatives	age	women	men	age women	men	major risk factors	high-risk groups		
Uterine Cervix (squamous carcinoma)	Cytology	In Situ 80-95	?	5-20	25-34	0.12*		25-34 12.2		Venereal diseases	Prostitutes	False negatives decrease with repeated screening and are least with the scraping smear.	Fidler, H.K., Boyes, D.A., and Worth, A.J. Screening for malignant disease by exfoliative cytology. *In* Sharp, C., and Keen, H., eds. *Presymptomatic Detection and Early Diagnosis.* Williams and Wilkins, Baltimore, 1968, pp. 295-333.
		Invasive 75-90 (increasing with increasing age)	50 (increasing with increasing age)	10-25	35-44 *in situ only	0.08*		35-44 11.4		Low socioeconomic class	Clinics treating venereal diseases	Peak age interval for prevalence of in situ is 30-45 years.	Kessler, I.I. Uterine cervix. *In* Schottenfeld, D., ed. *Cancer Epidemiology and Prevention: Current Concepts.* Charles C. Thomas, Springfield, Ill., 1974, pp. 263-317.
										Early age at first marriage	Family planning clinics	By directing a screening program to women married or pregnant before 20 yrs. of age, cost per case would be one-third less than screening never married and never pregnant women.	Christopherson, W.M., and Parker, J.E. Economic considerations of the control of cervix cancer in high risk patients. *CA 19:*107-111, 1969.
										Early age at first coitus	Women using oral contraceptive agents - self-selection vs. etiology?	Incidence of clinical invasive carcinoma in screened population in British Columbia has remained between 3-5/100,000 over the last 15 yrs., or one-seventh the expected incidence in an unscreened population.	Coppleson, L.W., and Brown, B. Estimation of the screening error rate from the observed detection rates in repeated cervical cytology. *Am. J. Obstet. Gynecol. 119:*953-958, 1974.
										Early age at first pregnancy		Very difficult to test the effectiveness of cytologic screening in diminishing uterine cervix cancer mortality. Age-specific mortality trends suggested that when compared with the rest of Canada, the decline in mortality during 1966-71 in British Columbia was greater only at 45-64 yrs. of age.	Worth, A.J. Cervical cytology screening (editorial). *Can. Med. Assoc. J. 110:*129-131, 1974.
										Cervical dysplasia, moderate to severe		The role of mass cytologic screening in altering age-specific mortality is confounded by: underutilization of available screening services by high-risk segments of the population, standardizing for socioeconomic class and age-specific prevalence of hysterectomy, geographic instability and incomplete ascertainment in record linkage studies in populations at risk, varying quality of diagnostic and therapeutic services, and degree of accuracy in certifying underlying cause of death by specific uterine site.	Richart, R.M., and Vaillant, H.W. Influence of cell collection techniques upon cytological diagnosis. *Cancer 18:*1474-1478, 1965.
										Abnormal vaginal bleeding or persistent discharge, despite normal cytology at initial exam			Kinlen, L.J., and Doll, R. Trends in mortality from cancer of the uterus in Canada and in England and Wales. *Br. J. Prev. Soc. Med. 27:*146-149, 1973.

TABLE 2 (Continued)

Site	Method	Validity			age-specific incidence at .05% or greater, U.S. 1969			% total population at risk, U.S. 1970			High-risk features		Comments	References
		percent sensitivity	percent specificity	percent false negatives	age	women	men	age	women	men	major risk factors	high-risk groups		
Uterine Corpus (endometrial carcinoma)	Vaginal pool cytology	70-80	?	20-30	45-54 / 55-64 / 65-74	0.05 / 0.07 / 0.08		45-54 / 55-64 / 65-74		11.5 / 9.4 / 6.7	Obesity—frequently a triad with diabetes and hypertension; Nulliparity; Increased stature(?); Late age at menopause; Family history; Frequent anovulatory cycles(?); Prior endometrial hyperplasia or polyps with cellular atypia	Nuns; Women using estrogens or other sex steroids - self-selection vs. etiology?	Endometrial aspiration is technically more difficult because of cervical and/or vaginal stenosis in patients over 60 yrs. of age, and particularly in nulliparous women.	Burk, J.R., Lehman, H.F., and Wolf, F.S. Inadequacy of Papanicolaou smears in the detection of endometrial cancer. *N. Engl. J. Med.* 291:191-192, 1974. Wynder, E.L., Escher, G.C., and Mantel, N. An epidemiological investigation of cancer of the endometrium. *Cancer* 19:489-520, 1966. Reagan, J.W., and Ng, A.B. *The Cells of Uterine Adenocarcinoma.* S. Karger, Basel, 1973. Abramson, D., and Driscoll, S.G. Endometrial aspiration biopsy. *Obstet. Gynecol.* 27:381-391, 1966.
	Endocervical and endometrial aspiration	80	?	20										
Breast	Clinical examination	82	78	18	35-44	0.09		35-44		11.4	Family history—breast cancer and benign breast disease; Nulliparity or age at first pregnancy 30 yrs. and older; Late age at menopause; Breast dysplasia-cellular atypia with ductal or lobular hyperplasia or papillomatosis; Previous carcinoma of opposite breast, ovary, endometrium or large intestine	Nuns	Sensitivity of clinical examination is greatest in women under age 50 yrs. Sensitivity of mammography is enhanced with increasing age. Clinical examination and mammography tend to select different subgroups of cases and their combination increases sensitivity at a cost of increasing the percentage of false positives. Among United States women 25-74 yrs. of age, breast cancer is the leading cause of cancer mortality, and in women 40-44 yrs. of age it is the leading cause of death. With the use of a molybdenum target (Senograph) and Lo-dose film, the average irradiation to the skin is 1.5 to 2.5 rads per exposure or 3.0 to 5.0 rads per examination with craniocaudal and lateral views. For X-irradiation exceeding 50 rads, the best estimate of absolute risk is 6.0 cases/10^6/yr/rad. Estimates may vary in relation to dose rate and type of irradiation as well as predisposing factors. The potential risk of radiation-induced cancers should be considered in the assessment of "costs." Specificity in rescreening with either mammography or clinical examination is increased to at least 99 percent.	Lilienfeld, A.M. Some limitations and problems of screening for cancer. *Cancer* 33J:1720-1724, 1974. Schottenfeld, D. Patient risk factors and the detection of early cancer. *Prev. Med.* 1: 335-351, 1972. Shapiro, S., Strax, P., Venet, L., et al. Changes in 5-year breast cancer mortality in a breast cancer screening program. In *Proceedings of the Seventh National Cancer Conference.* J. B. Lippincott, Philadelphia, 1973, pp. 663-678. Fraumeni, J.F., Jr., Lloyd, J.W., Smith, E.M., et al. Cancer mortality among nuns: Role of marital status in etiology of neoplastic disease in women. *J. Natl. Cancer Inst.* 42:455-468, 1969. MacMahon, B., Cole, P., and Brown, J. Etiology of human breast cancer: A review. *J. Natl. Cancer Inst.* 50:21-42, 1973. *The Effects on Populations of Exposure to Low Levels of Ionizing Radiation.* National Academy of Sciences-National Research Council, Washington, D.C., 1972, pp. 136-145.
	Thermography	74	60	26	45-54 / 55-64 / 65-74	0.17 / 0.20 / 0.24		45-54 / 55-64 / 65-74		11.5 / 9.4 / 6.7				
	Mammography	70	81	30										

TABLE 2 (Continued)

Site	Method	Validity — percent sensitivity	percent specificity	percent false negatives	High-risk features — age-specific incidence at .05% or greater, U.S. 1969 (age / women / men)	% total population at risk, U.S. 1970 (age / women / men)	major risk factors	high-risk groups	Comments	References
Lung and Bronchus	Sputum cytology, Chest X-ray	50–70, 42	98, 98	30–50, 58	45-54 / 0.09; 55-64 / 0.23; 65-74 / 0.37 / 0.05	45-54 / / 11.3; 55-64 / / 8.9; 65-74 / 6.7 / 5.5	Cigarette smoking; Previous squamous carcinoma of oral cavity, larynx, or esophagus; Family history; Prior X-ray showing diffuse pulmonary fibrosis; secondary to cigarette smoking, antecedent infection or of systemic connective tissue disease	Occupational exposure to: asbestos, uranium, nickel, chromate, arsenic trioxide and sulfur dioxide, hematite, mustard gas, alkylating agents, halo ethers	Attributable risk percent for tobacco inhalation has been estimated at 85%. Sensitivity of examining sputum cytology is enhanced when collecting multiple specimens of optimal quality from individuals at risk and in the presence of central as contrasted with peripheral lesions of the lung. Leading cause of cancer mortality in U.S. men between the ages, 35-74; has become the third leading cause of cancer deaths in U.S. women.	Lilienfeld, A.M., Archer, P.G., Burnett, C.H., et al. An evaluation of radiologic and cytologic screening for the early detection of lung cancer: A cooperative pilot study of the American Cancer Society and the Veterans Administration. *Cancer Res.* 26:2083-2121, 1966. Archer, P.G., Koprowska, I., McDonald, R.J., et al. A study of variability in the interpretation of sputum cytology slides. *Cancer Res.* 26:2122-2144, 1966. Lilienfeld, A.M., and Kordan, B. A study of variability in the interpretation of chest X-rays in the detection of lung cancer. *Cancer Res.* 26:2145-2147, 1966. Wynder, E.L., Mabuchi, K., and Hoffman, D. Tobacco. In Schottenfeld, D., ed. *Cancer Epidemiology and Prevention: Current Concepts.* Charles C. Thomas, Springfield, Ill., 1974, pp. 102-125. Dinman, B.D. *The Nature of Occupational Cancer.* Charles C. Thomas, Springfield, Ill., 1974. Hamilton, A., and Hardy, H.L. *Industrial Toxicology.* Publishing Sciences Group, Inc., Acton, Mass., 1974. Weiss, W., and Boucot, K.R. The Philadelphia pulmonary neoplasm research project. *Arch. Intern. Med. 134:* 306-311, 1974. Koss, L.G., Melamed, M.R., and Goodner, J.T. Pulmonary cytology – A brief survey of diagnostic results from July 1st, 1952 until December 31st, 1960. *Acta Cytol 8:*104-113, 1964.
Large Intestine	Occult blood in stool (method of Gregor)	?	97–99	?	55-64 / 0.10 / 0.12; 65-74 / 0.21 / 0.28	55-64 / 9.4 / 8.9; 65-74 / 6.7 / 5.5	Family history; Familial polyposis; Multiple polyps with family history; Gardner's syndrome; Previous carcinoma of colon or rectum-risk is further enhanced by association with adenomatous polyps or villous adenomas; Ulcerative colitis; Granulomatous colitis (?)	Asbestos (?)	Predictive value of positive hemoccult slide test (Gregor method) has been estimated at 10 percent. This will increase by selective testing in groups at high risk. The major identifiable conditions or risk factors probably account for less than ten percent of incidence of colorectal cancer. Two-thirds of colorectal cancers are within the view of the 25 cm proctosigmoidoscope. CEA false negativity diminishes with presentation of more advanced colorectal cancer. The relationship with the 'early' diagnosis of colorectal cancer is more quantitative than qualitative – with more false positives occurring around threshold level of 2.5 ng/ml. Diseases or conditions giving rise to positive test: 1. Cancer of pancreas, liver, lung, breast, testis, ovary, uterus, prostate, kidney, urinary bladder; neuroblastoma, osteogenic sarcoma, myeloma, lymphomas, leukemias 2. Benign diseases of digestive system: colorectal polyps, diverticulitis, pancreatitis, alcoholic cirrhosis	Fraumeni, J.F., Jr., and Mulvihill, J.J. Who is at risk of colorectal cancer? In Schottenfeld, D., ed. *Cancer Epidemiology and Prevention: Current Concepts.* Charles C. Thomas, Springfield, Ill., 1974, pp. 404-415. Gregor, D.H. Occult blood testing for detection of asymptomatic colon cancer. *Cancer* 28:131-134, 1971. Hastings, J.B. Mass screening for colorectal cancer. *Am. J. Surg.* 127:228-233, 1974. Berge, T., Ekelund, G., Mellner, C., et al. Carcinoma of the colon and rectum in a defined population. *Acta Chir. Scand. Suppl. 438:*1-76, 1973. Zamcheck, N. Carcinoembryonic antigen. *Advan. Int. Med. 19:*413-433, 1974. Livingstone, A.S., Hampson, L.G., Shuster, J., et al. Carcinoembryonic antigen in the diagnosis and management of colorectal carcinoma. *Arch. Surg. 109:*259-264, 1974. Stevens, D.P., and MacKay, I.R. Increased carcinoembryonic antigen in heavy cigarette smokers. *Lancet 2:*1238-1239, 1973.
	Carcinoembryonic antigen (CEA), a glycoprotein in serum (Gold assay) or plasma (Hansen and Todd assay)	62–83	?	17–38						

mine how and why men and women receive periodic physical examinations that include cancer tests was conducted by the American Cancer Society. The study sample consisted of 2,099 men and women, 21 years of age and older, from representative cities in major geographical regions in the United States. Whether the cancer tests were done periodically in the absence of symptoms as part of a general medical checkup or as a selective cancer examination, health-maintaining behavior was more common among women and was positively correlated with formal education and annual income. Older people without symptoms were less motivated to have regular cancer checkups. Those persons who went regularly for cancer checkups demonstrated greater awareness of the first "danger signals of cancer" [9].

As Kasl and Cobb discussed [10], the likelihood that a patient will engage in a particular kind of health behavior will be a function of how that individual perceives 1) personal susceptibility to a disease and its life-threatening consequences, and 2) the cost-benefits of preventive action in reducing susceptibility and limiting medical and social sequelae of a disease.

In a study of 1,201 adults in three United States cities, Hochbaum [11] identified some of the factors that determine whether a person will obtain voluntarily a chest X-ray for the purpose of detecting tuberculosis. He studied personal beliefs about susceptibility to tuberculosis and the benefits of early detection. Among those persons who believed that they were susceptible to tuberculosis, even without symptoms, and recognized the benefits of early diagnosis, 82 percent had obtained at least one routine chest X-ray during the previous 7 years. On the other hand, of the group exhibiting none of these beliefs, only 21 percent had obtained voluntarily a chest X-ray during a similar period. The external factors of availability, cost, and personal comfort determined the setting (e.g., mobile unit, clinic, physician's office, etc.) in which the chest X-ray was obtained. Hochbaum concluded that, in the interaction between perceived susceptibility and belief in a preventive program, perceived susceptibility was the more powerful motivating factor. Both the studies of Hochbaum and Tagliacozzo and Ima [12] suggested that the patient's knowledge of a disease process was a subtle motivating force which acted conjointly with past illness experiences and current perception of susceptibility.

Although past studies have been able to characterize the reluctant participant in a periodic cancer screening program in relation to age, education, socioeconomic status, current health attitudes, and past illness behavior, there is little evidence that changing health attitudes are correlated directly with changing health practices [13]. Other major forces inhibiting voluntary participation include situational and psychocultural factors. To facilitate the outreach of early detection services into low-income communities, Strax [14] explored the use of a mobile van and neighborhood examining centers for periodic mass screening for breast, uterine cervix, and lung cancer. The screening units are staffed with trained neighborhood personnel, and community health aides are serving to promote participation through home visits and individual counseling. Besides the role of informed community aides who are providing health education in a personalized setting, general large-scale public education is also being advanced through television, radiobroadcasting, and publications. This pilot program was made possible through private and public funds. Lynch et al. [15] developed a similar program which includes examination of the skin, uterus, breasts, oral cavity, and large intestine. The real challenge in providing community-based screening and early diagnostic services will be to broaden the base of participation in population groups at high risk and to maintain compliance with the prescribed rescheduling of examinations.

EVALUATING OUTCOME OF SCREENING

One important objective of epidemiology is to establish the natural history of a disease. As Hutchison stated [16], the natural history of a disease process and its morbid sequelae refer not only to the interaction of various etiologic agents and biologic host responses, but also to the effects of social, cultural, and behavioral factors. Assessment of the outcome over a period of time may be stated in terms of prevalence, incidence, mortality, residual disability, social restoration, and the ratio of benefits to costs. It is the array of unfavorable sequelae of a disease that we hope to prevent or alter through the screening and diagnostic process, subsequent therapeutic intervention, continuing care, and future surveillance. Note that screening is viewed as an extension of the medical-care process.

One assumption inherent in a program of early cancer detection is the concept of at least one "critical point" during the latent or early symptomatic stage of the disease. The application of treatment before any major critical point, rather than after, should result in a substantially better outcome. Indeed, the justification of periodic screening of patients at risk would be the availability of valid screening procedures to be introduced before the critical point, and where the critical point generally preceded the time of usual diagnosis in symptomatic patients.

In evaluation of any voluntary screening program, particularly one which includes repeated screening, there are interpretive pitfalls of self-selection and motivation in the screened population that bear on the measured outcome or prognosis. Individuals with a major disability (comorbidity) are unlikely to participate voluntarily in a screening program; consequently, the observed survival in those screened should exceed that expected in the general population, irrespective of the efficacy of the screening procedure. One expedient would be to compare the outcome in a population provided with readily accessible screening services with that in another reference population of demonstrated demographic similarity, which is not receiving preventive services. Ideally, total and age-specific mortality and morbidity and age-specific case fatality ratios during a given follow-up period in the randomly selected screened population should be compared with the outcome observed in a similarly selected control population. To assist in the assessment of the clinical effectiveness of randomized trials of cancer screening, the following criteria were advanced [17]:

1) How are patients allocated into screened and nonscreened groups? What characteristics determined whether individuals were to be excluded from the trial, and to what degree did this limit the ability to generalize the results to groups at high risk or to a total population?

2) Are the various subgroups comparable with respect to identifiable risk factors and associated diseases that may influence the frequency and prognosis of the target cancer site(s)? Randomization may not always ensure comparability, and it may be desirable to stratify prior to random allocation or to analyze the subsequent outcomes within equivalent subgroups at risk.

3) The criteria for allocating deaths by underlying cause should be applied uniformly to the study and comparison groups, and total mortality should be described. It is of interest that, although the number of breast cancer deaths in the Health Insurance Plan study were one-third lower in the experimental group having periodic mammographic and clinical examinations than among the controls, the mortality due to causes other than breast cancer was not significantly different. The reduction in breast cancer mortality occurred only among women aged 50 and over [18].

4) Did the observed increase in survival after "early" diagnosis and definitive treatment mean that the natural history was altered significantly? It might also mean that, although the time of diagnosis was advanced over that usually achieved by medical practice, this interval of "lead time" was not significantly less than the observed improvement in survival time. As noted by Feinleib and Zelen [19,20], the initial screening examination tends to select those individuals with longer mean duration of preclinical disease, and, in these instances, each subsequent stage of clinical disease would also be more indolent. For example, the lead time achieved in the Health Insurance Plan experimental group has been estimated to be from 1 to 2 years. Lead time will ultimately be derived for different age groups by examination of the time interval between the third or last annual reexamination and the point in time when the incidence of breast cancer among the study women reaches the frequency expected among women who have not been screened [21].

ECONOMIC ASPECTS OF SCREENING

With respect to the planning of cancer preventive services, it is important to estimate the burden of direct and indirect costs within different economic segments of the community. The direct costs (i.e., manpower, supporting services, equipment, and supplies) incurred from case-finding in an apparently healthy population include the costs of the screening procedures plus the costs required to provide diagnostic, therapeutic, and follow-up services. The indirect costs include those due to lost earnings and diminished productivity. The indirect costs within an indigent population are less and of a different nature than in the general population because of lower wage rates, greater unemployment, and dependency on income support through public programs. Utilization of screening and therapeutic services by the working poor, unless provided for under the prepaid benefits of employment contracts, may represent an intolerable hardship because of lost earnings [22] .

As Klarman described [23], a cost-benefit analysis compares costs and benefits between two programs competing for public funds. In a screening program, the cost of treatment of patients whose cancers were detected by screening would be compared with the usual cost of treatment of symptomatic patients. The benefits of early diagnosis and treatment include 1) savings in the use of health resources, 2) gains in economic productivity, and 3) enhancement of the quality of life. Indices of economic productivity, rather than social values, would tend to minimize the benefits of averting disability or premature death in the poor and in unemployed women. A cost-benefit analysis of a screening program for lung or oral cavity cancer may, therefore, suggest that the target population should include employed males of high income, whereas the epidemiologist would consider the screening of low-income (high-risk) groups. In program planning, humanitarian considerations and sound economic analysis enter into the formulation of policy decisions.

As suggested by Pole [24] in regard to screening, costs and benefits are related by the formula:

$$\frac{BN+BD+BL}{CS+CD+CT-CX} \times 100$$

where: BN=benefit to true negatives
BD=benefit from avoidance of disability
BL=benefit from gain in life-expectancy
CS=cost of screening test(s)
CD=cost of diagnostic test(s)
CT=cost of treatment following screening
CX=saving in usual cost for diagnosis and treatment
of symptomatic case

Dickinson [25] slightly altered this investment-benefits model by limiting the numerator of benefits to extended years of life, without assigning a monetary value to these years. The additional gain in productivity due to benefit from avoidance of disability (BD) is included in the denominator and subtracted from the costs of screening, diagnosis, and treatment. His "life" benefit model, like the "monetary" benefit model, does not assess quality of the added years of life. Cost-effectiveness analysis differs from cost-benefit analysis in that the costs of alternative programs for achieving a specified objective are compared. Commonly, the output is not expressed in dollars, but may be expressed in terms such as extended years of useful life. The cost-effectiveness of a program of early cancer detection that includes health education services may be translated into changing health behavior leading to enhanced recruitment, compliance, and reduction of patient delay.

SUGGESTIONS FOR FUTURE RESEARCH AND DEVELOPMENT

1) In the approach of Scandinavian countries to occupational medicine, sharp distinctions have not been made between occupational health and personal health services. Dolinsky [26] suggested that, in the United States, industrial and personal health services for employed persons and their families could be coordinated through neighborhood health centers or health maintenance organizations. The selective application of preventive services funded through prepaid health plans could be provided efficiently to employed persons and their families by industrial health clinics or the primary health care teams of neighborhood and public health centers. At least, demonstration programs in occupational and family medicine that explore the more effective provision and utilization of comprehensive health services, including those concerned with prescriptive screening and early detection, should be considered by the various comprehensive health planning agencies.

Programs of general health education and cancer education should be included in the industrial bargaining process as a program of benefit to both labor and management. Professionals in the industrial health field should provide leadership in developing effective methods for general health and cancer education.

2) A recent Gallup survey, sponsored by the American Cancer Society, of public attitudes and practices (e.g., self-examination) regarding breast cancer underscored important gaps in public information and physician communication. It showed that only 35 percent of adult women were instructed in breast self-examination, and less than 20 percent practiced it regularly or as a standardized procedure. We need to learn more about the attitudes and behavior of different segments of the general population, as well as of high-risk groups, that may

result in inappropriate health behavior such as inordinate delay or under-utilization of available cancer screening services. Various studies for applying conceptual models within defined populations should be coordinated into one national field effort.

There is a need for greater leadership by the educational establishment in our public elementary and secondary schools in general health and cancer education. A syllabus for a continuing program of cancer education needs to be developed and implemented cooperatively through the support of the National Cancer Institute, U.S. Office of Education, and the National Education Association. Such a program should enlist parental participation. Through this means, young men and women of different ethnic and sociocultural backgrounds will learn about the consequences of their personal health practices. Hopefully, this will lead to more effective health-maintaining behavior.

REFERENCES

1. Spratt, J.S., Jr., Spjut, H.J., and Roper, C.L. The frequency distribution of the rates of growth and the estimated duration of primary pulmonary carcinomas. *Cancer 16:* 687-693, 1963.

2. Spratt, J.S., Jr. The rates of growth of skeletal sarcomas. *Cancer 18:*14-24, 1965.

3. Dethlefsen, L.A., Prewitt, J.M.S., and Mendelsohn, M.L. Analysis of tumor growth curves. *J. Natl. Cancer Inst. 40:*389-405, 1968.

4. Wilson, J.M.G., and Jungner, G. Principles and practice of screening for disease. *In Public Health Papers 34.* W.H.O., Geneva, 1968, pp. 26-39.

5. Kirch, R.L.A., and Klein, M. Examination schedules for breast cancer. *Cancer 33:* 1444-1450, 1974.

6. Dunn, J.E., Jr. Epidemiology and possible identification of high-risk groups that could develop cancer of the breast. *Cancer 23:*775-780, 1969.

7. Shapiro, S., Goldberg, J., Venet, L., et al. Risk factors in breast cancer—a prospective study. *In* Doll, R., and Vodopija, I., eds. *Host Environment Interactions In The Etiology of Cancer In Man.* I.A.R.C. Scientific Publications No. 7, I.A.R.C., Lyon, 1973, pp. 169-182.

8. Schottenfeld, D. Patient risk factors and the detection of early cancer. *Prev. Med. 1:*335-351, 1972.

9. *A Study of Motivational, Attitudinal and Environmental Deterrents to the Taking of Physical Examinations That Include Cancer Tests.* Conducted for the American Cancer Society by Lieberman Research, Inc., 1966.

10. Kasl, S.V., and Cobb, S. Health behavior, illness behavior, and sick role behavior. *Arch. Environ. Health 12:*246-266, 531-541, 1966.

11. Hochbaum, G.M. *Public Participation in Medical Screening Programs. A Sociopsychological Study.* Public Health Service Publication 572, U.S. Govt. Print. Off., Washington, D.C., 1958.

12. Tagliacozzo, D.M., and Ima, K. Knowledge of illness as a predictor of patient behavior. *J. Chronic Dis. 22:*765-775, 1970.

13. Kegeles, S.S. Behavioral science data and approaches relevant to the development of education programs in cancer. *Health Educ. Monogr. 36:*18-33, 1973.

14. Strax, P. New techniques in mass screening for breast cancer. *Cancer 28:*1563–1568, 1971.

15. Lynch, H., Lynch, J., and Kraft, C. A new approach to cancer screening and education. *Geriatrics 28:*152–157, 1973.

16. Hutchison, G.B. Evaluation of preventive services. *J. Chronic Dis. 11:*497–508, 1960.

17. Sackett, D. Periodic examination of patients at risk. *In* Schottenfeld, D., ed. *Cancer Epidemiology and Prevention: Current Concepts.* Charles C. Thomas, Springfield, Ill., 1975, pp. 437–454.

18. Shapiro, S., Strax, P., Venet, L., et al. Changes in 5-year breast cancer mortality in a breast cancer screening program. *In Proceedings of the Seventh National Cancer Conference.* J. B. Lippincott Co., Philadelphia, 1973, pp. 663–678.

19. Feinleib, M., and Zelen, M. Some pitfalls in the evaluation of screening programs. *Arch. Environ. Health 19:*412–415, 1969.

20. Zelen, M., and Feinleib, M. On the theory of screening for chronic diseases. *Biometrika 56:*601–614, 1969.

21. Shapiro, S., Goldberg, J.D., and Hutchison, G.B. Lead time in breast cancer detection and implications for periodicity of screening. *Am. J. Epidemiol. 100:*357–366, 1974.

22. Muller, C. Cost-benefit evaluation of cancer screening. 1973. (Unpublished.)

23. Klarman, H.E. Present status of cost-benefit analysis in the health field. *Am. J. Public Health 57:*1948–1953, 1967.

24. Pole, J.D. Economic aspects of screening for disease. *In* Cohen, L. Williams, E.T., and McLachlan, G., eds. *Screening in Medical Care.* Oxford Univ. Press, London, 1968, pp. 141–158.

25. Dickinson, L. Evaluation of the effectiveness of cytologic screening for cervical cancer. III. Cost-benefit analysis. *Mayo Clin. Proc. 47:*550–555, 1972.

26. Dolinsky, E.M. Health maintenance organizations and occupational medicine. *Bull. N.Y. Acad. Med. 50:*1122–1137, 1974.

DISCUSSION

Dr. Cole emphasized that individual screening tests should be analyzed as well as the overall screening program. Program evaluation has been obscured by self-selection of individuals who come for screening and the participation of large but poorly delineated populations. **Dr. Cole** suggested we carefully assess the results of screening and determine its full impact on mortality and morbidity. Our attention should not be limited to the number of patients found with cancer. **Dr. S. Cutler** commented that the impact of screening programs can best be determined on defined communities with a central cancer-reporting system.

In designing cancer detection programs, **Dr. Bahn** discussed the criteria for periodicity testing and the use of allied health professionals; **Dr. Wynder** commented on the importance of testing also for nonneoplastic diseases such as hypertension; and **Mr. Shapiro** recommended a closer focus on "high-risk" populations for the sake of efficiency and cost benefit. Finally, **Dr. Lynch** urged that cancer screening be emphasized in medical school teaching and that health education be incorporated into screening programs.

Vincent F. Guinee

25

EDUCATION OF THE PUBLIC

John Wakefield, Ph. D.

University Hospital of South Manchester
Christie Hospital and Holt Radium Institute
Manchester, England

Education for people at high risk of cancer cannot be treated as something separate and distinct from general education of the public about cancer, although it has certain special features. Essentially, the aims of public education are:

1) To inform and educate about treatable forms of cancer and to reassure people that treatment is to their advantage.
2) To persuade people, particularly those at special risk, to undertake preventive action, to accept tests so that cancer can be detected at an earlier stage, or to seek appropriate medical advice quickly when recognizable signs of ill health occur.

Both aims are closely linked with professional education, because physicians and all other professionals involved in health care are an integral part of the network of communications by which people acquire information about cancer. Because they stand in a position of unique authority in the public eye, their responsibility is correspondingly heavy.

SPECIFIC OBJECTIVES OF PUBLIC EDUCATION

In practice, the first aim involves all the well-tried methods of large-scale public education—television, broadcasting, newspapers, magazines, films, lectures, posters, and brochures. Intensive work of this kind is an essential background to all the more clearly defined objectives of the second aim. Mass educational programs cannot be expected to have instant effects on a large proportion of the population, but without a widespread awareness—and acceptance—of the good results of prompt treatment, more substantial results cannot be achieved in groups at high risk. As long as cancer remains for many people the cause of deep-seated fears and anxieties, we should not be surprised if they resist blandishments to seek medical advice for still-tolerable symptoms or to accept tests designed to detect the disease. For people who are not convinced that cancer responds to treatment, early detection may signify no more than hearing a sentence of death sooner rather than later.

The second aim relates to more precise objectives:

1) *To alter well-established habits now known to be harmful.* Cigarette smokers are one of the most easily recognized and largest group of people at special risk. The literature and methods of tackling this problem have been assembled, evaluated, and published at considerable length by the National Clearinghouse for Smoking and Health. Other examples involve eating and drinking habits, which appear to be linked with high risk of cancer in some people but fall (as does cigarette smoking) into a category of personal habits that may relate as much to other serious health hazards as to cancer.

2) *To persuade people at special risk to undertake a defined course of action as a means of preventing frank cancer from developing or of detecting it before it progresses beyond the reach of curative treatment.* Current examples are the substantial campaigns to get women to have a regular Pap smear and mammographic examination, or to undertake breast self-examination. More limited have been efforts to persuade men previously employed in the manufacture of aniline dyes to accept urological examination for cancer of the bladder.

3) *To influence habits of seeking medical care in some sections of the population to enable them to get appropriate medical advice when certain warning signs occur.* This may not have obvious links with the problems of people at high risk of cancer. But since it is closely related to the success of cancer treatment, it bears heavily on how people see the relevance of prompt treatment to themselves if a threatening situation arises. This forum is not the place for a substantial discussion of how different ways of life affect a person's readiness or otherwise to seek medical advice. Two brief examples show how this wider question is part of the fabric of behavior of high-risk groups: a) the hard economic facts of life make it difficult for men with a small family business to leave it unattended for attention to some condition that would drive others to a doctor; b) the stoical tradition of people in isolated farming communities may make them less willing to "give in" to a complaint that others in their community would regard as trivial. In

these circumstances, exhortations to behave in ways that doctors would regard as sensible clash with entrenched beliefs and norms of behavior. Pinned down by the superior firepower of what their own society and way of life expect of them, people in this situation tend to keep their heads down and opt for the status quo. For this problem the current American Cancer Society (ACS) program [1] to take detection services to the people and let them learn by doing could be most helpful. This topic will be discussed later.

In some regions with large populations of subsistence farmers and poor people in arid areas (for instance, Mexico), where uterine and penile cancers dominate all other forms of the disease, cancer control is most properly and effectively regarded as a long-term problem of improving public health, hygiene, and water supply than as a matter of highly specific education about cancer. Until the root causes are dealt with, case-finding programs do no more than nibble at the problem and—as with all education about cancer—should only be an objective of public education if appropriate treatment facilities are available to all who are persuaded to seek them.

The three objectives can be distinguished for the purpose of clarifying thinking; in practice, they are indivisible. Cultural and social norms exert powerful pressures on individuals to conform to accepted patterns of behavior and to cling to established beliefs about health and disease. Susser and Watson [2] summed it up in this way:

> To health educators, as to most doctors, optimism and the conviction that professional knowledge is superior to lay beliefs are necessary to effective practice. This may lead to didactic educational programmes which are liable to evoke hostility and a failure of communication, particularly in controversial matters open to more than one interpretation . . . what is controversial for a given group is specific to its system of values, and can only be discovered by studying these values.

Public education cannot counter these pressures overnight. It has to be planned in the long term as what I have called elsewhere [3] "a process of gentle but unrelenting erosion of prejudice that will eventually reduce cancer in the public mind to the emotional level of other serious disease and so enable people to receive, accept and act on the practical advice that can save large numbers from untimely death."

THE MESSAGE OF PUBLIC EDUCATION

Perhaps the most powerful counterpressure to existing negative beliefs—and one not yet satisfactorily exploited—is to demonstrate that some forms of cancer can be averted by personal action. Into this category fall successful programs of early detection and prevention. An example was the dramatic elimination—although it was little publicized—of spinner's cancer in the cotton industry in northwest England [4]. Also worth mentioning is the significant fall in the mortality rates from lung cancer of British doctors [5,6] after they had markedly changed their cigarette-smoking habits; the rate continued to rise in the population at large, where cigarette consumption had not fallen. More recently, the work of Strax et al. [7] in New York has apparently reduced mortality from breast cancer in women over age 50.

In the same category, we might include population screening by cervical cytology, although reduction in mortality must be regarded as a potential, rather than a demonstrated, benefit. The kind of research that might have helped prove the case was swamped by an understandable public demand for facilities to be made available to all women. The efficacy of this test might still be confirmed by switching the emphasis to the women at highest risk, as discussed later. Whatever efforts may be deployed in informing and educating the public about detection and prevention, it has to be accepted that no program could be so decisively effective as primary or secondary prevention demonstrated and recognized as such among ordinary people.

CONTENT OF PUBLIC EDUCATION

If we do not have a sufficient body of self-evident (to the public) proof that measures of prevention and earlier detection reduce the mortality from cancer, what other directions must education take?

First must come continuing reassurance that *some* forms of cancer do respond well to treatment. There must be no exaggerated claims, because the evidence that cancer can kill is there for every citizen to see and experience at first hand. Overly optimistic claims may be a tempting ploy in countering excessive pessimism, but in the end they do no more than invite well-merited cynicism about the rest of the educational message. Even in countries where programs of public education are vigorous and well established, many people still have deep-seated fears and misconceptions about cancer and its etiology and doubts about the outcome of treatment, prompt or otherwise [8, 9]. In the United States, a recent ACS survey [10] of women's attitudes to breast cancer revealed strong evidence of residual fears, despite many years of public education on the subject and intensive special efforts to promote breast self-examination and regular checks by palpation and by mammography or thermography.

In public education, there is a peculiar difficulty in publicizing accurate epidemiological evidence of survival rates. Reports paint a satisfactorily optimistic picture of a hypothetical situation, but scarcely touch the individual suddenly confronted with alarming symptoms. To say, for example, that 80 percent of women whose breast cancers are treated while still localized will be alive and well 5 years after treatment may convince clinicians. For the public it may lighten the gloomier side of the picture painted in such somber colors by known deaths among relatives and friends. But, to the individual who suddenly finds in herself signs that she knows may indicate cancer, percentage survival rates cease to have personal relevance. Statistical probability takes on a new and harsher reality: her personal chances are no longer 8 out of 10, but either 100 percent or 0–to get well or to die. In this situation, as with most cancers that give rise to recognizable warning signs, the factual information acquired from careful programs of education does not necessarily make the individual act on what he knows. Knowledge can go hand in hand with deep-seated fears that influence behavior, even when the conscious mind is well aware of what ought to be done. A recent study in England [9] showed that between 80 and 90 percent of the female population was aware that a lump in the breast might mean cancer, but delay remains a problem. Even as far back as 1962, a national sample survey in the United States showed that only 12.3 percent still thought cancer could never be cured. But no one would be so foolhardy as to suggest that this encouraging body of knowledge of what can be done is always reflected in desirable behavior. Nor have studies of positive attitudes been able to show that they are accompanied by matching behavior [11–13]. Public education about cancer has been adequately shown in the United States, Canada, and England to be able to impart accurate knowledge of a kind that was lacking before. How to translate this hard-won knowledge into appropriate action at critical times remains a special problem that has proved much less amenable to solutions that can be applied on a large scale.

WHO IS TO EDUCATE?

There is much evidence that information or advice passed by one individual to another–the "one-to-one situation"–is most effective in triggering action. It is a cornerstone of all effective public education, but a warning is necessary. To preclude any general assumption that information diffused in this way is always beneficial, it needs to be stated that, coming from the ill-informed, it can equally well be harmful. A study in progress in schools in Manchester, England [14], suggests that a substantial body of unfounded beliefs on cancer causation is acquired early by young children from statements made by adults, whether directly or overheard. And these notions, along with subsequent personal experience of cancer, persist in the body of beliefs, scientific and otherwise, that can be traced in the adult population. Briggs and Wakefield [8] and Knopf [9] reported this in the United Kingdom recently, and there is a full summary of the world literature prior to these studies in Volume 5 of the *UICC Monograph*

Series [15]. Acknowledgment of the power of planned person-to-person education should not be taken as dismissing public education on a large scale. By its nature, the former reaches smaller numbers of the population over a longer period. In scope and speed, it can never match a program based on intelligent use of the mass media. The two have to be seen as complementary, with mass education and information providing the fertile soil in which the seeds of personal advice can bear fruit. With these provisos, it is beyond dispute that doctors, in particular [16, 17], and other health professionals [18] have the greatest potential for influencing people to undertake preventive tests. Their influence will be discussed.

Turning to the general public, research has shown that people with no special medical training can have a powerful influence for good or ill. Relatives and friends have triggered effective action by individuals both in cervical screening [19] and in self-referral for abnormal conditions of the breast [20]. This is particularly true of problems not yet accepted consciously as meriting resort to a doctor. This interaction between ordinary people, first described by Friedson [21] as the "lay-referral system," operates almost universally throughout the population. In the diagnostic process, the doctor, far from being the person of first resort, is often several links along the chain of referral.

For this reason, public education has as one of its most important tasks the creation of what I have called "informed nuclei" in the community [3]. These are people who, from whatever source, possess more than usually reliable information about cancer. It is at this point that the general program of mass information and education meshes with person-to-person education. In the particular matter of occupational high-risk groups, it is here that the potential of industrial unions can be brought to bear. General education has to be used, for instance, to disseminate information widely about the hazards of exposure to asbestos dust with the particular aim of reaching those people who are or have been exposed secondarily to asbestos dust. For those who work in primary contact with asbestos, the unions can make sure information on protection and health checks reaches every worker who is exposed. This applies with particular force to trades in which people work in the same setting, although less directly, with asbestos; this may include, for example, sweeping dust from the floors, above which well-protected asbestos workers are lagging pipes, and a multitude of workers involved in ship-breaking, where a good deal of old and highly dangerous asbestos insulation is being ripped apart. Such work is often done with little or no protection and often without clear knowledge that the dangers are other than those inherent in any dirty and dusty job.

There has been in Britain in recent years a striking example of the need for vigilance in industry and missed opportunities for initiative on the part of unions in seeing that workers at special risk were adequately briefed on protection. An occupational skin and scrotal cancer plagued the Lancashire cotton industry as a result of mineral oils that were thrown as a fine spray onto the operator's groin and forearms. From 1911 to 1943 the incidence of scrotal cancer [4] in male spinners was 422 per million of the population compared with 4 in the population at large. By the 1940's a noncarcinogenic lubricant had been introduced and hygiene arrangements had been improved. Now, this form of cancer, with a long latent period, is rare and occurs only in operators exposed many years before.

Curiously, all the knowledge and personnel education that helped wipe out scrotal cancer from the cotton textile industry has not prevented its arising in another industry, light engineering [22], particularly among the skilled setters of automatic machines [23]. It has not become a problem on a similar scale, presumably because of some residual awareness of the hazards among industrial medical officers, but much of the keen worker awareness that characterized the cotton industry is lacking. The lengthy exposure usually required for such skin lesions to occur is—as with the long-term effects of cigarette smoking to the young—one of the special obstacles to unremitting regard for safety precautions and hygiene by those at risk. Here is an obvious place for active union initiative in worker education, for those on the inside are always better placed than educators from outside the industry to influence their colleagues. Two examples illustrate this point, although the list of occupations at high risk where union support is vital could be greatly extended.

As noted, informed people without medical qualifications can influence others to take part in screening programs or to seek early detection. Other studies have shown that people can exert a powerful influence on one another in reaching group decisions to participate in screening. Fulghum's study [18] in Florida was a notable example of yet another form of what Kegeles [12] described as "public commitment." Fulghum showed in a study of cervical screening that a "statement of intention" led to full participation by every woman who had committed herself. The recent proposals by the ACS [1] to induce people to learn and to take part by doing—taking screening services directly to the community—are based on similar principles. In my own studies [17] and with Sansom et al. [24], these methods proved highly effective in northwest England. Mobile cytotest teams, closely following a priming visit by a nurse/educator, were extremely successful in the initial recruitment of women to the cervical screening program. In fact, none of the agencies doing Pap tests has equaled these mobile industrial teams in attracting women low on the social scale to have a first test.

Two cautionary notes must be introduced to modify this eulogy. One is that group decisions to have a Pap smear in an industrial setting may become a form of social behavior rather than a conscious health action [25], so there is little motivation to repeat the experience when it is time for the next routine reexamination. The second became apparent from our recent study [24] of 1,007 women invited to have a routine Pap test 3 years after their first. Women whose first test was done by a mobile industrial team had by far the worst rate of response to recall (a crude rate of 29 percent, compared with 62 percent whose first test was at an established local authority cytology clinic). There are several reasons for this lack of response: the first factor mentioned above; the high turnover of labor, particularly among the unskilled and semiskilled workers, which tends to scatter the original participants and to leave women in factories where access to reexamination is no longer easy; and the fact that some women married and no longer worked. All these women are left almost in the position of those who have never made arrangements to take a test. They are now confronted by the administrative details smoothed out for them by others when the mobile cytology team visited their factory. Since women low on the socioeconomic scale find it most difficult to cope with what they see as "authority," they never get around to arranging for a repeat test.

The paradox, then, is that taking population screening services to the people, particularly at their places of work, is both the *most* effective in recruiting the most vulnerable individuals and the *least* effective in bringing them back at regular intervals for reexamination. Sansom et al. [24] made it clear that lower rates of response to recall are not solely a feature of socioeconomic status. In fact, once women had been recruited to a cervical screening program, the response rate to recall was slightly better at the lower end of the socioeconomic scale. Once women had had an initial Pap test, the likelihood of their returning when invited 3 years later for reexamination depended more on whether they were working. Of women married to men in managerial and white-collar jobs, 50 percent of those who were housewives had a second test, but only 38 percent of those who were employed. For those married to men in semiskilled and unskilled jobs, the rates were higher—55 percent of the housewives and 49 percent of those who were working. The significance of having much of their day taken up by employment was also reflected in the difference between the proportion of working wives in full-time employment who had a second test (44 percent) and those who worked only part-time (55 percent). Not even the provision of evening clinic facilities greatly improved the response, presumably because the demands of home, family, and social life mortgage what is left of their day after leaving work.

These cautionary notes are in no way intended to negate the possibilities of taking detection programs into the community or into industry. The mobile teams in the Manchester region attempted to visit factories and other industrial establishments at regular intervals, but clearly the logistics of the operation were not entirely satisfactory. Any similar schemes undertaken in the United States will have to pay much closer attention to the practical difficulties inherent in the life style of working people. There is a great temptation, which we did not entirely avoid, to count success by the number of people initiated into a program. Many tests, however, demand regular repetition if they are to be effective.

People may learn by participating, but we cannot count on their continuing automatically to return unless their path is smoothed for subsequent visits as it was for their first.

These conclusions are based on a large cervical screening program, but similar findings are emerging from a feasibility study of breast screening in the same region. They may well apply with equal force to the campaign to encourage regular proctoscopic examination for men in the United States. In this case, another element must be taken into account. Careful research and assessment in the hospital setting may prove the effectiveness of a test. Publicity and medical enthusiasm, however, will not convince the people at risk to accept the test if they find it unpleasant, painful, or distasteful. Discovery of a possible threat to future well-being will never have as high a priority as the negative effects of an unpleasant procedure. And those who try a test once are sometimes discouraged from repeating the experience. Proving that proctoscopy is effective as a clinical procedure is a far cry from persuading the man in the street to overcome his natural revulsion against the action it involves. Hammerschlag [26] described the powerful psychological barriers that make acceptance of ano-rectal examination peculiarly difficult, even for those with symptoms that clearly justify the procedure.

The picture painted is pessimistic regarding the large-scale incorporation of regular proctoscopic examinations for men into programs of cancer detection, and figures on the extent of acceptance of the test in the United States tend to support this. No obvious solution suggests itself, but this special problem of public education has not always received the attention it deserves. The responsibility for "selling" a test to the general public cannot be handed over entirely to education and publicity experts. There are limits to what they can do, just as there are limits to what doctors can do. Acceptability should be as much a part of the preliminary research and evaluation process as reliability and specificity. If it is not, doctors should not be surprised if the educators can find no verbal alchemy to transform revulsion into acceptance or distaste into gratitude for the wonders of science.

HOW ARE HEALTH EDUCATORS TO TACKLE HIGH-RISK GROUPS?

Some possibilities for education were discussed in the previous section. Here, we examine the use of some of the high-risk profiles that epidemiologists have delineated in recent years. Stein [27] attempted to describe such possibilities in a form that health educators might use. The opportunities for addressing broad, easily identifiable groups in the population (e.g., women low on the socioeconomic scale for Pap tests) are obvious enough to educators; however, more attention should be given to differences in information sources relied on by people at different points on the socioeconomic scale. In England, Sansom et al.

[19] found that over 81 percent of women at the bottom of the social scale first learned about the Pap smear from some form of person-to-person communication, in contrast to 35 percent at the upper end. On the other hand, less than 19 percent of those at the bottom of the scale learned about it from the mass media and printed matter, against 57 percent of those at the upper end.

As Stein [27] explained, fat women between the ages of 40 and 44 and women who have had frequent sexual experience with several different partners confront educators with immediate difficulty. They are not specific groups, but descriptive categories of individuals distributed throughout the population. The same applies to workers who left their jobs and later were discovered to have been exposed to industrial carcinogens, e.g., men formerly employed in the manufacture of dyestuffs and chemicals involving contact with benzidine or 1- and 2-naphthylamine, and subsequently a wider range of workers in the rubber industry and in cablemaking. The problem of bringing home these hazards is compounded by the lengthy latent period (usually as much as 18 years, according to Case et al. [28]) before bladder tumors develop.

Those responsible for mass educational programs are in some difficulty with these descriptive categories. They can disseminate the information about hazards widely via the mass media, but the tools they use are not designed to be focused with precision on the individuals at risk. For the occupational hazards, the enforcement of safety precautions, regular examination, and systematic and thorough education of those still in the industry can be handled effectively by industrial unions for the reasons discussed earlier. For workers who have left the industry, especially before the full extent of the hazard was known, there are real problems. In England, the Department of Health and Social Security is proposing an extensive appeal by direct mailing to known ex-workers and their doctors, but the passage of time and the mobility of workers are obvious obstacles to the discovery of all individuals at risk.

For groups defined as being at special risk on medical grounds, we reach an area in which the role of professional health educators may be limited to making the hazard as widely and accurately known as possible, so that everyone affected will be aware of the actions recommended by doctors. When such information is made available, a certain amount of self-selection occurs among those at risk and they come forward for examination or consultation. The proportion who do act on this information is not high; about 10 percent of the population addressed is the most usual initial response. This proportion does increase with repetition and more personal stimuli, particularly if the cancer involved is a reasonably well-known threat in the public mind.

My current study of the records of 400,000 women examined by cervical cytology shows a remarkable degree of self-selection *within* those who came for a test: 24 percent had symptoms of some kind when examined, and this group accounted for 43 percent of all the positive/suspicious findings reported. Clearly these women were using the population screening program for a purpose quite different from that for which it was intended. The policy and the emphasis of all subsequent publicity had been on "well women" seeking continued assurance that all was well. Yet the existence of widely publicized facilities, freely and easily available—a vital requirement of any assault on risk populations—has produced an interesting shift in emphasis. Substantial numbers of women are using the facilities as a first stage in the diagnostic process, without the need to approach a doctor with a specific request to investigate this or that symptom.

There is evidence [29] that a similar trend toward self-referral is occurring in the breast screening study in Manchester, which is a departure from the original intention of examining symptomless women. Does it call for a change in the content of education? Almost certainly not. The present balance of information may be exactly right for encouraging women who might not otherwise "bother the doctor" to use the screening program as a way of having their as yet undramatic symptoms investigated.

In fact, these individuals may be a very important self-defined high-risk group. As Hammond and his colleagues [30] pointed out in the Toledo study, women who enter the screening program with complaints (spotting, bleeding, or discharge), but whose smears prove to have no abnormalities, have a much higher risk of developing uterine cancer in subsequent years than those without such complaints. Once identified, these women should be the subject of special educational efforts to persuade them to have regular reexamination. The special merit of having screening and detection facilities readily available is that women who use them, whatever their motives, have already entered the health-care system if some abnormality is found. They are, therefore, not as dependent on making a further decision for themselves to seek medical care as are, for example, those who discover a lump in the breast at home.

Self-selection as a result of publicity is, however, limited. As we have seen, knowledge does not always lead to action, and the challenge is how to bring more persuasive methods to bear. At this point fusion of the efforts of professional educators with those of doctors and others in primary health-care teams is needed.

Before passing on to this crucial aspect of educating people at high risk, certain particular problems must exercise the minds of those responsible for determining policy in public education. There are known risks to women in sexual promiscuity. Education and routine Pap smears in VD clinics are obvious possibilities, although they can only nibble at a problem that has much wider health and social implications. But can we publicize the relationship between promiscuity and cervical cancer as a strong feature of the program? The Florida study [18] of cervical screening among women low on the socioeconomic scale revealed that one factor against participation is the fear that the test will reveal past sexual adventures. In many minds, there are still prejudices about cancer and an element of stigma. Inverted logic is grafted onto prejudice and leads to the implication that women who get uterine cancer have been sexually promiscuous. Can the distress to women who develop cervical cancer after a moderate sexual life faithful to one partner be justified? To their concern at having the disease, are we to add the unhappy suspicion that others may think their lives have not been models of sexual rectitude? Deciding educational policy on this point is not easy, but there seems to be a strong case for moderating the general publicity and intensifying the efforts of doctors and community health-care teams to screen women under their care whom they know or suspect to be at risk.

A similar problem of policy arises with the discovery that the daughters of some women who received diethylstilbestrol (DES) during pregnancy are prone to adenocarcinoma of the vagina and cervix. Is this a case for intensive publicity throughout the population? Would it cause needless alarm and distress? Are most women reasonably well informed about the medication they have received in the past, or would substantial numbers become prey to unfounded doubts and fears because they do not remember whether DES was given when they were pregnant? There is no easy solution to these questions. From other studies of what people recall of even a recent regimen they were on, many probably will not be clear about the particular medication and dosages they received. Once we place ourselves in the care of a doctor, we transfer to him the responsibility for what we do and take and our memory of detail becomes highly selective. Thus, much of the responsibility for persuading and checking those at risk must rest with the gynecologists and other doctors who have access to the records of women known to have received DES during pregnancy.

ROLE OF THE MEDICAL PROFESSION

No education program so far has made enough of the unique opportunities of doctors and others involved in medical care. Much has been written on the subject, but the reality still falls woefully short of the potential. The key to much of what could be done is that they alone share with their patients the special relationship of consultation, where everyone is most susceptible to advice. Health educators can advise doctors and nurses on making the most of this situation; they can never intrude on it. The true strength of education by the medical profession lies in those situations where people at risk are identified largely or wholly by medical criteria rather than by features or characteristics recognizable to the outside world. The daughters of women treated with DES are a case in point. So are the relatives of those in whom polyposis is diagnosed. To determine whether the disease is inherited, a detailed family history must be compiled and attention focused on that side of the family in which the responsible parent is identified. Education of all the living relatives in a way that will lead them to accept the need for physical examination must be a matter for doctors and others in the health-care teams. It is a delicate business that can easily lead to alarm and resistance if too much pressure is applied; but as Dukes [31] pointed out, it is only when special attention is directed to the families of polyposis patients that cancer control assumes practical importance. Another example of a risk category that is defined by medical criteria emerges from the discovery that children born without irises (congenital aniridia) are prone to develop Wilms' tumor. This connection is still not sufficiently known among pediatricians and ophthalmologists, who are almost the only professionals in a position to maintain adequate surveillance over the affected children as regards cancer detection and to guide and counsel the parents.

Apart from these special instances are the more obvious examples of how doctors and others with medical training can be active in public education when conducting their professional routine. Not all are fully aware that their every word and action, especially in consultation with patients and their relatives, is a form of health education. The question is not whether they provide any health education: it is whether what they do is for good or ill. Professional education has a heavy responsibility for making sure the effect of what doctors say and do is more often of positive value. Advice to give up cigarette smoking is not always given with sufficient force to patients who are clearly at high risk of a number of health hazards, including various forms of cancer. As important as giving sound, vigorous advice, is the example doctors set in the matter of cigarette smoking. Fewer doctors now smoke cigarettes. But this is not enough, because every doctor who is seen to smoke is a powerful counter to the efforts of those who try to persuade others of the danger. Many medical schools still have far to go in teaching student doctors about the risks of cigarette smoking. The facts are presented, but usually in various parts of the curriculum. They are rarely brought together in a forceful way to present a rounded picture of all the health hazards. There appears to be a particular lack of special instruction about the future responsibility of student doctors as exemplars after graduation. In our recent study [32], students in a large medical school commented on the confusion generated by staff members who still smoke cigarettes despite the evidence that is presented in the medical curriculum. And the halfhearted enforcement of "no-smoking" rules within the medical school was taken as a further flaw in the argument that cigarette smoking is as hazardous as some of their teachers contend.

Nurses and other health professionals also have special authority in the eyes of the general public as experts in matters of health and disease. They can be potent persuaders in screening programs for people at risk. Often, as with nurses working in the community, they are seen as a more readily accessible source of expert information than are doctors. Nurses and other health professionals who work in hospitals or departments specializing in the treatment of cancer may be well informed, but we have found subtle differences in the attitudes of nurses working in different parts of the same cancer treatment center. Those in the departments that see patients on routine follow-up after successful treatment for cancer had a markedly more optimistic attitude to the disease than those who worked only in treatment departments and wards, who had much less opportunity to see the long-term successes among the patients in their care. Public health nurses [33], along with medical students and general practitioners [34], have a much more pessimistic view than the facts warrant of the prognosis for certain highly manageable forms of cancer. Add to this the large body of people whose work since their initial medical training has not kept them regularly in touch with up-to-date cancer treatment facilities, with cured patients, and with opportunities to see detection facilities in action, and we have a source of potential misinformation that is all the more dangerous because the general public believes it comes from an authoritative source. The meeting of a fearful public with ill-informed or pessimistic health-care professionals is a textbook example of how to reinforce old fears and prejudices. In fact, an investigation by Henderson et al. [35] in Canada led them to the even blunter conclusion that the fears and anxieties of the public are often no more than a reflection of the fears of their doctors. To find the beginnings of a solution will involve both an improvement of undergraduate education as regards cancer and—a perennial problem—an attempt to fill the empty slots in a doctor's medical knowledge that tend to grow in number with every year after leaving medical school. The eager specialist probably strives to keep abreast of his subject: he presents no serious problem. It is with the bulk of generalist doctors, nurses, and other paramedical workers, whose daily work is only occasionally concerned with cancer, that the difficulties of refresher education arise. It is axiomatic that those with most to gain from it are least likely to pay heed.

Easson [36] recently wrote persuasively on the role of the doctor in public education. He has a point of special interest that is often ignored in public education:

> Earlier, comment was made on those whom the public regard as "experts" on cancer simply because they work in the medical field. Some thought must be given to the education by doctors of the many types of paramedical worker, not in the sense of vocational training (as for medical physicists and radiotherapy technicians) but to equip them for their role as educators of the public. Everyone is involved whose work in hospitals and clinics brings them into regular contact with patients—nurses, physiotherapists, radiographers, social workers, pharmacists, physicists, and so on. It also involves supporting staff, whose opinions are often sought on medical matters—secretaries, receptionists, and administrators. Doctors with special knowledge should undertake to instruct these various categories of health workers about cancer, what it is and what it is not, its natural history, causation, treatment, and especially its prognosis and the controllable factors which can so influence prognosis. In addition, however, doctors must make very clear to all those health workers the importance of their role as educators of the public, and how they may best influence their family, friends, and acquaintances to take appropriate action when indicated.

This excerpt illustrates well the peculiar difficulty of separating public and professional education. To the oncologist, the group to which Easson refers is only barely distinguishable from the general public. And yet their special position as medically informed people in their own communities (even the hospital electrician is an "expert") makes them exceptionally suitable for the kind of education that was described earlier as "creating informed nuclei in the community." All hospitals specializing in the treatment of cancer should make sure that every member of their staff, down to the most recently hired records clerk or general porter, is given enough reliable facts about cancer, its treatment and prognosis, to assure that they move among their friends and relatives a little better informed than average. They will be more likely to give the kind of positive advice that research studies have shown to trigger appropriate action in people worried by symptoms or hesitating over making use of detection facilities. In promoting effective public education, I would rate the staffs of such oncological centers as one of the prime targets of any cancer control program aimed at high-risk people.

This is one area in which, to an outsider, the collaboration between the voluntary agencies in the United States and the hospitals and government health agencies concerned has seemed less effective than in other areas of public education. In northwest England, one of the strengths of the public education program (run by a voluntary organization) has been its extremely close association from the start with a major cancer treatment center (their organization's offices are located at the hospital). It has been particularly effective in stimulating research designed to improve the public education program and in evaluating educational activities in the areas of prevention, detection, and changes in knowledge. In the planned activities of the four "centers of excellence" (oncological centers or regional cancer organizations) recently established in England, public education has been cited as one of the responsibilities of the centers, along with appropriate research and evaluation. This concept is not new, and it is remarkable only insofar as it needed to be repeated in precise terms. In the past, the much advocated close collaboration between hospitals and health educators, particularly those from voluntary agencies, has been mostly a paper exercise. There has been collaboration, but not of the close day-to-day kind that makes for a truly effective symbiotic relationship. Doctors and other professionals can work as volunteers with voluntary agencies to great effect; voluntary agencies can offer practical and financial help to institutions and to patients. But, with the best of goodwill, there is inevitably a distance between expectation and reality on both sides. Any move that can link public education more closely to the treatment and detection service would be of inestimable value to both.

This section has shown that practicing doctors and health professionals have two distinct, though occasionally merging, roles in public education. One is to assist in the large-scale campaign of education to acquaint the public with hopeful, but accurate and unexaggerated, information about those forms of cancer that are responsive to early detection and treatment and about risk factors that can be avoided or kept under calm medical surveillance. In this sense, doctors and their colleagues might properly be regarded as volunteers in the public education program, whether they work in the program of the ACS or in a vital extension of their practice in special cancer centers or governmental agencies. The second role as educators is part of their more personal relationship with patients and their relatives. It is an educational process that necessarily reaches fewer people than do the mass media, but it is immensely more potent in triggering appropriate action. Perhaps a minor caveat may be entered here. It is comparatively easy for doctors to persuade people to accept an examination when it bears on what they currently consulted him for (e.g., a Pap test when a vaginal examination is called for on other grounds than suspicion of a uterine condition). But persuasion to act under these circumstances should not be equated too easily with education. Our study [19] showed quite clearly that women who had had a Pap test as an adjunct to another examination—postnatally, or when seeking contraceptive advice, for example—were much less aware than others of the need for regular repeat tests. Around 90 percent of those women who had asked for a Pap test, or had it suggested to them by a doctor or at a clinic, knew that the test needed regular repetition, but only 64 percent who were tested as an adjunct to another examination knew this. As we reported, "the results indicate that, although the family doctor was very successful in bringing women to have a test, and especially those in the 'hard-to-reach' groups, he was not as successful in educating them about the preventive nature of the test and its implications."

This illustration is useful in highlighting the pressing need for some better way of treating health education in the medical curriculum. Teaching it as a subject in its own right seems to relegate it in the minds of student doctors to the place of other topics of peripheral, but not obviously practical, interest. It becomes something others do, into which some doctors may later be drawn. Instead, it should be taught as part of the fabric of consultation and advice—as much a part of their training as where to prod, poke, and listen to discover bodily signs. The same might be said of much current teaching of the behavioral sciences to medical students. They cannot be expected to identify such bits of a mini-sociology course as being relevant to what they will do in the future as doctors. Unless concepts from the behavioral sciences can be shown to be useful and practical tools in their dealings with sick and healthy people, as tools that have already been used in particular clinical situations and might reasonably be applied in others, the chances of having these subjects accepted by students as a vital part of their training are slim.

Both the undergraduate and postgraduate training of medical professionals with respect to cancer and people at special risk must be regarded as essential elements in public education. The quality of public education will never be better than the quality of the health education learned and practiced in their daily work by doctors and their paramedical colleagues. Accurate information about special risks has to be disseminated to the public with as much tact, skill, and energy as the specialists in public education and information can command. In the end, the success of cancer control programs that aim to persuade specially vulnerable people to act on the best medical advice will depend largely on how seriously doctors, and others in the medical team, take their responsibility to persuade and to educate. In this face-to-face situation, the search for a special formula of education that will be effective in all situations for all kinds of people is as tempting, but as unrewarding, as the ancient search for the philosopher's stone.

SUGGESTIONS FOR FUTURE WORK

1) The effects of public education programs should be more carefully evaluated. Many past projects either have not been evaluated—or have not been evaluated in relation to prestated objectives. Often there was no clear statement of measurable objectives before education began.

2) Despite the many public education projects in the past, too few have found their way into the professional literature as reports that can be appraised critically and drawn on by other health professionals. There are opportunities for collaborative research studies that will link the vigorous and valuable fieldwork of the ACS with evaluative research that would eventually be reported in the literature.

3) The success or failure of public education per se must be measured by precise criteria. For example, the health educator may be asked, because of suggestive medical evidence, to persuade women below a certain point on the socioeconomic scale in a given population to accept Pap tests. The results of any consequent educational programs must be measured by the proportion of women who so act, not by changes in the pattern of survival. When public education is planned, there is almost always a tacit assumption that successful education will equal lower mortality. So it may, but the logical leap this involves has nothing to do with whether the educators have succeeded in doing what they were asked to do.

4) Few educational projects have been based on defined populations and scarcely any that involve controls. These are difficult to arrange, but the possibilities include trials of different methods of persuading people at high risk to accept certain procedures. One might use intensive but tactful publicity in one area to women who have had DES treatment

in pregnancy and compare it elsewhere with intensive tracing and persuasion by doctors of the people affected. An alternative might be to base responsibility for safety and preventive health checks in a risk occupation largely on labor union activity at some plants and compare it with personal persuasions by physicians and cancer control staff elsewhere.

5)   Projects developed from the simple model of Easson [34] might chart areas of unwarranted pessimism and unsatisfactory or out-of-date knowledge among doctors, particularly concerning the prognosis for cancers of certain sites. The results would provide a firmer basis for subsequent efforts to alleviate deficiencies in postgraduate professional education.

6)   This type of investigation could apply to nursing and paramedical personnel at all levels who have direct contact with and influence on the general public, whether at hospitals or centers specializing in cancer treatment. All are "experts" in the eyes of the lay public. At the special treatment centers in-service programs should be devised to ensure that all employees, even those with no medical responsibility, are well-informed about cancer when they come into contact with people in their own communities.

7)   Public education programs linked with or based on special cancer treatment and detection centers are needed. A particular strength of the program in Manchester, England—in the opinion of both the hospital and community physicians and the researchers and health-education professionals involved—is that it has been a unified program from the beginning. This gives it a special authority in the eyes of the public and of the nonspecialist medical profession. To be able to demonstrate the cooperation of doctors known to have special expertise and daily involvement in cancer treatment is of immeasurable value in having public education accepted as an integral part of cancer control.

8)   Implicit in several of these suggestions is the collaboration of medical, nursing, and paramedical professionals in public education. I would go further. So deeply are the professions involved, both in general programs of education and in the direct enlightenment and persuasion of individuals at risk in their care, that public education can never be better than professional education allows it to be. This fact calls for some vigorous rethinking of undergraduate and postgraduate professional education to ensure that everyone concerned sees public education not merely as something that merits occasional collaboration with the voluntary agencies, but as a crucial part of his daily business of consultation and advice with patients, whether worried or wholly unaware of the special risks they run.

REFERENCES

1. James, Walter G. Identifying our problems. *In Proceedings of the International Conference on Public Education about Cancer, 1974.* U.I.C.C., Geneva. In press.

2. Susser, M.W., and Watson, W. *Sociology in Medicine.* Oxford Univ. Press, London, 1962.

3. Wakefield, J. *Cancer and Public Education.* Pitman Medical Publishing Co. Ltd., London, 1963.

4. Henry, S.A. *Cancer of the Scrotum in Relation to Occupation.* Oxford Univ. Press, London, 1946.

5. Doll, R., and Hill, A.B. Mortality in relation to smoking: ten years' observations of British doctors. *Br. Med. J. i:*1399–1410 and 1460–1467, 1964.

6. Doll, R., and Pike, M.C. Trends in mortality among British doctors in relation to their smoking habits. *J. R. Coll. Physicians Lond. 6:*216–222, 1972.

7. Strax, P., Venet, L., and Shapiro, S. Value of mammography in reduction of mortality from breast cancer in mass screening. *Am. J. Roentgenol., Radium Ther. Nucl. Med. 117:* 686–689, 1973.

8. Briggs, J.E., and Wakefield, J. *Public Opinion on Cancer: A Survey of Knowledge and Attitudes Among Women in Lancaster 1966.* South Manchester Hospital Management Committee, Manchester, 1967.

9. Knopf, A. *Cancer: Changes in Opinion After 7 Years of Public Education.* Manchester Regional Committee on Cancer, Manchester, 1974.

10. Wakefield, J., and Read, C.R. eds. Public opinion about cancer. *U.I.C.C. Tech. Rep. Ser. 11:*68–73, 1974.

11. Kegeles, S.S. Attitudes and behavior of the public regarding cervical cytology: current findings and new directions for research. *J. Chronic Dis. 20:*911–922, 1967.

12. Kegeles, S.S. Behavioral science data and approaches relevant to the development of education programs in cancer. *Health Educ. Monogr. 36:*18–33, 1973.

13. McKinlay, J.B. Some approaches and problems in the study of the use of services—an overview. *J. Health Soc. Behav. 13:*115–152, 1972.

14. Charlton, A. Personal communication, 1974.

15. *Public Education About Cancer: Research Findings and Theoretical Concepts. U.I.C.C. Monograph Series 5.* Springer-Verlag, Berlin, Heidelberg, New York, 1967.

16. Breslow, L., and Hochstim, J.R. Sociocultural aspects of cervical cytology in Alameda County, California. *Public Health Rep. 79:*107–112, 1964.

17. Wakefield, J. ed. *Seek Wisely To Prevent: Studies of Attitudes and Action in Cervical Cytology Programme.* Department of Health and Social Security Report. Her Majesty's Stat. Off., London, 1972.

18. Fulghum, J.E. *Cervical Cancer Detection Through Cytology. Monograph Series No. 11.* Florida State Board of Health, Jacksonville, Fla., 1967.

19. Sansom, C.D., Wakefield, J., and Pinnock, K.M. Choice or chance? How women come to have a cytotest done by their family doctors. *Int. J. Health Educ. 14:*127–138, 1971.

20. Eardley, A. Triggers to action: A study of what makes women seek advice for breast conditions. *Int. J. Health Educ. 17:*256–265, 1974.

21. Friedson, E. Client control and medical practice. *Am. J. Soc. 65:*374–382, 1960.

22. Cruickshank, C.N.D., and Squire, J.R. Skin cancer in the engineering industry from the use of mineral oil. *Br. J. Ind. Med. 7:*1–11, 1950.

23. Fay, H.T. Personal communcation, 1974.

24. Sansom, C.D., MacInerney, J., Oliver, V., and Wakefield, J. Differential response to recall in a cervical screening programme. *Br. J. Prev. Soc. Med.* In press.

25. Sansom, C.D. The influence of social studies on a cytological screening programme in the United Kingdom. *Int. J. Health Educ. 12:*132–136, 1969.

26. Hammerschlag, E. *In* Bellak, L., ed. *Psychology of Physical Illness.* Churchill, London, 1952.

27. Stein, J.J. High-risk groups–opportunity to improve cancer survival. *Cancer News 28:* 1, 4–5, 1974.

28. Case, R.A.M., Hosker, M.E., McDonald, D.B., et al. Tumours of the urinary bladder in workmen engaged in the manufacture and use of certain dyestuff intermediates in the British chemical industry. *Br. J. Ind. Med. 11:*75–104, 1954.

29. Hobbs, P. Personal communication, 1974.

30. Hammond, E.C., Burns, E.L., Seidman, H., et al. Detection of uterine cancer: high and low risk groups. *Cancer 22:*1096–1107, 1968.

31. Dukes, C.E. Cancer control in familial polyposis of the colon. *Dis. Colon Rectum 1:* 413–423, 1958.

32. Knopf, A., and Wakefield, J. Effect of medical education on smoking behaviour. *Br. J. Prev. Soc. Med. 28:*246–251, 1974.

33. Davison, R.L. Opinion of nurses on cancer, its treatment and curability: A survey among nurses in public health service. *Br. J. Prev. Soc. Med. 19:*24–29, 1965.

34. Easson, E.C. Cancer and the problem of pessimism. *Ca–Cancer J. Clin. 17:*7–14, 1967.

35. Henderson, J.G., Wittkower, E.D., and Lougheed, M.N. A psychiatric investigation of the delay factor in patient to doctor presentation in cancer. *J. Psychosom. Res. 3:*27–41, 1958.

36. Easson, E.C. The role of the doctor in public education. *U.I.C.C. Tech. Rep. Ser. 10:* 14–20, 1974.

DISCUSSION

The complex ways in which the public in general, and individuals in particular, react to the threat of cancer remain an enigma. **Dr. Rothman** noted that the public apparently has received the message on cigarettes and lung cancer but has not acted appropriately. Two interpretations of this situation were offered by **Dr. Wynder.** First, there is an "illusion of immortality" which helps us cope with threats to life. Second, in our society a visit to the doctor carries with it an aura of being sick rather than healthy. These obstacles to preventive medicine must be confronted if public education programs are to be effective.

Dr. Wynder asked how society could be made to recognize and act upon what is already known about the causes of cancer. **Dr. Breslow** stated that much can be done to popularize available information and to persuade sensible persons, while acknowledging individual freedom. For such popularization, **Dr. Saffiotti** urged creating and publicizing a concise slogan for personal avoidance of carcinogens, such as the American Cancer Society did with the seven danger signs of cancer. For example, "Protect yourself from cancer: don't smoke, don't drink hard alcoholic beverages, adopt a prudent diet, avoid excessive sun (if you're fair-skinned), learn the cancer risks of substances you work with." However, **Dr. D. G. Miller,** as a clinical oncologist, challenged the practicality of advice that physicians can offer, beyond the avoidance of tobacco and excessive alcohol and sunlight. He pointed out that little can be done about certain risk factors, including the largest, namely age.

Vincent F. Guinee

26

OVERVIEW: PREVENTIVE ONCOLOGY

Michael B. Shimkin, M.D.

School of Medicine
University of California
San Diego, California

This forum is the right time and the appropriate occasion to propose a new specialty, *Preventive Oncology.*

It is no secret that in the United States preventive medicine has been talked about much more than practiced. It has no financial base, and it falls in the crack between public health and medicine. Some of us had hoped that preventive medicine could come of age under the Regional Medical Program, but that idea wound up on the shoals.

Preventive oncology can assume a leadership position for preventive medicine if it is developed as an integral, yet identified, component of the network of cancer centers that is being established under the National Cancer Plan. It would be my fervent hope that, under the flag of cancer, the plans would include not only other diseases, but also would be oriented to health rather than to disease. Since the objectives are broader than cancer, let us postpone creating an American Society of Preventive Oncology, or issuing an American Journal of Preventive Oncology!

Preventive oncology, and all preventive medicine, is not yet another clinical specialty. It involves different types of practitioners, and different practitioner-people relationships than those appropriate for the clinical branches of medicine.

The usual clinical patient is someone who hurts, or suspects he or she might hurt. Such a patient comes to a physician for help, and the roles of supplicant and grantor, or of consumer and provider, are immediate and obvious. In preventive medicine, there are no patients, but individuals, with different sets of

435

motivations and anticipations. People, in general, simply are not patients most of the time. To attract their attention and to motivate them to carry out recommendations said to be good for them require different techniques than are effective among the sick. Health education as it is practiced at present is not an exciting topic for the nonsick. Diagnostic procedures that are acceptable to a patient may be completely unacceptable, for reasons of time, expense, or discomfort, to an individual who feels well. And, finally, most of the practices and procedures used in preventive medicine are too simple and easy (otherwise they would not belong under preventive medicine) for highly trained physicians.

Clinical medicine is essentially a panic service; preventive medicine should be a maintenance service. A sharp division between the two is neither possible nor desirable. Nevertheless, preventive medicine has its own clientele and techniques, for which it needs its own practitioners and facilities. It cannot be practiced as a part-time adjunct of clinical medicine, yet it must be in close conjunction with clinical medicine. Here, again, a somewhat different pattern of relationships, of contracts, if you will, is required between client and practitioner in preventive medicine than in clinical medicine, and between preventive and clinical medicine than between clinical branches.

PREVENTIVE ONCOLOGY TASKS

Preventive oncology has three tasks:
1) The acquisition and validation of knowledge regarding prevention through research and field trials.
2) The transmission of such knowledge, through education, which also needs research and validation.
3) The use of knowledge, through development of motivation and compliance with health practices and procedures. This task also needs research, and the feedback of validation.

As you can see, these three tasks were the subjects of the papers presented by Higginson [1], Wakefield [2] and Schottenfeld [3]. To rephrase each, briefly, may be useful.

Task 1: Knowledge Acquisition and Validation

Essentially, there are two types of cancer prevention [4]: the prevention of occurrence (primary prevention) and the prevention of the consequences and sequelae of the disease or its precursors (secondary prevention). Information regarding primary prevention is obtained usually through epidemiologic research, which may go through the stages of description, analysis, and experimentation.

Table 1 summarizes our sparse knowledge regarding etiologic factors in cancer [5]. Additional knowledge must be sought, but for the practice of prevention

TABLE 1

Some factors related to occurrence of neoplasia

| Site | Causative or predisposing factors | | Premalignant states or lesions |
	Exogenous	Endogenous	
Mouth and pharynx	Tobacco Alcohol Nutritional deficiency	Plummer-Vinson syndrome (sideropenia)	Leukoplakia
Esophagus	Alcohol Tobacco Nutritional deficiency Stricture (lye)	Sideropenia Tylosis	Dysplasia?
Stomach	?	Achlorhydria Pernicious anemia	Atrophic gastritis Polyp
Colorectum	Diet	Familial (multiple) polyposis Ulcerative colitis Gardner's syndrome	Villous polyp
Liver	Alcohol Nutritional deficiency? Aflatoxin?	Hemochromatosis Cirrhosis	?
Larynx	Tobacco Alcohol	?	Leukoplakia
Lung	Tobacco Air pollution Occupational inhalation of chromate, asbestos, nickel, uranium, etc.	Family history	Cytologic atypia Bronchial adenoma
Urinary bladder	Tobacco *Schistosoma haematobium* Occupational: aniline dye products	Tryptophan metabolism abnormality?	Leukoplakia Papilloma

TABLE 1 (Continued)

| Site | Causative or predisposing factors | | Premalignant states or lesions |
	Exogenous	Endogenous	
Skin (incl. genitalia)	Actinic radiation Ionizing radiation Arsenic Petroleum, tar products Burn scars	Fair complexion Xeroderma pigmentosum	Senile keratosis Arsenical keratosis Leukoplakia
Leukemia (myelocytic)	Ionizing radiation Phenylbutazone? Benzol? Alkylating agents?	Mongolism Bloom's syndrome Fanconi's syndrome	Myeloproliferative states (preleukemia)
Lymphoma	Immunosuppression	Agammaglobulinemia Wiskott-Aldrich syndrome	?
Thyroid	Ionizing radiation Iodine deficiency	Family history	Adenoma?
Bone	Ionizing radiation (radium)	Paget's disease of bone Fibrous dysplasia Osteochondroma	?
Testis	Mumps orchitis?	Cryptorchidism	?
Uterine cervix	Early sexual intercourse Promiscuity Uncircumsized partner?	?	Leukoplakia Cytologic dysplasia
Endometrium	Diet?	Endocrine: obesity, infertility, diabetes Ovarian hyperfunction?	Cytologic atypia Hyperplasia?
Breast	Ionizing radiation Diet?	Nulliparity Family history Endocrine: obesity, diabetes	Intraductile papilloma Chronic cystic disease

it must also include validation. Thus, it is not sufficient to find a relationship between an environmental factor and an increased risk to some form of cancer. Further studies are necessary to validate that the withdrawal of the factor indeed reduces the risk to cancer.

Secondary prevention entails the definition and identification of high-risk groups and groups with precursor stages of disease (Table 1). There is, of course, no sharp break between primary and secondary prevention, nor between precursors and "early" stages of a disease. Thus, a woman who starts her sexual life early and continues intensive sexual activity increases her risk to cervical cancer; cervical dysplasia is a precursor of clinical cancer, and in situ carcinoma of the cervix is still our best example of biologically early cancer. In this continuum, intervention is preferable between dysplasia and morphological malignancy, through the use of cytologic techniques.

Two research areas in preventive oncology seem imperative but are conspicuous by their absence in the present cancer center plans. The first would encompass the study of the natural history and effect of treatment on the so-called premalignant lesions. We have but fuzzy knowledge of the actual quantitative risk of invasive cancer in patients with leukoplakia, keratoses, or polyps. Cohort studies are necessary to yield this information. The second is the study of the value of various suggested intervention procedures against cancer and its precursors. The model for this is the evaluation of X-ray mammography for breast cancer detection, performed by the Health Insurance Plan of New York [6]. We simply *must* have quantitative data from which we can draw conclusions regarding cost-benefit ratios, acceptance by the public, and similar mundane but essential matters. The determination of *cost* should not obscure *value,* but these considerations are complementary. We must know the value and the cost of what we are selling!

Task 2: Education

In regard to education, its purpose is to spread *accurate* information about cancer, and to discourage misinformation. Education should also include emphasis upon motivating the recipient to take the action implied in his education.

We must be sure that the products we purvey are correct and identify the areas of ignorance. We must clarify the thinking of teachers who continue to confuse "early" and "small" cancers. The term "early" is a misnomer for most situations regarding cancer, since we seldom have a measure of the time the lesion has existed. The size and extent of the lesion at first discovery by the patient or the physician do not measure the growth rate unless observed over time. "Late" also suggests that the prognosis in many cancers is related more closely to clinical delay than the facts support, and connotes guilt for the delay.

A recent paper [7] on patient delay in cancer used delay itself as the endpoint, rather than the effect of such delay, if any, on outcome. A flurry of letters [8] objecting to this was heartening. To reiterate for emphasis: Delay, from symptoms or signs to treatment, is meaningful only if it affects the outcome. Otherwise, reduction in delay merely lengthens the period of worry and expense.

How we educate in health is a field of special expertise. There has been disenchantment with hardware aids to education, and in ex cathedra spoonfeeding by professors. I suspect that what will prevail includes an early start of education, group participation, and peer and leadership examples.

Task 3: Motivation for Good Health Practices

One approach to the evaluation of education in cancer would be to analyze the stage distribution and outcome of cancer among physicians and other health personnel, as compared with appropriate patients without such medical background. Does a medical education motivate "earlier" reference for treatment of colorectal cancer? If it does not, a rigorous reappraisal of some of our educational concepts would be in order. A negative effect of too much education is not unknown.

PREVENTIVE ONCOLOGY FACILITY

The next component necessary for the development of preventive oncology is a facility staffed by men and women trained in preventive medical methodology [9]. The simpler predictive and screening procedures would be performed in the facility. They include a patient history and an abbreviated physical, blood pressure check, urinalysis, blood sample for the laboratory, electrocardiogram, and a hematest on a fecal sample, plus X-ray mammography and vaginal smear for women. A "checkup" physical, carried out by paramedical personnel, must be considered as a screening procedure, with those identified as abnormal being channeled immediately to appropriate medical clinics.

It must be admitted that cold analyses of the benefits of multiphasic screening are not exactly heartening in their conclusions [10]. With few exceptions, we lack data on the quantitative value and the cost of most procedures that are usually included in multiphasic screening. However, it is evident that in most settings the comparisons are not between groups getting the multiphasic screening versus groups not getting the procedures. The latter are also covered by some medical service scheme and receive many of the same procedures when they are considered to be indicated. Convenience and cost in time certainly should be considered as well as the more usual indices of beneficial medical effects.

It is neither economical nor medically sound to separate tests for cancer from tests for hypertension, diabetes, or habits that may be hazards to that individual. At this point we extend from cancer to the totality of risks that threaten health and life. The topic now is preventive medicine.

Risk to Life

The easiest risk to measure is risk to life. The insurance companies have been making good money on this measure for many decades.

Table 2 summarizes the total risk of mortality in four major groups that compose the population in the United States, expressed in 10-year periods. These are condensed from the Geller tables [11], based on 1968 data, and show the advantages of the female sex and the white skin.

TABLE 2

Chance in 100,000 of dying during next 10 years, U.S., 1968 [11]

Race and sex	Age (yr)				
	20	30	40	50	60
White male	1,810	2,220	5,490	14,290	31,840
Black male	4,070	6,730	12,220	23,000	44,350
White female	670	1,240	3,050	6,920	15,810
Black female	1,690	3,730	7,490	14,350	32,320

Table 3 indicates the major causes of death among white males, and Table 4, among white females. The relative risks for each age group are indicated in Roman numerals, as well as the absolute risks for 10-year periods. In the younger age group, our society profiles its violent nature.

Accidents, suicide, and homicide rank above all diseases. In older age groups, many of the diseases are self-induced. Lung cancer, the top neoplastic killer of men, and creeping up on the list for women, has cigarette smoking as its primary cause. Cirrhosis of the liver in 90 percent of cases is alcohol induced.

Traditional curative medicine is certainly not the answer to these societal life-style problems. As we learned recently, reduction in gasoline supplies and speed limits has saved more lives on our highways than could have been achieved by erecting and staffing first-aid stations on every crossroad of the nation. Automobile, alcohol, and arms make a particularly fatal triad.

Robbins et al. [12, 13] devised a systematic assay and guidance scheme that they call prospective medicine. I commend it to your attention. Table 5 [12] shows one step in the process, in which a 40-year old man, with a 5.5 percent chance of dying during the next 10 years on the basis of general age-sex-race risks, is analyzed for the risks relative to the first cause of anticipated death, arteriosclerotic heart disease, which accounts for one-third of the total risk.

TABLE 3

White male: Chance in 100,000 of dying during next 10 years [11]

Cause of death	Age (yr)[a]				
	20	30	40	50	60
All causes	1,810	2,220	5,490	14,290	31,840
Arteriosclerotic heart disease	22	II 310	I 1,861	I 5,874	I 13,759
Lung cancer		47	IV 291	II 1,040	III 2,165
Stroke	24	64	209	III 666	II 2,270
Auto accidents	I 762	I 376	II 339	V 373	400
Cirrhosis		86	III 304	IV 567	649
Emphysema			62	319	IV 1,164
Suicide	III 157	III 200	V 253	324	337
Pneumonia	V 28	45	114	297	722
Cancer of colorectum			88	303	V 747
Accidents	II 228	IV 174			
Homicide	IV 108	V 107			

[a]Roman numerals indicate relative importance in each age group.

TABLE 4
White female: Chance in 100,000 of dying during next 10 years [11]

Cause of death		20		30		40		50		60
All causes		670		1,240		3,050		6,920		15,810
Arteriosclerotic heart disease		8	V	62	I	355	I	1,483	I	5,448
Stroke	IV	23	IV	73	III	200	III	498	II	1,566
Cancer of breast		9	II	100	II	351	II	678	III	839
Cancer of colorectum						95	IV	289	IV	639
Auto accidents	I	170	I	119	V	127		148		204
Cirrhosis		8		51	IV	167	V	273		256
Lung cancer						99		237	V	325
Pneumonia	V	21		34		69		146		314
Suicide	II	59	III	94		126		129		
Homicide	III	28		29						

Age (yr)[a]

[a]Roman numerals indicate relative importance in each age group.

TABLE 5

White male at age 40: Risk factors for dying from arteriosclerotic heart disease during the next 10 years (Total risk = 5,560) [12]

Rank	Cause of death/injury	No.	Percentage	Prognostic characteristics		Low-Risk Factor	High-Risk Factor
1	Arteriosclerotic heart disease (ASHD)	1.877	33.8	Blood pressure			
				Systolic	200		3.2
					180		2.2
					160		1.4
					140	0.8	
					120	0.4	
				Diastolic	106		3.7
					100		2.0
					94		1.3
					88	0.8	
					82	0.4	
				Cholesterol level			
					280		1.5
					220	1.0	
					180	0.5	
				Diabetic			
				Yes			3.0
				Controlled			2.5
				No		1.0	
				Exercise habits			
				Sedentary work and leisure			2.5
				Some activity work or leisure		1.0	
				Moderate exercise		0.6	

444

TABLE 5 (Continued)

Rank	Cause of death: disease/injury	No.	Percentage	Prognostic characteristics	Low-Risk Factor	High-Risk Factor
1 (Cont.)	Arteriosclerotic heart disease (ASHD)	1.877	33.8	Family history of ASHD		
				Both parents died before 60		1.4
				One parent died before 60		1.2
				Neither, if now under 60	1.0	
				Neither, if now over 60	0.9	
				Smoking habits:		
				Cigarets daily average		
				½ pack or more		1.5
				under ½ pack		1.1
				Cigars or pipe	1.0	
				Stopped smoking within 10 years	0.7	
				Nonsmoker or stopped over 10 years ago	0.5	
				Weight		
				75% overweight		2.5
				50% overweight		1.5
				15% overweight	1.0	
				10% underweight	0.8	

There are at least six defined risk factors that are listed and to which rough numerical values can be given as they affect the risk. Thus, elevated blood pressure carries increased risk; it can be reduced by treatment. Other factors can be reduced only by changes in life-style, such as smoking. The importance of the analysis is that something can be done about many of the factors.

I would like to recommend that every cancer risk factor adduced at this conference be included in a health hazard appraisal scheme. Studies to obtain improved estimates of risk should have high priority for situations in which such data are dubious or crude.

Causes of mortality are the most obvious and most dramatic threats. With some disease entities we are also beginning to measure the cost in terms of incapacitation. We are still very far from objective approaches to the ultimate—the measure of the quality of life—but that day will come.

To return to the practitioners of preventive medicine and their clients, the public. This public service may well save medicine as well as improve the health of the people. Canada has recognized [14] that there can be no unlimited spending for personal health services, and that the legitimate way of controlling such demand is through education and health maintenance. This view makes medical as well as fiscal sense. Our main threats to life are now based primarily on life-styles and habits. Advice on healthy habits does not take highly specialized physicians or expensive hospital centers.

We should broaden health maintenance by teaching *body awareness*, including self-examinations and examinations of one's children or each other in conjugal or other pairings. Women's Lib has shown what can be done in this regard [15]. It needs some tidying up, but the approach is useful. It is a legitimate, useful concern for the preventive medicine units I am visualizing. Let us now designate them as *preventories.*

It is in the preventories that health education, health surveillance, and multiphasic screening would come together, where self-examinations and examinations of one's partners would be taught, where premarital and prenatal advice and guidance would be offered, all summarized in a neat packet for the individual as well as for any central recordkeeping. If automobiles have records placed on the door to indicate the date for the next lube job, a human machine deserves no less.

Another important role of preventories in the health scheme of the future is that they are natural units for community action for health. Here would be one of the groups that could discuss community health matters such as air pollution, water supplies, and industrial incursions.

The social contract between the members of a preventory and its professional staff would be different from one that is more appropriate between patients and doctors. The ideal, of course, is a full partnership, each in turn being a messenger into the community.

The relationship of preventories with clinical centers has to be intimately close. There is no point in picking up incipient disease if nothing can be or is done about it. There is also a serious limitation of the system if the fiscal arrangements of the preventory are separated from the clinical center. Here we are in that sticky area of unresolved national policy regarding national health insurance and health maintenance organizations, not to mention professional services review organizations. I assume that we accept the national consensus that medical care of all people is a right and no longer a privilege.

All segments of the medical care system would profit from inclusion of preventive medicine in the plans. The payoffs would be better health and better health-educated people.

We have now gone from preventive oncology to preventive medicine, to preventories, and thence to health maintenance for the population. For all these plans, the A_3M_3 matrix, as indicated in Table 6, has to be fulfilled. In turn, money, men (including women, of course), and matériel have to be available, acceptable, and accountable to the public. The people of the United States deserve no less than a health system that fulfills these characteristics.

TABLE 6

Requirements for health system: The A_3M_3 matrix:

	Money	Men	Matériel
Available			
Acceptable			
Accountable			

REFERENCES

1. Higginson, J. Cancer etiology and prevention. This volume, 1975.
2. Wakefield, J. Education of the public. This volume, 1975.
3. Schottenfeld, D. Cancer detection programs. This volume, 1975.
4. Breslow, L. The prevention of cancer. *In* Raven, R.W., ed. *Cancer.* Vol. 6. Butterworth, London, 1959, pp 464-493.
5. Shimkin, M.B. Primary prevention of cancer. *In* Holland, J.F. and Frei, E. III, eds. *Cancer Medicine,* Lea and Febiger, Philadelphia, 1973, pp. 382-390.
6. Shapiro, S., Strax, P., and Venet, L. Evaluation of the role of periodic breast screening in reducing the mortality from breast cancer. *J.A.M.A. 215:*1777-1785, 1971.
7. Hackett, T.P., Cassem, N.H., and Raker, J.W. Patient delay cancer. *N. Engl. J. Med. 289:*14-20, 1973.
8. Implications of delay in cancer (letters). *N. Engl. J. Med. 289:*810-811, 1973.

9. Martin, P.L. Cervical cancer. Use of a non-physician health team for screening procedures. *Calif. Med. 110:*463–467, 1969.

10. *Screening in Medical Care.* Oxford Univ. Press, London, 1968.

11. Geller, H. *Probability Tables of Deaths in the Next Ten Years from Specific Causes.* Methodist Hospital Graduate Medical Center, Indianapolis, 1972.

12. Robbins, L.C., and Hall, J.H. *How to Practice Prospective Medicine.* Slaymaker Enterprises, Indianapolis, 1970.

13. Sadusk, J.F., Jr., and Robbins, L.C. Proposal for health-hazard appraisal in comprehensive health care. *J.A.M.A. 203:* 1108-1112, 1968.

14. Somers, A.R. Recharting national health priorities: a new Canadian perspective. *N. Engl. J. Med. 291:* 415-416, 1974.

15. Boston Woman's Health Book Collective. *Our Bodies Our Selves.* Simon and Schuster, New York, 1971.

DISCUSSION

Dr. Wynder discussed the problems met in preventive medicine. The patients are asymptomatic and less motivated to receive care, and there is not a good explanatory phrase for "risk factor." The leading causes of death today are the result of lifestyle. The public must realize that the persons who are responsibly protecting their health are actually paying for the health care of those who behave irresponsibly.

John Cutler

FURTHER DELINEATION OF
HIGH-RISK GROUPS

27

SOURCES, RESOURCES, AND TSOURIS

Marvin A. Schneiderman, Ph. D.

Field Studies and Statistics, National Cancer Institute
Bethesda, Maryland

The material in this chapter concerns itself with many things that have been said earlier, where data can be found, where potential exists for using data not often exploited in cancer epidemiology, and some of the troubles involved in using these data.[1] It is intended to be a sampling, not an exhaustive review.

This chapter is oriented with an eye toward today's efforts at cancer control in the United States and, very likely, elsewhere. The tables follow a control-oriented pattern, too. The first section deals with mortality because current discussions about cancer often start (and sometimes end) with talking about deaths from cancer. The second section is in response to the question, "How can we reduce mortality?" The first obvious answer is, "Treat the disease better." In fact, the Conquest of Cancer Program was often referred to even by members of the Nixon Administration, which initiated the program, as the "Cure Cancer Program." Since first thoughts of others are usually directed at treatment improvement, and since much work is already going on in this area, only moderate attention will be paid to it here.

Whether or not treatment can be improved, better diagnosis will bring persons to treatment earlier in their disease, and they are likely to live longer

[1] The word "tsouris" in the title is from the Hebrew, meaning "troubles," or "aggravation." It has been defined by Leo Rosten in the *Joys of Yiddish* by means of a story (slightly modified): Two men, not well acquainted, talk with each other, socially. After awhile the first one realizes he's been doing most of the talking and mostly about his children. "Please, tell me about *your* children." "I don't have any." "You don't have any? What do you do for tsouris?"

451

afterward. The third section of the tables considers problems of early diagnosis, with some thought given to the selection of appropriate candidates for early diagnosis and screening efforts. If treatment is improved along with improvement in diagnosis, a double benefit will be realized.

Finally, it is obvious that fewer people will die of cancer if fewer people develop cancer, which raises issues of prevention. In turn, we face questions of what we know that we can use now to prevent cancer, what we need to know, and what we can do to get to know more of what we need.

POTENTIAL FOR CONTROL

In terms of current knowledge, it seems to me that one-fourth to one-third of all cancer deaths (about 330,000 in 1974) in the United States are now avoidable through the prevention or earlier diagnosis of cancer. The basis for these figures may be seen from the rough tabulations shown in Table 1.

TABLE 1
Estimated preventable deaths from cancer

	Type of Cancer	Expected deaths	Preventable deaths
Cancer associated with cigarette smoking	Lung & some larynx	80,000	70,000
With alcohol	Head & neck	7,500	5,000
	Esophagus	6,000	
With industrial exposure	Bladder	9,000	5,000
	Liver	9,800	
Cancer associated with aspects of diet	Breast	30,000	5,000 [a]
	Colon & rectum	30,000	10,000
Other factors	Uterine cervix	7,500	3,000 [a]
	Melanoma & other skin cancer [b]	5,000	1,500
			99,500

[a]Achievable mostly through earlier diagnosis by application of known techniques.
[b]Although melanomas were thought not to be associated with exposure to sunlight, findings of the *Third National Cancer Survey Advanced Three-Year Report,* 1969-71 Incidence (1974, National Cancer Institute) and a recent review of cancer deaths by county in the United States [3] showed a strong latitude gradient with a range of incidence in whites from 7.7 per 100,000 in Dallas to 3.0 per 100,000 in Pittsburgh and 3.1 per 100,000 in Detroit. By state, among white males, the highest mortality was recorded in Texas (2.29 per 100,000) and Alabama (2.19 per 100,000) and the lowest in the Dakotas, Wisconsin, Michigan, Minnesota, Montana, Washington, and Maine (0.86 per 100,000 to 1.19 per 100,000).

MORTALITY DATA

Existing mortality data, shown in Table 2, are broken down into four categories: country, states within the United States, smaller political subdivisions within states, and other identifiable geographic units, not necessarily within state political boundaries. The mortality data available for each of these breakdowns are of unequal quality. In general, the more developed countries have better death reporting and their mortality data are usually available. These have been gathered into the series of WHO "World Health Statistics Annuals." For cancer, however, the data compiled by Segi and Kurihara in the series *Cancer Mortality for Selected Sites in 24 Countries* have been most useful, although in recent years the WHO publications have contained data for more countries than the 24 Segi and Kurihara regularly report on. Number 6 in this series [3], covering mortality for 1966-67 based on the seventh revision of the *International Classification of Diseases (ICD)*, was published in November 1972. Although Professor Segi retired from Tohoku University in 1971, additional volumes are planned. Number 1 in the series covered the period 1950-57. In 1963 a supplemental volume of graphs showed trends in cancer mortality for the same sites and 24 countries for 1950-59. Number 5 carried limited data on 16 additional countries. Of the 10 (out of 40) countries showing the lowest cancer mortality rates in men, 9 were among the 16 not previously reported. In women, the 10 lowest were all drawn from those 16 additional countries. These data raise questions about the completeness of reporting for these additional countries. However, death rates are not uniformly low among the 16 countries for all sites. The major countries (in terms of population) missing from these tabulations are China (excluding Taiwan), India, U.S.S.R., Indonesia, Brazil, and Argentina.

The major strengths in the Segi compilations lie in their attempts at uniform reporting following the rules and the rubrics of the ICD. The data are clearly presented, population data are given, and both numbers of cases and rates are reported. The major difficulties with such data are their lack of detail. Histologic types are not given, although with the ninth revision of the ICD, histologic-type data will be given by many of the countries. Techniques for handling or reporting secondary and contributing causes of death still need to be worked out. Death certificates, the usual sources for mortality data, are sometimes in error. The data take a long time to compile, thus sharply limiting their use in "early warning" systems, or even in uncovering trends.

Finally, mortality as a measure of the effectiveness of cancer control is a catchall. It will reflect all the problems along the way to death: prevention—or the lack of it, early diagnosis—or the lack of it, improved treatment—or its absence, and delivery of medical care and its quality.

TABLE 2
Data needed for reducing mortality-morbidity from cancer: General

Measurement data	Data sources	Data assets	Data Improvement needed	Other troubles
Mortality data				
Countries	*World Health Statistics Annual*, Individual country reports.	Comparable data using ICD "causes of death."	More detailed area breakdowns.	
	Segi: *Cancer Mortality for Selected Sites in 24 Countries.*		Secondary and contributing causes of death.	
			More trend data.	
States	NCHS-Time Trends: Burbank.	Long-time series.	More timely data.	
			Histologic-type 9th revision data.	Mortality reflects both treatment and incidence.
Communities	NCI-*U.S. Cancer Mortality by County: 1950-69.*	Source of "hot spot" information.	Occupational data.	
Other identifiable units-nonpolitical boundaries.	Special population follow-up.			

Within the United States, the National Center for Health Statistics publishes extensive mortality tables each year that include all causes of death. To develop trends, one usually has to compile the data from the separate annual volumes. Burbank made such a compilation in 1971, tracing the patterns of U.S. cancer mortality, for the period 1950-67 [2]. The data are reported by state, sex, race, age group, and year. Time trends are graphed for 56 different tumor types, nine major "systems," and a total for all malignant neoplasms. Maps, by state, are given for each of these. There are three major deficiencies in the volume: 1) The numbers of cases are not given; 2) the graphs of time trends by age group are hard to read; and 3) the volume is now out of print. The Epidemiology Branch of the National Cancer Institute is planning to update this volume and correct any deficiencies.

An extension of the Burbank volume carrying the data to the county level was published in 1974 covering the period 1950-69 [3]. This volume does not give time trends but it does give numbers of cases. In addition to county data for the over 3,000 counties in the United States, this volume also gives data by state, sex, and race, including both numbers of cases and rates. This volume is not easy to use, because all data are given by county codes, using the Census Bureau identification numbers. A companion volume of maps has now appeared which should make it possible to visually identify the areas of high mortality.

Still missing from these compilations, but possible through existing computer technology, are tabulations and maps reflecting, not political aggregations, but rather, geologic and geographic assemblages. The tapes from which the county cancer mortality data were published can be merged with demographic, industrial, and similar data collected by the Census Bureau, to produce correlations and leads to further epidemiologic research. Crop, geologic, pesticide, chemical use, and similar data, if coded by the Census Bureau county codes, could also be merged.

None of these data identify individuals. Any work on a case-control basis will require working in the communities of interest to identify the cases. All the necessary precautions needed for the protection of the privacy of the individual's medical records can be taken at the local level; in general, the Federal Government is not likely to be involved.

TREATMENT DATA – SURVIVAL STATISTICS

In the application of improved treatment (Table 3), the major problem is identifying individuals to receive it. Many controlled trials are underway and the results, when carefully analyzed, should lead to the identification of which patients might benefit from what treatments. Where a treatment is overwhelmingly beneficial, or nearly useless, specific patient information is also not useful. However, where treatments are moderately useful and where there is controversy over the choice of treatment, it should often be possible to match treatments

TABLE 3

Data needed for reducing mortality-morbidity from cancer: Better treatment

Measurement Data	Data sources	Data assets	Data Improvement needed	Other troubles
Data on what is a "better" treatment.	Mostly medical literature; some *End Results, Report No. 4*, Randomized Controlled trials (RCT's).	Improvements seen in several sites. Evaluation is possible in the field.	Cervix, corpus, stomach, colon: nothing much yet developed.	
Data on who can benefit from specific treatments.	Holland and Glidewell (ALL in children) [5]; Byar, et al. (Cancer of the prostate) [4].	A whole new field opening up—better patient-oriented data.	Only one or two sites have been looked at.	Treatment involves large drain on resources and is usually most effective "early" in the disease.
Data on where better treatments are available. How much does it cost?	Lists of where RCT's are being conducted. TNCS cost data; NCHS cost data.	Most up-to-date people are represented.	Up-to-date people are not necessarily best	

456

to patient characteristics, providing the best treatment, given current knowledge, for each patient. Byar [4] has described such a technique and has applied it to patients with cancer of the prostate. Glidewell and Holland [5] have attempted a similar application for children with acute lymphocytic leukemia. I am not aware of whether their systems are being used.

To measure the overall effectiveness of cancer therapy in a noncontrolled real-world situation, one has to turn to general survival statistics. The National Cancer Institute has published a series of "End Results" volumes, the last one appearing under the title *End Results in Cancer, Report No. 4,* in 1972 as DHEW Publication No. (NIH) 73-272. A supplement, *Recent Trends in Survival of Cancer Patients –1960-71* has been published [6]. The data for these reports are gathered from three central (population-based) registries—California, Connecticut, and Massachusetts—and many individual hospital registries. The Massachusetts registry has since been discontinued. The sample from which these data are drawn is not a representative sample in the statistical sense. It may typify the better medical institutions associated with medical schools. Further, the data relate to white patients only (see Introduction to *End Results in Cancer, Report No. 4,* page 4). Survival for blacks is generally poorer than for whites. A report on black patient survival also has now appeared as part of the DHEW publication series [7]. These publications cover 48 cancer sites but, like all large series compilations, generally lack detailed information on histologic typing, its effect on stage at diagnosis, choice of treatment, and eventual survival.

These publications are similarly organized and give, by site and sex, the number of cases; the proportion diagnosed while localized, with regional or remote metastasis; and the form of initial treatment. Survival is given by age at diagnosis as well as by stage. Both actual and "relative" survivals (relative to survival of persons of the same age at time of diagnosis who are dying of other causes) are given. Time trends in survival and stage of diagnosis are given. In addition, the *Recent Trends* publication gives a listing of major sites in which survival has improved during the period 1950-1969. They include cancers of esophagus, pancreas (one year), larynx, lung, breast, prostate, testis, kidney, bladder, brain, thyroid, melanoma of the skin, reticulum cell sarcoma, lymphosarcoma, Hodgkin's disease, multiple myeloma, acute leukemia, and chronic leukemia. Major sites without recent improvement have been most cancers of the head and neck, stomach, colon, rectum, liver, uterine cervix (one-year survival is now 82 percent), and uterine corpus (one year survival, 87 percent).

Strongly affecting survival following treatment is the stage at which the disease is diagnosed. The *End Results* reports include this information, but not in the detail necessary to evaluate the effectiveness of different treatments in relation to stage of disease, or by age.

TABLE 4

Data needed for reducing mortality-morbidity from cancer: Better diagnosis

Measurement data needed	Data sources	Data assets	Data Improvement	Other troubles
Data on what constitutes "better" diagnosis.	Medical literature—HIP-breast study; Cervix—various studies; Current studies on lung cancer; Generalized tests—fetal antigens (e.g., carcinoembryonic antigen).	Rather good evaluations of current techniques.	Limited sites studied; Equivocal results so far—lung, stomach, colon/rectum, pancreas.	
		"There is something there." The early testing of the tests is encouraging.	Generalized tests are not "diagnostic" yet.	Economic problems in mounting "screening" studies, e.g., breast screening. $30 x 45 x 106 women.
Data to whom early diagnosis efforts should be directed—optimal utilization of resources—genetic or familial relations.	"High-risk" studies; Breast cancer-HIP studies; Lung cancer—many epidemiologic studies; Other cancers—some "genetic" studies, e.g., medullary cancer of the thyroid and pheochromocytoma; Occupation groups; Recovered cancer patients (registries);			Not all diagnostic procedures are without risk, e.g., mammography.

As a cancer control measure, the more extensive delivery of medical care of the quality given at the major cancer centers appears likely to improve survival after diagnosis. At present there is little detailed information about what treatments are actually being given. The Professional Standards Review Organizations (PSRO's) and/or the newly developing cancer centers may in the future generate some data along these lines, but they may often be in the anomalous position of having to make decisions that should be based on these data before the data have become available.

It is even difficult to know, except in some limited way, where the more current treatments are available. And, of course, it is not always true that current treatments are best. A tabulation of the groups conducting clinical therapeutic research with the support of the National Cancer Institute has been prepared [8]. Further tabulations will be made as part of the International Cancer Data Bank (ICDB) program. A registry of groups conducting experimental immunotherapy also has been developed [9]. Further work in developing standards for appropriate treatment will require substantial interdisciplinary cooperation with great care taken that "standards" set at any one time do not become rigid rules for treatment, making improvements difficult to develop.

Finally, while the man in the street often talks about discovering a "cure" for cancer, from the point of view of cancer control and the economical use of resources, a "cure" is probably the item of lowest priority. Prevention, if it can be accomplished by simple public health methods, is much more economical in its use of resources.

IMPROVING DIAGNOSIS

Table 4 deals with problems of diagnosis and the potentials for improvements leading to earlier diagnosis. Diagnosis, like treatment, is an expensive process. Screening is also expensive, even when adequate treatment is available after a "positive" has been discovered. In cancer this is not always true. The National Cancer Institute and the American Cancer Society are conducting a large number of breast cancer screening demonstration projects across the United States. These are modeled on the Health Insurance Plan (HIP) of New York City study [10] which showed about a 30 percent reduction in breast cancer mortality in the screened population. However, with an examination costing about $30, and about 45 million women over age 35 in the United States, the cost for a yearly examination for every woman would be over $1.3 billion—hardly a possible public health measure.

Substantial additional research still is needed in breast cancer screening. The optimal spacing of examinations is not known. The risks of radiation from mammography need to be weighed against the gains of earlier diagnosis. Some of the research should be of an operations research nature. For example, would there be fewer breast cancer deaths if examinations were made half as frequently but twice as many women were examined? The different pressures of ideal care for an individual versus the ideal care for a population of persons need to be evaluated.

The cervical screening techniques (Papanicolaou smears) have been extensively tested. Although questions still remain as to whether the extensive use of these techniques has caused the decline in mortality from cancer of the uterine cervix [11], there is no question that mortality from cancer of the uterine cervix has declined in the United States during the time the screening procedures have been used most extensively. The major problems in using these techniques are similar to those for screening for breast cancer—plus one other. The programs for screening have been least successful in reaching the highest risk populations—the poor, married-early woman who may have had many sexual partners.

All the other screening procedures now in use or under development suffer from one or more of the failings that Cochrane and Holland [12] have pointed out. For screening to be useful they suggested the following criteria:

1) The disease must be an important health problem or, if rare, have radical consequences.

2) After diagnosing the disease, there must be generally applicable ways of dealing with it successfully. It is important *not* to screen for conditions that cannot be treated.

3) The tests must be acceptable (i.e., noninvasive, not painful, not harmful in themselves) to the people undergoing them.

4) The tests must work; i.e., they must have high sensitivity, specificity, and accuracy.

To these, Holland has recently added a criterion that the tests must be economically justifiable in the context of total health expenditures.

To improve the "yield" of generalized diagnostic screening tests, screening high risk populations will be most economical. Holland notes with approval, mandatory screening of dyestuff and rubber workers for cancer of the bladder. Recovered cancer patients are certainly another high-risk group, as are persons receiving organ transplants, who should also be regularly screened thereafter.

REDUCING INCIDENCE

Prevention of cancer has the most appeal and yet is the least visible. A cured patient is known, but a prevented cancer case can never be known. Only in the statistical sense, by measuring changes in incidence, are we able to estimate cases prevented. As Table 5 indicates, there is little continuing incidence data that can be used to evaluate prevention programs in the United States. The major source of data used within the United States has been the Connecticut Cancer Registry [13]. This registry began collecting data in 1935. It attempts

TABLE 5

Data needed for reducing mortality-morbidity from cancer: Reducing incidence

Measurement Data	Data sources	Data assets	Data improvement	Other troubles
High risk groups, i.e. —smokers —industrial workers —urban dwellers —genetics, i.e. fairskinned —early pregnancy —diet, i.e. fats, bulk, etc. —animal data on carcinogenesis	Medical literature (epidemiological studies)—NCHS; TNCS and other data or skin cancer and melanoma. *Cancer in Five Continents* (other measures of incidence).	Smoking data are firm. Some chemcials and other hazards have been identified—urban/rural is real.	No brand data, or relationship to chemical constituents in man. Gross descriptions do not pinpoint things. How to extrapolate animal data to man.	"Personal" prevention is usually not effective. Public health measures are most meaningful. Some preventive measures are hardly possible to take; e.g. early pregnancy to reduce breast cancer risk.
—low economic groups (cervix) —high economic groups (breast)	Social Security continuous work history samples. Census Bureau industrial and manufacturing data. Special populations, e.g. rubber workers.			

461

to report on incidence by all major sites. Its deficiencies are obvious: histologic type data are scarce, reporting is slow, a user of the data often has to develop his own time trend materials from separate reports, and it covers mainly a white population in a largely industrial state in the high cancer northeastern part of the United States.

There are other state or area population-based registries that also suffer from similar defects. New York State has a cancer registry [14] that until last year excluded New York City. The Massachusetts registry is no longer in operation. There is a registry covering several areas in Texas [15], modeled on the Connecticut registry. Utah has a statewide registry, as does New Mexico. The Utah registry was extended to five other Rocky Mountain states, beginning in 1968. These states have small populations, but at least they include American Indians. There is a registry operated by the California State Department of Health that covers mainly the San Francisco Bay area (and thus includes Chinese and Japanese as well as whites and blacks). An incidence registry is developing in the Los Angeles area under the direction of Dr. Brian Henderson of the University of Southern California. Internationally, the compilation *Cancer Incidence in Five Continents,* Volume II, by Doll, Muir, and Waterhouse published by the UICC is the most comprehensive source. It is an excellent work, but suffers from the limitations of each of its national and regional sources.

Finally, within the United States, the National Cancer Institute has conducted three sampling surveys of cancer incidence, timed to coincide with a census year, to give a satisfactory population base for computing rates. The surveys were conducted in 1937, 1947, and 1969-71. The most recent, The Third National Cancer Survey (TNCS), is now in press [16]. This report will contain data on the nine areas studied—Atlanta, Birmingham, Colorado, Dallas-Ft. Worth, Detroit, Iowa, Minneapolis-St. Paul, Pittsburgh, and Oakland-San Francisco. Both numbers of cases and age standardized rates are given for males, females, whites and blacks, with some sex and race groupings, for 46 primary sites. Detailed histologic type data are available upon request but are not included.

The National Cancer Institute plans no additional incidence surveys, but will maintain an area incidence reporting system, known as the Surveillance, Epidemiology and End Result (SEER) Program, covering approximately 10 percent of the United States population. Like the surveys, it is not a random sampling, but includes areas where there is technical ability to carry on the work, plus an appropriate geographic and racial mix. Rural areas are underrepresented, while all nonwhite racial groups are (appropriately) oversampled. As a part of the TNCS, a special survey of skin cancer was conducted in four areas of the United States [17]. It indicated much higher levels of nonmelanotic skin cancer than previous studies, which is consistent with other recent studies showing increases in melanoma mortality. In whites in the United States, melanoma mortality has nearly doubled between 1950 and 1969. However, reported decreases in mortality for "other skin" cancers might indicate problems of classification confounding the apparent increases. There are, however, no plans by the National Cancer Institute to conduct other skin cancer surveys, nor do the SEER groups include superficial skin cancer in their reporting systems. A childhood cancer reporting system, on an international basis, is maintained by Dr. Robert W. Miller, in cooperation with the UICC [18].

There is obviously a need to relate incidence data to possible causal factors. For such things as skin cancer, ultraviolet radiation, genetic makeup, and some aspects of life style (Do people wear hats? Is much skin left uncovered? Is it fashionable to have a "tan" or to have pale skin?) are clearly important. For other environmental exposures, the elements to examine are not nearly so obvious. Some important data sources exist that have not been extensively used. The Social Security Administration maintains a continuous work history sample of workers. The disability certification data they maintain report approximately 10,000 cases of cancer per year. Specific cohorts, of course, can be followed through the use of Social Security numbers. This raises some questions about the possible invasion of privacy and problems of confidentiality that will be discussed later. The Census Bureau, both through its census of manufacturers and its extensive collection of occupational and industrial data, can provide the first layer of information if one wishes to attempt to correlate some gross economic-demographic data with cancer mortality (or incidence in a more limited way) by area. However, because of Census Bureau confidentiality requirements, it may be very hard to pinpoint sources of environmental carcinogens through these correlation techniques.

A few of the American labor unions have begun collecting data on the illnesses and the causes of mortality among their members. Several of the craft unions, particularly those associated with asbestos installation and dry wall construction, have provided the basis for the extensive follow-up study done by the Mt. Sinai group under Dr. Irving Selikoff. The Rubber Workers (AFL-CIO) have a "head tax" that has contributed to a health research fund now being used in at least two Schools of Public Health—North Carolina and Harvard—to investigate job-associated illnesses and causes of death. The Oil, Chemical, and Atomic Workers Union has a system of reporting illness and mortality among its members, but it has not been extensively used as yet.

In all the data systems involving the identification of individual persons, questions of confidentiality have been raised. It is interesting that this area is one in which the far ends of the political spectrum agree with each other and disagree with the middle. There are strong concerns that individual privacy should not be invaded. "Cured cancer" patients have reported job discrimination. Following Watergate and reports of military, FBI, and CIA surveillance of individuals, civil libertarians have become more concerned about undue Federal Government spying on individuals. At least one group in New Orleans—the Committee on Medical Staffs—opposed much of the TNCS, fearing that knowledge of patients' names might cause the Federal Government to interfere with the treatment of cancer patients by intruding into the patient-physician relationship. Of course, it is nearly impossible to avoid duplicate reporting if one does not know who is being reported. Similarly, it is difficult, if not impossible, to do follow-up studies if one does not know whom to follow.

There is no question that there have been circumstances under which confidentiality has been abused by Federal and other agencies. Techniques for minimum-invasive follow-up have been proposed, such as the National Death Index, and recent legislation, followed by administrative rules of the Department of Health, Education, and Welfare, have attempted to both safeguard privacy while not hamstringing appropriate medical research.

OTHER DATA

More Data Available (Resources)

Some data resources that have not been mentioned before, or which have been exploited only little in cancer epidemiology include:

Food consumption surveys of the United States Department of Agriculture
Twin-registry of National Academy of Sciences/National Research Council
International Cancer Data Bank (just beginning to become available)
Medicare and Medicaid data

Some New Data Possibilities (Sources)

Special population registries (transplant registries have been used): patients who have had the new treatments for psoriasis, frequent use of photo-sensitizing drugs plus intense ultraviolet light
"Cured" cancer patients
Persons with special genetic problems
Immune incompetents
Birth defect groups
National health data (if and when a national health scheme is developed in this country)
Special "in-bred" populations; e.g., the triracial isolate in Brandywine, Maryland
Autopsy series; problem: who comes to autopsy?
Low-risk groups: Mormons, Seventh-day Adventists, certain occupational groups

More Problems (Tsouris)

Occupational data as recorded on official documents are subject to "social creep" (the clerk is reported as an executive; the railway fireman is reported as an engineer; the janitor becomes a maintenance supervisor)

Confidentiality (again)

Biases in special populations. Who stays in the union long enough to become eligible for a pension?

Exposure information. How much, as well as what and who?

Time scale—latent periods. Today's cancers reflect conditions 20 to 30 years ago

High costs of prospective studies

Control populations

WHAT MORE CAN BE DONE?

Clearly much can be done in identification and follow-up of possible high-risk populations. There is not much question that all wisdom in cancer epidemiology does not lie in the National Cancer Plan and/or in the National Cancer Institute. Thus, there must be substantial "self-started" research, conducted by universities and similar groups, under their own stimuli, or following stimuli of labor unions and industry. Work is also essential where there are no labor unions, or in areas where one has not traditionally sought cancer hazards; e.g., clergymen, teachers, physicians, laboratory research workers, service trades (such as beauticians). Much of this work needs to be conducted as "microepidemiology"—recognition of unusual events in small groups moving on to larger populations. In many groups "precancers" should be identified and, where more good than harm will result, intervention may be in order. And we must find ways of telling each other what we know, or suspect, quickly.

Finally, it must be recognized that two sets of questions are always being asked in epidemiologic research that are not always compatible. The etiology set asks, "What has really caused this condition?" The control set asks, "What can be done?" Both sets of questions are meaningful, but the first does not always (or even often) have to be answered before the second can be answered. It is *not* necessary to know what individual or complex of chemicals in cigarette smoke causes cancer in order to take action now to reduce the risks of cigarette smoking by reducing cigarette smoking. Although some people may report that they are "dying for a cigarette," there is no case reported in the medical literature of anyone dying of the absence of cigarettes. Clean water and good sewers nearly eliminated cholera in Europe well before anyone knew what in dirty water or in sewage "caused" cholera. Controlling cancer must not get in the way of basic research, and the need for basic research must not delay controlling cancer.

REFERENCES

1. Segi, M., and Kurihara, M. *Cancer Mortality for Selected Sites in 24 Countries, No. 6 (1966-67).* Japan Cancer Soc. Nagoya, Japan, November 1972.

2. Burbank, F. Patterns in cancer mortality in the United States: 1950–67. *Natl. Cancer Inst. Monogr. 33.* May 1971.

3. Mason, T.J. and McKay, F.W. *U.S. Cancer Mortality by County: 1950-69.* DHEW Publication No. (NIH) 74-615, U.S. Govt. Print. Off., Washington, D.C., 1974.

4. Byar, D.P., and Corle, D.K. Selecting optimum treatment in clinical trials using covariate information. *J. Chron. Dis.* In press.

5. Holland, J.F., and Glidewell, O.J. Oncologists reply: survival expectancy in acute lymphocytic leukemia. *N. Engl. J. Med. 287:* 769–777, 1972.

6. Axtell, L.M., and Myers, M.H. *Recent Trends in Survival of Cancer Patients, 1960-71.* DHEW Publication No. (NIH) 75-767, U.S. Govt. Print. Off., Washington, D.C., 1975.

7. Axtell, L.M., Myers, M.H., and Shambaugh, E.M. *Treatment and Survival Patterns for Black and White Cancer Patients Diagnosed 1955 through 1964.* DHEW Publication No. (NIH) 75-712, U.S. Govt. Print. Off., Washington, D.C., 1975.

8. Cancer Cooperative Clinical Trials Program, Division of Cancer Research, Resources, and Centers. NCI: *Membership Roster: Cancer Clinical Cooperative Groups.* U.S. Dept. of Health, Education, and Welfare, NIH, Bethesda, Md. Sept. 1974.

9. Information can be obtained from Dr. Dorothy Windhorst, Natl. Cancer Inst. Bldg. 10, Rm. 4B11, Bethesda, Md. 20014.

10. Shapiro, S., Strax, P., and Venet, L.I. Periodic breast cancer screening. *Arch. Environ. Health 15:*547-553, 1967.

11. Cochrane, A.L. *Effectiveness and Efficiency.* The Nuffield Provincial Hospitals Trust, Cardiff, Wales, 1972.

12. Cochrane, A.L., and Holland, W.W. Validation of screening procedures. *Br. Med. Bull. 27:*3-8, 1971.

13. Christine, B., Flannery, J.T., and Sullivan, P.D. *Cancer in Connecticut, 1966-68.* Connecticut State Dept. of Health, Hartford, 1971.

14. Cancer Control and Registry Report, 1969. *N.Y. State Dept. of Health Monogr.* H. Ingraham, Director.

15. MacDonald, E.J. *The Survey of Cancer in Texas, 1944-66. Present Status and Results: June 30. 1–68.* Univ. of Texas M.D. Anderson Hospital and Tumor Institute, Houston, Tex., 1968.

16. The Third National Cancer Survey: Incidence Data. (Cutler, S. and Young, J., eds.) *Natl. Cancer Inst. Monogr. 41,* 1975.

17. Scotto, J., Kopf, A.W., and Urbach, F. Non-melanoma skin cancer among Caucasians in four areas of the United States. *Cancer 34:*1333-1338, 1974.

18. Miller, R.W. Interim report: UICC international study of childhood cancer. *Int. J. Cancer 10:* 675–677, 1972.

DISCUSSION

Dr. Goldsmith commented that for each group outlined for further study we should clearly keep in mind the population at risk. In occupational studies, for example, the "expected" values for cancer occurrence often are based upon the total white male population. Since a number of white males are not in the working force, expected values are overestimated. Social Security data on the working force would be more appropriate, and incidence data would be preferable to mortality data.

William A. Priester

28

MULTIPLE RISK FACTORS IN ENVIRONMENTAL CANCER

Irving J. Selikoff, M.D., and E. Cuyler Hammond, Sc. D.

Department of Community Medicine
Mount Sinai School of Medicine of the City of New York
and
American Cancer Society
New York, New York

For some environmental human cancer, it is now well established that inter-action of multiple factors may significantly influence the degree of risk. This observation suggests a number of considerations for prevention of these neoplasms; in addition, it may have more immediate relevance to current proposals for surveillance and control.

MULTIPLE INTERACTION OF TWO AGENTS
IN ETIOLOGY OF LUNG CANCER

Evidence of the carcinogenic potential of asbestos was provided over the period 1935-1965 for a number of neoplasms, including bronchogenic car-cinoma [1-3], pleural and peritoneal mesothelioma [4-6], and gastrointestinal cancer [7]. It was found in 1967, however, that for the most important of these neoplasms—lung cancer—the risk did not depend on asbestos alone. Rather, if there were not concordance of *two* agents—cigarette smoking and asbestos—the tumor was uncommon [8].

In 1963, prospective observation was begun of 370 long-exposed asbestos workers in the New York metropolitan area. By April 30, 1967, no death from lung cancer had occurred among the 87 men with no history of cigarette smoking, despite their many years of occupational exposure to asbestos. In

This research is supported by the National Institute of Environmental Health Sciences (ES 00928), National Institute for Occupational Safety and Health (OH 00320), New York City Health Research Council (U 1272) and the American Cancer Society (R 53).

467

contrast, 24 deaths from lung cancer occurred among the 283 men with a history of cigarette smoking [8], although only 2.98 such deaths had been expected, given their smoking habits [9]. We suggested that the combination of the two factors—asbestos greatly increasing the lung cancer risk of cigarette smoking—had a sharp, multiplying effect. It was calculated that an asbestos worker who smokes cigarettes has eight times the risk compared to smokers of the same age who do not work with asbestos, and 92 times the risk of men who neither work with asbestos nor smoke cigarettes [8].

These findings were based on limited observations, especially with regard to nonsmokers. Additional investigations confirm the original conclusions [10].

The survivors of the original group of 370 men were followed to December 31, 1973. Altogether, 191 died from 1963 to 1973. Among the 87 men with no history of cigarette smoking, two deaths (of 41) occurred from lung cancer; both men smoked pipes or cigars. Among the 283 with a history of regular cigarette smoking, there were 150 deaths, 45 of lung cancer (Table 1).

A second, much larger, study was undertaken to investigate whether asbestos exposure without cigarette smoking truly did not increase the risk of lung cancer significantly, especially since such exposure was clearly associated with increased cancer risk at other sites (e.g., peritoneum, gastrointestinal tract) in nonsmokers. On January 1, 1967, we registered the entire membership of the insulation workers' union in the United States and Canada[1] and have observed the group since. When the cohort was enrolled, each man was asked to record his lifetime smoking habits. Of those enrolled, 9,590 indicated that they were either then smoking cigarettes or had previously smoked regularly; 609 had a history of smoking pipes and/or cigars but no cigarettes; and 1,457 had never smoked regularly at all. Smoking habits were not recorded for 6,144 men. Analysis of lung cancer deaths among the 17,800 men to December 31, 1972, showed that increased risk of this neoplasm was limited to asbestos workers who also had a history of cigarette smoking. Among the 9,590 cigarette smokers, there were 179 deaths from lung cancer (of 640 all told); of the 2,066 men with no history of cigarette smoking, only 2 (of 93 total) died of lung cancer (Table 2). Unfortunately, data are not yet available detailing lung cancer risk specifically for amount and nature of smoking, as were available through 1965 [9]. Nevertheless, using the earlier tabulations, these new findings again demonstrate that asbestos workers who do not smoke, or smoke only pipe and/or cigars, have about the same lung cancer risk as men not occupationally exposed to asbestos dust. However, exposure to asbestos dust greatly increases the lung cancer risk among cigarette smokers [11].

There is evidence [12] that uranium mining and cigarette smoking also interact as multiple factors. Moreover, an association between smoking and

[1] International Association of Heat and Frost Insulators and Asbestos Workers, AFL-CIO, CLC.

TABLE 1

Expected and observed deaths among 370 New York–New Jersey asbestos insulation workers, January 1, 1963–December 31, 1973, by smoking habits

| | Number of men | Person-years of observation | Lung cancer | | | Pleural mesothelioma | Peritoneal mesothelioma | Asbestosis |
			Expected[a]	Observed	Ratio			
Cause of death								
History of cigarette smoking	283	2,195	4.07	45	11.06	7	14	19
Current smokers	181	1,443	2.48	32	12.09	6	7	12
Ex-smokers	102	752	1.59	13	8.18	1	7	7
No history of cigarette smoking	87	708	1.58	2	1.27	0	7	6
Never smoked	48	409	0.84	0	—	0	5	3
Pipe/cigar only	39	299	0.74	2	2.70	0	2	3

[a]Expected deaths are based upon age-specific white male death rate data of the U.S. National Office of Vital Statistics from 1963-71, disregarding smokings habits. Rates were extrapolated from 1972-73 from rates for 1967-71.

TABLE 2
Expected and observed deaths of lung cancer
among 17,800 U.S. and Canada asbestos insulation
workers, January 1, 1967-December 31, 1972;
relation to cigarette smoking

	No. of persons	Deaths from lung cancer		
		Expected[a]	Observed	Ratio
Smoking habits not known	6,144	16.76	94	5.6
History of cigarette smoking	9,590	31.60	179	5.7
No history of cigarette smoking	2,066	7.51	2	0.3
Never smoked	1,457	4.40	1	0.2
History of pipe and/or cigar only	609	3.11	1	0.3

[a]Expected deaths based upon age-specific U.S. mortality rates for white males, disregarding smoking. Lung cancer estimates based on U.S. rates for cancer of lung, pleura, bronchus and trachea, categories 162 and 163 of the International Classification of Diseases and Causes of Deaths, 7th Revision.

radiation has been noted [13] among Hiroshima and Nagasaki atomic-bomb survivors, with lung cancer disproportionately increased among the radiation-exposed individuals who also had a history of cigarette smoking.

FACTORS ASSOCIATED WITH MODIFICATIONS OF RISK OF OCCURRENCE OF ENVIRONMENTAL CANCER

Intensity of Exposure

Although it is widely assumed, probably correctly, that intensity of exposure strongly influences human cancer risk [14], there are comparatively few direct data apart from cigarette smoking [9] and radiation [15] that support this belief or establish that a linear relationship exists. In large part, this stems from the absence of exposure data during the period when the implicated agent was unsuspected of carcinogenicity. Nevertheless, broad approximations have some-times been made, either by reconstruction [16] or by comparison [17] of presumed exposures in occupational, neighborhood, and family contact circumstances. Despite this uncertainty, it is probably fair to conclude, at least over a considerable spectrum of exposure intensity, that cancer risk varies directly with exposure. In addition, this relationship may be used in predicting and defining high-risk groups, including the likelihood of a greater incidence of cancer and, often as a corollary, the appearance of some of the tumors after shorter induction periods.

Clearly the influence of exposure intensity is difficult to distinguish from variations in carcinogenic potential of agents or from multiplicative, additive, or less than additive effects of two or more coexisting agents. Further, some carcinogenic agents have nonneoplastic toxic effects that may be competitive with the cancer risk. Two important practical examples can be given. Verification of the cancer risk of occupational exposure to asbestos was delayed in Germany because of the extraordinary death rates from pulmonary fibrosis and cor pulmonale (asbestosis) resulting from the very poor hygiene conditions in East German (Dresden) factories in the difficult period immediately after World War II. More than 25 percent of deaths were caused by asbestosis, and many of the victims died before they reached the cancer-risk decades. Once industrial hygiene precautions were taken, deaths from asbestosis diminished to 3 percent, and workers lived well beyond the 20-year-from-onset point. Lung cancer then became common, with more than 20 percent of asbestos worker deaths so related [18].

We may see a similar competitive risk in the case of vinyl chloride angiosarcoma [19, 20], where nonneoplastic liver disease may be disabling or fatal [21-23] before the induction period of angiosarcoma has run its course.

In instances in which a carcinogenic agent can produce neoplasms at more than one site, again there can be variations in levels of risk for each tumor. Thus, the induction period for asbestos lung cancer seems shorter than for either pleural or peritoneal mesothelioma. We found this true in two cohorts of asbestos workers [24]. In one, shown in Table 3, composed of all 632 union asbestos insulation workers in the New York metropolitan area on January 1, 1943, and considering only deaths more than 20 years from onset of work, we found that in the first decade, 13 (15.7 percent) deaths were due to lung cancer and only 2 (2.4 percent) to mesothelioma. In the second decade, the percentages were much the same for the 170 deaths (29 cases or 17.1 percent vs. 5 cases or 2.9 percent). In the last 11 years, however, the percentages came closer together (191 total deaths, with 47 lung cancers or 29.8 percent, and 28 mesotheliomas or 14.7 percent).

The same tendency was observed in the experiences of another cohort, composed of 933 amosite asbestos factory workers first employed from 1941 to 1945 (Table 4). To 1962, there were 257 deaths with 31 or 12.1 percent from lung cancer; only one death from mesothelioma occurred. From 1963 to

TABLE 3

Expected and observed number of deaths among 623 New York-New Jersey asbestos insulation workers January 1, 1943-December 31, 1973, 20 or more years after onset of first exposure to asbestos.[a]

Cause of death	1943-1952			1953-1962			1963-1973			Total 1943-1973		
	Exp.	Obs.	Ratio	Exp.	Obs.	Ratio	Exp.	Obs.	Ratio	Exp.	Obs.	Ratio
Total deaths—all causes	88.22	83	0.94	111.05	170	1.53	101.38	191	1.88	300.65	444	1.48
Cancer—all sites	13.02	30	2.30	18.75	65	3.47	19.49	103	5.28	51.26	198	3.86
Lung cancer	1.83	13	7.10	4.20	29	6.90	5.65	47	8.32	11.68	89	7.62
Pleural mesothelioma[b]	n.a.	1	—	n.a.	2	—	n.a.	7	—	n.a.	10	—
Peritoneal mesothelioma[b]	n.a.	1	—	n.a.	3	—	n.a.	21	—	n.a.	25	—
Cancer of the stomach	2.13	2	0.94	1.87	10	5.35	1.10	6	5.45	5.10	18	3.53
Cancer of the colon, rectum	2.22	7	3.15	2.74	9	3.28	2.54	6	2.36	7.50	22	2.93
Asbestosis[b]	n.a.	1	—	n.a.	11	—	n.a.	25	—	n.a.	37	—
All other causes	75.20	52	0.69	92.30	94	1.02	81.89	63	0.77	249.39	209	0.84

[a]632 members were on the union's rolls on January 1, 1943. Nine died before reaching 20 years from first employment. All others entered these calculations upon reaching the 20-year from onset of first exposure point. Expected deaths are based on white male age-specific death rate data of the U.S. National Office of Vital Statistics from 1949-71. Rates were extrapolated for 1943-48 from rates for 1949-55, and for 1972-73 from rates for 1967-71.

[b]U.S. death rates not available, but these are rare causes of death in the general population.

TABLE 4

Expected and observed deaths among 933 amosite asbestos factory workers first employed 1941-1945, and observed to December 31, 1973, by time periods.[a]

Cause of death	Before 1953			1953-1962			1963-1973			Total 1941-1973		
	Exp.	Obs.	Ratio	Exp.	Obs.	Ratio	Exp.	Obs.	Ratio	Exp.	Obs.	Ratio
Total deaths—all causes	49.22	95	1.20	111.79	162	1.45	128.45	267	2.08	319.46	524	1.64
Cancer—all sites	11.90	15	1.35	19.36	50	2.58	24.13	98	4.06	54.58	163	2.99
Lung cancer	1.74	3	1.72	4.51	28	6.21	7.10	53	7.46	13.35	84	6.29
Pleural mesothelioma[b]	n.a.	1	–	n.a.	0	–	n.a.	4	–	n.a.	5	–
Peritoneal mesothelioma[b]	n.a.	0	–	n.a.	0	–	n.a.	6	–	n.a.	6	–
Cancer of the stomach	1.69	3	7.78	1.86	4	2.15	1.34	3	2.24	4.89	10	2.04
Cancer of the colon, rectum	1.82	2	1.10	2.74	5	1.82	3.09	9	2.91	7.65	16	2.09
All other cancer	5.25	6	1.14	9.11	13	1.12	11.53	23	1.99	25.89	42	1.62
Asbestosis[b]	n.a.	3	–	n.a.	8	–	n.a.	16	–	n.a.	27	–
All other causes	68.13	77	1.13	92.43	104	1.13	104.32	153	1.47	264.88	334	1.26

[a]Expected deaths are based upon white male age-specific death rate data of the U.S. National Office of Vital Statistics from 1949-71. Rates were extrapolated for 1941-48 from rates for 1949-55, and for 1972-73 from rates for 1967-71. 933 men were employed. In 5 cases, ages were not known and these men have been excluded from these calculations. 881 men were traced to death or to December 31, 1973. 47 men were partially traced and remain in the calculations until lost to observation.

[b]U.S. death rates not available, but these are rare causes of death in the general population.

1973 53 of 267 deaths were due to lung cancer (19.9 percent), but now 10
deaths were due to mesothelioma.

Duration from Onset of Exposure

By and large, cancers associated with exposure to identified environmental
agents do not become clinically evident for 20 or more years after first exposure;
often the elapsed period is 30, 40 or more years. There are exceptions, of course,
as with the broadened induction span seen with more intense exposure and consequent larger numbers of tumors [25], or perhaps with exposure at very early
ages. Despite such variations, the 20-plus year "rule" holds rather well, for
exposures as diverse as radiation [13], aniline bladder tumors [25], nickel
refining [26], or asbestos exposure [27]. Considerable data are now available
with regard to the latter. Thus, among the amosite asbestos factory workers,
cancer increased considerably after the first 20 years (Table 4). In the asbestos
insulation worker study (United States and Canada) mentioned above [27],
both total cancer and lung cancer increases were limited until after the 20-year
point (Tables 5 and 6); this limitation applied even when smoking was taken
into account (Table 7).

TABLE 5

Expected and observed deaths among 17,800 asbestos insulation workers
in the United States and Canada, January 1, 1967-December 31, 1972

| | Duration from onset of exposure | | | |
| | Less than 20 years | | More than 20 years | |
Cause of death	Expected[a]	Observed	Expected[a]	Observed
Total deaths—all causes	203.90	249	756.12	1,109
Cancer all sites	30.42	64	145.13	511
Lung cancer	8.40	28	47.47	247
Pleural mesothelioma[b]	n.a.	2	n.a.	27
Peritoneal mesothelioma[b]	n.a.	3	n.a.	60
Gastrointestinal cancer	4.64	5	33.15	56
All other cancer	17.38	26	64.51	121
Asbestosis[b]	n.a.	7	n.a.	94
All other causes	173.48	178	610.99	504
Number of persons	12,681		5,119	

[a]Expected rates are based on age-specific white male death rate data of the U.S. National
Office of Vital Statistics. Rates for 1972 were extrapolated from rates for 1967-71.
[b]U.S. rates are not available, but these are rare causes of death in the general population.

TABLE 6

Deaths from lung cancer among 17,800 asbestos
insulation workers in the U.S. and Canada,
January 1, 1967-December 31, 1972; relation
to elapsed period from onset of work exposure

	Lung cancer		
Years from onset	Expected deaths [a]	Observed deaths	Ratio
< 10	0.56	0	—
10-14	1.97	5	2.5
15-19	5.87	23	3.9
20-24	9.55	34	3.6
25-29	10.70	56	5.2
30-34	8.20	60	7.3
35-39	4.68	29	6.2
40-44	4.84	27	5.6
45-49	4.51	19	4.2
50+	4.97	22	4.4
Total	55.87	275	4.9 (average)

[a]Expected deaths are based upon age-specific white male death rate data of the U.S. National Office of Vital Statistics. Rates for 1972 were extrapolated from data for 1967-71.

It is likely that "duration from onset of exposure" is, in some instances at least, a composite effect and includes both the influence of total exposure and that of the passage of time from first exposure (or, perhaps more accurately, from the time sufficient exposure has occurred to result in increased cancer risk). Total duration of exposure has clear influence, as observed with uranium mining [28], aniline bladder cancer [25] and asbestos exposure. With regard to the latter, interesting data have recently become available. Among the amosite asbestos factory workers first employed in the period 1941 to 1945 (all in the same factory, during the same year, with the same exposure), approximately one-third worked for 3 months or less, one-third for 3 to 11 months, and one-third for a year or more. The group was traced through 1973. Both cancer of all sites and lung cancer showed their greatest increase in the last group (Table 8).

Our knowledge is still fragmentary concerning the mechanisms of cancer induction which influence these effects. We have inadequate information, for example, about tissue residence of various carcinogenic agents. Tissue burden

TABLE 7

Expected and observed deaths from lung cancer among 17,800 asbestos insulation workers in the U.S. and Canada, January 1, 1967-December 31, 1972, by duration from onset of work and cigarette smoking.

Years from onset of asbestos work

Smoking history	< 20 years			20 or more years			Total		
	Expected[a]	Observed	Ratio	Expected[a]	Observed	Ratio	Expected[a]	Observed	Ratio
Smoked cigarettes	4.95	13	2.6	26.65	166	6.2	31.60	179	5.7
Never smoked cigarettes	0.87	0	—	6.64	2	0.3	7.51	2	0.3
Unknown	2.59	15	5.8	14.17	79	5.6	16.76	94	5.6
Total	8.41	28	3.4 (avg.)	47.46	247	5.2 (avg.)	55.87	275	4.9 (avg.)

[a]Expected deaths based on age-specific U.S. mortality rates for white males, disregarding smoking. Lung cancer estimates based upon U.S. rates for cancer of lung, pleura, bronchus and trachea, categories 162 and 163 of the International Classification of Diseases and Causes of Death, Seventh Revision, World Health Organization, Geneva, 1957. Included 609 men who smoked pipes or cigars.

TABLE 8

Expected and observed deaths subsequent to first year after onset
of employment among 870 amosite asbestos factory workers
first employed in 1941-45 and observed to December 31, 1973.
Distribution of duration of employment [a]

Cause of death	3 months work or less			3-11 months work			1-year + work		
	Expected	Observed	Ratio	Expected	Observed	Ratio	Expected	Observed	Ratio
Total deaths, all causes	99.75	112	1.12	94.34	170	1.80	110.55	216	1.95
Cancer—all sites	16.92	28	1.65	16.29	46	2.82	18.99	81	4.27
Lung cancer	4.13	16	3.87	4.00	16	4.00	4.64	49	10.56
Pleural mesothelioma [b]	n.a.	0	–	n.a.	2	–	n.a.	2	–
Peritoneal mesothelioma [b]	n.a.	0	–	n.a.	1	–	n.a.	4	–
Cancer of stomach	1.46	1	0.68	1.47	3	2.04	1.73	5	2.89
Cancer of colon, rectum	2.38	4	1.68	2.27	7	3.08	2.67	5	1.87
Asbestosis [b]	n.a.	1	–	n.a.	2	–	n.a.	23	–
All other causes	82.83	83	1.00	78.05	122	1.56	91.56	112	1.22
Number of workers		249			294			327	
Person-years of observation		5,747			6,305			7,061	

[a]This table excluded 63 men. Ten died during first year of employment, 34 could not be traced after the first year, and 19 had prior occupational exposure to asbestos. Of the 870 men, 18 were partially traced and 16 had subsequent asbestos work. These remained in the calculations until lost to observation or until onset of subsequent asbestos work. Expected deaths are based on white male age-specific death rate data of the U.S. National Office of Vital Statistics, 1949-71. Rates were extrapolated for 1941-48 from rates for 1949-55 and for 1972-73 from rates for 1967-71.

[b]U.S. death rates not available, but these are rare causes of death in the general population.

of asbestos has been studied [29], and substances such as polychlorinated biphenyls, aldrin, dieldrin, and beryllium are found in tissues long after known exposure has ceased, but little can be concluded at present concerning the implications of such observations.

Specificity of Carcinogenic Effect

It is recognized, of course, that agents that classically produce neoplasms at one site may be potentially carcinogenic for other tissues as well. Cigarette smoking, for example, increases the risk of cancer of the larynx, buccal cavity, pharynx, esophagus, and bladder, as well as the lung. Bis(chloromethyl)ether affects the upper respiratory tract as well as the lung, and radiation can produce a number of neoplasms, sometimes varying with age at time of exposure, as with leukemia [30] and breast cancer [31]. Asbestos, as noted, is associated with a variety of tumors. Nevertheless, the various agents have predilections for certain sites. Mesothelioma brings asbestos to mind; nasal neoplasms, nickel carbonyl; and hemangiosarcoma, vinyl chloride. Skin cancer on the nose, hands, or ear lobes might suggest occupational exposure to coal tar. Indeed, such "signal" neoplasms have a long history, dating back to Percivall Pott's chimney sweeps' scrotal cancer [32], the precursor to more recent cancers of the same site with shale oil and mineral machine oils [33, 34]. Some investigators have even proposed that, in the case of asbestos, the specificity for mesothelioma is greater for some kinds of asbestos than for others [35, 36], although it has not been confirmed in extensive animal studies [37].

As expected, the converse is not true. Lung cancer may be associated with chromates [38], nickel, asbestos, hematite mining, bis(chloromethyl)ether [39], cigarette smoking, and radiation. Hemangiosarcoma of the liver may be associated with arsenic and thorotrast as well as vinyl chloride. Even mesothelioma, in at least 15 percent of instances, has no discernible asbestos etiology [40, 41].

Agent specificity may even extend to multiple factor interaction. Hammond and colleagues [11] recently observed in asbestos workers a suggestive difference between the effects of cigarette smoking and cigar and pipe smoking. The latter indicated an influence on the risk of buccal, pharyngeal, and laryngeal cancer, but not for cancer of the lung or esophagus (Table 9).

IMPLICATIONS FOR CONTROL OF CANCER AMONG HIGH-RISK GROUPS

Identification of Groups at Anticipated High Risk of Cancer

It is now possible to predict with some assurance the approximate incidence of cancers of several sites in a number of identified groups, and to focus sharply

TABLE 9

Ratio of observed to expected deaths among 17,800 asbestos insulation workers in the U.S. and Canada, January 1, 1967-December 31, 1972 [a]

Cause of death	History of Cigarette Smoking			History of Pipe and Cigar Smoking			Never Smoked		
	Expected[b]	Observed	Ratio	Expected	Observed	Ratio	Expected	Observed	Ratio
Lung cancer	31.60	179	5.7	3.11	1	0.3	4.40	1	0.2
Cancer of the esophagus	2.19	8	3.7	0.22	0	—	0.31	0	—
Cancer of the larynx	1.51	3	2.0	0.15	1	6.7	0.21	0	—
Cancer of the buccal cavity, pharynx	3.27	7	2.1	0.31	2	6.5	0.45	0	—
	6.97	18	2.6	0.68	3	4.4	0.97	0	—
Deaths all causes	521.15	765	1.5	54.27	54	1.0	65.82	24	0.4
Number of workers	9,590			609			1,457		
Person-years of observation	55,526			3,525			8,622		

[a] Includes 6,144 workers for whom smoking habits were not known, with 35,191 person-years of observation.

[b] Expected deaths based upon age-specific U.S. mortality rates for white males, disregarding smoking. Lung cancer estimates based on U.S. rates for cancer of lung, pleura, bronchus and trachea, categories 162 and 163 of the International Classification of Diseases and Causes of Deaths, Seventh Revision, World Health Organization, Geneva, 1957.

on subgroups likely to have particularly high incidence. Thus, it may be insufficient to say that asbestos workers have a high risk of lung cancer. One estimate has it that whereas now some 200,000 workers are in the asbestos trades, another 800,000 who previously worked in these trades may have gone to other work or retired [42]. It is possible, however, to define which asbestos workers are especially liable to have lung cancer: those more than 20 years from onset, with a history of cigarette smoking, especially if there has been longer work history (Tables 1, 2, 7, and 8). Using such discriminatory criteria, we estimate that 10 to 20 percent of some groups will be of immediate concern. Similar considerations obtain with other agents and other neoplasms. Thus, vinyl chloride hemangiosarcoma of the liver also appears to have something like a 20-year induction period [43], and promises to be more common with more intense exposure (as with polymerization exposure); subgroups of individuals exposed to vinyl chloride who are at higher risk can be identified. Similar approaches may be utilized for uranium miners, workers exposed to benzidine, 2-naphthylamine, or a variety of other occupational carcinogens.

Evaluation of multiple risk factors may be useful in other than occupational groups as with transplacental effects that are either known to occur, as with diethylstilbestrol (DES) [44], or are suspected [19]. Cancer risks related to occupational agents also have been observed in other populations, as among family contacts ("conjugal disease") or among residents of neighborhoods around specific industrial plants [45]. The exposure of individuals in such subgroups is less intense than occupational exposure, but the other multiple-risk factors apply (duration from onset, smoking). In some instances, it may be possible to utilize "exposure markers," such as pleural plaques denoting prior asbestos exposure [46], to delimit further subgroups at higher risk.

Surveillance

As high-risk groups are defined by discriminatory application of multiple risk factors, surveillance may become possible at reasonable cost in personnel and facilities for several purposes. First, of course, is early diagnosis and improved prospects of cure and management. Examples would include chest X-ray and cytological studies of bronchial secretions for lung cancer, urine cytology for bladder cancer, liver studies including scans in vinyl chloride workers, hematological observation for workers exposed to benzene, vaginal examinations for female offspring of women receiving DES during pregnancy, skin examinations where appropriate, and even simple hemoglobin determinations for the modest increase in gastrointestinal cancer seen in asbestos workers.

Such surveillance would include the opportunity for possible reversal of at least some of the multiple risk factors. It may be that cessation of cigarette smoking will ameliorate the lung cancer risk of asbestos workers, uranium miners, or atomic-bomb survivors. Alcohol may add to the liver stress of vinyl chloride [47]; guidance during surveillance may be valuable.

Prospective surveillance of high-risk groups may also have important theoretical benefits as well. The individuals in the groups under observation stand to gain by concomitant studies designed to investigate metabolic, serological and cytological changes which may be present long before the earliest evidence of clinical disease. For example, what chemical changes are in the urine of workers exposed to benzidine who develop bladder cancer as compared with those who do not [48]? Limited observations so far have indicated that one in eight deaths among vinyl chloride polymerization workers was due to angiosarcoma [22]. What biochemical peculiarities distinguish those who develop the neoplasm from those who do not? High-risk groups will also provide a practical opportunity for testing the likely utility of large-scale surveillance techniques before their general introduction, and perhaps even for trials of prophylactic therapeutic agents, as they become available.

The effectiveness of prospective surveillance in terms of reversal or diminution of risk or of earlier diagnosis and treatment is not known—few experiences are at hand. The identification of multiple-risk factors and consideration of their utilization only make feasible exploration of such effectiveness. Nevertheless, the possibility that they may result in significant improvement in cancer control suggests that appropriate programs are now warranted.

REFERENCES

1. Lynch, K.M., and Smith, W.A. Pulmonary asbestosis: Carcinoma of lung in asbesto-silicosis. *Am. J. Cancer 24:*56–64, 1935.

2. Doll, R. Mortality from lung cancer in asbestos workers *Br. J. Ind. Med. 12:*81–86, 1955.

3. Selikoff, I.J., Churg, J., and Hammond, E.C. Asbestos exposure and neoplasia. *J.A.M.A. 188:*22–26, 1964.

4. Wagner, J.C., Sleggs, C.A., and Marchand, P. Diffuse pleural mesothelioma and asbestos exposure in North Western Cape Province. *Br. J. Ind. Med. 17:*260–271, 1960.

5. Enticknap, J.B., and Smither, W.J. Peritoneal tumours in asbestosis. *Br. J. Ind. Med. 21:*20–30, 1964.

6. Selikoff, I.J., Churg, J., and Hammond, E.C. Relation between exposure to asbestos and mesothelioma. *N. Engl. J. Med. 272:*560–565, 1965.

7. Hammond, E.C., Selikoff, I.J., and Churg, J. Neoplasia among insulation workers in the United States with special reference to intra-abdominal neoplasia. *Ann. N.Y. Acad. Sci. 132:*519–525, 1965.

8. Selikoff, I.J., Hammond, E.C., and Churg, J. Asbestos exposure, smoking and neoplasia. *J.A.M.A. 204:*106–112, 1968.

9. Hammond, E.C. Smoking in relation to the death rates of 1,000,000 men and women. *In* Epidemiological Study of Cancer and Other Chronic Diseases. *Natl. Cancer Inst. Monogr. 19:*127–204, 1966.

10. Hammond, E.C., and Selikoff, I.J. Unpublished data.

11. Hammond, E.C., Selikoff, I.J., and Seidman, H. Multiple interaction effects of cigarette smoking: Extrapulmonary cancer. *In Proceedings of the 11th International Cancer Congress.* Excerpta Medica Int. Congr. Ser. In Press, 1975.

12. Lundin, F.E., Jr., Lloyd, J.W., Smith, E.M., et al. Mortality of uranium miners in relation to radiation exposure, hard-rock mining and cigarette smoking–1950 through Sept. 1967. *Health Phys. 16:*571–578, 1969.

13. Wanebo, C.K., Johnson, K.G., Sato, K., et al. Lung cancer following atomic radiation. *Am. Rev. Respir. Dis. 98:*778–787, 1968.

14. Ad Hoc Committee on the Evaluation of Low Levels of Environmental Chemical Carcinogens, *Evaluation of Environmental Carcinogens.* Report to the Surgeon General, USPHS, Bethesda, Md., April 22, 1970.

15. Harada, T., and Ishida, M. Neoplasms among A-bomb survivors in Hiroshima: First report of the Research Committee on Tumor Statistics, Hiroshima City Medical Association, Hiroshima, Japan. *J. Natl. Cancer Inst. 25:*1253, 1960.

16. Archer, V.E., and Lundin, F.E. Radiogenic lung cancer in man; exposure-effect relationship. *Environ. Res. 1:*370–383, 1967.

17. Committee on Biologic Effects of Atmospheric Pollutants. *Airborne Asbestos.* National Research Council, National Academy of Sciences, Washington, D.C., 1971.

18. Jacob, G., and Anspach, M. Pulmonary neoplasia among Dresden asbestos workers. *Ann. N.Y. Acad. Sci. 132:*536–548, 1965.

19. Maltoni, C., and Lefemine, G. Carcinogenicity bioassays of vinyl chloride. I. Research plan and early results. *Environ. Res. 7:*381–405, 1974.

20. Creech, J.L., and Johnson, M.N. Angiosarcoma of the liver in the manufacture of polyvinyl chloride. *J. Occup. Med. 16:*150–151, 1974.

21. Marsteller, H.J., Lelbach, W.K., Müller, R., et al. Unusual splenomegalic liver disease as evidenced by peritoneoscopy and guided liver biopsy among polyvinyl chloride production workers. *Ann. N.Y. Acad. Sci.* 1975. In press.

22. Nicholson, W.J., Seidman, H., Hammond, E.C., et al. Mortality experience of a cohort of vinyl chloride–polyvinyl chloride workers. *Ann. N.Y. Acad. Sci.* 1975. In press.

23. Thomas, L.B., Popper, H., Berk, P.E., et al. Vinyl chloride induced liver disease; from idiopathic portal hypertension (Banti's syndrome) to angiosarcomas. *N. Engl. J. Med. 292:*17-22. Jan. 1975.

24. Selikoff, I.J., Hammond, E.C., and Churg, J. Unpublished data.

25. Williams, M.H.C. Occupational tumors of the bladder. *In* Raven, R.W., ed. *Cancer,* vol. 3. Butterworth, London, 1958, pp. 333–380.

26. Pedersen, E., Hogetveit, A., and Andersen, A. Cancer of respiratory organs among workers at a nickel refinery in Norway. *Int. J. Cancer 12:*32–41, 1973.

27. Selikoff, I.J., Bader, R. A., Bader, M.E., et al. Editorial: Asbestosis and neoplasia. *Am. J. Med. 42:*487–496, 1967.

28. Wagoner, J.K., Archer, V.E., Lundin, F.E., et al. Radiation as the cause of lung cancer among uranium miners. *N. Engl. J. Med. 273:*181-188, 1965.

29. Langer, A.M., Ashley, R., Baden, V., et al. Identification of asbestos in human tissues. *J. Occup. Med. 15:*287–295, 1973.

30. Bizzozero, O.J., Johnson, K.G., and Ciocco, A. Radiation-related leukemia in Hiroshima and Nagasaki, 1946-1964: I. Distribution incidence and appearance time. *N. Engl. J. Med. 274:*1095-1101, 1966.

31. Wanebo, C.K., and Johnson, K.G. *Breast Cancer after Exposure to the Atomic Bombings of Hiroshima and Nagasaki.* Atomic Bomb Casualty Commission Technical Report 13–67.

32. Pott, P. Cancer of the scrotum. *In Chirurgical Observations.* Hawes, Clark and Collings, London, 1775, pp. 63-68.

33. Henry, S.A. *Cancer of the Scrotum in Relation to Occupation.* Oxford University Press, London, 1946.

34. Lee, W.R., Alderson, M.R., and Downes, J.E. Scrotal cancer in the northwest of England, 1962-68. *Br. J. Ind. Med. 29:*188–195, 1972.

35. McDonald, J.C., McDonald, A., Gibbs, G.W., et al. Mortality in the chrysotile asbestos mines and mills of Quebec. *Arch. Environ. Health 22:*677–686, 1971.

36. Wagner, J.C. Asbestos cancer. *J. Natl. Cancer Inst. 46:*v-ix, 1971.

37. Wagner, J.C., Berry, G., Skidmore, J.W., et al. The effects of the inhalation of asbestos in rats. *Br. J. Cancer 29:*252–269, 1974.

38. *Health of Workers in Chromate Industry.* PHS Publ. #192. Federal Security Agency, PHS, Washington, D.C., 1953.

39. Figueroa, W.G., Raskowski, R., and Weiss, W. Lung cancer in chloromethyl methyl ether workers. *N. Engl. J. Med. 288:*1096–1097, 1973.

40. Webster, I. Asbestos and malignancy. *S. Afr. Med. J. 47:*165–171, 1973.

41. Greenberg, M., and Lloyd Davies, T.A. Mesothelioma register 1967-68. *Br. J. Ind. Med. 31:*91–104, 1974.

42. National Institute for Occupational Safety and Health estimate, 1972.

43. Current intelligence: Angiosarcoma of the liver in vinyl chloride/polyvinyl chloride workers. *J. Occup. Med. 16:*809, 1974.

44. Herbst, A.L., Ulfelder, H., and Poskanzer, D.C. Adenocarcinoma of the vagina; association of maternal stilbestrol therapy with tumor appearance in young women. *N. Engl. J. Med. 284:*878–881, 1971.

45. Newhouse, M.L., and Thompson, H. Mesothelioma of pleura and peritoneum following exposure to asbestos in the London area. *Br. J. Ind. Med. 22:*261-269, 1965.

46. Kiviluoto, R. Pleural calcification as a roentgenologic sign of non-occupational endemic anthophyllite-asbestosis. *Acta Radio. 194:*1–67, 1960.

47. Lilis, R., Anderson, H., Nicholson, W.J., et al. Prevalence of disease among vinyl chloride and polyvinyl chloride workers. *Ann. N.Y. Acad. Sci.* In press.

48. Czygan, P., Grein, H., Garro, A.J., et al. Cytochrome P-450 content and the ability of liver microsomes from patients undergoing abdominal surgery to alter the mutagenicity of a primary and a secondary carcinogen. *J. Natl. Cancer Inst. 51:*1761–1764, 1973.

DISCUSSION

Dr. Higginson elaborated on the inappropriateness of average dose as a measure of carcinogenic effect. In Africa, for example, consumption of aflatoxin is either "spiking" or constant. Thus, residents of Kenya have an apparently steady intake of aflatoxin, while cultural differences in Swaziland produce sharp fluctuations in aflatoxin intake.

Dr. Rawson asked if patients with asbestosis are at poor risk for treatment because of impaired lung function. **Dr. Selikoff** responded that the tumors in asbestos workers tend to be peripheral, in the lower lobe, and sometimes operable. With mesothelioma, however, surgical intervention is often impossible and rarely attempted.

Dr. Nelson stressed the importance of studying the variables of intensity, duration of exposure, and postexposure intervals in evaluating groups at highest risk. Animal studies have revealed the dosage patterns most efficient in producing cancer, and these tend to fit the available human data.

W. Gary Flamm

29

INTERDISCIPLINARY AND EXPERIMENTAL APPROACHES: METABOLIC EPIDEMIOLOGY

Ernst L. Wynder, M.D., Dietrich Hoffmann, Ph. D., Po Chan, Ph. D., and
Bandaru Reddy, D.V.M., Ph. D.

American Health Foundation
New York, New York

Epidemiologic observations have been the principal means of obtaining new information on environmental carcinogens. Following an epidemiological lead, further study usually depends on 1) laboratory techniques involving chemical analyses of suspected carcinogens and bioassay experiments to determine carcinogenicity, and 2) metabolic epidemiological techniques that help to unravel the pathogenesis of a given cancer and the role of specific tumorigenic components.

This multidisciplinary approach is vital to the development of sound information on risk factors in many cancers, including marital, hormonal, and dietary factors in breast cancer, and marital, hygienic, and viral factors in cancer of the cervix. In this paper we will illustrate the application of the multidisciplinary approach to cancers of the upper alimentary and upper respiratory tracts and to cancer of the colon.

CANCERS OF THE UPPER ALIMENTARY AND UPPER RESPIRATORY TRACTS

The epidemiological patterns of cancer of the oral cavity, larynx (both glottic and supraglottic types), and esophagus are uniform throughout the Western world. Cigarettes, pipe tobacco, cigars, and chewing tobacco represent the principal stimulus for development of cancer at these sites. This stimulus is magnified,

485

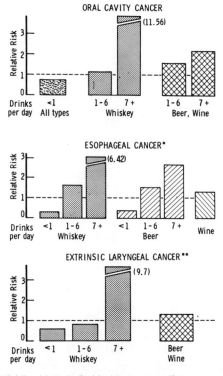

* Relative risk standardized for tobacco consumption.
** Relative risk compared with those smoking 16 – 34 cigarettes/day.

FIGURE 1.   Relative risks of developing cancers of the oral cavity, esophagus, and larynx by alcohol consumption.

as shown in Figure 1, by the heavy consumption of alcohol [1]. Our studies have indicated that, while tobacco use alone can lead to cancer in those regions, heavy intake of alcohol by itself does not lead to such carcinogenic activity.

A pertinent example is our most recent study on cancer of the larynx in which we found, among 259 male patients, only 5 (1.9 percent) who did not use tobacco, whereas 86 (38.2 percent) never or only occasionally used alcohol. In contrast, of 518 male controls, 105 (20.3 percent) did not use tobacco and 237 (57 percent) never or only occasionally used alcohol. On the other hand, heavy drinking, especially in the form of hard liquor, significantly increased the risk of cancer of the larynx among smokers (Figure 2). We found similar results for cancer of the mouth and esophagus [1]. Among ex-smokers, the risk for cancers of the upper alimentary and upper respiratory tracts declines slowly after an individual has smoked heavily for more than 25 years. In fact, for about 5 years, the rate remains relatively unchanged compared to the rate for those

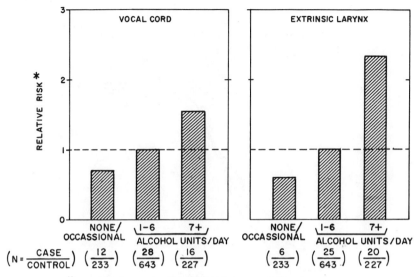

FIGURE 2. Relative risk of laryngeal cancer by current amount of alcohol
consumed by male smokers of 21+ cigarettes/day—ages 40-79;
New York, Los Angeles, and Houston, 1970-73.

who continue to smoke. Interestingly, this reduction in risk appears slower than
we have noted for lung cancer. Thus, if one were to test the effect of a less
harmful tobacco product in an individual who has smoked heavily for 25 years,
such a product would not show a significant reduction in risk for at least 10
years of "testing."

Laboratory studies are not required before recommendations are made regarding primary preventive measures, but the identification of specific carcinogenic components and their precursors in tobacco and tobacco smoke indicates
a means of producing a less carcinogenic tobacco product. A variety of tumor
initiators, promoters, and accelerators in tobacco smoke have been identified
and account for much of the biological activity of the particulate matter of
tobacco smoke when tested on mouse skin (Figure 3) [2]. Our studies showed
that the tumorigenic components tend to be higher in smoke particulates obtained from the lamina portion of the tobacco leaf than from tobacco stems
and that they also tend to be reduced in tar obtained from reconstituted tobaccos [3]. Dontenwill et al. [4] showed a good correlation of mouse skin data
to those of the larynx of hamsters exposed to smoke from different types of
cigarettes. Detailed studies [3] have been completed toward identifying the
tumorigenic substances and their precursors in tobacco with the aim of reducing

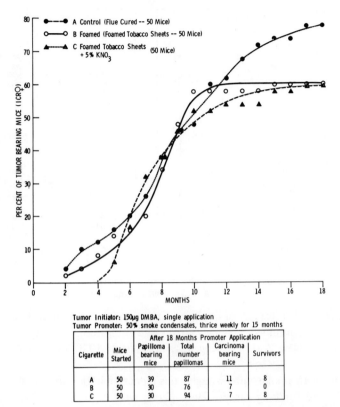

Tumor Initiator: 150µg DMBA, single application
Tumor Promoter: 50% smoke condensates, thrice weekly for 15 months

Cigarette	Mice Started	After 18 Months Promoter Application			Survivors
		Papilloma bearing mice	Total number papillomas	Carcinoma bearing mice	
A	50	39	87	11	8
B	50	30	76	7	0
C	50	30	94	7	8

FIGURE 3. Tumor-promoting activity of cigarette smoke condensates.

them. Among these components in smoke are polynuclear aromatic hydrocarbons (tumor initiators), phenol and substituted phenols (tumor promoters), and chlorostilbenes and catechols (tumor accelerators) [2, 3, 5]. These substances are in lower concentration in the smoke of today's cigarette, in line with lower carcinogenic activity of smoke condensates, compared to those 25 years ago.

Recently, nitrosonornicotine (NNN) was identified in tobacco, particularly in chewing tobacco [6]. Related investigations [7] showed that this component produces esophageal cancer in rats, as do certain related nitrosamines. NNN in chewing tobacco was found in high concentrations for an N-nitrosamine, up to 90 µg per gram of tobacco [8]. Furthermore, the carcinogenic NNN is found during the chewing of tobacco [9]. It remains to be shown whether this nitrosamine contributes to the higher risks of mouth and esophageal cancer in tobacco chewers. A key question, therefore, is whether the unusual organ specificity of certain nitrosamines for laboratory animals applies also to man. The type of study in which a specific agent in tobacco or tobacco smoke can be identified as an animal carcinogen can only be done in the laboratory. The multidisciplinary approach to tobacco carcinogenesis thus involves chemists and biologists. However, eventually the effectiveness of the reduction must be monitored through epidemiological studies of the type we are conducting in eight different cities in the United States. We have demonstrated for cancers of the lung (Figure 4), oral cavity (Figure 5), and larynx (Figure 6) that the long-term use of filter cigarettes, which are generally lower in tar content than nonfilter cigarettes, has already led to a decline in the risk of these tobacco-related forms of cancer. As yet, we do not know the risk for individuals who began their smoking careers with these new cigarettes. Today's cigarettes are not only lower in tar yield but, as we have shown, also are lower in carcinogenicity (as measured on mouse skin) compared to tar from cigarettes used 25 years ago. Thus, "managerial" measures made possible by the interaction of various scientific disciplines have led to a reduction of cancer risk in cigarette smokers.

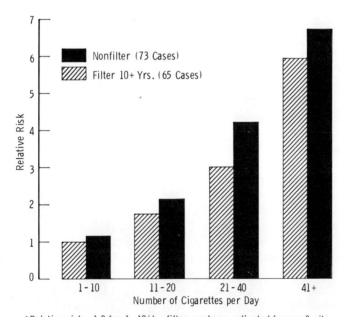

*Relative risk = 1.0 for 1 - 10/day filter smokers, adjusted for age & city

FIGURE 4. Relative risk* of lung cancer (Kreyberg I) in men
for current filter and nonfilter cigarette smokers;
New York, Los Angeles, and Houston, 1970-73.

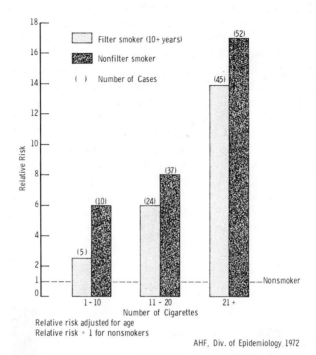

AHF, Div. of Epidemiology. 1972

FIGURE 5. Relative risk of oral cancer by type and number of cigarettes smoked per day; 304 male oral cancer patients and 2,300 controls; New York, Los Angeles, and Houston (1970-72).

Similar approaches are required to deal with the alcohol factor. How does heavy alcohol intake increase the risk of cancers arising in the upper alimentary and upper respiratory tracts of smokers, and how can this risk be reduced short of giving up drinking? Alcohol elevates the activities of an inducible microsomal oxidizing enzyme system [10]. This enzyme system also metabolizes drugs, steroids, and carcinogenic polycyclic hydrocarbons [11]. Recently, it was demonstrated that the activation of polycyclic carcinogens via the epoxide pathway involves the microsomal enzyme system [12]. Lieber [13] observed that the production of acetaldehyde in rats given alcohol induced impairment of mitochondria. Animal experiments by Kuratsune [14] in Japan showed an increased tumor yield in the esophagus induced with benzo[a]pyrene (BP) when ethanol was given in the drinking water. Whereas alcohol could act as a solvent for tobacco carcinogens, more likely heavy alcohol intake increases the risk for cancers of the upper alimentary and upper respiratory tracts by enhancing the activity of tobacco carcinogens in the cell where the respiratory enzymes have been impaired. Specifically, we propose that the key factor is nutritional, mainly

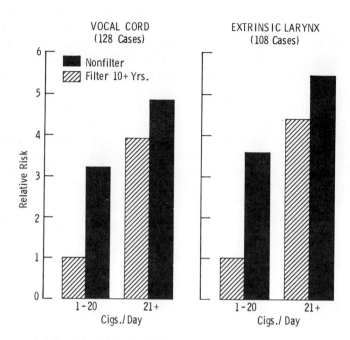

VOCAL CORD
(128 Cases)

EXTRINSIC LARYNX
(108 Cases)

Nonfilter
Filter 10+ Yrs.

Relative Risk

Cigs./ Day

Cigs./ Day

*Relative risk = 1.0 for 1-20/day filter smokers, adjusted for city and
educational level.

FIGURE 6. Relative risk* of laryngeal cancer in men for current
filter and nonfilter cigarette smokers—ages 40-79;
New York, Los Angeles, and Houston, 1970-73.

micronutrient deficiencies often associated with alcoholism that affect the
epithelium of the upper alimentary and upper respiratory tracts. How else
could one explain the increased risk among alcoholics for cancer of the vocal
cord? Alcoholics are believed to suffer primarily from a vitamin B deficiency,
and their nerve cells have shown a reduced activity of the respiratory enzymes
[15]. We are reminded of a similarity between this condition and Plummer-
Vinson syndrome, which results in part from a long-standing iron deficiency
and increases the risk of cancer of the upper alimentary tract in the absence
of tobacco and alcohol consumption [16]. Plummer-Vinson syndrome, inci-
dently, has dramatically declined in Sweden since flour was supplemented with
iron and other nutrients.

For a long time, we have believed that the epidemiological lead relative to
the Plummer-Vinson syndrome represents a critical clue to the mechanism by
which squamous cell epithelium may transform into neoplastic cells on the basis
of intracellular defect(s). Efforts have been made to duplicate this lead in mice.

We showed that in riboflavin-deficient animals, especially when fed a high-fat diet, the epithelium first undergoes atrophy, then hyperkeratosis, and finally hyperplasia [17]. We subsequently found that the skin of a riboflavin-deficient mouse is more susceptible to the effect of 7, 12-dimethylbenz[a]anthracene (DMBA) when followed by croton oil after an animal is returned to a normal diet (Figure 7) [18].

Subsequent experiments revealed that one of the respiratory enzymes, aryl hydrocarbon hydroxylase, may be responsible for the expression of the carcinogenic effects of polycyclic hydrocarbons such as BP and DMBA [19]. Tandler et al. [20] showed significant abnormalities in liver mitochondria in riboflavin-deficient mice. Similar studies on epithelial cells, though difficult, are needed. Since respiratory enzymes require riboflavin and iron to function, the activities of these enzymes are likely to fluctuate in accordance with the nutritional state. This, in turn, may activate or inactivate a carcinogen [18]. Thus, we hypothesize

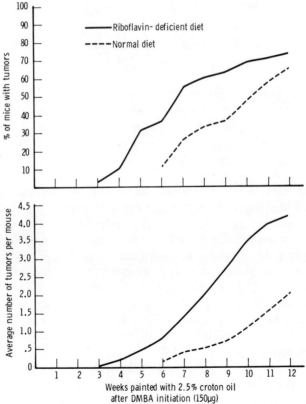

FIGURE 7. Skin tumor yield in riboflavin-deficient mice (Swiss ICR♀).

that alcoholism, iron deficiency, and riboflavin deficiency have a common denominator during carcinogenesis. An important question remaining to be solved is whether specific nutritional substances given to laboratory animals along with high doses of alcohol would reduce the risk of cancers of the upper alimentary and upper respiratory tracts in these test objects.

The epidemiology of the Plummer-Vinson syndrome and alcoholism—with deficiencies that tend to come and go, and in the presence of a high-fat diet, which at least in animals further depletes riboflavin and other essential micro-nutrients—is a lead that is difficult to explore biochemically in man and even more difficult to duplicate in animals. In man we need to study the biochemistry of the epithelial cells in the upper alimentary and upper respiratory tracts— a far more pertinent target of study than the liver cells. We should not act like the drunk who looks for his lost keys under the lantern simply because that is where the light is and look only at the liver cell because it is relatively an easy system to investigate biochemically. We believe that an understanding of the biochemical framework of the squamous cell of the upper alimentary tract of an alcoholic and knowledge of why it is more susceptible to tobacco carcinogens will provide major clues to the biochemical parameters controlling the transformation of a squamous cell into a neoplastic cell.

It is apparent from the foregoing that a full understanding of carcinogenesis affecting the upper alimentary and upper respiratory tracts requires a team of epidemiologists, biochemists with various subspecialties, biologists, and electron-microscopists to work in unison on the intriguing epidemiologic leads. However, it is also evident that, from the practical point of view of preventive medicine, the mechanistic studies are not required to prevent a group of cancers that are very uncommon (except for certain geographic areas such as Iran and China) in a nonsmoking and nondrinking population. Thus, to this multidisciplinary team that is "tackling" tobacco-alcohol factors as they relate to cancer of the mouth, larynx, and esophagus, we must add the discipline of public health.

CANCER OF THE COLON

The etiology of cancer of the colon represents another example which is unlikely to be fully unraveled by classical epidemiologic techniques alone. The major leads for colon cancer emerge from these observations: It is more prevalent in the Western world, its sex ratio is near unity, its worldwide distribution is different from cancer of the lower part of the rectum, its incidence is higher in the first and second generation of Japanese migrants to Hawaii and California than in Japan, and a close correlation exists between its incidence and total fat consumption (Figure 8) [1]. It is somewhat less common among Seventh-day Adventists [21], a group that has a lower fat intake than other Americans.

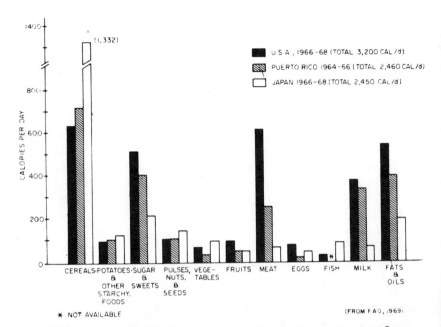

FIGURE 8. Per capita food consumption in U.S.A., Puerto Rico and Japan.

In an epidemiologic study in 1967 [22], we confirmed the increased risk of colon cancer in patients with familial polyposis and ulcerative colitis, although these conditions cannot account for the overall incidence of colon cancer. This study did not uncover a positive association with any other variable. We did not obtain dietary information because, in a population such as exists in North America, the dietary intake is not uniform and the historical information too inaccurate to expect meaningful results.

The above study, in a limited number of cases, showed no relation to serum cholesterol levels. In a recent prospective study, Rose et al. [23] also found no association with serum cholesterol levels, although colon cancer has shown a positive correlation with myocardial infarction. In addition, our studies did not link large-bowel cancer with constipation. Burkitt [24] has suggested rapid intestinal transit time as a protective factor. If constipation were an important variable, the risk of colon cancer would be considerably higher in women, since they are constipated significantly more often than men. However, the sex ratio of colon cancer is near unity, so we do not consider transit time as an important factor of etiologic significance.

In 1969, a retrospective study of colon cancer in Japan [25] again did not suggest relationships with serum cholesterol levels or constipation. However, we did find an association with westernization of the diet. A study by Correa and Llanos [26] in Colombia showed that the higher the income group, the greater the rate of colon cancer.

Selikoff et al. [27] reported that asbestos workers have a higher-than-expected rate of large-bowel cancer. A case-control study of colon cancer by Haenszel et al. [28] among the Japanese immigrants to Hawaii showed a positive relationship with the intake of beef, the major source of saturated fat in the United States. Since meat contributes about 45 percent of the total fat calories in the adult population of the United States, we have proposed that total fat intake is the important etiologic factor in colon cancer. These retrospective studies suggest that a correlation exists between increased income and increase in total dietary fat intake, and that a specific dietary component such as beef plays some role, the nature of which remains to be determined.

The results have raised questions about the specific function of dietary factors in the etiology of colon cancer. Logically, the intraluminal constituents of large bowel having tumor-promoting and tumor-accelerating activity could stem from dietary habits and be involved in carcinogenesis. These constituents include bacteria and, among other chemicals, acid and neutral steriods, amino acids, and fatty acids. Some acid and neutral sterols have tumor-promoting activity in animal models. Thus, the diet may exert its effect both by altering the supply of the amount and type of substrates for cocarcinogen and/or carcinogen production, and by changing the composition of intestinal bacteria available to act on such substrates.

It is obvious that we have been limited by classical etiologic approaches, in view of the difficulty of duplicating our dietary hypothesis in experimental animals. Indeed, in laboratory animals the metabolic pathways of many nutrients and metabolites may be quite different from those in man. Until now, most laboratory animals have not been shown to have the type of bacterial flora existing in man. Hill et al. in England [29], as well as our group [30], investigated this problem from the point of metabolic epidemiology. Our studies supported the hypotheses that populations on a mixed Western diet, among whom the rate of large-bowel cancer is high, degrade and excrete cholesterol and bile acid metabolites to a greater degree than those populations in which the rate of colon cancer is relatively low (Figures 9 and 10).

In searching for a biochemical marker useful in uncovering the causative factors of colon cancer in man, we found a positive correlation between the bacterial β-glucuronidase activity and the excretion of bacterial metabolites of cholesterol and bile acids. Fecal excretion of microbially modified bile acids and cholesterol, anaerobic bacteria, and the activity of bacterial β-glucuronidase were decreased when populations on a high-meat diet transferred to a nonmeat diet for 4 weeks [31].

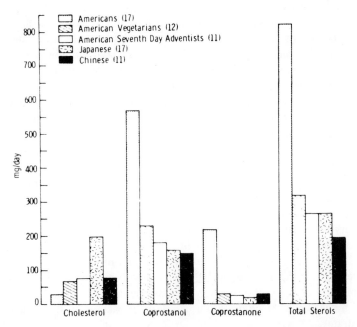

FIGURE 9. Daily fecal neutral sterol excretion of various population groups.

It was important to demonstrate next whether the fecal composition of colon cancer patients differed from that of control patients in the same population. Hill [32] studied single stool specimens from colon cancer patients in England, and discovered not only high levels of microbially modified bile acids, but also a relatively high number of *clostridia*, as compared with control patients. We have examined 48-hour fresh stool specimens from patients with colon cancer, familial polyposis, and ulcerative colitis. Preliminary data indicate that patients with colon cancer excrete higher levels of microbially modified acid and neutral sterols, *clostridia*, and 7-α-dehydroxylase than do the controls.

As part of our multidisciplinary approach to this problem, we then explored some of these variables in experimental animals. In planning animal experiments, it is important to determine to what extent animals can contribute to our knowledge of colon carcinogenesis. As stated before, there are many limitations in the use of these animals, particularly rodents.

In a series of experiments, bile acids were tested as possible tumor promoters for the colon. We instilled lithocholic acid and taurodeoxycholic acid intrarectally into rats, after an initiating dose of *N*-methyl-*N*'-nitro-*N*-nitrosoguanidine (MNNG). The colon tumor yield increased in these rats, compared to the

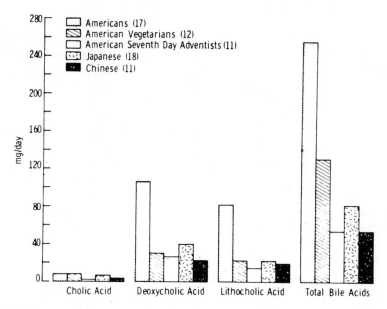

FIGURE 10. Daily fecal bile acid excretion of various population groups.

group being given MNNG only. A number of animal studies are in progress to determine whether the quality and quantity of dietary fat and protein as well as intestinal microflora can influence the susceptibility of colon tissues to chemical carcinogens. Since human populations usually remain on comparable regimens over generations, and since the incidence of colon cancer is comparatively high in second-generation Japanese immigrants to the United States, we designed dietary experiments so that animals are exposed to a given regimen for two generations before treatment with a carcinogen. Preliminary results show that rats on a high-fat diet are more sensitive. Intestinal microflora also seem to have a modifying function in colon carcinogenesis in animal models. Among other projects, we are injecting a large-bowel carcinogen and applying asbestos topically to the colon, in an effort to duplicate the epidemiologic suggestion that asbestos workers have a higher-than-expected incidence of colon cancer.

THE MULTIDISCIPLINARY APPROACH

We have given two examples stressing the need for interrelating and coordinating various groups of experts in an attempt to elucidate the role of environmental factors in the development of cancer. We must recognize that classical epidemiological techniques have their limitations, as do metabolic epidemiological studies in man and laboratory investigations in animals. Fortunately, we deal with different limitations. The initial lead to an environmental risk factor in man has usually come from classical epidemiological techniques, while further specifics about such a factor have been elucidated in an experimental setting. Recently, we have begun to understand that, particularly with carcinogens requiring metabolic activation, small laboratory animals may not provide the proper mechanistic understanding. Indeed, such animals may not exhibit the same anatomic or metabolic capacity as man. Thus, it has become increasingly evident that man himself, in terms of hormonal profile, microflora, serum lipids, or fecal constituents, needs to become part of our total epidemiological survey. In our view, a comparative program involving the various scientific parameters, such as reviewed here, is required not only to identify exogenous and endogenous environmental factors that increase the risk of cancer, but also to investigate the specific elements peculiar to man that will clarify the entire process of carcinogenesis. Of course, a full understanding of carcinogenic mechanisms is not necessarily required to apply broad preventive measures, such as a reduction in fat content of our diet.

Finally, as in the case of etiologic factors for cancer of the endocrine-related organs, it is suggested that the public should adopt the *Prudent Diet* (Figure 11). This diet is thought to lower the incidence of myocardial infarction, and hopefully can also reduce those types of cancer that we now believe are caused by high dietary fat intake. The educational measures and most steps involving the "managerial" reduction of the fat content of the American diet through production of leaner meats and low-fat dairy products fall into the category of public health, which, as we have noted before, should become an integral part of a total approach to environmental carcinogenesis.

SUMMARY

As illustrated in this review, the multidisciplinary approaches to environmental carcinogenesis can best be conducted within a given institute. Our organization has the capacity to interrelate the activities of the epidemiologist with those of laboratory investigators of varied degrees of specialization. We believe that such an interrelationship, on a day-to-day basis, is necessary to fully develop the various epidemiological and experimental leads available in environmental carcinogenesis. At the same time, we recognize that a mechanistic understanding is not always a prerequisite for recommending and implementing appropriate preventive measures. The approach of preventive medicine, which has been so successful in reducing disease in general, should now be applied to environmental cancer in particular. Such a reduction, after all, is the ultimate goal of everyone involved in the conquest of cancer.

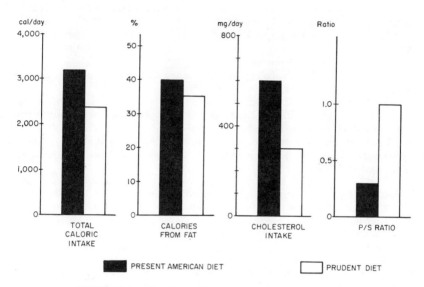

FIGURE 11. Prudent diet and present American diet.

REFERENCES

1. Wynder, E.L., and Mabuchi, K. Etiological and preventive aspects of human cancer. *Prev. Med. 1*:300-334, 1972.

2. Wynder, E.L., and Hoffmann, D. *Tobacco and Tobacco Smoke: Studies in Experimental Carcinogenesis.* Academic Press, New York, 1967.

3. Hoffmann, D., and Wynder, E.L. Selective reduction of tumorigenicity of tobacco smoke. II. Experimental approaches. *J. Natl. Cancer Inst. 48*:1855-1868, 1972.

4. Dontenwill, W., Chevalier, J.J., Hacke, H.P., et al. Investigations on the effects of chronic cigarette-smoke inhalation in Syrian golden hamster. *J. Natl. Cancer Inst. 51*:1781-1832, 1973.

5. Van Duren, B.L., Katz, C., and Goldschmidt, B.M. Carcinogenic agents in tobacco carcinogenesis. *J. Natl. Cancer Inst. 51*:703-705, 1973.

6. Hoffmann, D., Hecht, S.S., Ornaf, R.M., et al. *N'*-nitrosonornicotine in tobacco. *Science 186*:265-267, 1974.

7. Hoffmann, D., Maronpot, R., Raineri, R., et al. A study in tobacco carcinogenesis. XIII. On the carcinogenicity of N'-nitrosonornicotine and N-nitrosoanabasine (unpublished).

8. Sen, N.P. Nitrosamines. *In* Liener, I.E., ed. *Toxic Constituents in Animal Foodstuffs.* Academic Press, New York, 1974, pp. 131-194.

9. Hecht, S.S., Ornaf, R.M., and Hoffmann, D. *N'*-nitrosonornicotine in tobacco. Analysis of possible contributing factors and biological implications (unpublished).

10. Von Wartburg, J.P. The metabolism of alcohol in normals and alcoholics: Enzymes. *In* Kissin, B., and Begleiter, H., eds. *The Biology of Alcoholism. vol. 1. Biochemistry.* Plenum Press, New York, 1971, pp. 63-102.

11. Conney, A.H., and Burns, J.J. Metabolic interactions between environmental chemicals and drugs. *Science 178*:576-586, 1972.

12. Conney, A.H. Carcinogen metabolism and human cancer. *N. Engl. J. Med. 289*: 871-873, 1973.

13. Lieber, C. Personal communication.

14. Kuratsune, M. Test of alcoholic beverages and ethanol solutions for carcinogenicity and tumor-promoting activity. *Gann 62*:395-405, 1971.

15. Wallgren, H. Effect of ethanol on intracellular respiration and cerebral function. *In* Kissin, B., and Begleiter, H., eds. *The Biology of Alcoholism. vol 1. Biochemistry.* Plenum Press, New York, 1971, pp. 103-159.

16. Wynder, E.L., Hultberg, J., Jacobsson, F., et al. Environmental factors in cancer of the upper alimentary tract: A Swedish study with special reference to Plummer-Vinson (Paterson-Kelly) syndrome. *Cancer 19*:470-487, 1957.

17. Wynder, E.L., and Klin, U.E. The possible role of riboflavin deficiency in epithelial neoplasia: I. Epithelial changes in mice in simple deficiency. *Cancer 18*:167-180, 1965.

18. Wynder, E.L., and Chan, P.C. The possible role of riboflavin deficiency in epithelial neoplasia: II. Effect on skin tumor development. *Cancer 26*: 1221-1224, 1970.

19. Wynder, E.L., and Chan, P.C. The possible role of riboflavin deficiency in epithelial neoplasia: III. Induction and microsomal aryl hydrocarbon hydroxylase. *J. Natl. Cancer Inst. 48*:1341-1345, 1972.

20. Tandler, B., Erlandson, R.A., and Wynder, E.L. Riboflavin and mouse hepatic cell structure and function. *Am. J. Pathol. 52*:69-78, 1968.

21. Phillips, R.L., Kuzma, J.W., Lemon, F.R., et al. Mortality from colon-rectal cancer among California Seventh-Day Adventists. Annual Meeting of the American Public Health Association, San Francisco, November 8, 1973.

22. Wynder, E.L., and Shigematsu, T. Environmental factors of cancer of the colon and rectum. *Cancer 20*:1520-1561, 1967.

23. Rose, G., Blackburn, H., Keys, A., et al. Colon cancer and blood cholesterol. *Lancet 1*:181-183, 1974.

24. Burkitt, D.P. Epidemiology of cancer of the colon and rectum. *Cancer 28*:3-13, 1971.

25. Wynder, E.L., Kajitani, T., Ishikawa, S., et al. Environmental factors of cancer of the colon and rectum. II. Japanese epidemiological data. *Cancer 23*:1210-1220, 1969.

26. Correa, P., and Llanos, G. Morbidity and mortality from cancer in Cali, Colombia. *J. Natl. Cancer Inst. 36*:717-745, 1966.

27. Selikoff, I.J., Churg, J., and Hammond, E.C. Asbestos exposure and neoplasia. *J. Am. Med. Assoc. 188*:22-26, 1964.

28. Haenszel, W., Berg, J.W., Segi, M., et al. Large bowel cancer in Hawaiian Japanese. *J. Natl. Cancer Inst. 51*:1765-1779, 1973.

29. Hill, M.J., Crowther, J.S., Drasar, B.S., et al. Bacteria and aetiology of cancer of the large bowel. *Lancet 1*:95-100, 1971.

30. Reddy, B.S., and Wynder, E.L. Large bowel carcinogenesis: fecal constituents of populations with diverse incidence rates of colon cancer. *J. Natl. Cancer Inst. 50*:1437-1442, 1973.

31. Reddy, B.S., Weisburger, J.H., and Wynder, E.L. Fecal bacterial β-glucuronidase: Control by diet. *Science 183*:416-417, 1974.

32. Hill, M.J. Bacteria and the etiology of colon cancer. *Cancer 34*:815-818, 1974.

DISCUSSION

Dr. Bahn asked if differences in the various metabolic determinations between cancer and noncancer patients might result from the cancer or its therapy, rather than the etiologic event. **Dr. Wynder** responded that the associations are not necessarily causal in nature but provide useful leads for future studies, particularly collaborative and interdisciplinary investigations. He suggested, for example, the possibility of studying the influence of diet modification on the regression of colonic polyps. **Dr. Hananian** asked about the influence of diet in childhood on the risk of certain cancers, particularly the colon, in later life. **Dr. Wynder** agreed that the childhood experience may be crucial, and he cited migrant studies showing that certain populations retain to some extent the cancer patterns of their native land. He also pointed out that childhood eating patterns produce habituation, so that diet modification in later life is difficult.

Dr. Schneiderman observed that Norway is taking deliberate action to modify the diet of the entire country. **Mr. Haenszel** responded that such an experiment could be incorporated into the ongoing migrant studies in Norway to assess its impact on cancer risk. Finally, **Dr. Wynder** pointed out that his group, the American Health Foundation, has contacted the U. S. Department of Agriculture on various aspects of the prudent diet and the Department is taking notice, especially in relation to reducing the fat content in meat.

Frederick P. Li

30

OVERVIEW: TOWARD THE UNDERSTANDING
AND CONTROL OF CANCER

Alfred G. Knudson, Jr., M.D., Ph. D.

Graduate School of Biomedical Sciences
University of Texas Health Science Center
Houston, Texas

This conference has provided a splendid opportunity to achieve a broad view of factors operating in carcinogenesis and of the possible approaches to the control of cancer that emerge therefrom. Unfortunately, because the conference has ranged so widely, I find it necessary to simplify what has been said to accomplish an overview. To this end, I refer to Figure 1, which presents a model of the origin of a cancer from a normal cell [1]. I have illustrated the sequence in two broad phases: the first involves the transformation of a normal cell into a cancer cell; the second, the subsequent proliferation of the cancer cell into a cancer. Two steps are indicated for transformation because some people are born with a dominant mutation that makes them very susceptible to cancer, and yet only a very rare cell ever becomes a cancer cell. Some other event must occur for such people to develop cancer; as, for example, in retinoblastoma or in polyposis of the colon. Whether the second step of the transformation phase is a mutation cannot be stated as a certainty; but the fact that, in certain diseases, agents thought to act as mutagens increase disease frequency suggests that it may be. The second phase, growth, may also involve more than one step. It has been observed, for example, that small tumors are sometimes karyotypically normal and that chromosomal abnormalities increase as a tumor grows. This characteristic is generally believed to result from selection of newly emerging clones that are better able to grow in a particular host. Such a change undoubtedly is a factor in tumor progression. I would like, then, to refer to this model in discussing the relationship between host and environmental factors, which were the subjects of the first two conference sessions.

503

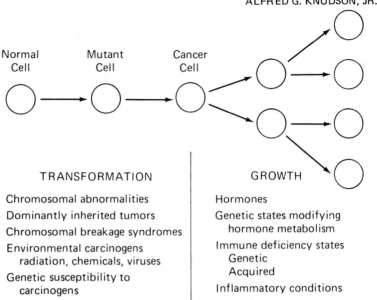

TRANSFORMATION	GROWTH
Chromosomal abnormalities	Hormones
Dominantly inherited tumors	Genetic states modifying
Chromosomal breakage syndromes	hormone metabolism
Environmental carcinogens	Immune deficiency states
radiation, chemicals, viruses	Genetic
Genetic susceptibility to	Acquired
carcinogens	Inflammatory conditions

FIGURE 1. A model for carcinogenesis. A normal cell is converted to a cancer cell in two mutational steps in a transformation phase which can be accelerated by the means listed thereunder. The cancer cell than proliferates to form a tumor in a growth phase which can be accelerated by other means.

GENETIC AND ENDOCRINE FACTORS

Mulvihill discussed chromosomal and single-gene abnormalities associated with cancer. Particularly important to our understanding of cancer has been the Philadelphia chromosome (Ph[1]). The presence of this chromosome in most cases of chronic myelocytic leukemia argues in favor of the clonal origin of cancer. It has also made possible an understanding of the progression of leukemia as new chromosomal abnormalities evolve. Although it cannot be proved that the Ph[1] chromosome precedes the occurrence of leukemia, most likely its presence is involved in the conversion of a normal cell to a cancer cell. One case of such a relationship is in the 13-deletion syndrome, in which a deletion in chromosome 13 is found in all cells of the body and in which an undue number of subjects develop retinoblastoma. This suggests that the gene mutation that frequently causes retinoblastoma in the absence of the 13-deletion syndrome involves a point mutation or other submicroscopic change on chromosome 13. It is hoped that these diseases will be the first of a series demonstrating the relationship between specific chromosomal defects and specific cancers.

In discussing single-gene abnormalities associated with cancer, Mulvihill emphasized those abnormalities that seem to be mediated by chromosomal breakage, namely, the syndromes of Bloom and Fanconi and ataxia-telangiectasia (Figure 1). These abnormalities are presumed to increase the probability that mutation of a normal cell into a cancer cell will occur, a condition also operative in xeroderma pigmentosum. Mulvihill urged the careful screening of entire families in delineating genetic states predisposing to cancer.

Single-gene predisposition to cancer was pursued further by Anderson in discussing dominantly inherited tumors and genetic predisposition to cancer in adulthood. He noted that virtually all human cancers include a dominantly inherited subgroup. A classic example is retinoblastoma, in which approximately 60 percent of cases are not heritable and about 40 percent are associated with a dominant mutation. All cells in the target tissues of those who have inherited such a dominant mutation are at the mutant step rather than at the normal step of other individuals (Figure 1). In nongenetic cases, both steps are regarded as somatic mutations. Family studies in adult cancers, such as breast cancer, are much more complicated. Some pedigrees suggest a dominant gene, but others suggest a recessive predisposition to breast cancer. Anderson proposed that recessively inherited anomalies of estrogen metabolism might predispose to breast cancer, and emphasized further study along this line. He repeatedly emphasized the need to view the adult cancers as genetically heterogeneous in origin. Henderson et al. pursued the matter of breast cancer further in an attempt to explain the large difference in incidence between Oriental and Caucasian females. It was pointed out that excretion levels of estrone and estradiol are higher among American females. Whether such differences are causative and whether they result from genetic or environmental differences remain unknown. The carcinogenic effect of female hormones was also discussed by Hoover and Fraumeni in reviewing the incredible occurrence of vaginal clear cell carcinoma in young females born to women who had received diethylstilbestrol (DES) during pregnancy. One burning question, which some investigators feel has been settled positively, is whether contraceptive hormones cause hepatoma.

ENVIRONMENTAL CARCINOGENESIS

In reviewing radiation carcinogenesis, probably mediated via mutagenesis, Jablon pointed out that the latent period of leukemia is approximately 5 years, whereas that for epithelial cancers is 15 years or longer. Data on atomic-bomb survivors indicate a particular increase in cancers of the respiratory tract, breast, and gastrointestinal system, except stomach. No excesses were noted with respect to gastric cancer or cancer of the uterus, both of which are very common in Japan. This high background incidence may preclude the possibility of observing a relatively small fractional increase resulting from radiation. Among British spondylitis patients treated with radiation, gastric cancer was significantly increased. In discussing the unsettled relationship between prenatal radiation and childhood cancer, Jablon noted that it is generally agreed there is an excess of leukemia among children who were exposed as fetuses, but there is not general agreement on solid tumors.

Radiation, whether ionizing or from ultraviolet light, can also be an occupational hazard with respect to carcinogenesis. Cole noted that such occupations as farming, radiology, and certain types of mining involve such exposure. Even more important as occupational hazards are chemicals, such as the organic hydrocarbons found in coal and petroleum products, the aromatic amines in the dye and rubber industries, vinyl chloride in the plastic industries, metals in various mining and manufacturing processes, and asbestos in mining, processing and use. Carcinogenicity of these agents is most apparent when the agents cause a very rare tumor, such as asbestos-induced mesothelioma. A relatively small, but considerably important, absolute increase in common cancers could easily go undetected. In some instances, the agents probably produce their effects via mutation and increase the probability that normal cells will be converted to cancer cells (Figure 1). In other cases, particularly with respect to asbestos, it is much less clear. The great increase in lung cancer produced by asbestos is associated with smoking, since nonsmoking asbestos workers are not at increased risk of lung cancer. Quantitative risk estimates are difficult to establish with many occupational exposures because of the extremely long latent periods. Such variables as age at onset of exposure and duration of exposure are also very important.

The strongest case for the importance of chemical carcinogenesis in man is shown in the clear relationship between cigarette smoking and lung cancer. Hammond noted the gradually decreasing risk for lung cancer in individuals who stop smoking and the diminished risk among those who smoke cigarettes with reduced tar and nicotine content. It is believed the carcinogenic effect of tobacco increases the probability that normal cells will be converted into cancer cells (Figure 1). Nonspecific changes may also occur in the lung that increase the probability of mutant cancer cells actually growing into fully developed cancers. If we continue to be unsuccessful in persuading cigarette smokers to stop their habit, then perhaps the best prospect for the future is to produce cigarettes free of the carcinogenic effect. Chemical carcinogenesis is also thought to be an important aspect of air pollution in modern cities, as summarized by Pike et al. Here there are many uncertainties: The movement of people from urban to rural areas, the modifications of industrial practices through the years, the exponential growth of automobiles in cities, and the long latent periods for environmental carcinogenesis are all complications impeding the analysis of cancer produced by air pollution. The strongest evidence of a carcinogen in polluted air is in areas where coal is used. Under conditions of incomplete oxidation, there can be large amounts of polycyclic hydrocarbons in the atmosphere. Benzo[a]pyrene (BP) has been used as an indicator of pollution, but its content is poorly correlated with particulate content of air. Some cities known to have serious air pollution, such as Los Angeles, actually have very low BP levels. What is not known, however, is whether other pollutants, perhaps ozone or other chemicals found in such smog, may be carcinogenic.

Rothman summarized the role of alcoholism in carcinogenesis; he noted the clearest associations are for cancer of the mouth, pharynx, and larynx. Further work needs to be done to clarify possible associations with cancers of the esophagus, stomach, liver, rectum, prostate, and pancreas. At those sites where the association has been established, it is heavily dependent upon an interaction with smoking. The combination of smoking and drinking produces a great excess of cancer over that expected from each separately. Analysis of the associations with alcohol suggests that the alcohol itself may be operating as a cocarcinogen, or possibly not at all. Certain alcoholic beverages such as vodka, which is not usually associated with cancers, and whiskey, which is, indicate a congener in alcoholic beverages that is carcinogenic and not the alcohol. Such an association would have obvious implications in cancer prevention.

A potential for chemical carcinogenesis also lies with diet as analyzed by Berg. In some cases, a definite carcinogen has been found in food. The most outstanding example is aflatoxin, which has been found as a fungal product in peanuts. Polycyclic hydrocarbons can also be contaminants of human food, but the extent to which these may cause cancer is almost totally unevaluated. Highly suspicious are nitrosamines, which are known to be powerful carcinogens in animals and which in foods can be found frequently in both active and precursor forms. Most challenging is the possible relationship between normal dietary products and cancer of the digestive tract, notably carcinomas of the stomach, colon, esophagus, and liver. Much work needs to be done on the problem of fats in relation to cancer.

INFECTION AND PRECANCEROUS STATES

The possibility that viruses may produce human cancer was discussed by Heath et al., and by Templeton, both of whom emphasized the importance of herpes simplex virus type 2, the Epstein-Barr virus, the feline leukemia virus, and hepatitis virus B. Despite intense investigation, we still do not have one proven case of a human malignant tumor caused by a virus. Transmission could be primarily vertical, with generation-to-generation transmission of an integrated viral genome that might only rarely, or never, yield infectious virus. Such elements might be indistinguishable from Mendelian mutations. Templeton categorized acquired disorders, including viral infections, that are thought to cause cancer. Among parasitic infections, that produced by *Schistosoma haemat-*

obium is notable for the high risk of bladder cancer it imparts. Infection with *Clonorchis sinensis* has been associated with an increase in biliary tract cancer. Among noninfectious inflammatory conditions, two repeatedly associated with an increased risk of cancer are ulcerative colitis and cirrhosis of the liver. Templeton stressed that there are still many associations that have not been established and that quantitative risk has been provided for only a few. One hindrance is lack of information on the incidence of the predisposing disease, particularly in different parts of the world. There is also virtually no understanding of the mechanism whereby these conditions predispose to cancer. Some inflammatory conditions could influence cell division and stimulate the growth of cancer cells already formed (Figure 1). In viral infection, the conversion of normal cells to cancer cells seems to be involved.

Koss extended the discussion of predisposing conditions to precancerous lesions, again noting the relationship between infection with herpes simplex virus type 2 and cervical carcinoma. He gave particular attention to carcinoma in situ and other histologic abnormalities closely resembling cancer itself. Such lesions may represent small clones of cancer cells with little malignant potential, but from which additional malignant clones may emerge through any of various epigenetic phenomena, such as chromosomal nondisjunction. The rate at which these lesions progress to cancer varies considerably, and the delineation of the risks need to be refined.

IMMUNE DEFICIENCY AND SUSCEPTIBILITY TO CANCER

The general subject of immune deficiency and cancer was discussed by Kersey and Spector. The findings of The Immunodeficiency Cancer Registry suggest an excessive risk of cancer among afflicted subjects. For the more serious, and frequently fatal, immune deficiency conditions of childhood, there has been primarily an excess of lymphoreticular neoplasms and leukemia. In some conditions more frequently observed in adults, however, not only is this group greatly increased but epithelial cancers of adult type are also noted. This suggests that immune deficiency predisposes not only to lymphoid neoplasms, but to cancer generally. It is not known whether the great excess of lymphoid neoplasms is because they are simply seen earlier than others or whether the mutations involved in creating the immune deficiency also increase the probability that lymphoid neoplasms will occur (Figure 1). Of course, immune deficiency may also arise environmentally, most notably among individuals who receive immunosuppressant drugs for kidney transplantation.

HEREDITY AND ENVIRONMENT IN CARCINOGENESIS

Host factors involved in carcinogenesis might be either genetic or environmental according to Schoenberg. In directing our attention to multiple primary neoplasms, he classified them according to one-way and two-way associations. In one-way associations, there is an increased risk of a second cancer when a first occurs, but not of the first cancer when the second occurs. One manner in which this is known to be caused is by treatment of a first cancer with an agent that has carcinogenic potential and is capable of causing a second cancer. Such agents include radiation and some chemicals. In two-way associations, the association is increased in both directions suggesting a common etiology. The basis is evidently genetic when various cancers occur together in certain dominant pedigrees, such as those with multiple endocrine adenomatosis. Sometimes two cancers are associated together in demographic groups, as has been noted in women for cancers of the breast, uterine corpus, ovary, and colon. Further study of multiple primary neoplasms should clarify the carcinogenic potential of various treatment modalities and aid our understanding of pathogenesis.

The discussions of host and environmental factors in the etiology of cancer repeatedly demonstrated an exquisite interaction between the two. Such an interaction is illustrated in a problem that does not involve cancer—or perhaps it does—namely, consumption of milk. The use of milk by Japanese and Americans is strikingly different. However, one would necessarily be cautious in attributing this difference to environmental factors, because the adult genetic form of digestive lactase deficiency has a 90 percent incidence among Japanese and a 10 percent incidence among Caucasian Americans. Demographic variation in cancer incidence was, in fact, the topic of the third segment of the conference. Muir gathered together the maximal and minimal incidences for a large number of cancers around the world and emphasized that the differences were far too great not to be real. Such differences sometimes result from genetic and environmental factors, as with the low rates of skin cancer among African blacks. Some differences, such as the very high incidence of hepatoma in this same region compared to the low incidence among American blacks, are almost certainly environmental in origin; hopefully, further study will reveal the nature of the agent. There are also significant differences in rates within the United States, as demonstrated by Cutler and Young and Hoover et al. In some instances, as with skin cancer or certain occupational cancers, the differences have apparent causes. A survey of the nation by counties has demonstrated that stomach cancer is highest in counties with large Scandinavian populations and bladder cancer is highest in industrial counties. This geographic methodology will hopefully provide new etiologic leads, as could be true with the high incidence of cancer of the colon in the Northeast. In reviewing the study of migrant populations, Haenszel showed that rates for most cancers among migrants shift toward the rates characteristic of the populations in the areas to which migration occurs, which suggests that environmental influences are largely responsible for observed differences. The exceptions, notably stomach cancer for all high-risk migrants and breast cancer for Japanese migrants, suggest that host factors are of great importance in these cases.

THE EVALUATION OF CANCER RISK

Viewing all these genetic and environmental factors brings us to the questions: Who are the people at risk and what are the risks? Many of you will do as I did and personalize the consideration. I, for example, thought of the facts that I have one first-degree relative and seven second-degree relatives who died of cancer; that I have Scandinavian ancestry; that I have lived in Los Angeles, New York, and Texas; and that I have worked with radioactivity, with tumor viruses, and with children with cancer. I don't know what all this adds up to: Can one quantitate it in some meaningful way? Occasionally, we can quantitate it rather accurately. For example, the retinoblastoma gene changes the probability of getting that disease from 1 in 30,000 to 0.95. This fact does not help us a great deal, because most of the genetic cases result from new germinal mutations we do not know how to monitor. We really gain nothing by discriminating between these two groups, one of which is extremely low risk and one of which is extremely high risk. The best course is to examine the eyes of all children carefully and periodically if we want to pick up retinoblastoma very early.

In going over this high-risk group, it suddenly occurred to me that I was about to address a high-risk audience. According to national statistics, one-sixth of the people in this room will die of cancer; therefore, in a sense it is a high-risk group. The question then is, what is it we are trying to do? What are the alternatives? One is to decrease mortality, and we can do that by becoming immortal, or we could do it by dying from something else. The second possibility is that we can defer mortality and die later of cancer, or maybe die so much later of cancer that we would die of something else, which brings us full circle. When Higginson, Schottenfeld, and Wakefield discussed the general problem of identifying high risks, the great difficulty of detection, and of educating the public and physicians, we faced such questions as how many cases warrant the labor and what is the absolute risk versus relative risk. We also imply we are not only interested in the numbers of people who are detected, but also in the number of person-years we save. For example, if we save a 20-year-old 40 years of life, that must have a different meaning from saving 5 years in an 80-year-old person. Although examining older people will bring more cases, examining younger people will add more years per case.

Schneiderman reviewed the state of our knowledge regarding high-risk groups and the problems associated with reducing incidence even when we have accomplished their identification. The well-known example of asbestos workers was used by Selikoff and Hammond to demonstrate the dissection of responsible and interacting factors in etiology and the enormous problem posed for a surveillance program by a long latent period. Wynder et al. cited examples to show that laboratory investigation can be combined with epidemiology to develop a foundation for prevention.

Finally we come to the point of what is to be done from among the many possibilities. I shall conclude with an overview of the overviewers. Miller said that he would like to see more people who would be called etiologists, and see more etiologic thinking in hospitals as we work with cancer patients. It does not matter if we are in a radiotherapy unit or a pathology unit but it certainly should be more at the bedside than is generally the case. MacMahon addressed the very difficult problem of resources at our disposal; he pointed out that record linkage is especially troublesome and getting worse with time. Our nation must clearly understand the losses sustained under a system of excessive privacy. This problem is particularly acute because there are long latent periods in carcinogenesis. Davies was interested in action, and he rightly pointed out that sometimes action can come without understanding. For example, one solution to the problem of cancers caused by smoking would be to prohibit smoking; we do not have to understand how tobacco produces it. On the other hand, if we want to face the problem that people may not stop smoking, then we have to understand what is in cigarettes and try to remove it. He also pointed out that we have some bad practices in teaching students about cancer. We should spend more time in talking about the optimistic side of cancer and the beneficial effects of prevention. Finally, Shimkin reminded us that we are talking about people and not patients; if we are trying to preserve life, we should be looking at people before they are patients. That is the essence of preventive medicine.

REFERENCE

1. Knudson, A.G. Heredity and human cancer. *Am. J. Pathol.*, 77:77–84, 1974.

FUTURE PROSPECTS

31

OPPORTUNITIES FOR CANCER CONTROL

Lester Breslow, M.D., M.P.H.

School of Public Health
University of California at Los Angeles
Los Angeles, California

INTRODUCTION

Passage of the National Cancer Act of 1971 and its approval by the President constituted a renewed and expanded national commitment to conquer cancer initially made by the National Cancer Act of 1937. The goal of the National Cancer Program, based on the 1971 Act, is:

> To develop, through research and development efforts, the means to significantly reduce the morbidity and mortality from cancer by:
> Preventing as many cancers as possible
> Curing patients who develop cancer
> Providing maximum palliation to patients not cured
> Rehabilitating treated patients to as nearly normal a state as possible.

Cancer control was made an expanded element of the National Cancer Program in 1971. Its importance was heightened by a series of conferences specifically on cancer control during late 1973 and early 1974; by specific provision in the Cancer Act Amendments of 1974; by specific budgetary provision for cancer control beginning in 1973 and increasing thereafter; and by establishment of

---

This chapter is based in part on suggestions from a discussion group that met during the conference. The participants were Drs. Anita K. Bahn, Peter Greenwald, Sam Shapiro, and Michael B. Shimkin.

the Division of Cancer Control and Rehabilitation as the fifth division of the National Cancer Institute.

MEANING OF CANCER CONTROL

Cancer control consists of many activities, with the following aims:
1) To identify potential cancer control methods or techniques that have been developed by research
2) To conduct necessary testing of those methods and techniques in community settings
3) To evaluate their applicability for widespread community use
4) To promote the appropriate widespread community use of methods and techniques that are found applicable.

Cancer *research* seeks to find the means for combating cancer, whereas cancer *control* is concerned with identifying, community testing, evaluating, and promoting the application of these means.

Cancer control thus includes developmental research—the identification of new methods and techniques and their field testing and evaluation in limited community settings; and community demonstration and application activities— the promotion of community-tested cancer control methods and techniques to assure their appropriate application and use.

INTERVENTION POINTS FOR CANCER CONTROL

The plan of action for cancer control may be visualized as a chain of activities directed at certain intervention points that are critical to making progress against cancer. These intervention points and their attendant activities are as follows:

Prevention
  I. Increase the understanding of the public and health professionals of measures that would reduce the risk of cancer.
 II. Motivate people to take steps to reduce the risk, morbidity, and mortality of cancer.

Screening and Detection
III. Identify, field test, and evaluate screening tests with the greatest potential for detection at a stage that leads to reduced morbidity and mortality.
 IV. Demonstrate and promote the widespread application of practical and effective screening methods.

Diagnosis and Pretreatment Evaluation
  V. Aid professional groups in the assessment of current practices and in the development of principles for the optimal diagnosis and pretreatment evaluation of cancer.

VI.   Field test, evaluate, demonstrate, and promote measures for the opti-
      mal diagnosis and pretreatment evaluation of persons with precancerous
      or cancerous lesions.
      Treatment
VII. Promote optimal, comprehensive, and continuous treatment and fol-
      low-up care for each cancer patient.
      Rehabilitation
VIII. Identify, field test, evaluate, demonstrate, and promote widespread ap-
      plication of measures for the optimal rehabilitation of cancer patients.
      Continuing Care
IX.   Identify, field test, evaluate, demonstrate, and promote the widespread
      application of methods for the optimal continuing care of patients with
      recurrent or disseminated cancer.

CANCER CONTROL OPPORTUNITIES CREATED BY
KNOWLEDGE OF HIGH-RISK GROUPS

For centuries it has been known that cancer affects certain segments of the
population with particular force: chimney sweeps of the eighteenth century,
Schneeburg miners in the nineteenth century, and cigarette smokers in the twentieth century. During the latter half of the twentieth century, an explosion of
knowledge is highlighting the fact that increased risk of cancer is affecting not
just a few isolated groups but large segments of the population.

What are the implications for cancer control? First, consider three identifying characteristics of groups at high risk: 1) known host factors, such as genetic
and other congenital defects and immunologic deficiency disorders; 2) exposure
to known cancer-producing agents, such as tobacco, alcohol, and radiation; and
3) certain demographic features, which reflect unknown endogenous or exogenous factors, such as place of residence and migration.

Throughout history, man has ultimately controlled diseases by understanding causation sufficiently to prevent them. This same sequence appears likely
to be true for cancer. Knowledge is rapidly accumulating that permits certain
forms of cancer to be prevented. They include the great majority of lung cancers that are recognized as resulting from cigarette smoking, a substantial portion
of bladder cancers that are caused by occupational exposures, and some infrequently occurring cancers from genetic defects that can be identified. To avoid
these factors depends first of all upon identifying persons who are at high risk
because of exposure to them, and then undertaking to avoid exposure.

Knowledge is being pursued and applied that will permit the ultimate form
of cancer control—prevention. Increasingly available information about high-risk
groups enhances our ability to intervene effectively at other points. For example, screening and detection may be applied with greater benefit among people

known to be at high risk of a particular form of cancer than among others at lesser risk. Thus, women of low socioeconomic status who started sexual activity early in life are more likely to benefit from the Papanicolaou smear for cervical cancer than women of higher socioeconomic levels who started sexual activity later in life.

To proceed systematically with knowledge about high-risk groups for the control of cancer, it is necessary to:

1) Analyze the opportunities for cancer control, using data from this conference and other sources.

Consideration needs to be given to: a) the level and trend in the incidence and mortality of various kinds of cancers; b) the ability to identify groups and individuals at high risk; and c) the effectiveness and feasibility of intervention. On the basis of such criteria, lung cancer would be selected in the United States for control activities during the 1970's rather than stomach cancer, and Hodgkin's disease rather than glioblastoma.

2) Establish the concept and practice of health maintenance as the basis of health care.

Cancer control will be most effective when, guided by knowledge of endogenous and exogenous risk factors, it proceeds actively as a regular health maintenance endeavor rather than waiting for serious symptoms to arise. This concept will require reorienting health care as a whole toward the kind now given mothers and children. Control based on current knowledge should be applied to the risks of cancer as well as to the risks of eclampsia and poliomyelitis. It will entail a new partnership between people and their doctors, with individual responsibility for health behavior and professional responsibility for health-maintenance procedures. It will also mean incorporating preventive medical services into health insurance and other plans for payment of medical care.

Cancer control should be linked with efforts to control other diseases: screening for hypertension as well as for cancer; joining activities for control of genetic factors in cancer with activities for control of other genetic disease; and campaigning against cigarettes as a factor in several diseases. Such linkage will enhance cancer control economically and by promoting the idea of health maintenance.

3) Provide for the development of lifetime careers in preventive medicine and health maintenance applied to cancer control.

Preventive medicine should have opportunities comparable with those in the specialties of curative medicine. This development will require expanding training resources, and encouraging young physicians and other health-care professionals to undertake the training provided. It will also be necessary to extend into undergraduate training emphasis on potential health achievements based on knowledge about individuals and groups at high risk of cancer.

4) Proceed with studies and demonstration projects designed to achieve behavior modification necessary for cancer control among persons at high risk of cancer.

This area should include attention to personal habits such as cigarette smoking; seeking care and following advice from health-care professionals; and avoiding cancer hazards in industry.

Current methodology for influencing behavior is not sufficiently effective in taking advantage of knowledge about high risk of cancer. It is increasingly important to link individual volition in this matter to regulation; for example, minimizing exposure to carcinogens in industry and requiring certain screening tests for individuals employed in certain situations.

5) Proceed with development and testing of cancer screening and detection procedures, for application particularly among high-risk groups.

Such development and testing should include carefully designed evaluation studies; the aim is to assess the effectiveness of screening detection programs in reducing cancer mortality especially among high-risk groups.

Screening and detection activities for cancer should be directed to the maximum extent possible toward multiple sites. For example, cervical cytology and mammography should be combined for appropriate risk groups and be incorporated into multiphasic screening.

6) Involve cancer centers and their affiliated medical facilities and educational institutions in community cancer control.

Such centers have great potential for facilitating community demonstrations of cancer control. Their expertise, joined with that of health departments and other agencies traditionally engaged in preventive medicine, would add not only the latest knowledge and possibly a more effective evaluation, but also direct feedback to the centers concerning community need.

7) Popularize what is known about high-risk groups and what has been said about and could be achieved among such groups.

Prudent behavior on the part of individuals, as well as their doctors, is increasingly an important basis for the control of cancer. The disease is to a considerable extent man-made, in the sense that exposure to cigarette smoke, chemical carcinogens, radiation, and other factors controlled by man are the causative agents of cancer. Individuals and groups at high risk need to know the implications and what can be done about their situations, either by prevention or by intervention at other points along the spectrum of cancer control.

8) Develop systematic monitoring of persons exposed to high risk of cancer from technological changes introduced into industry, medicine, and other aspects of modern life, whenever there is any basis for suspecting carcinogenic potential.

The introduction of new chemical and physical agents whose potentially harmful characteristics are not fully known into industry and medicine already has increased the frequency of some forms of cancer.

9) Establish a framework for cancer control that continues to incorporate new knowledge about high-risk groups and how these risks can be controlled.

Those responsible for community cancer control efforts should be constantly alert for new knowledge about host and environmental factors that may be useful. This endeavor also entails refresher courses and continuing education.

10) Incorporate the concept of health benefit versus health cost, as well as social cost, into health care generally.

In cancer control and in other aspects of modern health care, such powerful drugs and devices (e.g., X-ray procedures) are being used that one must carefully evaluate one risk being exchanged for another.

Finally, it should be noted that cancer control, especially as it pertains to high-risk groups, requires an interdisciplinary approach with maximum interchange of knowledge and viewpoint for greatest effectiveness.

32

OPPORTUNITIES FOR CANCER ETIOLOGY

A. B. Miller, M.B.

National Cancer Institute of Canada
Toronto, Ontario, Canada

INTRODUCTION

In general, this chapter does not attempt to repeat the suggestions for further work made by each author in this monograph. General themes, however, may be detected, and they are summarized here as follows:

1) In many cancers, both common and uncommon, insufficient knowledge is available on risk factors; nevertheless, with additional study, risk factors for the majority of human cancers would be identifiable.

2) Except for smoking and lung cancer, the risk factors identified so far explain only a small proportion of the cases of cancer. We expect that further work will correct this deficiency and provide information on absolute risks for factors where only relative risk estimates have been established.

3) Evidence for the interaction of host susceptibility and environmental agents is becoming available. Data are required on the nature of these interactions and the relative contribution of individual factors.

This chapter is based in part on suggestions from a discussion group that met during the conference. The participants were Drs. J.N.P. Davies, Takeshi Hirayama, Irving I. Kessler, Alfred G. Knudson, Brian MacMahon, Robert W. Miller, Norton Nelson, and Alan S. Rabson.

4) Collaboration between epidemiologists (plus other etiologists) and other disciplines is an increasing necessity at the conceptual and execution stages of research.
5) Resources (scientific, accessible subjects and finance) are limited, and work must be directed to promising areas for etiology studies using promising methods.
6) Substantial advances in knowledge will come from existing cancer centers and others to be established, but it is essential to continue adequate research support for *individual*, innovative investigators.
7) Continued and increasing support for the training of epidemiologists and other etiologists should be assured, especially at the postdoctoral level.

The balance of this chapter outlines opportunities for research under five functional headings: Definitions, Host Factors, Environmental Factors, Resource Requirements and Funding Needs, and Methodology. The final section, Conclusions, summarizes the scope of cancer etiologic research and relates it to cancer control endeavors.

DEFINITIONS

The concept of the high-risk group should be defined more clearly using techniques of descriptive or analytic epidemiology. *Descriptive epidemiology* will identify groups at high risk by demographic markers. *Analytic epidemiology* will identify groups:

1) In a high-risk environment
2) With a high-risk habit
3) With predisposing and precancerous conditions
4) With genetic, immunologic, metabolic, and endocrinologic high-risk characteristics
5) With exposure to specified environmental agents.

Interactions between each group should also be clarified. For many cancers, North Americans appear to have uniformly high risk compared to other parts of the world. However, this homogeneity may well prove spurious when the responsible interactions have been worked out, notwithstanding the different exposures and genetic backgrounds of migrant groups.

HOST FACTORS

Further delineation is necessary for clinical and laboratory manifestations of syndromes predisposing to neoplasia. Among the means to achieve this are:

1) Searches for biologic markers associated with the cancer (and the underlying syndrome) that could be used as markers in relatives and in the presumed normal population; such markers could be cytogenetic, enzymatic, immunologic, or hormonal

2) Application of new laboratory techniques, such as chromosomal banding and cell and nucleic acid hybridization, to the syndromes.

Establish registries for rare cancer events, presumed genetic predispositions, and familial aggregations to further evaluate causative mechanisms (e.g., ascertain the risk of cancer in heterozygotes of certain recessively inherited disorders).

Study familial aggregations of cancer for associated anomalies that might help to determine whether the cause was genetic or environmental. These studies could include:

1) Immunologic status

2) Hormonal status (e.g., estrogen metabolism in breast cancer families).

Characterize preneoplastic states and obtain more information on their naural history. This effort will require accurate prevalence and incidence data, both cross-sectional and cohort, that may well need synthesizing by computer simulation studies.

Establish reliable incidence data on "acquired" diseases that predispose to cancer (such as chronic ulcerative colitis).

Pursue virus studies using new techniques in specially defined risk groups, including patients with congenital or acquired immunodeficiency for:

1) Epstein-Barr virus cell-mediated immunity (CMI)

2) Serologic and CMI responses to newly discovered human papova viruses

3) Evidence of primate oncornaviruses (e.g., specific virion proteins) in tumors that develop in such patients.

Study hormonal metabolism for specific abnormalities (possibly genetically determined) in patients with cancer other than of the breast (e.g., endometrium, ovary, and prostate).

Search for animal models of human genetic neoplasms and preneoplastic states.

ENVIRONMENTAL FACTORS

Attention should be devoted to establishing etiologic factors by site and histological type for different geographic areas and, where present, for specific populations within areas.

Recently developed in vitro tests for mutagenicity should be applied to food and other substances implicated in epidemiologic studies; e.g., alcoholic beverages of various kinds, beef, and beef-related substances.

Continued surveillance is necessary to assess the health effects of oral contraceptives and other mass chronic medications. Many cancers possibly affected by exogenous hormones have long latent periods, and oral contraceptives have not been available long enough for us to be confident that we know all the hazards associated with them.

Create registries of individuals exposed to known or strongly suspect cancer risks; e.g., individuals who work with tumor viruses, known chemical carcinogens, or occupations that involve radiation exposure.

Confirm or refute the hypothesis that some or all cases of Hodgkin's disease have an infectious basis.

Pay more attention to occupational groups than in the past, since:

1) They are often the highest risk group with respect to carcinogenic exposures and will be efficient sources of information on etiologic factors in general

2) The information derived will often enable interaction of different factors to be evaluated for the benefit of both occupational and general population groups.

Evaluate the implications of transplacental carcinogenesis, which involves the necessity for long-term surveillance, using birth registers and record-linkage techniques, of individuals exposed to medications and other environmental agents in utero.

Obtain further information on the effect of cessation of exposure to an agent. This area has considerable theoretical interest relating to carcinogenesis.

Evaluate the indicator value of acute or semiacute toxicity of an agent as a predictor of carcinogenicity after the expected latent period.

RESOURCE REQUIREMENTS AND FUNDING NEEDS

The National Cancer Institute should stimulate, encourage, and help to finance the establishment of a National Death Index within the National Center for Health Statistics.

The National Cancer Institute should designate support funds for etiologic and epidemiologic studies and encourage and support collaborative epidemiologic studies.

It is important that concerted efforts are made to link laboratory and epidemiologic research more closely. This step may require special efforts to strengthen the weak component (epidemiologic or experimental studies as the case may be) in those centers where interest exists in both.

All responsible agencies should collaborate towards developing special national and international networks composed of motivated epidemiologists and other oncologists to obtain the necessary information within the shortest time period (consider use of newsletters and/or Telex).

Specialization of approach within groups should be encouraged and attempts made to avoid fruitless competition for similar projects. Support of innovative teams should be encouraged.

Teachers of epidemiology of cancer at medical and public health schools should be supported and opportunities created for the exposure of medical students to research in cancer epidemiology.

Attempts should be made to identify persons with an aptitude to think etiologically at the bedside, in the factory, and in the community. These individuals will be students as well as practitioners.

Positions for bedside and clinic etiologists should be established on the faculties of appropriate clinical departments and cancer centers to search for new clues.

Support for epidemiologic fellowships and postdoctoral training programs should be encouraged.

METHODOLOGY

Our ability to follow high-risk patients throughout life should be improved by developing record-linkage techniques and applying them to suitable resources (twin registers, inbred groups, and birth defect registers for host factors and occupational groups, prescription registers, and geographically exposed populations for environmental factors).

Methods for establishing new data should be evaluated, for example:

1) Checklists for etiologic information
2) Rapid, appropriate case-history retrieval
3) Periodic survey for special suspect risk items.

Our ability to obtain relevant nutritional and dietary information should be developed further, both in case-control and cohort studies; in the latter, the problems of periodic updating should be given special consideration.

The efficiency of cancer registration needs to be improved as does further evaluation of the correct dividing line between sufficient data to adequately identify the individual, characterize his disease, and define his position in the spectrum of risk, and the danger that too detailed a requirement will result in inaccurate compilation and incomplete registration.

The appropriate dividing line between confidentiality and the need to carry out epidemiologic and other research should, in cooperation with the public, be defined appropriately. The public is dangerously ignorant of the immediate and long-term benefits of etiologic investigations that depend on the identification of individuals.

Methods of monitoring occupational and general population groups for unsuspected hazards using both cancer registries and death indices should be refined.

CONCLUSION

A substantial endeavor is required to obtain the necessary data to assure that individuals at high risk can be identified with precision. In some respects the barrier between etiology and control is artificial; control endeavors, even when based on incomplete etiologic information, may well help to clarify etiologic relationships either by their effect or lack of effect (when primary prevention is attempted) or through the opportunities such programs provide to obtain etiologic data. Nevertheless, while recognizing that sometimes action based on relative ignorance may be unavoidable, etiologists in general would argue for the sequence: research on etiology followed by appropriate control based on the knowledge gained. Much etiologic research therefore is vital before our control colleagues can be completely unleashed.

SUBJECT INDEX

A

Acquired diseases, cancer risk and, 69-84
Acrokeratosis verruciformis, 22
Adenomatosis, multiple endocrine, 112
Adenovirus, 245
Aflatoxin, liver cancer and, 202-203, 214-215, 299, 388
Africa, liver cancer in, 96
Air pollution
  automobile sources, 226
  aromatic hydrocarbons in, 205, 226-228, 233-234
  carcinogenic substances in, 225-239
  industrial sources, 226
  lung cancer, 178, 230-234
Albinism, skin cancer and, 21
Alcohol
  cancer control, 146
  cancer mortality, 144-145
  carcinogens in, 139-140, 146
  esophageal cancer, 76, 142-143, 416, 486, 490
  laryngeal cancer, 76, 140-142, 352, 486-487, 491
  liver cancer, 76, 144
  malnutrition, 140, 491
  nitrosamines, 76
  oral cancer, 76, 140, 352, 486
  pancreatic cancer, 76, 144
  pharyngeal cancer, 76, 140, 352
  prostatic cancer, 144
  rectal cancer, 144
  stomach cancer, 143
  tobacco smoking, 76, 140-142, 286, 486-487, 490-493
Aldrin, 208
Alkylating agents, 173
α_1-antitrypsin deficiency, 26
American Cancer Society

breast cancer demonstration project, 459
health-maintaining behavior, study of, 407
public attitudes and practices, survey of, 411
public education, role in, 417-418, 421
4-aminodiphenyl, bladder cancer and, 94, 173, 388
Amphetamines, Hodgkin's disease and, 187-189
Androgenic-anabolic steroids, hepatocellular carcinoma and, 15, 187-188
Androgens, breast cancer, role in, 271
Aniline dye workers, bladder cancer in, 168, 416, 424, 474-475
Aniridia, congenital, Wilms' tumor and, 9, 427
Antibiotics, 208
Antioxidants, 210, 213
Aplastic anemia, 15
Appendectomy, 77
Aromatic amines, bladder cancer and, 94
Arsenic, 174
  drinking water, in, 208-209, 211
  hemangioendothelioma of liver, 188
  lung cancer, 188, 388
  skin cancer, 187-188
Arteriosclerotic heart disease, risk factors in, 441, 444-445
Artificial colorings, 206-207
Artificial sweeteners, 207
Aryl hydrocarbon hydroxylase, lung cancer and, 49, 235-236, 395, 492
Asbestos
  drinking water, in, 208-209, 353
  gastrointestinal cancer, 208, 467, 474, 480, 495-497
  lung cancer, 171, 388, 467-483, 510
  mesothelioma, 298, 389, 392, 467-483
  public education, 420
  tobacco smoking, 171, 394, 467-468, 476,